COMPLICATIONS OF CARDIOVASCULAR PROCEDURES

Risk Factors, Management, and Bailout Techniques

MAURO MOSCUCCI, MD, MBA

Clinical Vice Chairman
Department of Medicine
Chief, Cardiovascular Division
Professor of Medicine
University of Miami Miller School of Medicine
Miami, Florida

Wolters Kluwer | Lippincott Williams & Wilkins
Health

Philadelphia · Baltimore · New York · London
Buenos Aires · Hong Kong · Sydney · Tokyo

Acquisitions Editor: Frances DeStefano
Development Editor: Grace Caputo, Dovetail Content Solutions
Product Manager: Leanne McMillan
Production Manager: Alicia Jackson
Senior Manufacturing Manager: Benjamin Rivera
Marketing Manager: Kimberly Schonberger
Creative Director: Doug Smock
Production Service: Aptara, Inc.

Printed in China

Library of Congress Cataloging-in-Publication Data

Complications of cardiovascular procedures : risk factors, management, and bailout techniques / [edited by] Mauro Moscucci.
   p. ; cm.
   Includes bibliographical references and index.
   Summary: "Provides interventional cardiologists, endovascular interventionalists, and physicians in training with a comprehensive resource on the prevention and management of complications in interventional cardiology. The book focuses specifically on risk factors, prevention, and management with conventional and/or with bailout techniques and devices. The textbook includes images of devices and other resources. The first section, on general principles, includes quality assurance, training requirements, legal considerations, adjunctive pharmacotherapy, and conscious sedation. Subsequent sections cover general complications of invasive procedures and complications of specific coronary interventions, noncoronary cardiac interventions, peripheral vascular procedures, pediatric interventions, and electrophysiology procedures. A companion website includes videos of over 100 complications and bailout techniques"—Provided by publisher.
   ISBN-13: 978-0-7817-7588-5 (alk. paper)
   ISBN-10: 0-7817-7588-4 (alk. paper)
   1. Heart–Surgery–Complications.   2. Cardiac catheterization–Complications. I. Moscucci, Mauro.
   [DNLM: 1. Cardiovascular Diseases–surgery.   2. Cardiovascular Surgical Procedures–adverse effects.   3. Heart Catheterization–adverse effects.
4. Intraoperative Complications–prevention & control. WG 168]
   RD598.C545 2011
   617.4′12—dc22

                                    2010028320

Care has been taken to confirm the accuracy of the information presented and to describe generally accepted practices. However, the authors, editors, and publisher are not responsible for errors or omissions or for any consequences from application of the information in this book and make no warranty, expressed or implied, with respect to the currency, completeness, or accuracy of the contents of the publication. Application of the information in a particular situation remains the professional responsibility of the practitioner.

   The authors, editors, and publisher have exerted every effort to ensure that drug selection and dosage set forth in this text are in accordance with current recommendations and practice at the time of publication. However, in view of ongoing research, changes in government regulations, and the constant flow of information relating to drug therapy and drug reactions, the reader is urged to check the package insert for each drug for any change in indications and dosage and for added warnings and precautions. This is particularly important when the recommended agent is a new or infrequently employed drug.

   Some drugs and medical devices presented in the publication have Food and Drug Administration (FDA) clearance for limited use in restricted research settings. It is the responsibility of the health care provider to ascertain the FDA status of each drug or device planned for use in their clinical practice.

To purchase additional copies of this book, call our customer service department at (800) 638-3030 or fax orders to (301) 223-2320. International customers should call (301) 223-2300.

Visit Lippincott Williams & Wilkins on the Internet: at LWW.com. Lippincott Williams & Wilkins customer service representatives are available from 8:30 am to 6 pm, EST.

                                          10 9 8 7 6 5 4 3 2 1

RRS1007

To my mentor – Donald Baim – in recognition of his charismatic role in shaping modern interventional cardiology and of his full support in this endeavor.

And to my wife, Adriana, and my children, Alessandra and Matteo. I thank them for their patience, understanding, love and support, and for adapting their life around the work schedule that was required to create this book.

CONTENTS

SECTION VI: Specific Complications of Pediatric Interventions

SECTION VII: Electrophysiology Procedures

CONTRIBUTORS

Alex Abou-Chebl, MD
Associate Professor
Department of Neurology
University of Louisville School of Medicine
Director
Neurointerventional Services
University of Louisville Hospital
Louisville, Kentucky

Imran N. Ahmad, MD
Fellow
Interventional Cardiology
Cleveland Clinic
Cleveland, Ohio

Ranjit Aiyagari, MD
Assistant Professor
Department of Pediatrics and Communicable Diseases
University of Michigan
Pediatric Interventional Cardiologist
Michigan Congenital Heart Center
C.S. Mott Children's Hospital
Ann Arbor, Michigan

Mamata M. Alwarshetty, MD
Fellow
Department of Medicine
Rush University
Chicago, Illinois

Aimee K. Armstrong, MD
Assistant Professor
Department of Pediatrics and Communicable Diseases
University of Michigan
Assistant Professor
Department of Pediatrics and Communicable Diseases
C.S. Mott Children's Hospital
Ann Arbor, Michigan

Gio J. Baracco, MD, FACP
Associate Professor of Clinical Medicine
Division of Infectious Diseases
University of Miami Miller School of Medicine
Acting Chief
Medical Service
Miami VA Healthcare System
Miami, Florida

Amy C. Blackwell, JD
Claims Process Manager
Office of Clinical Affairs
University of Michigan Health System
Ann Arbor, Michigan

Richard C. Boothman, JD
Associate Professor
Department of Surgery
University of Michigan Medical School
Chief Risk Officer
Office of Clinical Affairs
University of Michigan Health System
Ann Arbor, Michigan

Qi-Ling Cao, MD
Associate Professor
Department of Pediatrics
Rush University
Research Scientist
Rush Center for Congenital & Structural
    Heart Disease
Rush University medical Center
Chicago, Illinois

John D. Carroll, MD
Professor
Department of Medicine/Cardiology
University of Colorado Denver
Aurora, Colorado

Stanley J. Chetcuti, MD
Assistant Professor
Department of Cardiovascular Medicine
University of Michigan Medical School
Director, Cardiac Catheterization Laboratory
Department of Medicine, Cardiovascular Division
University of Michigan Medical School
Ann Arbor, Michigan

Kyung J. Cho, MD, FACR
Professor of Radiology
Department of Interventional Radiology
University of Michigan
Ann Arbor, Michigan

Mauricio G. Cohen, MD, FACC
Associate Professor of Medicine
Cardiovascular Division
University of Miami Miller School of Medicine
Director, Cardiac Catheterization Laboratory
Department of Medicine
University of Miami Hospital
Miami, Florida

Andre D'Avila, MD, PhD
Associate Professor
Department of Medicine
Mount Sinai School of Medicine
Co-Director—Cardiac Arrhythmia Service
The Leona M. and Harry B. Helmsley
    Charitable Trust Center for Cardiac
    Electrophysiology
The Zena and Michael A. Wiener Cardiovascular
    Institute
Mount Sinai Medical Center
New York, New York

Jonathan L. Eliason, MD
Assistant Professor of Vascular Surgery
Department of Surgery
University of Michigan Health System
Ann Arbor, Michigan

Stephen G. Ellis, MD
Professor of Medicine
Lerner College of Medicine
Section Head of Invasive/Interventional
    Cardiology
Department of Cardiology
Cleveland Clinic
Cleveland, Ohio

Guillermo A. Escobar, MD
Assistant Professor
Department of Vascular Surgery
University of Michigan
Ann Arbor, Michigan

Valerian L. Fernandes, MD, MRCP, FACC
Associate Professor
Department of Medicine
Medical University of South Carolina
Director
Cardiac Catheterization Laboratory
Ralph H. Johnson VA Medical Center
Charleston, South Carolina

Avi Fischer, MD, FACC
Assistant Professor
Department of Medicine
Mount Sinai School of Medicine
Director—Pacemaker and Defibrillator Therapy
The Leona M. and Harry B. Helmsley Charitable Trust
    Center for Cardiac Electrophysiology
The Zena and Michael A. Wiener Cardiovascular Institute
Mount Sinai Medical Center
New York, New York

Dheeraj Gandhi, MBBS, MD
Assistant Professor
Radiology, Neurosurgery, Neurology
Johns Hopkins School of Medicine
Baltimore, Maryland

C. Michael Gibson, MS, MD
Associate Professor
Department of Medicine
Harvard Medical School
Associate Physician
Department of Medicine, Cardiology Division
Beth Israel Deaconess Medical Center
Boston, Massachusetts

Eric D. Good, DO
Assistant Professor
Department of Cardiovascular
    Medicine/Electrophysiology
University of Michigan—Cardiovascular Center
Ann Arbor, Michigan

P. Michael Grossman, MD
Assistant Professor
Department of Internal Medicine, Division of
    Cardiovascular Medicine
University of Michigan School of Medicine
Director, Cardiac Catheterization Laboratory
Department of Internal Medicine, Division of
    Cardiovascular Medicine
University of Michigan and Veterans Administration
Ann Arbor Healthcare Systems
Ann Arbor, Michigan

Hitinder S. Gurm, MD
Associate Professor
Department of Cardiovascular Medicine
Director, Inpatient Cardiology Services
Department of Cardiovascular Medicine
University of Michigan
Ann Arbor, Michigan

Elias V. Haddad, MD
Fellow
Department of Medicine
Vanderbilt University School of Medicine
Nashville, Tennessee

Jonathan W. Haft, MD
Assistant Professor of Surgery & Anesthesia
Department of Cardiac Surgery
University of Michigan
Ann Arbor, Michigan

Alan W. Heldman, MD, FSCAI
Professor of Medicine, Interventional Cardiology
Interdisciplinary Stem Cell Institute
Cardiovascular Division
University of Miami Miller School of Medicine
Miami, Florida

Ziyad M. Hijazi, MD, MPH
Professor
Department of Pediatrics & Internal Medicine
Rush University
Chief
Rush Center for Congenital & Structural Heart Disease
Rush University Medical Center
Chicago, Illinois

John W. Hirshfeld Jr., MD
Professor of Medicine
Cardiovascular Division
University of Pennsylvania School of Medicine
Director, Interventional Cardiology Training Program
Cardiovascular Division
University of Pennsylvania Medical Center
Philadelphia, Pennsylvania

Ashequl M. Islam, MD, MPH, FACC
Assistant Professor
Department of Medicine
Tufts University School of Medicine
Boston, Massachusetts
Interventional Cardiologist
Division of Cardiology, Department of Medicine
Baystate Medical Center
Springfield, Massachusetts

Samir R. Kapadia, MD
Associate Professor
Department of Medicine
Case Western Reserve University
Director
Sones Cardiac Catheterization Laboratory
Cleveland Clinic
Cleveland, Ohio

Sudhir Kathuria, MBBS, MD
Assistant Professor
Department of Radiology, Interventional Neurology
Johns Hopkins University
Director of Spine Interventions
Department of Radiology, INR Division
Johns Hopkins Hospital
Baltimore, Maryland

Clifford J. Kavinsky, MD, PhD
Professor
Department of Internal Medicine
Rush University
Chief
Department of Medicine
Rush University Medical Center
Chicago, Illinois

Michael S. Kim, MD
Assistant Professor
Department of Medicine/Cardiology
University of Washington School of Medicine
Seattle, Washington

Aaron D. Kugelmass, MD, FACC
Instructor
Department of Medicine
Tufts University School of Medicine
Boston, Massachusetts
Chief, Division of Cardiology
Medical Director, Heart and Vascular Center
Baystate Medical Center
Springfield, Massachusetts

Thomas R. Lloyd, MD
Professor
Department of Pediatrics and Communicable Diseases
University of Michigan
Chief
Cardiac Catheterization Laboratory
C.S. Mott Children's Hospital
Ann Arbor, Michigan

David J. Malenka, MD
Professor of Medicine
Department of Medicine
Dartmouth Medical School
Hanover, New Hampshire
Associate Director, Cardiac Ultrasound
Department of Medicine, Section of Cardiology
Dartmouth-Hitchcock Medical Center
Lebanon, New Hampshire

Claudia A. Martinez, MD
Instructor
Medicine, Cardiovascular Division
University of Miami Miller School of Medicine
Miami, Florida

Ricardo Martinez-Ruiz, MD
Assistant Professor of Clinical Anesthesiology
Anesthesiology, Perioperative Medicine, and Pain
    Management
University of Miami Miller School of Medicine
Medical Director, Surgical Intensive Care Unit
Chief, Division of Cardiovascular and Thoracic
    Anesthesia, VAMC
Department of Anesthesiology
Bruce W. Carter Veterans Affairs Medical Center
Miami, Florida

Christina M. Matadial, MD
Assistant Professor of Clinical Anesthesiology
Anesthesiology, Perioperative Medicine, and Pain
    Management
University of Miami Miller School of Medicine
Chief, Anesthesiology Service
Department of Anesthesiology
Bruce W. Carter Veterans Affairs Medical Center
Miami, Florida

Roxana Mehran, MD
Chief Scientific Officer
Clinical Trial Center
Cardiovascular Research Foundation
Associate Professor
Center for Interventional Vascular Therapy
Columbia University
New York, New York

Lewis B. Morgenstern, MD
Professor
Neurology, Neurosurgery and Emergency Medicine
University of Michigan Medical School
Director of the Stroke Program
University of Michigan Health System
Ann Arbor, Michigan

Mauro Moscucci, MD, MBA
Clinical Vice Chairman, Department of Medicine
Chief, Cardiovascular Division
Professor of Medicine
University of Miami Miller School of Medicine
Miami, Florida

William W. O'Neill, MD
Executive Dean for Clinical Affairs
Professor of Medicine and Cardiology
Department of Medicine
Chief Medical Officer, University of Miami Health
    System
Department of Medicine
University of Miami Miller School of Medicine
Miami, Florida

Hakan Oral, MD
Professor of Internal Medicine
Department of Cardiovascular Medicine
University of Michigan
Ann Arbor, Michigan;
Director, Cardiac Electrophysiology Service
Department of Cardiovascular Medicine
University of Michigan, Cardiovascular Center
Ann Arbor, Michigan

Carlo Pappone, MD, PhD
Chief
Department of Arrhythmology
The Villa Maria Cecilia Hospital
Cotignola (Ravenna), Italy

Robert N. Piana, MD
Professor of Medicine
Division of Cardiovascular, Department of Medicine
Vanderbilt University;
Director, Adult Congenital Interventional Program
Division of Cardiovascular, Department of Medicine
Vanderbilt University Medical Center
Nashville, Tennessee

Yuri B. Pride, MD
Clinical Fellow in Medicine
Department of Medicine
Harvard Medical School
Cardiology Fellow
Department of Medicine, Cardiovascular Division
Beth Israel Deaconess Medical Center
Boston, Massachusetts

John E. Rectenwald, MD, MS
Assistant Professor of Surgery
Department of Surgery
University of Michigan
Ann Arbor, Michigan

Joseph S. Rossi, MD
Assistant Professor
Division of Cardiology
University of North Carolina
Chapel Hill, North Carolina

Solomon Sager, MD
Fellow, Cardiovascular Division
Department of Medicine
University of Miami/Jackson Memorial Hospital
Miami, Florida

Vincenzo Santinelli, MD
Scientific Director
Department of Arrhythmology
The Villa Maria Cecilia Hospital
Cotignola (Ravenna), Italy

James J. Shields, MD
Clinical Assistant Professor
Department of Radiology
University of Michigan;
Division Director
Vascular and Interventional Radiology
University of Michigan Health System
Ann Arbor, Michigan

William H. Spencer III, MD
Professor of Medicine
Department of Medicine
Medical University of South Carolina
Charleston, South Carolina

Eron Sturm, MD
Fellow in Interventional Cardiology
Cardiovascular Division
University of Pennsylvania School of Medicine
Philadelphia, Pennsylvania

Gilbert R. Upchurch Jr., MD
Professor of Surgery
Department of Surgery
University of Michigan
Ann Arbor, Michigan

Frank C. Vandy, MD
Resident in Vascular Surgery
Section of Vascular Surgery
University of Michigan Medical School
Ann Arbor, Michigan

Jay S. Yadav, MD, IACC
Chairman of Innovation Center
Innovation Center
Piedmont Heart Institute
Atlanta, Georgia

PREFACE

Despite advancements in technology that have resulted in a significant increase in the safety of invasive diagnostic and therapeutic cardiovascular procedures, prevention and management of complications continue to be imperative components of the current practice of interventional cardiology. Given the relatively rare frequency of certain complications, there is little opportunity to include a "how to manage" approach during formal training of cardiovascular interventionalists. Thus, it is not uncommon that the first time a physician becomes aware of a particular complication is, unfortunately, only when he or she faces it in the interventional suite.

Since completing my training in interventional cardiology at the Beth Israel Hospital in Boston in 1994, my clinical and research interest has focused on complications of cardiovascular procedures and on factors that might relate to their development. My goal has incessantly been to reduce complication rates through changes in process of care, and to minimize their adverse consequences through prompt recognition and management.

This project started following a visit from my mentor, Dr. Donald Baim, to the University of Michigan, where I was director of the Cardiac Catheterization Laboratory. After that visit, I approached him with an idea that had been brewing for several years about a comprehensive textbook on complications. To my delight, Don was very enthusiastic in endorsing the project. He promptly agreed to participate as a coeditor and to help as a liaison with Lippincott Williams & Wilkins. His unexpected and premature death in late 2009 was a major loss for the interventional community and a major personal loss for me.

The purpose of *Complications of Cardiovascular Procedures: Risk Factors, Management, and Bailout Techniques* is to provide a comprehensive resource for practicing interventional cardiologists, endovascular interventionalists (vascular surgeons, radiologists, and neurosurgeons), and physicians on training for the prevention and management of complications. A particular emphasis has been placed on providing information on risk factors, prevention, and management with conventional and bailout techniques and devices.

The book is divided into seven sections. The first section is on general principles, and it addresses issues surrounding quality assurance, training requirements, and legal considerations. Two chapters on adjunctive pharmacotherapy and conscious sedation are also included in this section. The second and third sections cover general complications and complications of coronary interventions, whereas the fourth and fifth sections include specific noncoronary cardiac and endovascular procedures and their complications. The sixth section is dedicated to pediatric interventions, and the seventh section covers electrophysiology procedures.

I hope that the information provided in this book will help interventionalists in avoiding complications and that it will provide them with useful suggestions regarding management. Ultimately, I hope that the great work done by all the contributors to this endeavor will benefit our patients.

Mauro Moscucci, MD, MBA
Miami, Florida

ACKNOWLEDGMENTS

First and foremost, I would like to thank my mentor, Dr. Donald Baim, who enthusiastically supported my initial proposal for this textbook.

I would also like to thank Fran DeStefano, from Lippincott Williams & Wilkins, for her enthusiasm and support as we first presented the project, and for her patience through the development phase. In addition, I would like to thank Grace Caputo, from Dovetail Content Solutions, for her skillful editorial assistance and project management, and Leanne McMillan, from Lippincott Williams & Wilkins, for her careful supporting role as managing editor.

Finally, I am immensely grateful to all the contributing authors and to the many colleagues who over the years have given me tips and shared their experience, leading to the idea for the development of this textbook.

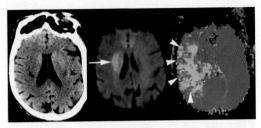

FIGURE 9-2 A. See page 128 for this figure legend.

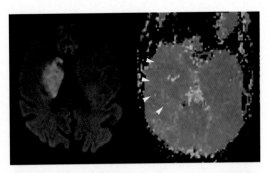

FIGURE 9-2 D. See page 128 for this figure legend.

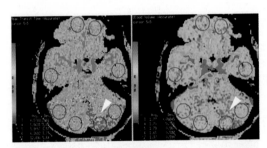

FIGURE 9-4 A. See page 130 for this figure legend.

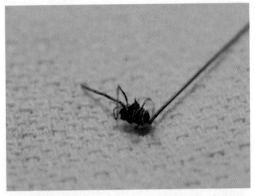

FIGURE 9-4 C. See page 130 for this figure legend.

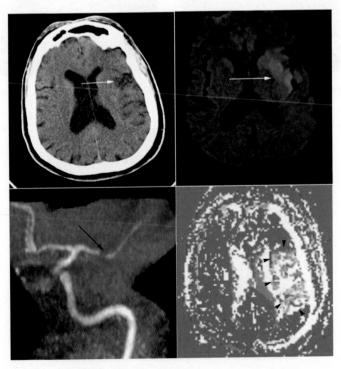

FIGURE 9-5 A. See page 133 for this figure legend.

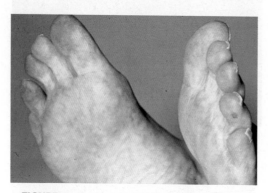

FIGURE 13-6. See page 186 for this figure legend.

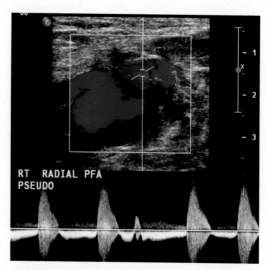

RT RADIAL PFA
PSEUDO

FIGURE 14-15 A. See page 224 for this figure legend.

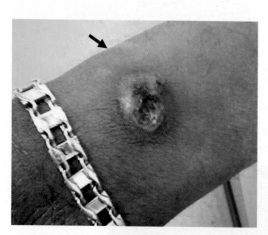

FIGURE 14-17. See page 225 for this figure legend.

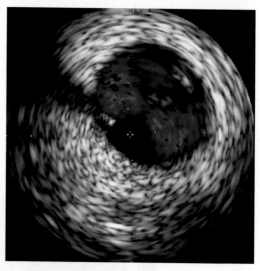

FIGURE 15-3 C. See page 246 for this figure legend.

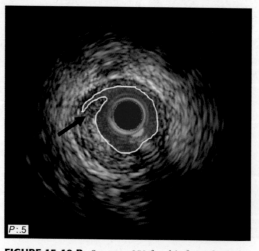

P:.5

FIGURE 15-10 B. See page 250 for this figure legend.

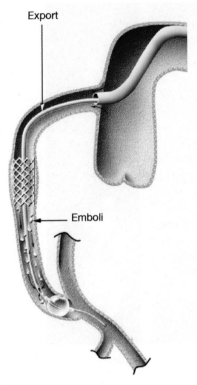

Export

Emboli

FIGURE 17-9 B. See page 283 for this figure legend.

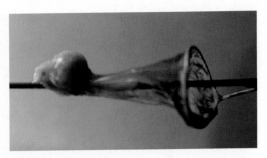

FIGURE 17-11 D. See page 284 for this figure legend.

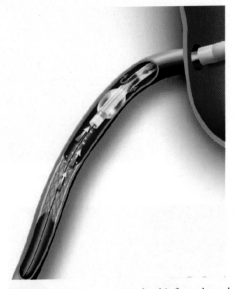

FIGURE 17-15. See page 288 for this figure legend.

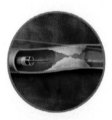

The Proxis sealing balloon is positioned proximal to the lesion, The interventional device is advanced to the distal end of the Proxis catheter.

Treat

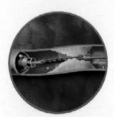

The guidewire is advanced acroos the lesion and the interventional device is delivered, while the vessel is protected.

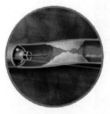

The Proxis sealing balloon is inflated, temporarily suspending antegrade blood flow and protecting all downstream vessels during lesion crossing.

Aspirate

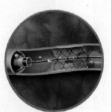

Fluid and embolic debris are aspirated from the vessel.

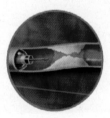

With the blood flow suspended, contrast medium can be injected into the vessel to provide better visualization and give you a visual "road map" for the intervention.

Restore

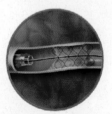

Balloon is deflated and antegrade blood flow is restored.

FIGURE 17-16. See page 288 for this figure legend.

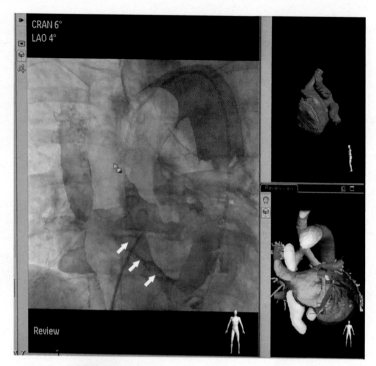

FIGURE 19-4. See page 326 for this figure legend.

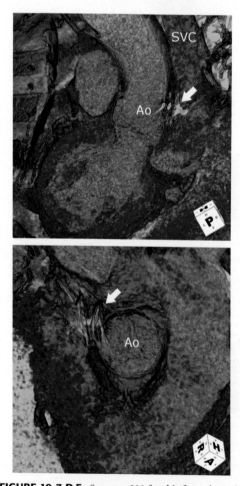

FIGURE 19-7 D,E. See page 330 for this figure legend.

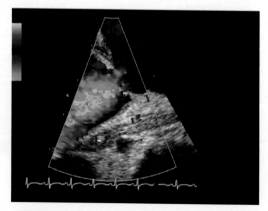

FIGURE 19-12 D. See page 335 for this figure legend.

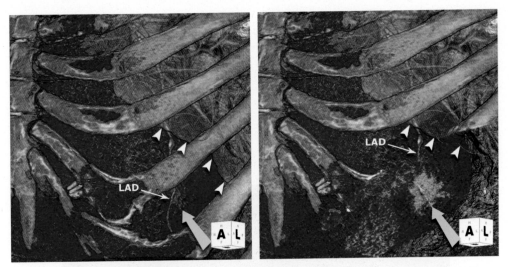

FIGURE 19-13 A,B. See page 338 for this figure legend.

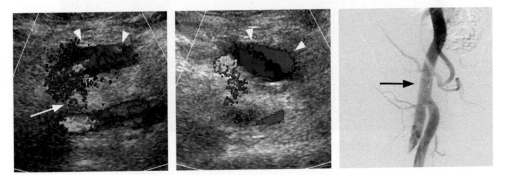

FIGURE 20-1 A-C. See page 344 for this figure legend.

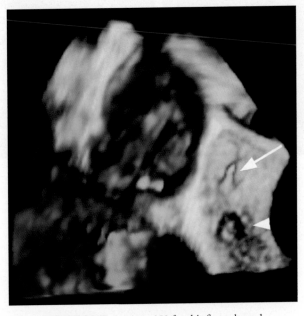

FIGURE 20-7. See page 350 for this figure legend.

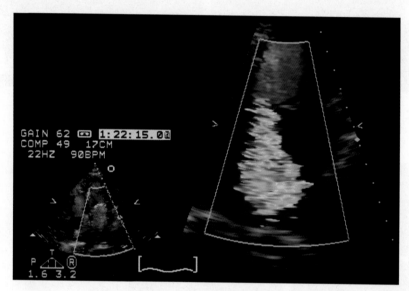

FIGURE 20-11. See page 352 for this figure legend.

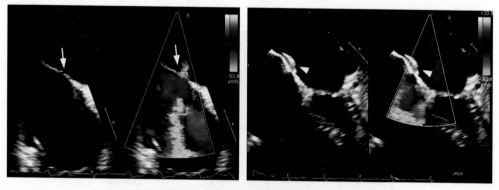

FIGURE 20-14 A,B. See page 353 for this figure legend.

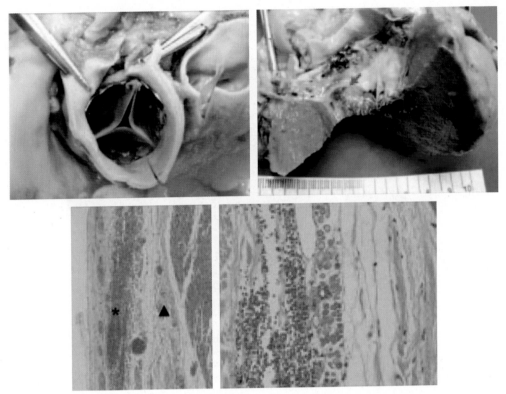

FIGURE 21-6 A-D. See page 372 for this figure legend.

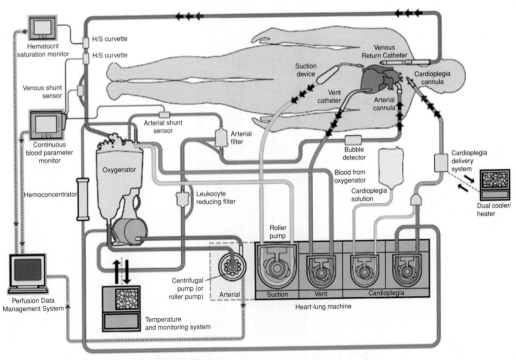

FIGURE 24-1. See page 404 for this figure legend.

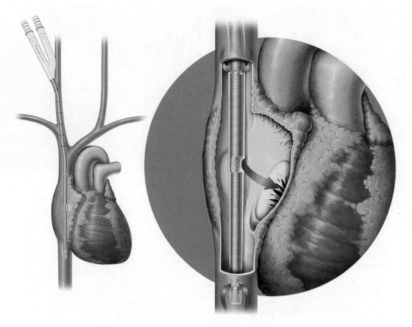

FIGURE 24-6. See page 407 for this figure legend.

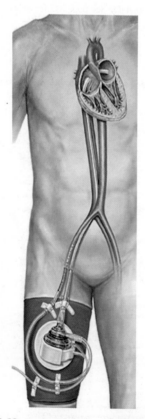

FIGURE 24-12. See page 413 for this figure legend.

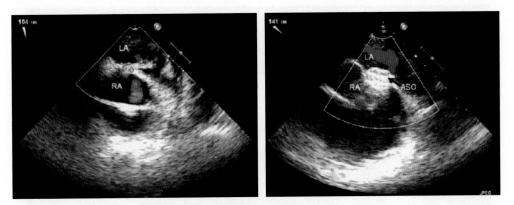

FIGURE 24-14 A,B. See page 414 for this figure legend.

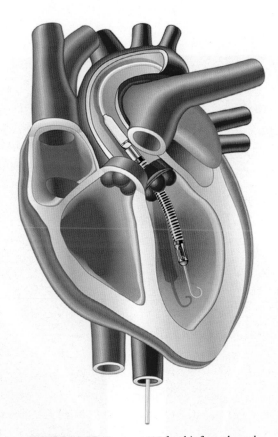

FIGURE 24-15. See page 415 for this figure legend.

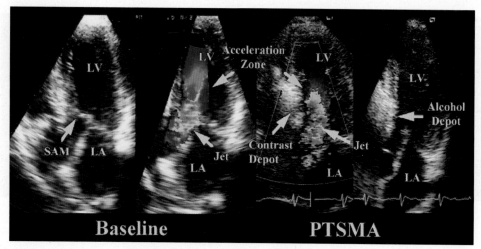

FIGURE 25-4. See page 420 for this figure legend.

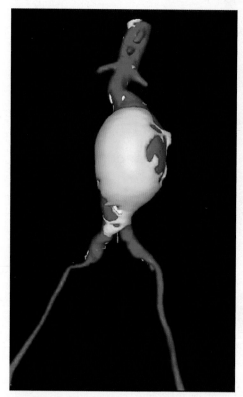

FIGURE 27-2. See page 463 for this figure legend.

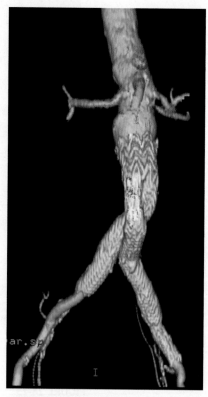

FIGURE 27-8 A. See page 469 for this figure legend.

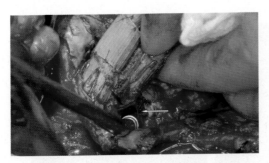

FIGURE 27-12. See page 470 for this figure legend.

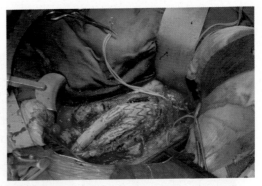

FIGURE 27-14. See page 471 for this figure legend.

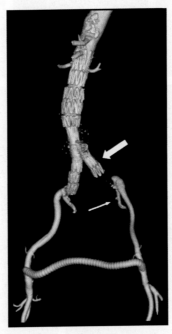

FIGURE 27-18 C. See page 473 for this figure legend.

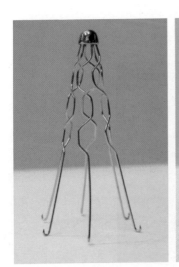 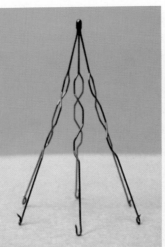 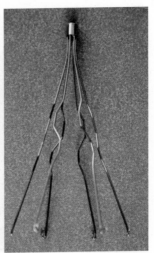

FIGURE 29-2 A-C. See page 513 for this figure legend.

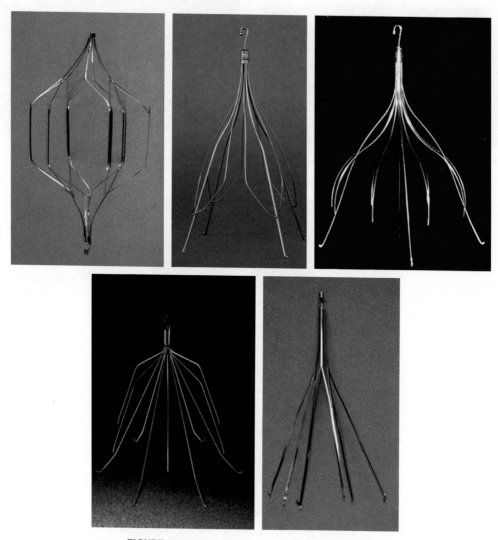

FIGURE 29-9 A-E. See page 519 for this figure legend.

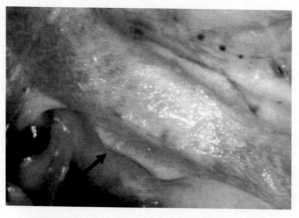

FIGURE 29-12 C. See page 524 for this figure legend.

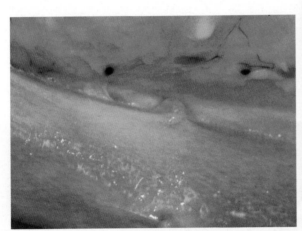
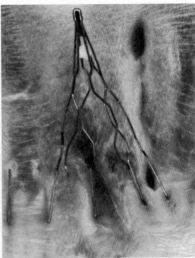

FIGURE 29-19 A,B. See page 533 for this figure legend.

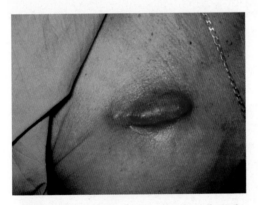

FIGURE 33-7. See page 600 for this figure legend.

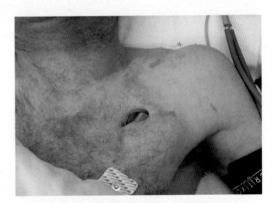

FIGURE 33-8. See page 601 for this figure legend.

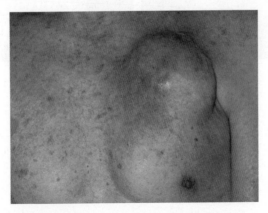

FIGURE 33-9. See page 601 for this figure legend.

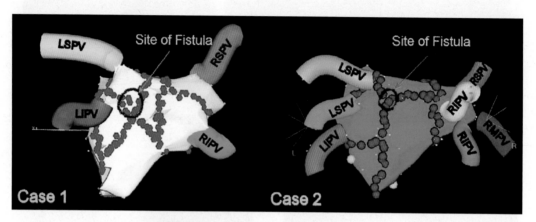

FIGURE 34-6. See page 615 for this figure legend.

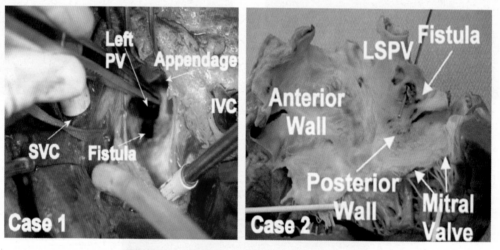

FIGURE 34-7 A,B. See page 615 for this figure legend.

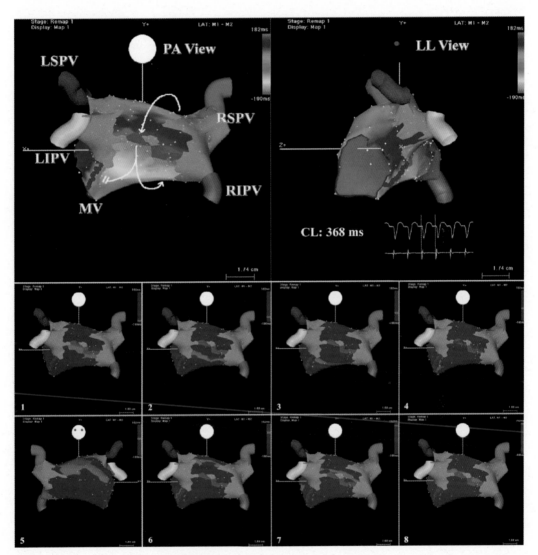

FIGURE 34-9. See page 618 for this figure legend.

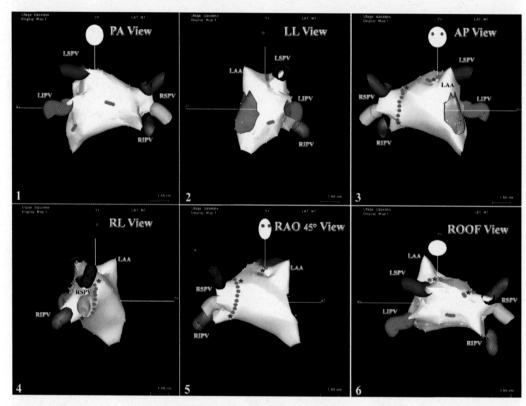

FIGURE 34-14. See page 623 for this figure legend.

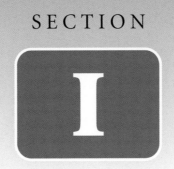

SECTION

I

General Principles

1

Risk Assessment

DAVID J. MALENKA AND MAURO MOSCUCCI

A percutaneous coronary revascularization is not risk free, and as such, no patient should undergo a percutaneous coronary intervention (PCI) without understanding the risks of the procedure. This is not just good patient-centered care, but the elements of a truly informed consent process (1) mandate that the risks of treatment be specified. Furthermore, it is likely that an informed consent process that adheres to these guidelines and speaks specifically to the procedural risk offers the practitioner some element of legal protection from malpractice litigation (2).

Assessing patient-specific risk is challenging. The more knowledgeable and experienced physicians are, the better they should be able to predict a patient's risk. However, studies have shown that clinicians' predictions of risk may be inaccurate (3–5). In addition, as elegantly described by Kahneman et al., (6) and more recently highlighted in the popular work of Dan Ariely (7), most people make use of mental shortcuts or heuristics that may lead them astray when predicting risk. For physicians, an obvious example is the impact of the availability heuristic, or last-case bias, which may lead a physician to overestimate the risk of a treatment if a recent patient undergoing that treatment had a complication. Though this book focuses on the myriad complications of PCI, the total risk of a PCI is actually quite low. As a consequence, few physicians (or for that matter institutions) ever have enough experience with adverse outcomes to be able to predict with much precision patient-specific risk for an adverse event.

Given the need to estimate risk more precisely, there has been a growing interest in the development and use of clinical prediction rules. Clinical prediction rules are mathematical models that use elements of the history, physical findings, and sometimes test results to derive a patient-specific estimate of the probability of an outcome. While they can be used to estimate the probability of disease, the utility of diagnostic testing, or even as decision aids (8), in the context of this chapter we are speaking of their use to predict outcomes following a PCI. As such, they make use of past experience with PCI from observational registries or randomized trials to determine how patient characteristics relate to the risks of specific outcomes and to predict future risk.

■ METHODS FOR DEVELOPING CLINICAL PREDICTION RULES

Clinical prediction rules can be developed using many different multivariable modeling techniques including linear regression, logistic regression, discriminant function analysis, recursive partitioning, Cox proportional hazards regression, and neural networks. Each technique has its strengths and weaknesses. A rich discussion of their relative merits is beyond the scope of this text. Rules to predict outcomes following PCI have relied mainly on logistic regression and rarely on Cox proportional hazards regression.

Logistic regression (9) is particularly appropriate for predicting risk following PCI because most of the outcome variables of interest are binary events (e.g., death, myocardial infarction) and physicians are interested in the probability they will occur at a fixed time interval, such as during the index hospitalization or within 30 days. The logistic model for the probability of an outcome (the dependent variable) always yields a value that is between 0 and 1. It incorporates the assumption that an individual variable in the model (the independent variable) multiplies the odds of disease by an amount that is the same regardless of the values for other variables (unless interactions are also modeled). The independent variables may be continuous (e.g., age) or categorical (e.g., sex). An intercept and coefficient for each independent variable that significantly contributes to the prediction are reported. These are the values that maximized the likelihood of reproducing the relationships between dependent and independent variables in the data (the so-called maximum likelihood estimates). The intercept and variable coefficients can be used to calculate a patient-specific probability of the outcome using the following formula:

Probability of the outcome

$$= \frac{1}{1 + \exp[-(a + b1 \times 1 + \cdots brxr)]}$$

where a is the intercept, b are the coefficients, x are the predictor variables, and r is the number of predictor variables.

Solving a clinical predication rule from a logistic equation requires a calculator or a spreadsheet. In an effort to increase their use in the routine process of care, a simple scoring system is sometimes created in which regression coefficients are divided by the lowest regression coefficient in the model and then rounded to their nearest whole number. All that needs calculating is a simple sum based on the weight given to each variable (10,11). A nomogram or table is then provided relating any given score to the probability of the endpoint of interest (Fig. 1-1 and Table 1-1).

Although this introduces some minor imprecision into the calculation of risk, the imprecision is not clinically significant (11,12) and the ease of use more than compensates for this.

Cox proportional hazards regression (13) is a form of survival analysis. The dependent variable is the time to occurrence of a binary event during follow-up. Thus, in the setting of a PCI, Cox regression is well suited for predicting long-term survival and repeats revascularization, whether it is target lesion revascularization, target vessel revascularization, mode of revascularization (PCI or CABG), or any revascularization. Using maximization of a partial likelihood, it determines the relative contribution of a group of independent variables to the risk or "hazard" of the outcome. The proportional hazards assumption is that the risk/hazard associated with any independent variable is constant throughout the period of observation. Cox models are reported out as a constant with adjusted hazard ratios. This information can be used to determine the probability of any binary endpoint throughout the period of follow-up (14).

■ EVALUATING PREDICTION RULES

Methodological standards have been proposed for developing and evaluating clinical prediction

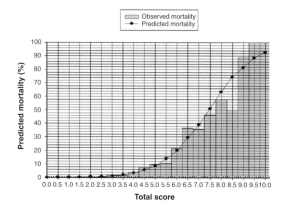

Variable	Score
Acute MI	1
Shock	2.5
Creatinine 1.5 mg dL	1.5
History of cardiac arrest	1.5
# Diseased vessels	0.5
Age ≥ 70	1.0
EF < 50%	0.5
Thrombus	0.5
PVD	0.5
Female gender	0.5
Total score	

FIGURE 1-1. Example of a risk prediction rule for PCI mortality. For the estimation of risk, the total score can be calculated by adding individual scores if the comorbidity is present. For number of diseased vessels, a score of 0.5 should be added for each major epicardial vessel that has >70% stenosis. The total score can then be transferred to the horizontal axis of the plot, and the corresponding probability of death can be estimated on the vertical axis. Scores ≤2.5 are associated with a risk of death <0.8%, whereas scores >7 are associated with a risk of death >40%. MI, myocardial infarction; EF, ejection fraction; PVD, peripheral artery disease. (From Moscucci M, Kline-Rogers E, Share D, et al. Simple bedside additive tool for prediction of in-hospital mortality after percutaneous coronary interventions. *Circulation.* 2001;104:263–268.)

| TABLE 1-1 | NCDR CathPCI Risk Score System for In-Hospital Mortality |

Variable	Scoring Response Categories				Total Points	In-Hospital Mortality
Age	<60	60–69	70–79	≥80	0	0.0%
	0	4	8	14	5	0.1%
Cardiogenic shock	No	Yes			10	0.1%
	0	25			15	0.2%
Prior CHF	No	Yes			20	0.3%
	0	5			25	0.6%
PVD	No	Yes			30	1.1%
	0	5			35	2.0%
CLD	No	Yes			40	3.6%
	0	4			45	6.3%
GFR	<30	30–60	60–90	>90	50	10.9%
	18	10	6	0	55	18.3%
NYHA Class IV	No	Yes			60	29.0%
	0	4			65	42.7%
STEMI priority	Elective	Urgent	Emergent	Salvage	70	57.6%
	12	15	20	38	75	71.2%
Non-STEMI priority	Elective	Urgent	Emergent	Salvage	80	89.2%
	0	8	20	42	85	89.2%
					90	93.8%
					95	96.5%
					100	98.0%

CHF, congestive heart failure; PVD, peripheral vascular disease; CLD, chronic lung disease; GFR, glomerular filtration rate; NYHA, New York Heart Association; STEMI, ST-segment elevation myocardial infarction; PCI, percutaneous coronary intervention.

(Reprinted from Peterson ED, Dai D, DeLong ER, et al. Contemporary mortality risk prediction for percutaneous coronary intervention: results from 588,398 procedures in the National Cardiovascular Data Registry. *J Am Coll Cardiol*.2010; 55(18):1923–1932, with permission from Elsevier.)

rules (15–17). Several of them deserve mention. One of the more important is determining the generalizability of the prediction rule. Were the patients, physicians, hospitals, and the technical details of care sufficiently similar to the practice setting in which the rule might be used to suggest that the rule will work well? A rule developed in the era of balloon angioplasty might not perform as well in the era of coronary stenting with its lower rate of acute closure and need for emergency coronary artery bypass surgery. Another relates to whether the variables included in the model were sufficiently well defined to ensure that others could identify these characteristics in their patients? There are many definitions of an "urgent" PCI. To maximize the accuracy of the prediction rule, the user needs access to a clear definition to ensure they identify similar patients as urgent. Were the performance characteristics of the rule described? This may include the familiar descriptions of test performance such as sensitivity, specificity, likelihood ratios, and predictive values or less familiar measures such as discrimination and calibration, two of the more frequently reported metrics. Discrimination refers to the ability of the rule to distinguish between patients with versus without the outcome of interest. It is reported out as the area under the receiver operator characteristic curve (the plot of sensitivity vs. 1-specificity), is bounded between 0.5 and 1.0, with 1.0 indicating perfect discrimination, and is equivalent to a c statistic (18). Calibration refers to how well the model predicts across the range of risk and can be assessed by comparing the observed versus expected numbers of adverse events by decile of predicted risk in probability plots and using the Hosmer–Lemeshow goodness-of-fit statistic (9). Most importantly, has the rule been validated? Internal, or statistical, validation is frequently performed using a bootstrapping technique in which rule performance is tested on numerous subsets of random samples of the dataset from which the rule was derived (19). Prospective validation is less often performed, as it requires that rule performance be evaluated in a group of patients different from the group in which it was derived. This can be a validation dataset drawn from the same data source in the derivation dataset or data from an entirely different source, such as a different set of hospitals (20). The latter is the gold standard for assessing rule performance as several studies have reported a decline in the calibration of rule with prospective external validation (21–24). One caveat is that there is no need for external validation if one is practicing in the care system in which the rule was developed.

■ PCI PREDICTION RULES

For this purposes of this text, we have decided to reference prediction rules that are likely to have the greatest generalizability. They reflect reasonably current practice and for the most part were derived from a spectrum of patients, hospitals, and interventionists. Variable definitions, discrimination and calibration, and internal validation have been reported for all. For some, there has been external validation. We report only the most recent version of the model. For ease of use, we have tried to include models that report an integer score that can be used at the bedside. For mortality we do not include rules derived solely from a primary PCI experience.

Short-Term Mortality

Although short-term mortality following PCI is uncommon, it is an outcome of concern to both patients and physicians and an important consideration when choosing among medical management versus surgical revascularization versus a PCI. Models predicting in-hospital mortality are summarized in Table 1-2.

Likely to become a widely used model for predicting PCI mortality is one recently derived from the National Cardiovascular Data Registry Cath/PCI Registry using data on 181,775 patients who underwent a PCI between 1/2004 and 3/2006 at >800 sites in the United States (25). Standard data definitions were available to all sites (http://www.acc.org/ncdr/cathlab.htm). The model discriminated well (c statistic = 0.929) and was well calibrated. The 181,775 patients represented a two-thirds random sample of patients who underwent a PCI from 1/2004 to 3/2006. The other one-third ($n = 121,183$) were used to prospectively validate the model (c statistic = 0.925; good calibration), as was data on 285,440 additional patients (c statistic = 0.924; good calibration) who underwent their procedure after the derivation cohort, from 4/2006 to 3/2007. External validation in a group of hospitals that do not contribute to the NCDR CathPCI registry has yet to be done, though it is hard to question the generalizability of a dataset that has such broad participation in hospitals across the nation.

The full NCDR CathPCI model contains 21 variables. To their credit, the investigators showed that a more parsimonious model that excluded angiographic data had good performance characteristics (with c statistics of 0.912 and 0.914 in the two validation cohorts). This is likely a more relevant model than the full one because most PCIs occur ad hoc, which means that the details of the coronary anatomy are not known at the time informed consent is obtained, and, therefore, are not available to help predict risk. A simple scoring system was derived from this model, which performed well (c statistic = 0.890), and is reproduced in Table 1-1.

Other prediction rules that are likely to be generalizable include those derived from the Mayo Clinic (26), the Blue Cross Blue Shield of Michigan Cardiovascular Consortium (11), the Northern New England Cardiovascular Disease Study Group (27), the New York State PCI Reporting System (28), and the British Columbia Cardiac Registry (29). While the Mayo Clinic Risk Score could be criticized for being developed on the select Mayo Clinic population, it has undergone external validation and recalibration using NCDR CathPCI data from 309,351 patients who underwent a PCI from 1/2004 to 3/2006 (23). It had

TABLE 1-2 Prediction Rules for Post-PCI Short-Term Mortality

Reference	Peterson et al. (25) Full	Simplified	Moscucci et al. (11)	Singh et al. (23,26)	Wu et al. (28)	O'Connor et al. (27)	Hamburger et al. (29)
Data Source	NCDR CathPCI	NCDR CathPCI	Blue Cross Blue Shield of Michigan Cardiovascular Consortium	Mayo Clinic	New York State PCI Reporting System	Northern New England Cardiovascular Disease Study Group	British Columbia Cardiac Registry
Dates/N	1/2004–3/2006 $N = 181,775$	1/2004–3/2006 $N = 181,775$	7/1997–9/1999 $N = 10,796$	1/2000–4/2005 $N = 7,640$	1/2002–12/2002 $N = 46,090$	1/1994–12/1996 $N = 15,331$	1/2000–12/2004 $N = 26,350$
Mortality	In-hospital	In-hospital	In-hospital	In-hospital	In-hospital	In-hospital	30 Day
Internal validation	No —	No —	No —	Yes $c = 0.90$	No —	Yes $c = 0.88$	No —
Prospective validation	Yes $c = 0.924$	Yes $c = 0.905$	Yes $c = 0.91$	No —	Yes $c = 0.905$	No —	Yes $c = 0.911$
External validation	No	No	NHLBI Dynamic Registry (38) $c = 0.86$ APPROACH (39) $c = 0.94$ Toronto University Health Network (40) $c = 0.868$	NCDR CathPCI (23) $c = 0.885$	Toronto University Health Network (40) $c = 0.865$	Moscucci University of Michigan PCI Data $c = 0.88$ NHLBI Dynamic Registry (38) $c = 0.89$ Toronto University Health Network (40) $c = 0.923$	No
Calibration	Yes	Yes	Yes	Yes	Yes	Yes	Yes
Uses Angiographic Data	Yes	No	Yes	No	Yes	Yes	Yes
Risk Score	Yes (Table 1-2)	Yes (Table 1-2)	Yes	Yes	Yes	No	No

(continued)

TABLE 1-2 Prediction Rules for Post-PCI Short-Term Mortality (*Continued*)

Reference	Peterson et al. (25) Full	Peterson et al. (25) Simplified	Moscucci et al. (11)	Singh et al. (23,26)	Wu et al. (28)	O'Connor et al. (27)	Hamburger et al. (29)
Variables							
Demographic							
Age	×	×	×	×	×	×	×
Sex	×	—	×	—	×	—	×
BMI or BSA	×	—	—	—	—	—	—
Comorbidities							
Diabetes	×	—	—	—	—	—	—
PVD[a]	×	×	×	×	×	×	—
COPD	×	×	—	—	—	—	—
Renal Function	×	×	×	×	×	×	×
Cardiac History & Function							
CHF	×	×	—	×	×	×	×
NYHA Class	×	×	—	—	—	—	×
Prior PCI	×	—	—	—	—	×	—
Priority (elective, urgent, Emergent, salvage)	×	—	—	—	—	—	×
Indication (STEMI, no-STEMI)	×	×	×	×	×	×	×
Shock and/or VF Arrest	×	×	×	×	×	×	×
IABP	×	—	—	—	—	×	—
Cardiac anatomy and function							
Ejection fraction	×	—	×	×	×	×	×
No. disease vessels and/or lesion location	×	—	×	—	×	×	×
Lesion type	×	—	—	—	—	×	—
TIMI flow	×	—	—	—	—	—	—
Thrombus	×	—	×	—	—	—	—

[a]Could include cerebrovascular disease.

excellent discrimination (c statistic = 0.885) and calibration in a validation set of 433,045 patients who underwent a PCI from 4/2006 to 3/2007. Like the simplified NCDR CathPCI risk score, it does not include angiographic data.

The remaining prediction rules for in-hospital PCI mortality all make use of angiographic data. Their clinical utility is limited to patients having a cardiac catheterization at a different time from their PCI. Among them the Blue Cross Blue Shield of Michigan Cardiovascular Consortium and the Northern New England Cardiovascular Disease Study Group PCI mortality prediction rules have been the most extensively externally validated and shown to perform well. The former has the advantage of a published risk score, whereas the latter slightly better discrimination and calibration in some studies. The New York State Cardiovascular Consortium rule is based on the relatively recent statewide experience with PCI, but its performance in other patient populations waits testing. The British Columbia Cardiac Registry prediction rule predicts 30-day mortality, which would seem a more relevant endpoint than in-hospital mortality. Like the New York State Cardiovascular Consortium prediction rule, it has not been externally validated. Although a risk score was not developed, an online calculator for solving the logistic equation and obtaining a probability of death is available at www.bcpci.org (accessed 7/1/2010).

Predicting Nonfatal PCI Outcomes

Prediction rules for nonfatal PCI outcomes tend to have lower discrimination when compared with prediction rules for short-term mortality. Incomplete ascertainment of the outcome assessed, different definitions and sometime different interpretations of the same definition, and management bias are among the limitations leading to lower discrimination power of prediction rules for nonfatal outcomes. Yet, these predictions rules can still be quite helpful in identifying patients at increased risk, and in introducing modifications of the procedure strategy aimed toward reducing that risk. As an example, the identification of an increased risk of contrast nephropathy for an individual patient should lead the interventionalist to institute appropriate preprocedure hydration, to select the appropriate contrast media, and to

modify the procedure strategy in order to minimize the total amount of radiocontrast used (Fig. 1-2). The following is an outline of prediction rules for nonfatal PCI outcomes that have been proposed on the basis of registries analysis.

Bleeding

Bleeding is the most common complication following PCI and is associated with an increased risk of other adverse outcomes. Using NCDR CathPCI data from an 80% sample of 309,351 patients who underwent a PCI between 1/2004 and 3/2006 at 484 hospitals, Mehta et al (30). developed a risk score to predict post-PCI bleeding. Bleeding was defined as occurring at percutaneous entry site, during or after catheterization laboratory visit until discharge, which may be external or a hematoma >10 cm for femoral, >5 cm for brachial, or >2 cm for radial access or retroperitoneal or gastrointestinal or genitourinary or other/unknown origin during or after catheterization visit until discharge and required a transfusion, prolonged hospital stay, and/or a drop in hemoglobin >3.0 g/dL. The bleeding risk score is shown in Table 1-3, as is the risk of bleeding for three categories of scores. In a validation dataset consisting of the other 20% of patients, the score had reasonable discrimination (c statistic = 0.73) and calibration. Caveats include the fact that in the NCDR CathPCI bleeding is not an adjudicated outcome and the model has yet to be externally validated. Patients identified at high risk of bleeding might receive more careful dosing of anticoagulants, a smaller size sheath, radial access, and/or the use of a direct thrombin inhibitor and avoidance of a glycoprotein IIb/IIIa inhibitor.

Bleeding and Access Site Complications

Access site complications, which include but are not limited to bleeding, are another common complication of PCI. Piper et al. (31) used data on a consecutive series of 18,137 patients who underwent PCI in northern New England between 1/1997 and 12/1999 to develop a prediction rule for the combination of vascular complications, defined as an access site injury requiring procedural or surgical intervention or any bleeding requiring a transfusion. Internal validation was good (c statistic = 0.77) and the

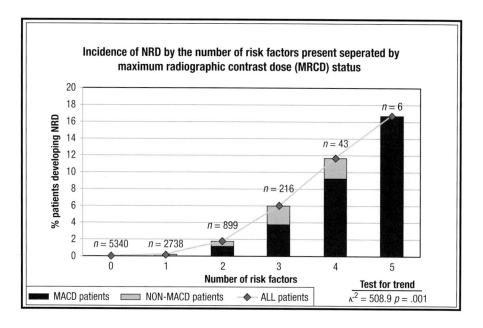

**High-risk patient characteristics
for contrast nephropathy**

Diabetes
Creatinine ≥2 mg/dL
Peripheral vascular disease
Cardiogenic shock
Congestive heart failure

Proposed guidelines for high-risk patients

A) Aggressive hydration **before** contrast administration. Measuring the LVEDP or PCWP before contrast administration might help in further determining volume status. It is not uncommon to find low PCWP/LVEDP in patients who have been admitted for preprocedure "I.V. Hydration."

B) Determine "maximum allowed contrast dose" according to the following formula:

5cc × kg body weight/creatinine

C) Avoid exceeding this amount. Use of biplane coronary angiography and avoidance of unnecessary images (i.e., left ventriculogram or other images) might help in minimizing total amount of contast used.

D) Consider staged procedures. When planning a staged procedure, current recommendations are to perform the second procedure several days after the first.

E) Use of smaller catheters might help in decreasing amount of contrast.

F) Use of low osmolar or nonionic contrast might decrease the risk in high-risk patients.

G) In view of a recent study showing a significant benefit from acetylcysteine, and given its safety, consider acetylcysteine 600 mg bid on the day before and on the day of contrast administration (*NEJM* 2000;343:180–184).

FIGURE 1-2. BMC (2) bedside risk prediction tool for the prediction and prevention of nephropathy requiring dialysis. (From Moscucci M, Rogers EK, Montoye C, et al. Association of a continuous quality improvement initiative with practice and outcome variations of contemporary percutaneous coronary interventions. *Circulation.* 2006;113(6):814–822. ©2001 University of Michigan Board of Regents. All Rights Reserved.)

model was well calibrated. They created a risk score (Table 1-4) and nomogram (Fig. 1-3) for ease of use. The score has not been prospectively or externally validated. One weakness of the score is that it was calibrated based on knowl-edge of the coronary anatomy and the proposed intervention. Use of this risk score is immedi-ately actionable. Patients identified at high risk might be candidates for more careful use of anticoagulants, radial or ultrasound-guided

TABLE 1-3   **NCDR CathPCI Risk Score for Bleeding**

Variable	Points Assigned	Risk Score	Risk of Bleeding
STEMI	10	≤7	0.63%
NSTEMI-USA	3	8–17	1.77%
Shock	8	≥18	5.08%
Female	6		
History of CHF	5		
No prior PCI	4		
NYHA Class IV	4		
PVD	2		
Age 66–75	2		
Age 76–85	5		
Age >85	8		
EGFR	1 (per 10 unit decrease if <90)		

(From Mehta SK, Frutkin AD, Lindsey JB, et al. Bleeding in patient undergoing percutaneous coronary intervention; the development of a clinical risk algorithm from the National Cardiovascular Data Registry. *Circ Cardiovasc Interv.* 2009;2:222–229.)

access, access by an experienced operator, as well as for more careful postprocedure monitoring.

Acute Kidney Injury

Post-PCI acute kidney injury (AKI) requiring dialysis is a devastating consequence of the procedure, but even AKI not requiring dialysis has been associated with increased short-term and long-term mortality (32). Identifying patients at increased risk for this complication should alert the health care team to any of a number of interventions that likely decrease the risk of this complication (33).

In 2002, Freeman et al. (34) described a clinical prediction rule to identify a patient's risk of AKI requiring dialysis. Their derivation dataset consisted of 9,242 consecutive patient in the Blue Cross Blue Shield of Michigan Cardiovascular Registry who underwent a PCI from 7/1997 to 9/1999, of whom 0.44% required dialysis. They identified baseline renal insufficiency, diabetes mellitus, congestive heart failure, and cardiogenic shock as the five risk factors predictive of AKI requiring dialysis. The model was validated in 5,382 patients undergoing a PCI from 9/1999 to 8/2000 and discriminated well (c statistic = 0.89). A simple sum of risk factors

correlated well with an increased risk of dialysis. Of most interest, they showed that exceeding the maximum radiographic contrast dose ($5 \times$ kg body weight/serum creatinine [mg/dL]) was strongly related to the risk of dialysis, the latter being a variable potentially under the control of the interventional cardiologists. This rule was then used in a multicenter continuous quality improvement project aimed to reduce contrast nephropathy and nephropathy requiring dialysis among other complications of PCI (35).

Bartholomew et al. used data from 10,481 PCI patients who underwent PCI at William Beaumont Hospital from 1/1993 to 12/1998 to identify predictors of radiocontrast-induced nephropathy (RCIN), defined as a >1.0 mg/dL increase in serum creatinine from the baseline level, which occurred in 2.0% of the cohort. Risk factors included baseline creatinine clearance <60 mL/min, intra-aortic balloon pump use, urgent or emergent procedures, diabetes mellitus, congestive heart failure, hypertension, peripheral vascular disease, and contrast volume >260 mL. In the prospective validation dataset of 9,998 patients undergoing PCI from 1/1999 to 12/2002, the model discriminated well (c statistic = 0.89) and was well calibrated.

TABLE 1-4	Northern New England Risk Score for Bleeding and Access Site Complications

Variable	Score
Age 60–69	1.5
Age 70–79	2.5
Age >80	3
Female	2
BSA 1.6–1.8 m^2	1.5
BSA <1.6 m^2	2
CHF	1.5
Bleeding disorder	1.5
PAD	1.5
COPD	1.5
Dialysis or CR > 2 mg/dL	2
Urgent procedure	1.5
Emergent procedure	2
Primary PCI	1.5
Cardiogenic shock	2
2 Lesion PCI	1.5
≥3 Lesion PCI	1.5
ACC B2 lesion	1.5
ACC C lesion	1.5
Preprocedure clopidogrel	1.5
Glycoprotein IIb/IIIa inhibitor	2

(Reprinted from Piper WD, Malenka DJ, Ryan TJ Jr, et al. Predicting vascular complications in percutaneous coronary interventions. *Am Heart J.* 2003;145:1022–1029, with permission from Elsevier.)

Mehran et al. published one of the more frequently cited prediction rules in 2004 (36). The derivation cohort consisted of a two-thirds random sample of 5,571 patients who underwent PCI over a 6-year period and were included in the Cardiovascular Research Foundation interventional registry. Contrast-induced nephropathy (CIN) was defined as an increase of ≥25% or ≥0.5 mg/dL in pre-PCI serum creatinine at 48 hours post-PCI, occurring in 13.1% of the derivation cohort. The other one-third of patients, 2,786, was used for validation of the model that had acceptable discrimination (c statistic = 0.67) and calibration. The predictors of CIN, the risk score and weights derived from the logistic model, and the risk of both CIN and post-PCI dialysis are shown in Figure 1-4.

Brown et al. (37) recently published a clinical prediction rule for AKI that did not incorporate any procedural variables, and as a consequence could be used to predict preprocedural risk that might lead to changes in management strategy. Their dependent variable was serious renal dysfunction (SRD) defined as new onset dialysis or ≥50% increased in creatinine from baseline. The model was developed on 11,141 consecutive patients who underwent PCI in northern New England from 1/2003 to 12/2005 with a SRD rate of 0.7%. The model was validated on 2006 PCI data and was found to discriminate well (c statistic = 0.84). Age ≥80, female, diabetes mellitus, urgent priority and emergent priority, congestive heart failure, baseline renal function, and preprocedure placement of an intra-aortic balloon pump were significantly predictive of SRD. A risk score was derived and a nomogram relating it to the probability of SRD provided (Fig. 1-5).

As should be apparent, one of the major problems with this literature is the varied definitions of contrast-induced kidney injury. The Acute Kidney Injury Network has proposed a definition (an abrupt increase in serum creatinine within 48 hours of ≥0.3 mg/dL or ≥50% increase from baseline) that they are hoping will gain traction. Another issue is the lack of routine surveillance for post-PCI AKI that frequently occurs several days following the procedure at a time when many patients have already been discharged. The incidence of this adverse event will only be known when there is standardized assessment of renal function at fixed time intervals following procedures requiring intravenous contrast.

Long-Term Survival

Despite growing data on long-term survival following PCI, little work has been done on predicting patient-specific estimates of survival. This is becoming increasingly important as it is apparent from a growing number of studies that medical management and surgical revascularization are reasonable alternatives to the treatment of patients with coronary artery disease

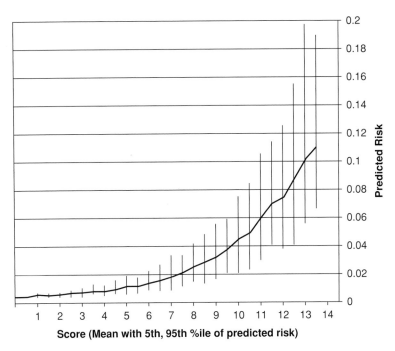

FIGURE 1-3. Northern New England risk score nomogram for bleeding and access site complications. (Reprinted from Piper WD, Malenka DJ, Ryan TJ Jr, et al. Predicting vascular complications in percutaneous coronary interventions. *Am Heart J.* 2003;145:1022–1029, with permission from Elsevier.)

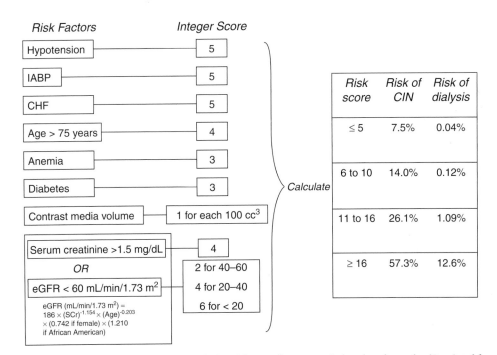

FIGURE 1-4. Cardiovascular Research Foundation risk score for contrast induced nephropathy. (Reprinted from Mehran R, Aymong ED, Nikolsky E, et al. A simple risk score for prediction of contrast-induced nephropathy after percutaneous coronary intervention: development and initial validation. *J Am Coll Cardiol.* 2004;44:1393–1399, with permission from Elsevier.)

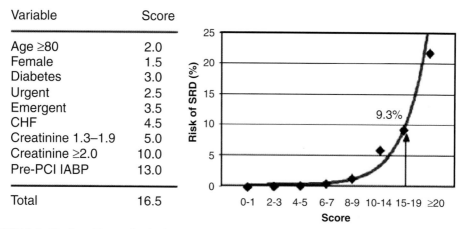

Variable	Score
Age ≥80	2.0
Female	1.5
Diabetes	3.0
Urgent	2.5
Emergent	3.5
CHF	4.5
Creatinine 1.3–1.9	5.0
Creatinine ≥2.0	10.0
Pre-PCI IABP	13.0
Total	**16.5**

FIGURE 1-5. Northern New England risk score and nomogram for serious renal dysfunction. Calculation of predicted risk. (Reprinted from Brown JR, DeVries JT, Piper WD, et al. Serious renal dysfunction after percutaneous coronary interventions can be predicted. *Am Heart J.* 2008;155:260–266, with permission from Elsevier.)

but carry with them different short-term risks and benefits, as well as different long-term risks and benefits. Truly informed consent and appropriate use of procedures require a rich discussion of these tradeoffs and, to the extent that patient-specific estimates of outcomes can be provided, higher quality decision making and a more satisfied patient population should be the result. In this regard, we mention a recent publication by MacKenzie et al. (14) who used data on 32,672 patients who underwent PCI in northern New England from 1987 to 2001 and 15,245 patients who underwent CABG in the same time period to develop clinical prediction rules for survival out to 5 years using Cox's model. Discrimination and calibration for survival at 3 months, 1 year, and 5 years are reported with c statistics of 0.80 for all three time periods, and a good match of expected-to-observed survival. Guidance for estimating survival for each of the procedures is provided in an appendix (14).

■ CONCLUSION

The science of prediction is sound and there are a growing numbers of high-quality clinical prediction rules and high-quality data sources for developing new clinical prediction rules, or for recalibrating and improving existing ones. The real hurdle is creating the infrastructure and expectation to get clinical prediction rules used in the routine process of care. This will likely require integrated informatics to populate the prediction rules and to relatively seamlessly provide these probabilities at points of care where they are needed. It may require their use as a quality metric. Until such time, pocket or web-based calculators or cards with risk scores, and nomograms are available to make it relatively easy to predict a patient's risk for a number of important adverse events following PCI. Physicians who want to help their patients make really informed decisions, and minimizing the risk of the procedure will make the effort to use them.

References

1. American Medical Association Patient Physician Relationship Topics. http://www.ama-assn.org/ama/pub/physician-resources/legal-topics/patient-physician-relationship-topics/informed consent.shtml. Accessed July 1, 2010.
2. Hurwitz B. How does evidence based guidance influence determinations of medical negligence? *BMJ.* 2004;329:1024–1028.
3. Perkins HS, Jonsen AR, Epstein WV. Providers as predictors: using outcome predictions in intensive care. *Crit Care Med.* 1986;14:105–110.
4. Poses RM, Smith WR, McGlish DK, et al. Physician's survival predictions for patients with actue congestive heart failure. *Arch Intern Med.* 1997;157:1001–1007.
5. Reilly BM, Evan AT, Schaider JJ, Wang Y. Triage of patients with chest pain in the emergency department: a comparative study of physicians' decisions. *Am J Med.* 2002;112:95–103.

6. Kahneman D, Slovic P, Tversky A. *Judgment Under Uncertainty: Heuristics and Biases.* Cambridge, MA: Cambridge University Press; 1982.

7. Ariely D. *Predictably Irrational: the Hidden Forces that Shape Our Decisions.* New York, NY: Harper; 2008.

8. Reilly BM, Evan AT. Translating clinical research into clinical practice: impact of using prediction rule to make decisions. *Ann Intern Med.* 2006; 144:201–209.

9. Hosmer DW, Lemeshow S. *Applied Logistic Regression.* New York, NY: Willey; 1989.

10. Sullivan LM, Massaro JM, D'Agostino RB Sr. Presentation of multivariate data for clinical use: the Framingham Study risk score functions. *Stat Med.* 2004;23:1631–1660.

11. Moscucci M, Kline-Rogers E, Share D, et al. Simple bedside additive tool for prediction of in-hospital mortality after percutaneous coronary interventions. *Circulation.* 2001;104:263–268.

12. Resnic FS, Ohno-Machado L, Selwyn A, Simon DI, Popma JJ. Simplified risk score models accurately predict the risk of major in-hospital complications following percutaneous coronary intervention. *Am J Cardiol.* 2001;88:5–9.

13. Cox DR, Oakes D. *Analysis of Survival Data.* London, UK: Chapman & Hall; 1984.

14. MacKenzie TA, Malenka DJ, Olmstead EM, et al. Prediction of survival after coronary revascularization: modeling short-term, mid-term, and long-term survival. *Ann Thorac Surg.* 2009;87: 463–472.

15. Wasson JH, Sox HC, Neff RK, Goldman L. Clinical prediction rules. Applications and methodological standards. *N Engl J Med.* 1985;313(13): 793–799.

16. Laupacis A, Sekar N, Stiell IG. Clinical prediction rules: a review and suggested modifications of methodological standards. *JAMA.* 1997;277: 488–494.

17. Concato J, Feinstein AR, Holford TR. The risk of determining risk with multivariable models. *Ann Intern Med.* 1993;118:201–210.

18. Hanley JA, McNeil BJ. The meaning and use of the area under a receiver operating characteristic (ROC) curve. *Diagn Radiol.* 1982;143:29–36.

19. Harrell F, Lee K, Mark D. Multivariate prognostic models: issues in developing models, evaluating assumptions and adequacy, and measuring and reducing errors. *Stat Med.* 1996;15:361–387.

20. Moscucci M, O'Connor GT, Ellis SG, et al. Validation of risk adjustment models for in-hospital percutaneous transluminal coronary angioplasty mortality on an independent data set. *J Am Coll Cardiol.* 1999;34(3):692–697.

21. Kizer JR, Berlin JA, Laskey WK, et al. Limitations of current risk-adjustment models in the era of coronary stenting. *Am Heart J.* 2003;145: 683–692.

22. Matheny ME, Ohno-Machado L, Resnic FS. Discrimination and calibration of mortality risk prediction models in interventional cardiology. *J Biomed Inform.* 2005;38(5):367–375.

23. Singh M, Peterson ED, Milford-Beland S, Rumsfeld JS, Spertus JA. Validation of the Mayo Clinic risk score for in-hospital mortality after percutaneous coronary interventions using the National Cardiovascular Data Registry. *Circ Cardiovasc Interv.* 2008;1:36–44.

24. Ivanov J, Tu JV, Naylor CD. Ready-made, recalibrated, or remodeled? Issues in the use of risk indexes for assessing mortality after coronary artery bypass graft surgery. *Circulation.* 1999;99: 2098–2104.

25. Peterson ED, Dai D, DeLong ER, et al. Contemporary mortality risk prediction for percutaneous coronary intervention: results from 588, 398 procedures in the National Cardiovascular Data Registry. *J Am Coll Cardiol.* 2010;55(18):1923–1932.

26. Singh M, Rihal CS, Lennon RJ, Spertus J, Rumsfeld JS, Holmes DR Jr. Bedside estimation of risk from percutaneous coronary intervention: the new Mayo Clinic risk scores. *Mayo Clin Proc.* 2007;82(6):701–708.

27. O'Connor GT, Malenka DJ, Quinton H, et al. Multivariate prediction of in-hospital mortality after percutaneous coronary interventions in 1994–1996. Northern New England Cardiovascular Disease Study Group. *J Am Coll Cardiol.* 1999; 34:681–691.

28. Wu C, Hannan EL, Walford G, et al. A risk score to predict in-hospital mortality for percutaneous coronary interventions. *J Am Coll Cardiol.* 2006; 47:654–660.

29. Hamburger JN, Walsh SJ, Khurana R, et al. Percutaneous coronary intervention and 30-day mortality: the British Columbia PCI risk score. *Catheter Cardiovasc Interv.* 2009;74:377–385.

30. Mehta SK, Frutkin AD, Lindsey JB, et al. Bleeding in patient undergoing percutaneous coronary intervention; the development of a clinical risk

algorithm from the National Cardiovascular Data Registry. *Circ Cardiovasc Interv.* 2009;2:222–229.

31. Piper WD, Malenka DJ, Ryan TJ Jr, et al. Predicting vascular complications in percutaneous coronary interventions. *Am Heart J.* 2003;145:1022–1029.

32. McCullough PA, Adam A, Becker CR, et al. Epidemiology and prognostic implications of contrast-induced nephropathy. *Am J Cardiol.* 2006;98:5K–13K.

33. Stacul F, Adam A, Becker CR, et al. Strategies to reduce the risk of contrast-induced nephropathy. *Am J Cardiol.* 2006;98:59K–77K.

34. Freeman RV, O'Donnell M, Share D, et al. Nephropathy requiring dialysis after percutaneous coronary intervention and the critical role of an adjusted contrast dose. *Am J Med.* 2002;90:1068–1073.

35. Moscucci M, Rogers EK, Montoye C, et al. Association of a continuous quality improvement initiative with practice and outcome variations of contemporary percutaneous coronary interventions. *Circulation.* 2006;113(6):814–822.

36. Mehran R, Aymong ED, Nikolsky E, et al. A simple risk score for prediction of contrast-induced nephropathy after percutaneous coronary intervention: development and initial validation. *J Am Coll Cardiol.* 2004;44:1393–1399.

37. Brown JR, DeVries JT, Piper WD, et al. Serious renal dysfunction after percutaneous coronary interventions can be predicted. *Am Heart J.* 2008;155:260–266.

38. Holmes DR, Selzer F, Johnston JM, et al. Modeling and risk prediction in the current era of interventional cardiology: a report from the National Heart, Lung, and Blood Institute Dynamic Registry. *Circulation.* 2003;107:1871–1876.

39. Hubacek J, Galbraith PD, Gao M, et al. External validation of a percutaneous coronary intervention mortality prediction model in patients with acute coronary syndromes. *Am Heart J.* 2006;151:308–315.

40. Chowdhary S, Ivanov J, Mackie K, Seidelin PH, Dzavik V. The Toronto score for in-hospital mortality after percutaneous coronary interventions. *Am Heart J.* 2009;157:156–163.

2

Quality Assurance, Peer Review, and Quality Improvement

MAURO MOSCUCCI

From an operational and organizational perspective, interventional cardiovascular programs can be classified as "complex systems," defined as systems which require the complex integration and interaction of multiple independent units and health care providers, and the characteristics and requirements of which are not necessarily evident from the characteristics and requirements of individual components. For example, the development of a program for primary percutaneous coronary intervention for acute myocardial infarction requires the coordination of different areas within and outside the institution, including transportation services, emergency department, cardiac catheterization suite, coronary care unit, and all the way to long-term follow-up care. Importantly, additional characteristics of complex systems include a constant evolution over time that can be sensitive to small changes and that can follow multiple pathways. The continuous introduction of new devices and of new procedures, the multiple options available within clinical protocols, and the horizontal characteristics of interventional care across different units well apply to the concept of "complex system" and support the need of a detailed quality assurance and quality improvement program.

Quality assurance requires a systematic approach toward the assessment of various aspects of interventional cardiovascular care ranging from credentialing to outcome assessment and compliance with quality indicators and recommended guidelines. Table 2-1 lists key areas pertaining to quality assurance in interventional cardiovascular care.

■ CREDENTIALING

A well-defined credentialing process is the first component for setting quality standards. With advancements in technology and with the development of cross-training, the boundaries between subspecialties for specific procedures are not as defined as they used to be. It is common today to have within the same institution cardiologists, vascular surgeons, interventional radiologists, and more recently cardiac surgeons performing the same procedures. Therefore, in order to ensure high standards and to avoid conflicts, it is important to thoroughly define the credentialing requirements for each procedure using a multidisciplinary approach and available guidelines. Table 2-2 lists minimum volume standards as recommended by consensus statements and as endorsed by the American Council of Graduate Medical Education (ACGME) for training in diagnostic cardiac catheterization and in percutaneous coronary intervention (1). Criteria for training and credentialing (2) include a dedicated 4th year of training and a detailed curriculum on topics ranging from vascular biology to clinical management strategies. During this 4th year the trainee should perform a minimum of 250 coronary interventional cases. Similar training requirements have been recommended for electrophysiology procedures (3) (Table 2-3) and for peripheral vascular intervention (4) (Table 2-4). Importantly, the joint American College of Cardiology/American College of Physicians/ Society of Coronary Angiography and Intervention/ Society of Vascular Medicine and Biology/ Society of Vascular Surgery (ACC/ACP/

TABLE 2-1	Key Areas Pertaining to Quality Assurance in Interventional Cardiovascular Care

Credentialing
Focused review
Peer review
Catheterization laboratory and periprocedural protocols
Informed consent process
Training and proficiency of cardiac catheterization laboratory personnel
Radiation safety
Equipment maintenance
Assessment of clinical appropriateness of procedures performed
Compliance with quality indicators
Outcome assessment

SCAI/SVMB/SVS) clinical competence statement on vascular medicine and catheter-based peripheral vascular interventions recommends similar pathways and training requirements for cardiovascular physicians, for interventional radiologists, and for vascular surgeons (see Table 2-3). The adoption of these recommendations will ensure laying a fair playing ground in the credentialing committee given that this recommendation has been endorsed by all the major societies.

Noncoronary Cardiac Procedures and Structural Heart Disease

There are currently no defined training requirements for structural heart disease or noncoronary cardiac procedures. Unfortunately, exposure of trainees to these procedures during training tends to be low, and there is definitely a learning curve for procedures such as alcohol ablation, mitral valvuloplasty, and repair of atrial septal defects. While recognizing the lack of data on minimum volume standards, the American college of Cardiology/Society of Coronary Angiography and Intervention (ACC/SCAI) Clinical Competence Statement on Cardiac Interventional Procedures recommends that a minimum of 10 cases are proctored by an interventional cardiologist trained in these procedures. In addition, the Statement strongly recommends the development of a multidisciplinary program for assessment of appropriateness, triaging toward the appropriate treatment modality (i.e., surgery vs. percutaneous management vs. medical therapy) and for outcome assessment. The statement also recommends a minimum of 10 cases/year for operators and for laboratories to maintain competency (5). Institutions can incorporate the general recommendations from the Competence Statement when developing internal credentialing criteria for structural heart disease.

Alternative Pathways

It is recognized that for individuals who were not able to achieve training within a formal training

TABLE 2-2	Training Requirement for Operators Performing Adult Diagnostic Cardiac Catheterization and Coronary Intervention

Level	Proficiency Level	Training Time	Number of Diagnostic Cardiac Catheterization	Number of Coronary Interventions
1	Basic training required of all trainees to be competent, consulting cardiologists	4 mo	100	
2	Additional training required to perform diagnostic procedures	12 mo	300, with 200 as primary operator	
3	Advanced training in interventional cardiac catheterization	12 mo		250 as primary operator

TABLE 2-3   **Invasive Electrophysiologic Studies (EPS): Recommendation for Training to Achieve Competence**

Source	Training (yr)	EPS (n)	EPS in Patients With Supraventricular Tachycardia (n)	Catheter Ablation (n)	Antiarrhythmic Devices (n)
ACP/ACC/AHA, 1994 (61)	1	100	NS	NS	NS
Canadian Cardiovascular Society (55)					
Level 2	1–2	100	NS	NS	NS
Level 3	1–2	NS	NS	NS	NS
British Cardiac Society (56)	1	70	NS	50	NS
COCATS (57)	1	100	50	50	50
ACGME (58)	1	150	NS	75	25
ABIM	1	150	NS	75	25
ACC/AHA/ACP Clinical (3) Competence Statement	1	100	>50	50–75	NS

ACP, American College of Physicians; ACC, American College of Cardiology; AHA, American Heart Association; COCATS, Core Cardiology Training Symposium; ACGME, Accreditation Council for Graduate Medical Education; ABIM, American Board of Internal Medicine

(From Tracy CM, Akhtar M, DiMarco JP, et al. American College of Cardiology/American Heart Association 2006 update of the clinical competence statement on invasive electrophysiology studies, catheter ablation, and cardioversion: a report of the American College of Cardiology/American Heart Association/American College of Physicians Task Force on Clinical Competence and Training: developed in collaboration with the Heart Rhythm Society. *Circulation*. 2006;114: 1654–1668.)

TABLE 2-4   **Formal Training to Achieve Competence in Peripheral Catheter-Based Interventions**

	Cardiovascular Physicians	Interventional Radiologists	Vascular Surgeons
Duration	12 mo	12 mo	12 mo
Diagnostic coronary angiograms	300 (200 as primary operator)		
Diagnostic coronary angiograms	100 (50 as primary operator)	100 (50 as primary operator)	100 (50 as primary operator)
Peripheral interventional cases	50 (25 as primary operator)	50 (25 as primary operator)	50 (25 as primary operator)
Aortic aneurysm endografts			10 (5 as primary operator)

(Adapted from Creager MA, Goldstone J, Hirshfeld JW Jr, et al. ACC/ACP/SCAI/SVMB/SVS clinical competence statement on vascular medicine and catheter-based peripheral vascular interventions: a report of the American College of Cardiology/ American Heart Association/American College of Physician Task Force on Clinical Competence (ACC/ACP/SCAI/SVMB/ SVS Writing Committee to develop a clinical competence statement on peripheral vascular disease. *J Am Coll Cardiol.* 2004;44:941–957.)

TABLE 2-5	Alternative Route to Achieve Competence in Peripheral Catheter-Based Interventions

Common requirements	• Completion of required training within 24-mo period
	• Training under proctorship of formally trained vascular interventionalist competent to perform full range of procedures
	• Written curriculum with goals and objectives
	  • Regular written evaluations by proctor
	  • Documentation of procedures and outcomes
	  • Supervised experience in inpatient and outpatient vascular consultation settings
	  • Supervised experience in inpatient and outpatient consultation settings

Procedural requirements for competency in all areas	• Diagnostic peripheral angiograms—100 cases (50 as primary operator) • Peripheral interventions—50 cases (25 as primary operator) • No fewer than 20 diagnostic/10 interventional cases in each area, excluding extracranial cerebral arteries • Extracranial cerebral (carotid/vertebral) arteries—30 diagnostic (15 as primary operator)/25 interventional (13 as primary operator) • Percutaneous thrombolysis/thrombectomy—five cases
Requirements for competency in subset of areas (up to three, excluding carotid/vertebral arteries)	• Diagnostic peripheral angiograms per area—30 cases (15 as primary operator) • Peripheral interventions per area—15 cases (eight as primary operator) • Must include aortoiliac arteries as initial area of competency

(Adapted from Creager MA, Goldstone J, Hirshfeld JW Jr, et al. ACC/ACP/SCAI/SVMB/SVS clinical competence statement on vascular medicine and catheter-based peripheral vascular interventions: a report of the American College of Cardiology/American Heart Association/American College of Physician Task Force on Clinical Competence (ACC/ACP/SCAI/SVMB/SVS Writing Committee to develop a clinical competence statement on peripheral vascular disease). *J Am Coll Cardiol.* 2004;44:941–957.)

program there are available alternative routes to achieving competency in the area of electrophysiology, catheter ablation, and peripheral vascular interventions (3,4). The requirements for achieving competency through an alternative pathway have been well defined and include the completion of required training within a 24-month period, training under the proctorship of a formally trained electrophysiologist or vascular interventionalist with a well-defined written curriculum, a regular written evaluation by the proctor, documentation of procedures and outcomes, and the same procedure volume standards recommended for formal training (Tables 2-5 to 2-7).

Board Certification

Current board certification indicates that the interventionalist is at least current with the standard of care in his/her subsubspecialty and that has met the training requirements. Although no study has thoroughly evaluated whether there is any direct relationship between board certifica-

tion and outcomes of cardiovascular procedures, intuitively board certification should result in higher quality of care, or at least in a higher likelihood of evidence-based practice. Thus, most hospitals require current board certification to maintain privileges in cardiology, interventional cardiology, electrophysiology, and other subspecialties. The recommended credentialing criteria for a catheterization laboratory director and for a training program director include a minimum of 5 years in practice and board certification in cardiovascular disease and interventional cardiology. In addition, all faculty members actively participating and officially listed in a subspecialty training program such as interventional cardiology or electrophysiology must maintain current board certification (ACGME criteria (1)).

Minimum Volume Standards to Maintain Proficiency

The relationship between operator volume and outcomes has been well documented in

TABLE 2-6	Alternative Route to Achieve Competence in Clinical Cardiac Electrophysiology

Training should still be completed in a structured environment

The operator should perform the same number of listed procedures as recommended for U.S. trainees in a formal training program

The operator should participate in courses designed to provide specific instructions in clinical cardiac electrophysiology

A minimum of 30 hr of continuous medical education should be obtained every 2 yr

Training should be performed under the supervision and mentorship of a recognized expert in the field of cardiac electrophysiology who has achieved board certification by the ABIM or an equivalent degree of training in countries outside the United States

Trainees completing the program in a non-ACGME-approved program will not be eligible to take the ABIM examination

ABIM, American Board of Internal Medicine; ACGME, American Council of Graduate Medical Education. (From Tracy CM, Akhtar M, DiMarco JP, et al. American College of Cardiology/American Heart Association 2006 update of the clinical competence statement on invasive electrophysiology studies, catheter ablation, and cardioversion: a report of the American College of Cardiology/American Heart Association/American College of Physicians Task Force on Clinical Competence and Training: developed in collaboration with the Heart Rhythm Society. *Circulation*. 2006;114:1654–1668.)

numerous registry analyses. Although blunted by recent advancements in technology, this relationship still exists with contemporary Percutaneous Coronary Intervention (PCI) (6,7). Thus, current guidelines recommend a minimum of 75 PCI/year to maintain proficiency. For operators performing less than 75 procedures/year, a case-by-case review including case selection and outcomes is currently recommended (8). In relation to diagnostic cardiac catheterization, in the absence of any supporting data, minimum volume standards have been removed from recent guidelines (2). Similar minimum volume standards have been recommended for peripheral vascular interventions and for other procedures such as lead extraction and electrophysiology procedures (Table 2-8).

Focused Review

According to the Joint Commission of Hospital Accreditation, a period of focused review (Focused Professional Practice Evaluation) is required for all new privileges, meaning all privileges for new applicants and all new

TABLE 2-7	Alternative Route to Achieve Competence in Catheter Ablation for Board Eligible or Certified Electrophysiologists Desiring to Learn Ablation

Mentoring by an electrophysiologist trained in ablation should be pursued

Documentation of satisfactory completion of such training should be kept in a log book

A minimum of 75 procedures will be required

Participation in courses designed to provide specific instruction in the cognitive and technical skills required for catheter ablation is also required

(From Tracy CM, Akhtar M, DiMarco JP, et al. American College of Cardiology/American Heart Association 2006 update of the clinical competence statement on invasive electrophysiology studies, catheter ablation, and cardioversion: a report of the American College of Cardiology/American Heart Association/American College of Physicians Task Force on Clinical Competence and Training: developed in collaboration with the Heart Rhythm Society. *Circulation*. 2006;114:1654–1668.)

TABLE 2-8 Recommended Minimum Procedure Volume Standards to Maintain Proficiency

Procedure	Minimal Annual Volume
PCI (8)	75
Peripheral interventions (4)	25
Electrophysiologic studies	100
EP ablation (3)	20–50
ASD/PFO closure (8)	10
Alcohol ablation (8)	6

PCI, percutaneous coronary intervention;
EP, electrophysiology; ASD, atrial septal defect;
PFO, paten foramen ovalis.

privileges for existing practitioners. The following "principles" should be applied to the focused review (9):

1. No exemption for board certification, documented experience, or reputation. All applicants for new privileges must have a period of focused review.
2. The components for design include, but are not limited to
   a. criteria for conducting performance evaluations
   b. method for establishing the monitoring plan specific to the requested privilege
   c. method for determining the duration of performance monitoring
   d. circumstances under which monitoring by an external source is required
3. The organization may choose to use the methodologies for collecting information, which can include
   a. periodic chart review
   b. direct observation
   c. monitoring of diagnostic and treatment techniques
   d. discussion with other individuals involved in the care of each patient including consulting physicians, assistants at surgery, nursing, and administrative personnel
4. In general, a multitiered/level approach may be needed and the type of review for different privileges can be different, that is, direct observation in some cases and chart audits in other cases.
5. The process should be predefined in accordance with the criteria and requirements defined by the organized medical staff, and although there is no requirement that it be included in the medical staff bylaws, the organization may wish to put it in writing.
6. In general, there is no required provisional period, and it might be appropriate to consider a different approach for high-volume versus low-volume privileges or high-risk versus low-risk privileges, for example, performing a focused review for a defined number of procedures, such as 5, 10, 20, and so forth, or for a short period of time such as 1 month or 3 months. For an infrequently performed privilege, numbers might work better than a time period especially if the privilege is not performed in that time period.
7. The duration could also be different for different levels of documented training and experience, for example:
   a. practitioners coming directly from an outside residency program
   b. practitioners coming directly from the organization's residency program
   c. practitioners coming with a documented record of performance of the privilege and its associated outcomes
   d. practitioners coming with no record of performance of the privilege and its associated outcomes

The Joint Commission also requires an "Ongoing Professional Practice Evaluation (OPPE)," the intent of which is to evaluate data on performance for all practitioners with privileges on an ongoing basis rather than at the 2-year reappointment process (10) (for more information, see reference number 10).

■ PEER REVIEW

Peer review indicates a critical and judicious evaluation which is performed by one of equals. The first documentation of a peer review process can be traced back to the eighth century in Syria. According to information published in a book called *Ethics of the Physician* by Ishap bin Ali Al Rahwi (CE 854 to 931), it was the duty of a visiting physician to make duplicate notes of the condition of the patient treated (11). The notes of the physician and his work would then be examined by a local Council who would determine whether the physician had treated patients according to the standard of the time. On the basis of the ruling of the Council, the physician could be sued for damages by a patient who had been mistreated.

Since then, the peer-reviewed process has evolved, and it is unquestionable that the past 30 years have been characterized by a further major transformation. One turning point was a lawsuit which was filed by a general surgeon against his peers who had removed him from a hospital medical staff following "peer review." The allegation was that the removal from the medical staff was not based on quality of care, but rather on market competition. The lawsuit resulted in a multimillion-dollar award against the physicians performing the peer review (12). After that case, a reluctance toward participation in peer review committees ensued. To address an evolving crisis and to protect medical peer review bodies from liability while preventing incompetent practitioners from moving from state to state, in 1986 Congress passed the Health Care Quality Improvement Act (HCQIA). The purpose of the Act was to encourage "good faith professional review activities." The principles behind the act included a recognition of the evolving medical malpractice crisis and of the need to improve the quality of medical care, the recognition of a *"national need to restrict the ability of incompetent physicians to move from State to State without disclosure or discovery of the physician's previous incompetent performance,"* and a belief that the problem could be addressed through effective professional peer review (13). Importantly, a driving force was the realization of a threat of private damage liability under Federal laws, discouraging physicians from participating in effective professional peer review, and the belief of an overriding national need to provide incentive and protection for physicians engaging in effective professional peer review. Many states today provide legal protection for physicians involved in peer review. Legal protection ranges from immunity for peer reviewers, immunity for individuals providing information to peer review committee, and immunity for hospitals acting in response to recommendations of peer review committee. In addition, some states, to enhance the peer review process, have included protection from the use of information obtained during peer review in medical malpractice cases. The same type of protection is provided at the Federal level. Several recent federal court decisions document how the principles on which the Health Care Quality Improvement Act was based to provide immunity are applied in practice. In some cases, the federal court not only ruled that the disciplinary action against physicians was conducted according to the HCQIA procedural requirements but also ordered the plaintiff to pay the defendant's attorney fees.

From a hospital administration point of view, the peer review process is a mean to ensure quality of care. The problem with the current peer review system is that it has evolved toward a punitive process. Clinical outcomes are reviewed, and if the practice is considered unsafe the physician can be suspended or his/her privileges can be revoked. The peer reviewers are protected by the immunity provided by the HCQIA, but protection of physicians been reviewed is not as clear. In addition, economic factors and market competition can lead to conflicts and potential for abuses.

The same principles that apply to the focused review process for new privileges can be applied to the continuous peer review process. Some organizations have taken a nonpunitive, educational approach, and institute sanctions only for recurrent patterns or serious deviations from the standard of care.

National Practitioner Data Bank

The development of the National Practitioner Data Bank (NPDB) was a key component of the Health Care Quality Improvement Act. The NPDB was developed to provide an alert or flagging system to facilitate a comprehensive review of health care practitioners' professional credentials (14). It provides a resource to assist state licensing boards, hospitals and other health care entities in conducting extensive, and independent investigation of the qualification of health care providers who seek a license or are seeking clinical privileges. The NPDB includes information on specific areas of licensure, professional society memberships, medical malpractice payments, and records of clinical privilege. The information is considered confidential and its release or disclosure is regulated by specific rules. The NPDB also contains information regarding practitioners who have been declared ineligible to participate in Medicare or Medicaid under the Social Security Act. Information required to be reported to the NPDB includes (15) the following:

1. All licensor actions taken against all health care practitioners, not just physicians and dentists, and health care entities.
2. Any negative action or finding taken against health care practitioners and organizations by peer review organizations and private accreditation organizations.
3. Any medical malpractice payment reports.
4. Any adverse action report.
5. Any adverse licensor action including relocation, suspension, censor, reprimand, probation, and surrender must be reported within 30 days from the date of the action.
6. Any professional review action that adversely affects a physician or a dentist clinical privilege for a period of more than 30 days.
7. Any acceptance of a physician or dentist to surrender or restriction of clinical privilege while under investigation for possible professional incompetence or improper professional conduct.

Any entity that makes a medical malpractice payment for the benefit of a physician, dentist, or other health care practitioner in settlement or in satisfaction of a written claim or a judgment against the petitioner, must report certain payment information to the NPDB. A payment made as a result of a suit or claim solely against an entity and that does not identify the name of a practitioner is not reportable. Eligible entities must report when a lump sum payment is made or when the first of multiple payments is made.

The regulation also includes voluntary reporting for adverse action taken against clinical privileges of licensed health care practitioners other than physicians and dentists. Importantly, the regulation includes sanctions for failing to report to the NPDB.

Organization of Peer Review Committees

Cases referred for peer review should be assigned to the physician or the group of physicians with the highest expertise in that particular field. The committees should include members of the quality department and of the risk management team. From an organizational perspective, two models can be followed. The first model includes a single, hospital-wide multispecialty peer review committee. The second model includes individual service line or department specific committee or councils. In general, it has been suggested that the following characteristics are required for a successful peer review process (16):

1. **Physician lead process.** Physicians' buy in and physicians' leadership are key components of a successful program. In addition, when external consultants or facilitators are brought in by the hospital administration, it is critical that those consultants work closely with the physicians' group and broker a transition program to the hospital medical staff.
2. **High level of consistency.** Expectation, criteria for peer review, and parameters to follow when making recommendations should be clearly stated. In addition, it has been suggested that rotation through the committee should be staggered to avoid sudden and sweeping changes in the process.
3. **Disciplinary actions.** Given that each case is different, it has been suggested that disciplinary actions should be set on a case-by-case basis rather than on preset levels.
4. **Focus on educational actions.** A focus on educational responses can have a tremendous effect on enhancing the value of the peer review process. As previously stated, major concerns about current peer review processes are related to the fact that they tend to focus on punitive actions rather than on educational and quality improvement actions. A focus on punitive actions can reduce the likelihood that employees will refer their peers for review, and it will increase the risk that the process is used for purposes other than quality issues. The development of a nonpunitive morbidity–

mortality conference, where cases are discussed anonymously in an open forum, although not part of the peer review process, can provide additional value. In summary, shifting the focus on learning, education, and on quality improvement can go a long way toward enhancing quality of care within the institution, and toward gaining physicians' buy in.

■ CLINICAL PROTOCOLS AND INFORMED CONSENT PROCESS

Variability and lack of standardization result in inefficiency, worse outcomes, and increased cost. The periprocedure management of patients referred for cardiovascular procedure can benefit in terms of cost, efficiency, and outcomes from the institution of periprocedural protocols and algorithms. Table 2-9 lists examples of areas that can benefit from the development of such standardized protocols.

Issues surrounding the informed consent process are discussed in details in Chapter 3.

■ TRAINING AND PROFICIENCY OF CARDIAC CATHETERIZATION LABORATORY PERSONNEL

In the modern interventional cardiovascular suite, laboratory personnel usually includes cardiovascular technicians who have undergone specific training and have passed the cardiovascular technicians examination, nurses, nurse practitioners, physician assistants, radiology technicians, and technicians who have been trained "on the job." The increasing complexity of patients treated, advancements in technology, and the continuous introduction of new devices and new procedures require a well-structured training and proficiency assessment program. The program should be tailored toward promoting a thorough understanding of complex cardiovascular conditions, procedures and complications, and toward the achievement of proficiency in the use of devices and of diagnostic and monitoring equipment. It is of critical importance to provide specific targeted training of catheterization laboratory personnel with the

---

TABLE 2-9   **Examples of Areas that Can Benefit from the Development of Standardized Periprocedural Protocols for Patients Undergoing Cardiovascular Procedures**

Area	Protocols
Management of oral anticoagulant	• Standardized protocol for last dose of oral anticoagulant, timing of the procedure, and assessment of INR prior to the procedure • Assessment of INR • Development of bridging protocols depending on reason for oral anticoagulants and available guidelines
Prevention of contrast nephropathy	• See Chapter 13
Use of antithrombotic in the catheterization laboratory	• Weight-adjusted heparin dosing • Timing of ACT • Routine measurement of ACT in patients receiving bivalirudin to ensure that the patient received the drug • Dosage adjustment of GP IIb/IIIa receptor blockers (i.e., eptifibatide) in patients with chronic renal failure
Use of vascular closure devices	• Assessment of proficiency • Routine angiographic assessment prior to use of closure device • Exclusion criteria • Protocols to ensure sterile technique
Patients with diabetes	• Insulin dosing • Metformin (see Chapter 13)
Management of arterial sheaths	• Sheath removal protocols • Duration of bed rest

INR, international normalized ratio; ACT, activated clotting time.

introduction of any new protocol, new technology, or new procedures, regardless of whether the new procedures might include the use of "old" or "new" technology. A "clinical ladder" providing recognition of clinical expertise and a corresponding financial compensation ladder can provide an incentive toward professional growth and excellence. The designation of a technical leader in charge of training and of quality assurance plays a key role in the development of the appropriate environment. As part of proficiency assessment and maintenance, most institutions also require Advanced Cardiac Life Support certification for all catheterization laboratory personnel involved with direct patient care.

■ RADIATION SAFETY

The effects of ionizing radiation can be classified into two major categories—deterministic and stochastic effects. Deterministic effects are the acute results of exceeding a threshold dose to the affected tissue leading to cell death (17). They range from early transient erythema, which occurs within hours from radiation exposure at a threshold dose of 2 Gy, to ischemic dermal necrosis, which occurs at a dose threshold of 18 Gy with a delayed presentation at more than 10 weeks from exposure. Stochastic or "random" effects relate to injury to the DNA resulting in an increased risk of cancer in the subject radiated or of genetic disorders in the offspring. While deterministic effects are seen within days to months from radiation exposure, stochastic effects typically manifest years after the exposure. In contrast to deterministic effects, the magnitude of stochastic effects is independent of the dose, but the probability of their occurrence increases with the dose and it is cumulative over time.

It is worth noticing that radiation control programs were initially based on the belief that all radiation injuries were due to a deterministic effect, thus leading to the development of dose limits and of maximum permissible doses (MPD) (18). The identification of stochastic effects has led to the development of the "As Low As Reasonably Achievable" (ALARA) principle to reduce the total dose to a fraction of the MPD and to minimize the risk of stochastic effects (cancer and genetic defects) to levels that are similar to other risks of general workers (19). Training on the use of optimal angiographic and

fluoroscopic techniques and on the optimal use of shielding, including the use of mobile shielding (20), is a key component of such program.

Table 2-10 shows MPD recommended by the National Council on Radiation Protection and Measurement (17–21). Currently, the MPD is 50 millisieverts (mSv) in any 1 year for radiation workers and 1 mSv/year for nonradiation workers (19–21). The cumulative dose for radiation workers should not exceed 10 mSv × age. Thus, in general radiation workers should not exceed 10 mSv/year.

The ALARA principle should be applied to reduce radiation exposure of workers and patients to fractions of those doses.

The radiation safety quality assurance program should include

1. ongoing educational programs on radiation safety and on appropriate use of x-ray equipment
2. accurate monitoring and timely reporting of personnel exposure
3. modification of procedural conduct in cases in which exposure levels are of concern (2,22)
4. optimization of mobile and fixed radiation shielding in the catheterization laboratory

All staff members and trainees should be required to wear radiation dosimeters, have monthly dosimeters readings, and have monitoring performed by the radiation safety depart-

TABLE 2-10 **Maximum Permissible Radiation Doses for Medical Radiation Workers and General Public (21,59)**

Whole body	50 mSv/yr
Skin	300–500 mSv/yr
Hands, feet	500–750 mSv/yr
Lens	50–150 mSv/yr
Others (including thyroid)	150 mSv/yr
Fetus (pregnant workers)	5/ms/yr (0.5 mSv/mo)
Cumulative exposure	10 mSv × age
General public dose limit for continuous exposure	1 mSv/yr
U.S. average background	1 mSv/yr

ment. All staff must wear protective lead at all times during the procedures, including a thyroid collar. Lead apron should be annually inspected under fluoroscopy to ensure no breakdown in the lead barrier (20). The need for using leaded glasses is controversial, as the lens is relatively insensitive to radiation. However, the development of cataract has been reported, and eyeglasses can provide a protective barrier against body fluids splashes (20). Protective shields should be used whenever it is possible. In particular, protective shields should be applied under and above the table to protect from scatter radiation.

Compliance with wearing dosimeters can often be an issue. The compliance issue can be addressed from a QI perspective by establishing a simplified process for distribution and collection of dosimeters. A board that includes names of all personnel involved with the use of x-ray equipment, including trainees can be posted in the cardiac catheterization laboratory. New dosimeters are attached to the names at each cycle and can be easily picked up by the catheterization laboratory personnel. The used dosimeters are returned in a bin located near the board. Operators who have not returned their used dosimeters are reminded repeatedly until they have returned their dosimeter by a staff member in charge of ensuring compliance. A policy of suspending cardiac catheterization laboratory privileges of noncompliant personnel has also been used in some institutions.

■ EQUIPMENT MAINTENANCE

The complexity of the equipment and of procedures performed in the cardiac catheterization laboratory requires a rigorous and detailed equipment maintenance program to prevent unscheduled down times and equipment failures resulting in adverse outcomes. In general, the Joint Commission standard requires organizations to follow manufacturer's recommendations for equipment maintenance.

The x-ray equipment and the hemodynamic monitoring system should be checked at the beginning of each day to ensure appropriate operation. In a recent study evaluating two measures of fluoroscopic image quality in 64 interventional cardiology catheterization laboratories, both measurements showed significant variation and limitation in performance (23). Thus, maintenance should include sched-

uled assessment of the image quality and of the image chain, evaluation of natural wear, and recalibration or preventive replacement of components of the image chain (24,25).

Routine calibration of coagulation monitoring devices, blood gas analysis devices and other monitoring devices, and the routine assessment of appropriate operation of diagnostic and therapeutic devices such as intravascular ultrasound equipment, rheolytic thrombectomy devices, rotational atherectomy, left ventricular assist devices, automatic external defibrillators, and other devices are other areas pertaining to the equipment maintenance and quality assurance.

■ COST CONTAINMENT

Methods to improve efficiency and to reduce costs of PCI can focus on process and on supplies. From a process perspective, implementation of critical pathways and protocols for the reduction of complications and of postprocedure length of stay (26,27), percutaneous revascularization performed at the same time of diagnostic catheterization (28,29), reduced anticoagulation and early sheath removal (leading to shorter length of hospital stay) (30,31), the use of new pharmacological interventions to reduce acute complications, and a focus on scheduling, cross-training of staff members, turnover time, and patient flow can play an important role in improving efficiency and reducing cost.

From a supply chain perspective, the use of consignment, reuse of equipment (32,33), the implementation of competitive bidding for catheterization laboratory supplies (26,27,34), and a reduction in supplies to avoid overstocking leading to expiration of products on the shelves can result in further marked reductions in costs.

Providing feedback to physicians on resource utilization and procedure costs, and a close partnership between hospital administrators and physicians should be incorporated in cost reduction efforts.

■ APPROPRIATE UTILIZATION OF PROCEDURES

The importance of appropriateness of surgical and percutaneous cardiovascular procedures cannot be overemphasized. As shown in this textbook, despite advancements in catheter technology and despite the introduction of pharmacological interventions aimed toward reducing complications, each cardiovascular procedure is still associated with a low although not insignificant risk of complications, some of which can be serious and potentially fatal. For example, PCI are associated with an approximately 2% risk of vascular complications, a 0.5% risk of emergency CABG (35), and a 0.8% to 1.6% risk of in hospital death. In addition, subacute stent thrombosis continues to occur in approximately 1% of cases, and it is associated with a 15% rate of Q-Wave myocardial infarction and a 20% 6-month mortality rate (36). In a retrospective analysis of data from the American College of Cardiology National Cardiovascular Data Registry, Anderson et al. found that up to 8% of 412,617 procedures could be classified as a class III indication, which is defined as a "condition for which there is evidence and/or general agreement that the procedure/treatment is not useful/effective, and in some cases may be harmful" (37). In that analysis, there was a less than benign association between inappropriate procedures and outcomes, as documented by a 1.7% mortality rate, a 1.5% incidence of myocardial infarction, and a 0.4% emergency CABG rate in the group of patients undergoing inappropriate procedures. It is estimated that approximately 1,000,000 stenting procedures are performed each year in the United State alone. On the basis of the study by Anderson et al. and on the basis of expected complications of PCI, an 8% inappropriate procedure rate could result in a total of 400 cases of emergency CABG, 800 subacute stent thrombosis, approximately 900 deaths (38), and 160 deaths secondary to subacute stent thrombosis alone. Thus, performance of inappropriate procedures will expose patients to the risk of potential complications in the absence of any expected benefit.

Regional variations in the utilization of procedures in the absence of improved outcomes and of differences in comorbidities, and the report of an association between a proliferation of heart hospitals and a sharp increase in utilization of procedures in areas where those heart hospitals are built (39), have raised concerns about overutilization and perhaps inappropriate utilization of cardiac procedures. Recent news media headlines about inappropriately high use or coronary artery bypass surgery, PCI and coronary angiography, and recent legal cases

leading to civil and criminal charges brought by the Federal Government against physicians, hospitals, and hospital administrators have further fueled those concerns (40,41). A brief discussion on appropriateness criteria and guidelines for PCI and for peripheral vascular interventions is included in Chapter 5. While assessment of adherence to guidelines might be challenging, and while it is recognized that there might be many "grey zones," a quality assurance program for interventional cardiology should incorporate some assessment of clinical appropriateness. Such assessment can include random review of cases, at least to evaluate the severity of disease treated, and a prospective discussion of cases in which clinical decisions might be controversial. The development of a combined cardiac surgery/interventional cardiology conference where cases can be discussed prospectively is an ideal setting for such evaluation. In addition, as recommended by the ACCF/AHA/SCAI Clinical Competence Statement on Cardiac Interventional Procedures, the quality assurance program for procedures such as atrial septal defect closure, alcohol ablation, and other low volume procedures for structural heart disease could benefit from regular case conferences to discuss indications, procedural techniques, and outcomes (8).

■ POSTPROCEDURE AND LONG-TERM FOLLOW-UP CARE

The beneficial effects of statins, beta-blockers, ACE inhibitors, and the importance of compliance with dual antiplatelet therapy have been well documented in numerous studies. In addition, adherence to these quality indicators has been included in several measurements of quality of care and in programs of "Pay for performance." Therefore, it is highly recommended to include in quality assurance programs the development of processes, such as standardized order sets and discharge planning, aimed toward ensuring the highest compliance possible with these quality indicators.

■ DATA COLLECTION, OUTCOME ASSESSMENT, AND BENCHMARKING

It is only through a prospective evaluation of clinical outcomes and through a systematic data collection process that programs can ensure full capture of adverse events, and a fair assessment of the quality of care provided within the program by individual operators. Data collected should include comorbidities, procedure variables, and clinical outcomes variables (42). In addition, participation to a national or a regional registry is a must for any interventional cardiology program that seeks to measure, to maintain, and to improve quality of care. Participation to national and regional registries and the use of available data collection tools facilitate the process, and they provide the added benefit of having comparative data with a regional or a national benchmark. There are several procedure-based regional and national registries for PCI, peripheral vascular interventions, carotid stenting, and Automatic Implantable Cardioverter Defibrillators (AICD). In the United States, participation to the national ACC Cath/PCI data registry is currently voluntary, although it is now requested by many third-party payers and by the Leap Frog group as an indirect measurement of quality (43–45). The New York State Data Registry is a regional registry with mandatory participation in New York State (46) which has been publicly reporting outcome data by facility and by individual operator. Mandatory reporting to statewide registries is also required in Massachusetts, New Jersey, and in Washington State. In addition, in the Unites States, mandatory reporting to a national registry is required by Medicare for reimbursement of AICD implantation and for Carotid Artery Stenting. The Northern New England Cardiovascular Consortium (47) and the Blue Cross Blue Shield of Michigan Cardiovascular Consortium (48) are two regional registries that were developed with the primary goal of improving outcomes of percutaneous coronary interventions. The Michigan registry has recently been expanded to peripheral vascular interventions. It is important to underscore that participation in the national registries and participation in regional registries are not mutually exclusive. While participation in national registries provides access to a national benchmark, the regional registries traditionally include direct quality improvement programs, a data-monitoring process, and promote exchange of information across institutions in a rapid cycle that involves bench-marking, data feedback, working group meetings, and site visits (49).

■ QUALITY IMPROVEMENT

The past two decades have been characterized by the development of quality indicators aimed to assess quality of care. Measurements such as beta-blockers use following myocardial infarction, use of ACE inhibitors in patients with left ventricular systolic dysfunction, aspirin use, and the use of other pharmacological interventions that have been shown to improve acute and long-term outcomes are easy to collect and to report. Measuring clinical outcomes is, however, more complex. In most industries, the assessment of the quality of a product requires measurement of failure rates and of prespecified characteristics of the product. The added complexity of measuring the quality of care through an assessment of clinical outcomes relates to the need of factoring in additional variables such as patient's comorbidities, age, and clinical presentation which can affect those same outcomes. For decades we have known that the relation between an outcome variable such as death or bleeding, and a procedure such as coronary artery bypass graft surgery or PCI can be modified by other "explanatory" variables such as advanced age, renal failure, or anemia. The development of mathematical or "risk adjustment" statistical models that can correct for patient's comorbidities and patient's severity has led to a major progress in understanding and measuring the relationship between comorbidities and outcomes. These models have been used for the evaluation of individual patient prognosis and for the comparison of outcomes across different operators and institutions. In addition, they can be used to better understand procedure variables that can relate to adverse outcomes and that are potentially modifiable, thus leading to improved care. Chapter 1 describes in details the characteristics of risk adjustment models, and how they can be applied in clinical practice.

Six Sigma

Six Sigma is a process developed by Motorola in the mid-1980s aimed toward identifying and removing the causes of defects (50). The initial concept of Six Sigma was based on the normal Gaussian distribution of the characteristics or specifications of a product. According to a normal distribution, the individual values will be distributed symmetrically around the mean (μ). The word sigma stands for standard deviation, which is a measurement of variability. In a normal distribution, 68% of values will be within ± 1 standard deviation from the mean μ, about 95% of the values will be within ± 2 standard deviations, and 99.73% will lie within ± 3 standard deviations. When the upper and lower limits of tolerance of a product are set and the process is centered at the middle of the specifications, for a company that works with upper and lower specifications at 3 sigma, the overall defect rate will be 0.27% or 2,700 per million which corresponds to the *3-sigma rule*. Unfortunately, manufacturing a product requires usually more than one step. The yield of the full process will be equal to the product of the yield of each step (51). For a process including 10 steps, each at 3 sigma, the yield will be $(0.9973)^{10}$ or 0.973326. That will correspond to a defect rate of 26,674 per million. From a statistical perspective, the 6-sigma process introduces the concept of working within 6 sigma from the mean. At 6 sigma, with a centered mean, the defect rate will be only 2 units per million units. However, Motorola has added a conservative correction by allowing that the mean might deviate ± 1.5 standard deviations from the center. Thus, allowing for a 1.5 sigma shift, a 6-sigma process even if not perfectly centered will result in producing 3.4 defective units per million units. At the same upper and lower limit of tolerance, a 6-sigma process will require much lower standard deviation and variability.

As an example, the mathematical modeling behind 6-sigma can be applied to door-to-balloon time for patients undergoing PCI for STEMI. The gold standard is currently set at 90 minutes. Let us assume that total door-to-balloon time is the sum of just two steps, door to EKG time and EKG to balloon time. The gold standard for door to EKG time is 10 minutes, which can be set as the upper limit of tolerance for door to EKG time. To achieve a total door-to-balloon time of less than 90 minutes, the EKG to balloon time should be 80 minutes, which we can set as the upper limit of tolerance for this second step of the process. If the mean door to EKG time is 8 minutes, and the standard deviation is 2 minutes, the yield will be 0.84 given that this step of the process is at 1 sigma, and that we

are not concerned for values that are equal to μ-σ. Thus, 84% of patients will have a door to EKG time of 10 minutes or less. The same estimate can be applied to the EKG to balloon time. If the mean of this step is 70 minutes and the standard deviation is 10 minutes, the yield of this second step with an upper limit of 80 minutes will be once again 0.84. However, when combining the two steps, the overall yield of the process will be $0.84 \times 0.84 = 0.7056$. Thus, only 70% of patients will reach the gold standard of 90 minutes. Therefore, from a quality improvement perspective, in addition to reducing mean times, the goal should be to reduce variability or the standard deviation of each individual step. Reducing the mean door to EKG time to 7 minutes and its standard deviation to 0.8 minutes and reducing the mean EKG to balloon time to 65 minutes and its standard deviation to 5 minutes will move the upper limit for each step within 3 standard deviations from the mean. This will result in an overall yield for the process of 0.994 (0.997×0.997) corresponding to 99% of patients having a door-to-balloon time of less than 90 minutes.

The use of statistical methods is only one of several components of Six Sigma. Overall, Six Sigma is based on a top down approach focused on reducing variations and waste and in creating an output that fully meets costumer's expectations. Variation leads to inconsistent and unpredictable results over time, it leads to defects, and defects lead to unsatisfied customers and increased costs. The basic concepts are process and defect, and the philosophy which is embraced by companies adopting Six Sigma is based on a passion for achieving perfection as practically as possible. Six Sigma uses different general programs, depending whether the goal is focused on process improvement or on product development. Table 2-11 lists the different steps included in two-process improvement programs, the DMAIC and the DMADV.

Since its initial development, Six Sigma has further evolved through the incorporation of the Lean process, it has moved from just a focus on defects toward a focus on strategy execution and value creation, and it has branched toward other applications and industries, including the health care industry (50).

TABLE 2-11   **Six Sigma Methodologies**

DMAIC Improving Existing Process	DMADV Create New Process
Define the problem	Define the project goal, which must be consistent with customer's expectation and desire
Measure key components and collect data	Measure customer needs and specifications, product capabilities, and production process capabilities
Analyze the data collected	Analyze process options to meet customer's needs
Improve the current process	Design the process, optimize details
Control the process following implementation of changes	Verify the design to ensure that it meets customer's needs

Application of Six Sigma and Similar Methodologies in Improving Clinical Outcomes

Borrowing from the concepts introduced by the DMAIC project methodology listed in Table 2-11, in general, quality efforts toward improving clinical outcomes can be divided into five major phases.

Phase 1. Identification of the problem. Typical examples that we can apply to cardiovascular procedures include excess complications, prevention of contrast nephropathy, vascular complications, and reducing the use of blood products.

Phase 2. Measurement. Baseline data collection for measurement of the outcome of interest. Benchmarking for the comparison of clinical outcomes and process of care and the use of the risk adjustment methodology are key components of this phase.

Phase 3. Thorough analysis of the process of care. The process of care should be broken down into detailed components so that areas for changes can be identified. As an example, reducing bleeding complications following PCI involves an analysis of the various steps in the process including among others vascular access techniques and sites, use of antithrombotic agents, protocols for the use of vascular closure devices, protocols for manual removal of arterial sheath, and identification of patients at high risk.

Phase 4. Implementation of changes. Application of critical pathways and standing orders, modification of procedural proto-cols, training of physicians and cardiac catheterization laboratory personnel, and providing continuous feedback on data are among the interventions that can be introduced to modify the incidence of adverse outcomes. Examples of protocols and technical tips that can be used to reduce complications rates and improving outcomes are included in several of the following chapters. As supporting material pertinent to the example made for the mathematical modeling surrounding 6 sigma, Table 2-12 includes steps that have been found to be effective in reducing door-to-balloon time in patients undergoing primary PCI for ST segment elevation myocardial infarction.

Phase 5. Follow-up. Collection of follow-up data and analysis of risk adjusted data to assess the results of the intervention. The follow-up phase should also ensure that there are no deviations from the newly established process.

Blood transfusion and contrast nephropathy can be used as an example of outcome variables which might be modified through the application of the process previously described.

In 1998, the University of Michigan interventional cardiology program performed an analysis of transfusion practices on the basis of guidelines for blood transfusion recommended by the American College of Physicians (52). Based on that retrospective analysis, up to 67% of transfusion events could be classified as inappropriate (53) (Fig. 2-1). Not surprising, when comparative data became available through the

TABLE 2-12 **Strategies to Reduced Door-to-Balloon Time for Patients Undergoing Primary PCI**

Strategy	Minutes Saved[a]
Catheterization laboratory activated by emergency physician	−8.2
Activation through a single page	−13.8
Catheterization laboratory activation while the patient is still en route	−15.4
Expected interval from page to arrival of catheterization laboratory staff >30 min	+19.3[b]
Attending cardiologists always in the hospital	−14.6
Real time feedback to staff in the emergency department and catheterization laboratory	−8.6

[a]Numbers corresponds to minutes saved when compared to no strategy in place (60).
[b]Expected interval from page to arrival of catheterization laboratory staff >30 min results in an increase in door-to-balloon time of 19.3 min.

development of a multicenter registry, the University of Michigan was clearly an outlier with regard to the use of blood transfusion (54). A bedside tool with guidelines for blood transfusion was therefore developed (Fig. 2-2) and distributed through an educational program across different health care providers including residents and attending physicians. Over the following 3 years, there was a progressive decrease in the use of blood transfusion, and in the last year, the transfusion rate at the University of Michigan was the lowest within a multi-center consortium (Fig. 2-3). This example, although derived from observational, nonrandomized data, suggests that the application of an aggressive quality improvement process with inclusion of feedback on risk adjusted outcomes and modification of the processes of care can result in improved outcomes. A similar process can be applied toward the reduction of other adverse outcomes such as contrast nephropathy or vascular complications (also see Chapters 13 and 14).

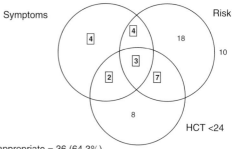

Inappropriate = 36 (64.3%)
Appropriate = 20 (35.7%)

FIGURE 2-1. Venn diagram illustrating the number of appropriate and inappropriate transfusion according to the criteria used in a retrospective analysis of transfusion practice following PCI in a single institution (53). In that analysis, a hematocrit of less than 24% was included as an additional appropriate trigger for blood transfusion in asymptomatic patients at risk of ischemia. Transfusions that fulfill only one criterion are enclosed by one circle. Transfusions that fulfill two criteria are enclosed by three circles, whereas transfusions that fulfill three criteria are enclosed in all circles. Transfusions that do not meet any criteria are outside the circles, whereas appropriate transfusions are enclosed in the framed areas. HCT, Hematocrit. (Reprinted from Moscucci M, Ricciardi M, Eagle KA, et al. Frequency, predictors, and appropriateness of blood transfusion after percutaneous coronary interventions. *Am J Cardiol.* 1998;81(6):702–707, with permission from Elsevier.)

FIGURE 2-3. Standardized transfusion ratios for the index hospital versus all other hospitals during the 4 years of follow-up. The data represent the ratio of observed over predicted transfusion rates. Predicted transfusion rates were estimated using multivariate logistic regression modeling. A ratio above 1 indicates that the observed rate is higher than predicted. As shown in figure, in the first year the index hospital was clearly an outlier, with a transfusion rate much higher than expected. During the following 3 years, there was a progressive reduction in observed transfusion rate, resulting in the last year in a standardized ratio of less than 1. (Reprinted from Chetcuti SJ, Grossman PM, Kline-Rogers EM, et al. Improving outcomes of percutaneous coronary intervention through the application of guidelines and benchmarking: reduction of major bleeding and blood transfusion as a model. *Clin Cardiol.* 2007;30(10 suppl 2):II44–II48, with permission from John Wiley and Sons.)

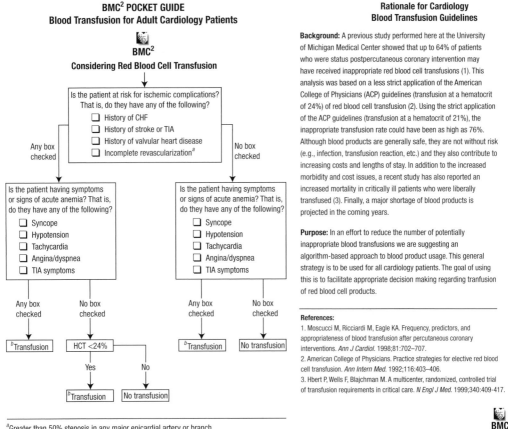

FIGURE 2-2. Clinical algorithm with guidelines for blood transfusion developed to aid the decision-making process for administering blood transfusion. The other side of the index card includes reference and a brief explanation with the rational for the guideline for blood transfusion. The algorithm is printed on a laminated index card that was distributed to each physician rotating on the cardiology service. The proposed guidelines are based on adaptation of the guidelines developed by the American College of Physicians in 1992 (52). CHF, congestive heart failure; TIA, transient ischemic attack. (© 2001 University of Michigan Board of Regents. All rights reserved.)

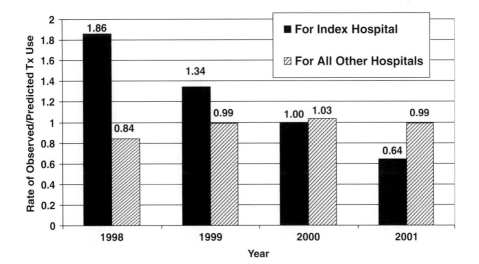

■ CONCLUSION

The development of an effective quality assurance and quality improvement program surrounding cardiovascular procedures goes beyond the interventional cardiovascular suite and requires a multidisciplinary team approach with the inclusion of physicians leaders, technical staff leaders, nursing leaders, and hospital administrators. It is only through this multidisciplinary approach that institutions will be able to assure and improve quality of care for patients undergoing cardiovascular procedures.

References

1. ACGME Program Requirements for Graduate Medical Education in Interventional Cardiology. http://www.acgme.org/acWebsite/home/home.asp Accessed June 29, 2010.
2. Bashore TM, Bates ER, Berger PB, et al. American College of Cardiology/Society for Cardiac Angiography and Interventions Clinical Expert Consensus Document on cardiac catheterization laboratory standards. A report of the American College of Cardiology Task Force on Clinical Expert Consensus Documents. *J Am Coll Cardiol.* 2001;37(8):2170–2214.
3. Tracy CM, Akhtar M, DiMarco JP, et al. American College of Cardiology/American Heart Association 2006 update of the clinical competence statement on invasive electrophysiology studies, catheter ablation, and cardioversion: a report of the American College of Cardiology/American Heart Association/American College of Physicians Task Force on Clinical Competence and Training: developed in collaboration with the Heart Rhythm Society. *Circulation.* 2006;114(15):1654–1668.
4. Creager MA, Goldstone J, Hirshfeld JW Jr, et al. ACC/ACP/SCAI/SVMB/SVS clinical competence statement on vascular medicine and catheter-based peripheral vascular interventions: a report of the American College of Cardiology/American Heart Association/American College of Physician Task Force on Clinical Competence (ACC/ACP/SCAI/SVMB/SVS Writing Committee to develop a clinical competence statement on peripheral vascular disease). *J Am Coll Cardiol.* 2004;44(4):941–957.
5. Hirshfeld JW Jr, Ellis SG, Faxon DP. Recommendations for the assessment and maintenance of proficiency in coronary interventional procedures: statement of the American College of Cardiology. *J Am Coll Cardiol.* 1998;31(3):722–743.
6. Moscucci M, Share D, Smith D, et al. Relationship between operator volume and adverse outcome in contemporary percutaneous coronary intervention practice: an analysis of a quality-controlled multicenter percutaneous coronary intervention clinical database. *J Am Coll Cardiol.* 2005;46(4):625–632.
7. Hannan EL, Wu C, Walford G, et al. Volume-outcome relationships for percutaneous coronary interventions in the stent era. *Circulation.* 2005;112(8):1171–1179.
8. King SB III, Aversano T, Ballard WL, et al. ACCF/AHA/SCAI 2007 update of the clinical competence statement on cardiac interventional procedures: a report of the American College of Cardiology Foundation/American Heart Association/American College of Physicians Task Force on Clinical Competence and Training (writing Committee to Update the 1998 Clinical Competence Statement on Recommendations for the Assessment and Maintenance of Proficiency in Coronary Interventional Procedures). *J Am Coll Cardiol.* 2007;50(1):82–108.
9. Focused Professional Practice Evaluation. The Joint Commission. http://www.jointcommission.org/AccreditationPrograms/CriticalAccessHospitals/Standards/09_FAQs/MS/Focused_Professional_Practice.htm. Accessed June 29, 2010.
10. Ongoing Professional Practice Evaluation (OPPE). Joint Commission. http://www.jointcommission.org/AccreditationPrograms/CriticalAccessHospitals/Standards/09_FAQs/MS/Ongoing_Professional_Practice_Evaluation.htm. Accessed June 29, 2010.
11. Spier R. The history of the peer-review process. *Trends Biotechnol.* 2002;20(8):357–358.
12. Patrick v Burget 486 U.S. 94 (1988). 05/16/88 PATRICK v. BURGET ET AL. SUPREME COURT OF THE UNITED STATES No. 86-1145.
13. The Health Care Quality Improvement Act of 1986, as amended 42 USC Sec. 11101 01/26/98. http://www.npdb-hipdb.hrsa.gov/legislation/title4.html. Accessed June 29, 2010.
14. http://www.npdb-hipdb.hrsa.gov/npdb.html. Accessed June 29, 2010.
15. National Practitioner Data Bank Healthcare Integrity and Protection Data Bank. FACT SHEET ON THE NATIONAL PRACTITIONER DATA BANK. www.npdb-hipdb.hrsa.gov. Accessed June 29, 2010.
16. Johston, A and Brown, K. Examples of Physician Peer Review Process. Washington DC: The Advisory Board Company; 2006.

17. Balter S. Radiation safety in the cardiac catheterization laboratory: basic principles. *Catheter Cardiovasc Interv.* 1999;47(2):229–236.

18. Balter S. An overview of radiation safety regulatory recommendations and requirements. *Catheter Cardiovasc Interv.* 1999;47(4):469–474.

19. Sinclair WK. Radiation protection recommendations on dose limits: the role of the NCRP and the ICRP and future developments. *Int J Radiat Oncol Biol Phys.* 1995;31(2):387–392.

20. Balter S. Radiation safety in the cardiac catheterization laboratory: operational radiation safety. *Catheter Cardiovasc Interv.* 1999;47(3):347–353.

21. National Council on Radiation Protection and Measurements. *Report 116: Limitation of Exposure to Ionizing Radiation.* Bethesda, MD: National Council on Radiation Protection and Measurement; 1993.

22. Hirshfeld JW Jr, Balter S, Brinker JA, et al. ACCF/AHA/HRS/SCAI clinical competence statement on physician knowledge to optimize patient safety and image quality in fluoroscopically guided invasive cardiovascular procedures. A report of the American College of Cardiology Foundation/American Heart Association/American College of Physicians Task Force on Clinical Competence and Training. *J Am Coll Cardiol.* 2004;44(11):2259–2282.

23. Laskey WK, Stueve R, Wondrow M, et al. Image quality assessment in contemporary interventional cardiology laboratories: spatial and low-contrast video resolution. *Catheter Cardiovasc Interv.* 2000;50(2):257–263.

24. Laskey WK, Holmes DR, Kern MJ. Image quality assessment: a timely look. *Catheter Cardiovasc Interv.* 1999;46(2):125–126.

25. Wondrow MA, Laskey WK, Hildner FJ, et al. Cardiac catheterization laboratory imaging quality assurance program. *Catheter Cardiovasc Interv.* 2001;52(1):59–66.

26. Eagle KA, Moscucci M, Kline-Rogers E, et al. Evaluating and improving the delivery of heart care: the University of Michigan experience. *Am J Manag Care.* 1998;4(9):1300–1309.

27. Moscucci M, Muller DW, Watts CM, et al. Reducing costs and improving outcomes of percutaneous coronary interventions. *Am J Manag Care.* 2003;9(5):365–372.

28. Rozenman Y, Gotsman MS, Penchas S. Single-stage coronary angiography and angioplasty: a new standard. *Am J Cardiol.* 1995;76(17):1321.

29. O'Keefe JH Jr, Gernon C, McCallister BD, et al. Safety and cost effectiveness of combined coronary angiography and angioplasty. *Am Heart J.* 1991;122(1 pt 1):50–54.

30. Friedman HZ, Cragg DR, Glazier SM, et al. Randomized prospective evaluation of prolonged versus abbreviated intravenous heparin therapy after coronary angioplasty. *J Am Coll Cardiol.* 1994;24(5):1214–1219.

31. Rabah M, Mason D, Muller DW, et al. Heparin after percutaneous intervention (HAPI): a prospective multicenter randomized trial of three heparin regimens after successful coronary intervention. *J Am Coll Cardiol.* 1999;34(2):461–467.

32. Plante S, Strauss BH, Goulet G, et al. Reuse of balloon catheters for coronary angioplasty: a potential cost-saving strategy? *J Am Coll Cardiol.* 1994;24(6):1475–1481.

33. Rozenman Y, Gotsman MS. Reuse of balloon catheters for coronary angioplasty. *J Am Coll Cardiol.* 1995;26(3):840–841.

34. Eagle KA, Knight BP, Moscucci M, et al. Competitive bidding for interventional cardiology supplies: lessons learned during round 2. *Am J Manag Care.* 2002;8(4):384–388.

35. Seshadri N, Whitlow PL, Acharya N, et al. Emergency coronary artery bypass surgery in the contemporary percutaneous coronary intervention era. *Circulation.* 2002;106(18):2346–2350.

36. Cutlip DE, Baim DS, Ho KK, et al. Stent thrombosis in the modern era: a pooled analysis of multicenter coronary stent clinical trials. *Circulation.* 2001;103(15):1967–1971.

37. Anderson HV, Shaw RE, Brindis RG, et al. Relationship between procedure indications and outcomes of percutaneous coronary interventions by American College of Cardiology/American Heart Association Task Force Guidelines. *Circulation.* 2005;112(18):2786–2791.

38. Moscucci M. Behavioral factors, bias, and practice guidelines in the decision to use percutaneous coronary interventions for stable coronary artery disease. *Arch Intern Med.* 2007;167(15):1573–1575.

39. Nallamothu BK, Rogers MA, Chernew ME, et al. Opening of specialty cardiac hospitals and use of coronary revascularization in medicare beneficiaries. *JAMA.* 2007;297(9):962–968.

40. The Department of Health and Human Services and the Department of Justice Health Care Fraud and Abuse Control Program Annual Report for FY 2006. November 2007. (Available at: oig.hhs.gov/publications/docs/hcfac/hcfacreport2006.pdf. Accessed June 29, 2010.

41. U.S. Department of Justice United States Attorney Northern District of Illinois. Edgewater Medical Center management firms to pay $2.9 million in resolving related criminal and civil health care fraud cases. www.justice.gov/usao/iln/pr/chicago/2003/pr011503_01.pdf. Published 2003.

42. Kline-Rogers E, Share D, Bondie D, et al. Development of a multicenter interventional cardiology database: the Blue Cross Blue Shield of Michigan Cardiovascular Consortium (BMC2) experience. *J Interv Cardiol.* 2002;15(5):387–392.

43. Brindis RG, Fitzgerald S, Anderson HV, et al. The American College of Cardiology-National Cardiovascular Data Registry (ACC-NCDR): building a national clinical data repository. *J Am Coll Cardiol.* 2001;37(8):2240–2245.

44. Shaw RE, Anderson HV, Brindis RG, et al. Development of a risk adjustment mortality model using the American College of Cardiology-National Cardiovascular Data Registry (ACC-NCDR) experience: 1998–2000. *J Am Coll Cardiol.* 2002;39(7):1104–1112.

45. Shaw RE, Anderson HV, Brindis RG, et al. Updated risk adjustment mortality model using the complete 1.1 dataset from the American College of Cardiology National Cardiovascular Data Registry (ACC-NCDR). *J Invasive Cardiol.* 2003;15(10):578–580.

46. Hannan EL, Arani DT, Johnson LW, et al. Percutaneous transluminal coronary angioplasty in New York State. Risk factors and outcomes. *JAMA.* 1992;268(21):3092–3097.

47. Malenka DJ. Indications, practice, and procedural outcomes of percutaneous transluminal coronary angioplasty in northern New England in the early 1990s. The Northern New England Cardiovascular Disease Study Group. *Am J Cardiol.* 1996;78(3):260–265.

48. Moscucci M, Share D, Kline-Rogers E, et al. The Blue Cross Blue Shield of Michigan Cardiovascular Consortium (BMC2) collaborative quality improvement initiative in percutaneous coronary interventions. *J Interv Cardiol.* 2002;15(5):381–386.

49. Moscucci M, Rogers EK, Montoye C, et al. Association of a continuous quality improvement initiative with practice and outcome variations of contemporary percutaneous coronary interventions. *Circulation.* 2006;113(6):814–822.

50. Six Sigma through the years. http://www.motorola.com/Business/US-EN/Motorola+University/About/Inventors+of+Six+Sigma?globalObjectId = 3079. Accessed June 29, 2010.

51. Thomas Pyzdek and Paul Keller. The Six Sigma Handbook. McGraw-Hill Professional; New York, 2006.

52. Practice strategies for elective red blood cell transfusion. American College of Physicians. *Ann Intern Med.* 1992;116(5):403–406.

53. Moscucci M, Ricciardi M, Eagle KA, et al. Frequency, predictors, and appropriateness of blood transfusion after percutaneous coronary interventions. *Am J Cardiol.* 1998;81(6):702–707.

54. Chetcuti SJ, Grossman PM, Kline-Rogers EM, et al. Improving outcomes of percutaneous coronary intervention through the application of guidelines and benchmarking: reduction of major bleeding and blood transfusion as a model. *Clin Cardiol.* 2007;30(10 suppl 2):II44–II48.

55. Mitchell LB, Dorian P, Gillis A, et al. Standards for training in adult clinical cardiac electrophysiology. Canadian Cardiovascular Society Committee. *Can J Cardiol.* 1996;12(5):476–480.

56. Guidelines for specialist training in cardiology. Council of the British Cardiac Society and the Specialist Advisory Committee in Cardiovascular Medicine of the Royal College of Physicians. *Br Heart J.* 1995;73(4 suppl 1):1–24.

57. Josephson ME, Maloney JD, Barold SS, et al. Guidelines for training in adult cardiovascular medicine. Core Cardiology Training Symposium (COCATS). Task Force 6: training in specialized electrophysiology, cardiac pacing and arrhythmia management. *J Am Coll Cardiol.* 1995;25(1):23–26.

58. ACGME Program Requirements for Graduate Medical Education in Electrophysiology. http://www.acgme.org/acWebsite/home/home.asp. Accessed June 29, 2010.

59. Limacher MC, Douglas PS, Germano G, et al. ACC expert consensus document. Radiation safety in the practice of cardiology. American College of Cardiology. *J Am Coll Cardiol.* 1998;31(4):892–913.

60. Bradley EH, Herrin J, Wang Y, et al. Strategies for reducing the door-to-balloon time in acute myocardial infarction. *N Engl J Med.* 2006;355(22):2308–2320.

61. Akhtar M, Williams SV, Achord JL, et al. Clinical competence in invasive cardiac electrophysiological studies. A statement for physicians from the ACP/ACC/AHA Task Force on Clinical Privileges in Cardiology. *Circulation Apr.* 1994;89(4):1917–1920.

3

Legal Considerations: Informed Consent and Disclosure Practices

RICHARD C. BOOTHMAN AND AMY C. BLACKWELL

R isk of injury infiltrates nearly every aspect of a medical professional's work. A physician prescribing an antibiotic for the first time has little way to know if the medicine may send his or her patient to an emergency department fighting for his life with fulminant liver failure. A small percentage of the time, a seemingly benign gastrointestinal complaint actually signals a fatal myocardial infarction and caregivers get no second chance to understand. By definition, piercing the femoral artery to insert a catheter causes injury and bleeding to that vessel wall and exposes the patient to infection, nerve injury, and clots, whereas deciding not to insert the catheter may risk death by coronary artery occlusion. Intrinsic to nearly everything a caregiver offers to do, or suggests not to do, the patient is expected to choose among potential injuries of varying magnitude and significance to their lives.

When patients experience unplanned outcomes, some accept the complication and its ramifications without question. Other patients move at light speed directly to the lawyer's office. What separates one group from the other? Studies exploring reasons why some patients choose to sue their physicians yield common themes: (1) the need for an explanation, (2) a desire to ensure the safety of others, (3) sense of accountability, and (4) compensation (1). A common thread among this group clearly is the element of surprise; being effectively forewarned diminishes the sense of surprise and softens the demand for answers. Physicians who understand the development of the duty to obtain informed consent will not only better comprehend how to satisfy this important legal requirement but will also appreciate its value as an effective risk management strategy.

Humans quickly become desensitized to risk, especially in repetitive activities or commonplace settings. How many of us heed the ubiquitous warning and actually "close cover before striking" a match? Or check the oil levels and air pressure in our cars every time we refuel as most owner's manuals direct? Medical professionals are quickly, and probably necessarily, desensitized to the dangerous world in which they live and work. Desensitization can be useful—without it, cardiologists may be handcuffed by the magnitude of the risk they take when they place stents or open occluded blood vessels with angioplasty. The relatively low complication rate dulls concern, appreciated perhaps on an intellectual level, but is only foremost on the cardiologist's mind when that single patient in a thousand dies from a contrast dye reaction or exsanguinates after a friable blood vessel ruptures during an otherwise routine procedure.

In the same way, the physician's awareness of danger is easily and quickly desensitized, different human factors lead patients to dismiss the risks and find false comfort in statistics. Physicians can easily rationalize that a complication rate of 1% is completely acceptable, even laudatory in a busy practice. Fueled by the idea that 99 of 100 patients escape complication, patients, already willing to believe the proffered procedure will cure all that ails them, easily become certain that "it" won't happen to them—until they realize that when "it" does happen to them, the percentage risk turns out to be 100%. Statistics, of course, are completely irrelevant to individuals. It is easy to see how a physician, naturally downplaying dangers he or she confronts daily, combined with a patient who willingly suspends concern for the serious risks of the procedure he or she believes will solve all medical problems, results in a surprised patient, a stunned family, demands for answers, and deep suspicion that someone must have erred in order for the adverse event to have occurred.

Procedures are certainly not the only occasion in which informed consent arises as an issue in the practice of cardiology, but interventional cardiologists are most definitely in the line of fire. Review of the University of Michigan's Cardiology Division's claims record from 1996 to 2006 reveals that 35% of its claims for that period were procedure related (18 of 51), and the average payment ($99,527) was twice that of nonprocedure-related claims ($50,875) for the same division over the same time frame. All claims arising from procedures had some informed consent component to the allegations and salient facts. Careful cardiologists take time to prepare their patients through an informed consent discussion that effectively educates their patients to the challenges of the procedure being proposed and reasonably adjusts expectations so that when something bad happens, the element of surprise does not drive them to the lawyer's office.

■ INFORMED CONSENT: HURDLE OR OPPORTUNITY?
The Legal Requirements and Reasons for Them

Informed consent is most often viewed by interventional cardiologists as a legal obligation that must be fulfilled, a hurdle to be cleared in order to perform the procedure requested. It is that, of course, but seen as more of a hindrance, it is generally not effectively accomplished and often delegated to subordinates as just another paper to be signed. The most intuitive cardiologists understand the duality of this exercise: first, that it is a serious legal obligation inextricably linked to a physician's ethical obligations to his or her

patient, and second, that it represents an important opportunity for managing risk.

The Origins of the Duty to Obtain Informed Consent

The legal requirement derives from well-established legal and behavioral norms in our culture: we may touch only those who consent to be touched. Touching without consent of the patient is called battery, even where the battery does not cause physical injury. Criminal assault and battery differs in one serious respect from a civil action based in assault and battery: criminal intent. For a person who is kissed against her wishes, for instance, the intrusion represents a compensable civil offense. A person kissed against his wishes by someone with a communicable disease intent on passing it on has an action for both a civil and criminal assault and battery.

One of the earliest known American cases clearly established the claim of battery in the context of medical care. In *Mohr v. Williams* (2), an opinion issued in 1905, the Supreme Court of Minnesota considered a case in which the patient complained of problems with her *right* ear and consented to surgery after a clinic examination revealed a large perforation of her tympanic membrane and the presence of a large polyp. After the patient was anesthetized, however, the surgeon undertook an examination of her *left* ear and concluded that it was more seriously diseased than the right: the eardrum was perforated, but in addition, it appeared that the bones of the middle ear were "diseased and dead." After consultation with the patient's primary care physician while the patient was still anesthetized, the surgeon elected to operate on the *left* ear, not the right as previously planned. Although the operation was deemed a success, the patient sued claiming that the surgery was "wrongful and unlawful, constituting an assault and battery." The court disregarded that the surgery was deemed successful, rejected as disingenuous the suggestion that the surgery was performed under emergency circumstances, but considered whether the surgeon had "implied consent" to operate on the other ear. The question, as framed by the court, was simple:

> In the case at bar, as we have already seen, the question whether defendant's act in performing

the operation upon plaintiff was authorized was a question for the jury to determine. If it was unauthorized, then it was, within what we have said, unlawful (2).

The court elaborated on the relationship between the physician and the patient and the physician's legal boundaries.

The medical profession has made signal progress in solving the problems of health and disease, and they may justly point with pride to the advancements made in supplementing nature and correcting deformities, and relieving pain and suffering. The physician impliedly contracts that he possesses, and will exercise in the treatment of patients, skill and learning, and that he will exercise reasonable care and exert his best judgment to bring about favorable results. The methods of treatment are committed almost exclusively to his judgment, but we are aware of no rule or principle of law which would extend to him free license respecting surgical operations (2).

The court rejected the surgeon's arguments and characterized his actions bluntly: "It was a violent assault, not a mere pleasantry; and, even though no negligence is shown, it was wrongful and unlawful." The distinction between the surgeon's actions in this case and the criminal assault and battery was a fundamental, albeit slim one: "The case is unlike a criminal prosecution for assault and battery, for there an unlawful intent must be shown." The difference between a civil assault and battery charge and a criminal one remains even today a question of the physician's intent alone.

In another legal opinion often quoted as one of the earliest expressions of the importance of informed consent in the context of medical care, one of America's most celebrated jurists and US Supreme Court Justices, Justice Benjamin Cardozo (sitting at the time on the New York Court of Appeals) explained:

In the case at hand, the wrong complained of is not merely negligence. It is trespass. Every human being of adult years and sound mind has a right to determine what shall be done with his own body; and a surgeon who performs an operation without his patient's consent, commits an assault, for which he is liable in damages. This is true

except in cases of emergency where the patient is unconscious and where it is necessary to operate before consent can be obtained (3).

Because medical "touching" poses intrinsic risks that mostly are not understood by patients, the concept of *informed* consent logically developed, the law reasoning that one cannot truly consent in the absence of some appreciation of the consequences. The reality of the disparate positions occupied in the conversation between the patient and the physician has long been recognized and acknowledged by the courts to place a greater burden on the physician to clarify the complicated medical risks sufficiently to inform the medically unsophisticated patient. Springing from Justice Cardozo's axiom that every human being has a right of self-determination in the context of receiving medical care, one court wrote:

True consent to what happens to one's self is the informed exercise of a choice, and that entails an opportunity to evaluate knowledgeably the options available and the risks attendant upon each. The average patient has little or no understanding of the medical arts, and ordinarily has only his physician to whom he can look for enlightenment with which to reach an intelligent decision. From these almost axiomatic considerations springs the need, and in turn the requirement, of a reasonable divulgence by physician to patient to make such a decision possible.

* * *

The context in which the duty of risk-disclosure arises is invariably the occasion for decision as to whether a particular treatment procedure is to be undertaken. To the physician, whose training enables a self-satisfying evaluation, the answer may seem clear, but it is the prerogative of the patient, not the physician, to determine for himself the direction in which his interests seem to lie. To enable the patient to chart his course understandably, some familiarity with the therapeutic alternatives and their hazards becomes essential (4).

The legal right of every patient to make the choice for himself is clear. The next logical question then concerns the scope of information that is required. Clearly, the courts and common sense do not require encyclopedic disclosure of every known possibility, but it is equally "evident that it is normally impossible to obtain a consent worthy of the name unless the physician first elucidates the options and the perils for the patient's edification" (4). Courts have not however expected physicians to know with certainty what questions exist in any individual patient's mind or the things that any individual patient considers material. Several considerations influence the scope of the disclosure required under any given circumstance, and understanding the logical and legal underpinnings of the requirement provides guidance for the physician. The legal right to self-determination and the concomitant trust any patient must have in the physician proposing the therapy, the universe of information any reasonable patient would need to make an intelligent choice, a judgment about what information is material to the decision, and the urgency of the circumstances all play a role. Thus, the scope of the disclosure required to constitute legally adequate informed consent is described ultimately as

> The scope of the standard is not subjective as to either the physician or the patient; it remains objective with due regard for the patient's informational needs and with suitable leeway for the physician's situation. In broad outline, we agree that "(a) risk is material when a reasonable person, in what the physician knows or should know to be the patient's position, would be likely to attach significance to the risk or cluster of risks in deciding whether or not to forgo the proposed therapy (4).

■ DOCUMENTING INFORMED CONSENT AND THE ROLE OF THE CONSENT FORM

Any basic discussion about the informed consent process must include the importance of documentation. Studies have established convincingly that patients' memories of the details of consent discussions are highly unreliable. Patients are influenced by subsequent events, human factors, the effects of anesthesia, and organic changes in short-term and long-term memory caused by the surgery or procedures themselves. In one early study of 20 cardiac surgery patients, all were provided meticulous informed consent preoperatively and none

remembered those consent discussions adequately only 4 to 6 months later (5). The memories of care providers may even be worse: for the patient, the event is usually unique and perhaps more likely to be remembered. The care provider may do thousands of procedures before being called upon to remember one from years before. In most cases, the interventional cardiologist will have no previous or continuing relationship with the patient to reinforce what actually transpired in their conversations before the procedure. With no clear documentation, the old saw, "If it isn't documented, it didn't happen" becomes an evidentiary reality in a courtroom. Although the provider may be allowed to talk about his or her habit and custom, the weight of that testimony pales in comparison to the direct, albeit often flawed, testimony of the patient.

So, how should an interventional cardiologist synthesize these considerations into understandable legal boundaries and solid, smart practices? First, a word of warning: there is variability in these legal requirements from jurisdiction to jurisdiction and possibly even from procedure to procedure. The following represents reasonable advice that should be valid nationally, but caregivers must check and know the specific state requirements for their location. That said, the following represents a sensible distillation of most legal requirements and recommended practices:

■ **What is informed consent?** It is NOT simply securing a signature on a consent form. It IS the education of the patient that should occur in conversation between the physician and the patient in which the patient obtains sufficient information to make a knowing decision. This includes minimally a comprehensive discussion of the proposed treatment and the alternatives, the relative risks and benefits of each, and culminates in an agreement obtained from an informed patient.

■ **Who should obtain it?** The duty is generally considered a nondelegable one of the physician proposing the therapy. Ideally, clinical programs would be constructed so the physician performing the procedure would be the person obtaining the patient's informed consent. Often, surrogates such as residents, fellows, physician assistants, and nurses are expected to secure the patient's consent, but the physician doing the procedure will be bound by the adequacy of that conversation. Any clinical workflow should allow for a meaningful conversation between the person set to perform the procedure and the patient.

- **When should it be obtained?** Because the idea is to enable a patient to make an informed decision, the conversation in which the patient is informed and after which the patient makes a decision must happen before the procedure and under circumstances that are not coercive and when the patient is clearheaded. Clinic workflow designed to obtain consent in the minutes before the procedure is usually worthless and easily attacked on the grounds that permission was coerced or because the patient was already sedated. When evaluating the validity of a clinic or practitioner's practice, ask how one might attack the practice later— Are patients under any pressure to sign? Are patients already medicated? Did the patient have time to listen to the conversation and read the form presented? Did the patient have a chance to ask questions? Was there an opportunity to change his or her mind?

- **How should it be delivered?** If approached consciously with the legal and ethical considerations in mind, programs and practitioners should construct practices and a workflow that are reasonably calculated to accomplish the purpose of arming most patients to make an intelligent choice. Practices must be flexible enough to recognize and respond to individual needs for departures from the usual in order to accomplish the purposes of informed consent. Marginally competent, illiterate, foreign, elderly, hearing-impaired patients are examples of individuals who may present challenges, small and large, to the usual process; ultimately, it is the nondelegable duty of the proceduralist to make sure reasonable efforts are made to effectively achieve informed consent, given the specific needs of each patient. Involving families as a patient's permission is obtained is usually a very good idea—family members may not have unrealistic expectations or be seized with the same level of anxiety as the patient. Family reaction to consent is also a good gauge of reasonableness of the conversation, whether the information is being delivered in a way that the patient can

reasonably understand, or that the material questions have been raised and answered.

A novel, more interactive manner of securing informed consent was recently promoted by the nonprofit patient safety organization National Quality Forum (NQF) in its "Safe Practices for Better Healthcare—2009 Update" (6). Noting that communication failures are at the root of medical errors that lead to injury and that the informed consent process was greatly lacking, NQF's "Safe Practice" focuses on the nature of the communication between the patient and the caregiver, as opposed to consent forms. The NQF informed consent "Safe Practice Statement" urges that the patient or legal surrogate be asked to "teach back" key information discussed in the informed consent conversation. This interactive model is aimed at ensuring the patient truly understands important information and increases the chance the patient will remember the discussion later. The personal involvement of the patient or family member would also foster better recall of the informed consent discussion afterward. The value and feasibility of this "teach back" approach to the informed consent discussion is something clinicians should consider in developing their informed consent habits.

- **What should be divulged?** Information that a reasonable patient would likely need under the circumstances to make an informed choice represents a threshold. There is no black and white answer to this question. The risks material to the patient, procedure, and situation are important. What other similarly situated practitioners do for the same procedure is a good gauge but not the end of the analysis. The physician should consider what most patients reasonably need to know to make an informed decision. Questions received from other patients are flags-try to anticipate those in informed consent discussions. Ultimately, the standard is what was reasonable under the circumstances to create an adequately informed patient.

There are two components to proper informed consent: content and documentation. The content, as described in the preceding sections, is the substantive discussion that occurs with patients aimed at educating them about their condition, the proposed treatment and its accompanying risks, benefits, and alternatives. Just as the process of securing informed consent is much more than obtaining a signature on a paper form, documentation ideally would be more than a mechanical act as well. A signed consent form is not by itself informed consent; it importantly memorializes the discussion and education that is the informed consent. The signed form actually benefits the caregiver more than the patient. It stands as *evidence* that the caregiver fulfilled his or her legal obligation and the quality of that evidence, the impact it has later at a trial, for instance, rises and falls with the documentation's credibility. As is noted earlier, patients' memories are fickle, uncertain and vary subject to recreation, suggestion, and a host of other forces that make memory highly variable and unreliable. Hence, much as it is important to document pertinent physical and diagnostic findings about the patient, it is important to document informed consent in a credible, contemporary record.

Standardized consent forms are generally viewed as the "permit" allowing the physician to perform the proposed procedure. Standardized consent forms are practical, simple and require little time and effort on the part of the clinician. When used to their best advantage, they can ensure that informed consent is documented in the patient's chart reliably. To be most useful, standardized consent forms should be concise and written in language patients will understand and have a hard time disavowing later. Forms heavy with medical jargon, legalese, and terms that the average patient cannot understand are easily dismissed as just another hospital form that was presented and signed with no explanation. They carry little weight in discussions with the patient afterward, or with a jury down the road. The consent form used must be consistent, up-to-date, and an accurate reflection of the proposed procedure and risks and benefits to the particular patient. Inaccuracies easily render the form irrelevant when compared to the patient's recall, and gross inaccuracies reinforce the idea that consent was not seriously pursued at all. In general, standardized consent forms should include the following:

- The nature of the patient's condition, illness, or diagnosis.
- The proposed treatment plan.

- The risks, side effects, and complications. It is not necessary that the standardized consent form list each and every possible risk or complication that may theoretically occur. In general, a standardized form should specifically list those risks or complications most commonly associated with the procedure and those that are perhaps rare but have grave consequences. The standardized form should be formatted to encourage the caregiver to think about and list other, less common risks or complications that may uniquely apply to a particular patient.
- A description of the risks and benefits of reasonable alternatives to the proposed treatment plan (including the alternative of nontreatment).
- A record of any brochures, pamphlets, or other written or audiovisual information relating to the procedure that were given to the patient.
- That the patient had an opportunity to ask questions and that those questions were answered to his or her satisfaction before signing the form.

A common misconception related to standardized consent forms is that "if the complication is listed, I should not be able to be sued for its occurrence." The simple response is "Yes, but the patient never consented to a negligently performed procedure." Health care providers are not immune from a claim of negligence merely because the patient was told of the risk beforehand and still agreed to the procedure. For example, a standardized consent form for a cardiac catheterization might include retroperitoneal bleeding as a risk. This does not mean that a patient who suffers a retroperitoneal bleed as a result of a negligently performed catheterization cannot successfully sue. Conversely, if a patient sustains a complication that is not listed on the standardized consent form, it does not necessarily follow that this is proof the procedure was done negligently. Some complications may be unknown, unforeseen, and not discussed with the patient in advance. These exceedingly rare, unforeseen complications are not the type that should be itemized on a standardized consent form for a particular case. There are likely valid reasons why a certain complication was neither foreseen nor emphasized in advance, and these reasons can be shared with the patient or the patient's family after the unforeseen complication occurs. To itemize every theoretical complication on a standardized consent form would water down the impact of those that should be highlighted: the risks or complications that are generally relevant and encountered with a particular procedure.

Standardized consent forms have their limitations. They are often flippantly presented to the patient along with many other forms for signing. With the clinician who presented the form hovering over the patient, impatiently waiting for signature, the patient may not take the time to read, understand, and digest what is written, let alone ask questions. The forms are typically written in technical, medical terms that are beyond the understanding of most patients. The forms can easily become outdated and do not encourage documentation or discussion of risks, benefits, and alternatives that may be unique to that particular patient. This is why a detailed, contemporaneous clinic note outlining the informed consent discussion is valuable.

A tailored clinic note in the patient's chart memorializing that the informed consent conversation occurred, identifying the participants to that conversation, the salient points made and the patient's agreement, coupled with a statement that all the patient's questions were answered resulting in the patient's agreement and request to proceed is a very valuable compliment to the usual operative or procedure permit. A good clinic note that accurately reflects the conversation between the clinician and the patient is strong evidence that the patient was adequately informed and that the physician fulfilled his or her legal obligation. The note does not have to be *War and Peace*, but it should reflect the basic elements that comprise the informed consent discussion: that the proposed treatment and its risks, benefits, and alternatives were discussed with the patient, that the patient understood the risks and benefits, that any questions the patient had have been answered satisfactorily, and that the patient agrees to the proposed treatment. The note is also a better vehicle for the physician to recount risks, benefits, and alternatives that are unique to that particular patient, and ideally, these should be documented as well. A signed, dated, and witnessed standardized consent form, coupled with a contemporaneous clinic note, is powerful evidence of the carefully obtained consent.

■ THE OPPORTUNITY TO MANAGE RISK WITH INFORMED CONSENT

Practically speaking, most patients seek legal help after they were surprised by an outcome and explanations they could trust were not offered as they struggled to understand what happened to them. Solid risk management begins *before* a problem develops. Obtaining informed consent remains the most underutilized opportunity to set reasonable expectations and sensitize the patient to the difficulties and potential adverse outcomes. Logically, a patient who is well informed before a problem occurs will more easily understand what happened if a problem develops later. Although they may need assistance to remember the consent discussion and process what happened to them, thoughtful informed consent will have prepared them better to embrace the idea that the complication alone does not mean that the practitioner was negligent. Trying to make that point afterward in the absence of forewarning sounds to patients like self-serving coverup. If the possibility was clearly raised before the problem, it is far easier for a patient to embrace the idea that bad things can happen in the face of reasonable care. Think of this from the patient's perspective as a cycle: beginning with the patient's expectations, progressing through the patient's actual experiences, passing then to the patient's access to information after the complication, and ending with help to process the experience. If the cycle remains intact, if the patient's expectations presage his actual experience, if warning beforehand about the complication was clearly made, and when it happened, the patient had ready access to caregivers willing to explain and help the patient process the new reality, the likelihood that the patient will feel the need to have an advocate (read: lawyer) drops significantly (7).

Few interventional cardiologists use the informed consent conversation as an opportunity to establish reasonable expectations. In fact, the obligation to provide informed consent becomes for many an opportunity to create unrealistic expectations. Practitioners who find themselves saying things such as "you'll be up and running in no time," "you're in good hands—I've got the best complication rate in the state," and "you'll feel better as soon as you wake up" are really communicating: "It won't happen to you." Statistics grease this slippery slope. Reciting remote statistical chances deceives patients into believing their personal risk is the same as the risk of a large study population. No individual patient experiences 0.3% death or complication. If the complication occurs to your patient, he or she experiences 100% of that complication. Statistics may have bearing in an informed consent discussion, but any recitation of a statistical risk should be placed in context and balanced with strong personal reminders that regardless of a population's risk, if a complication happens to your patient, it could change the patient's life dramatically.

INTERVENTIONAL CARDIOLOGY FELLOW TO CARDIAC

CATHETERIZATION PATIENT (as her groin is being shaved by one nurse and another is starting an IV in her arm, and after her glasses have been surrendered): "I need your signature on this form and we'll get you in and out."

PATIENT: "Well, what is this?"

FELLOW: "It's just a formality—I just need your signature down here."

PATIENT: "Well, don't you think I should read it before I sign it?"

FELLOW (impatiently): "You can if you want, but we can't take you back until I get your signature."

PATIENT: "I don't have my glasses—what does it say?"

FELLOW: "It just lists some potential complications—nothing to worry about really—this is very safe. Your risks are about the same as the risk you'll be struck by lightning."

PATIENT (very irritated now): "That's not very comforting! *I was struck by lightning when I was 13 years old!*"

Although amusing, the true case example above occurs only too frequently. Not only was the patient uninformed but also the risks were minimized to the point of absurdity, and the opportunity to set realistic expectations was lost. Moreover, because the duty to obtain informed consent is generally regarded as a nondelegable duty for the person actually about to do the procedure, the fellow's cavalier handling places the attending personally at risk. Why can't physicians say, "I'm not going to kid you, Mrs. Jones. The percentage chance you'll have a serious

problem is low, but if it happens to you it's 100%. Some of these complications could seriously alter your life. You should carefully consider these risks and options, including the risk of doing nothing. There's no guarantee. I can't even guarantee I won't make a mistake. All I can promise you is that I'll do my best. Do you have any questions?" A patient who participates in a discussion like this would be far more prepared for an adverse outcome than the patient in the example above. It is important to balance the discussion such that you do not scare your patient out of the procedure altogether, but frankly, if all it takes to dissuade a patient from having a procedure is an honest disclosure of the relative risks, the proceduralist probably should not do it anyway. Few procedures are being done without documented medical need and with some thought and sensitivity, this balance should be easily struck.

An example of an ideal consent documentation in a clinic follows. Note that this would be in addition to the forms that the patient signs.

This is a note to document the current plans at the Interventional Cardiology Clinic for Robert L. For my records, Mr. L. is a 69-year-old man who was referred from outside hospital X with reported 100% occlusion of his right coronary artery, and 70% blockage of his left main. I have examined the cath lab films that were sent down to me, and indeed these reveal these blockages. I think that angioplasty with drug-eluding stent placement as had been suggested by Dr. B. is indeed the best option in my opinion. I discussed my assessment thoroughly with Mr. L. by phone, explained my feelings and recommendations, together with his other options and attendant risks of each, and he agrees to proceed. The procedure is scheduled for October 2007, and we will keep you apprised of our progress. I encouraged Mr. L. to call me should he have any other questions or concerns in the interim.

■ INFORMED CONSENT AND OFF-LABEL MEDICAL DEVICE USE

Surprise after the fact, as we have discussed earlier, is a major reason patients look to professionals other than their caregivers (lawyers predominantly) for answers; when a complication occurs and the patients discover a material fact afterward about their care that was not disclosed beforehand, they quickly conclude the care giver was not honest and cannot be trusted presently and they instinctively turn to those whose credibility and loyalty to them is not in question. Dr. Gerald Hickson, a noted researcher who has for years examined the factors that prompt some patients to sue and others not, concluded a long time ago that a sizeable percentage of patients who hired lawyers did so when they suspected that their physician had not been honest with them (8). The discovery, after a complication, that a device untested, unproven, and unapproved played a role in their postprocedure difficulties is almost guaranteed to provoke a feeling in the patient or family that something improper occurred and a coverup followed. Caregivers need to tailor the manner in which they handle the off-label use of devices in individual circumstances, but in every case the informed consent process should be viewed especially critically as a means by which that pivotal element of surprise can be diffused to ameliorate the risk that subsequent discovery sparks a trip to the lawyer's office.

Given the painstakingly time-consuming process for securing Food and Drug Administration (FDA) approval of a device for a specific use, it has been, and is becoming more common for physicians, and interventionalists in particular, to use FDA-approved devices "off-label" (i.e., for a use other than one specifically approved by the FDA). It is instructive to understand exactly how this happens. The FDA admittedly does not have the authority, and does not want the authority, to regulate the practice of medicine. The Federal Food, Drug and Cosmetic Act specifically states that "nothing in this Act shall be construed to limit or interfere with the authority of a health care practitioner to prescribe or administer any legally marketed device to a patient for any condition or disease within a legitimate health care practitioner–patient relationship" (9). The FDA has recognized that

> Good medical practice and the best interests of the patient require that physicians use legally available . . . devices according to their best knowledge and judgment. If physicians use a product for an indication not in the approved labeling, they have the responsibility to be well informed about the product, to base its use on

firm scientific rationale and on sound medical evidence, and to maintain records of the product's use and effects. Use of a marketed product in this manner when the intent is the "practice of medicine" does not require the submission of an Investigational New Drug Application (IND), Investigational Device Exemption (IDE) or review by an Institutional Review Board (IRB). However, the institution at which the product will be used may, under its own authority, require IRB review or other institutional oversight (10).

Thus, it has become generally accepted that physicians may use devices off-label, provided the use is consistent with the "best interests of the patient," and is based on "firm, scientific rationale and on sound medical evidence." The use should be recognized as within the standard of care for the specific specialist, which means in the case of an interventional cardiologist that "a reasonably prudent cardiologist of the same education, training, and expertise would have used the device in that manner under the same or similar circumstances." It is the responsibility of the interventionalist to ensure the use is safe, effective, and supported by medical literature, scientific rationale, and patient need. Assuming the physician is well informed about the device and is basing its use on something founded in science and medical evidence, the question then becomes: when using approved devices off-label, what should patients be told about the regulatory status of the device as part of the informed consent process? Or, more to the point, how can advising the patient ahead of time avoid the kind of surprise and discovery afterward that would make the patient think something inappropriate or even illegal occurred in the procedure?

There is nothing in the Federal Food, Drug and Cosmetic Act that requires that patients are advised of the regulatory status of a device, not surprising given the explicit exclusion in the Act of any pretense that it regulate the practice of medicine. But the absence in the Federal Food, Drug and Cosmetic Act does not mean physicians are absolved of any preprocedure disclosure and certainly does not mean no preprocedure disclosure is a good idea. Importantly, nothing in the Act or regulations prohibits states or courts (via case law) from requiring disclosure of the regulatory status of a device in the informed consent process.

Courts across the country have held that physicians are not required to address the regulatory status of a device in the informed consent process and that the regulatory status of the device is not *necessarily* material to informed consent. In a courtroom, whether the regulatory status is material to informed consent may be driven by the specific facts of the case at issue. Bottom line: there is no hard and fast legal maxim as to what must be shared with the patient about a device during the informed consent discussion. Identifiable factors may drive the decision as to whether to overtly seek a patient's approval before proceeding with a procedure planned to involve an off-label use of a device approved for other uses:

- How close to the approved purposes is the off-label use being considered?
- How widespread is the off-label use within the community of specialists across the country?
- How controversial is the off-label use within your specialty and other overlapping specialties?
- How significant is the device to the procedure being proposed?
- How necessary is the off-label use to the success of the procedure? And, related: Are there accepted alternatives to achieve the same results?
- Are there studies underway specifically to examine the safety and efficacy of the off-label use?
- Does the individual caregiver have a track record with the off-label use that would suggest both skill and experience and the comfort of a record of safety?
- Is the caregiver tied financially or otherwise to the device manufacturer, or the expansion of the device use?

In general, the closer the off-label use is to the approved use, the lower the perceived need to make a special disclosure in the preprocedure visits. The less widespread the use nationally, the harder it will be to convince the patient after the fact that it was appropriate. The existence of robust controversy in the literature almost guarantees that absent full disclosure ahead of time and specific informed consent by the patient, the patient will both believe it was wrong AND have no problem finding physicians to validate this belief, as they offer their services as experts in

the ensuing malpractice case. While off-label use of a device that is only incidental to the procedure may warrant no attention at all in the informed consent discussion, off-label use of a device for an essential purpose to the procedure takes on more importance in the preprocedure discussions, especially if there are less-controversial alternatives that will accomplish the same purpose. There is probably nothing like the specter of personal gain to cement a sense in an injured patient or grieving family that the caregiver's motives for the off-label use were improper. Whether to mention an intended off-label use or not in the conversation before the procedure at least should be considered against these and other considerations, but it is a choice ultimately left to the sound discretion of the physician, as informed by the standard of care.

That being said, if there is any question about the wisdom of doing so, cardiologists should err on the side of disclosure. Presumably, off-label use of the device is being considered because the patient's physician has concluded that the patient will benefit from its use; if that's true, there should be no harm in sharing that judgment with the patient. Before the caregiver decides what form the disclosure should take and its content, he or she should consider a number of factors that would include the sophistication of the patient, the significance of the role the device will play, and the potential complications among them. The manner of the disclosure and education may range from making it a part of the informed consent discussion to use of special information sheets and a specific written consent form. Controlling the tenor and content of the message and documenting exactly what was discussed is important and reducing it to writing, augmented with an opportunity for discussion, is an excellent way of protecting the clinicians involved in these situations.

Although not exactly on point, the manner in which the University of Michigan chose to address a new FDA concern about a dermatology drug will illustrate the value of a written information sheet and consent form. In March 2005, the FDA issued a black box warning expressing concerns that animal studies suggested an increased risk of lymphoma, among other problems, with a class of medications used for many years in the treatment of eczema. The American Academy of Dermatology disagreed with the FDA's concerns and the University's physicians, drawing on years of experience with the drug, strongly favored its continued use. Rather than ignore the FDA's concerns and determined not to succumb to the threat of potential liability by discontinuing its use, the University elected to confront the problem head-on with patients and families. Working with Dermatology faculty, legal counsel for the University drafted an information sheet that alerted the patients and families to the controversy, described the position held by the American Academy of Dermatology, and explained the University's collective experience and recommendations. The letter was distributed to patients and families, with recommendations and patients and families were asked to indicate in writing whether they were willing to receive the medication over the FDA's concerns. Contrary to fears that patients would be scared away from using the medication, the letter allowed the University to describe the issue in objective and balanced terms, before patients read about it on the Internet or saw it on television. The University was able to control the message and at the same time document the information given, the permission received, and create excellent evidence of informed consent.

Protecting the caregiver is important, especially when the device being used off-label is an important part of the procedure or therapy being proposed. It is typically important to document the disclosure of the off-label use of anything significant to the procedure or posing a serious threat to the patient, not just to avoid a legal pitfall but also to ensure the patient's involvement in his or her own medical treatment and decision making.

■ DISCLOSURE OF ADVERSE OUTCOMES AND THE ROLE OF INFORMED CONSENT

Bad things can and do happen during procedures, often despite appropriate care. The ubiquitous risk that these bad things might happen establishes the need for informed consent in the first place. Informing a patient (and family) well about these risks makes the conversation afterward much easier. And yet, human nature being

what it is, many health care providers run for cover when a bad outcome occurs, apparently hoping that the consequences of the complication, and perhaps the patient, will just go away. Although understandable, deep avoidance is unethical, an abdication of the physician's responsibility to his or her patient, and counter to the wishful thinking, actually invites litigation. Adverse outcomes should be addressed head-on, disclosed in a factual way to patients and families with honesty and in a manner devoid of defensiveness. Why?

1. Patients are always entitled to understand the status of their health and their medical options after a complication. It is the ethical, right thing to do—for the patient/ family and caregiver.
2. Disclosure affords the health care provider the chance to maintain the patient's trust. Avoidance only guarantees a bad ending to the patient–caregiver relationship.
3. Disclosure makes practical sense— patients and families need information to make knowledgeable, informed decisions about future care.
4. Disclosure is the caregiver's opportunity to help the patient understand what actually happened. It is natural for people to try to make sense of what happens to them—if patients are not given the true facts, the caregiver risks that his or her patient will assume the worst about the situation.
5. Disclosure is a necessary precursor to learning from mistakes and improving patient safety. We must acknowledge the error in order to learn from it.
6. While this may be counterintuitive to some, open and honest disclosure makes sense from a claims management perspective, allowing the caregiver to intercept the patient before the patient even feels the need to see a lawyer.
7. Disclosure is now mandated by the Centers for Medicare & Medicaid Services and accrediting agencies such as The Joint Commission.

Study after study demonstrates the same point: patients seek legal advice when they find they cannot get honest answers they can trust, when they sense the absence of accountability, and when no one is there to help them put the pieces together in a credible way. Answering questions directly leads to credibility and offers an opportunity to clarify misconceptions. In one study, it was found that 24% of patients sued their physicians because they felt that their physicians were not being honest (11).

Disclosure of an unanticipated outcome is a process, not a single event. We do not recommend that any caregiver handle disclosure of a serious complication without first getting good advice. When adverse consequences happen as a result of well-intended medical care, caregivers experience a complex set of emotions and it is prudent to get an independent view of the situation and advice before undertaking a full disclosure. Committing to disclose once the facts are clear, but reserving a time frame to consult with resources such as a risk management office or counsel and gather facts, not simply expressing assumptions and uninformed opinions, is always a good idea. The process of disclosure should begin as soon as the adverse outcome is appreciated, if only to promise full disclosure once the facts are in. As additional facts and information about the event are accumulated, further discussions with the patient and families need to occur. Well-executed and well-documented informed consent before the procedure sets the stage for these difficult conversations later, allowing the caregiver and the risk manager to build on what was established before the problem developed.

Disclosure of an Acute Patient Event

The importance of a solid informed consent discussion to a disclosure of an adverse event is apparent from the following clinical example. A 62-year-old man was admitted for a cardiac catheterization for unstable angina. As it happened in this case, both the fellow and the attending together met with the patient and the family for the usual informed consent drill, except in this case, the attending cardiologist had a specific motivation to role model the consent discussion for his brand new fellow. He spent time with the patient and the patient's spouse and daughter, outlining all of the potential risks. He later recalled that he made a point of sitting on their level, speaking in nonmedical

language, and reviewing the more common complications led by, of course, allergic reaction to dye.

The events of the case unfolded as every cardiologist's nightmare. The following is an excerpt from the clinic note on this patient:

> After injection of LCA, developed severe anaphylactic reaction with laryngeal edema, severe stridor and hypoxia, followed by hypotension. Emergently intubated and given IV Solu-Medrol, IV Benadryl and IV epinephrine with some improvement in BP; however continued to be hypoxic and developed non-cardiogenic pulmonary edema; multiple episodes of hypotension treated with IV vasopressors; BP continued to spiral down and placed on ECMO with restoration of flow and restoration of oxygenation.

The brevity of this description belies the magnitude of this complication and one can only imagine the complex mix of emotions running through the minds of all involved. This patient ultimately died from severe hypoxic ischemic brain injury. At some point in this horrible chain of events, someone needed to talk with the family.

Evidencing the same care and social sensitivity that made the informed consent process so meaningful, the attending found a moment to inform the family what was happening. At that point, the family had a general feeling things had not gone well. Too much time had passed and though they were unaware of the specific actions being taken, they sensed that the mood had changed substantially within the cath lab waiting area. They remember being taken to a private place and they remember that the cardiologist, clearly shaken, minced no words. He said he wanted time to gather more information, but it appeared to him that their husband and father may have had a serious reaction to the dye. He emphasized that he himself had a lot of questions but that the focus at that point had to be on giving the patient every chance to survive—there would be time to answer questions once the patient was stabilized. In that first conversation, he made reference to the informed consent discussion and the link was made in the family's mind. Later, they remembered discussing that specifically while they waited to know if their loved one would survive. When the cardiologist had to break the news that the brain damage was so severe the patient was not likely to make it, the family was already processing what had happened in an accurate way, the groundwork having been laid in that clinic visit before the cardiac catheterization occurred.

The cardiologist's response to this situation is educational to our point:

- He responded as best he could to the emergency and stayed with the patient until he got the patient relatively stable. His first instinct was to attend to the patient's medical needs.
- At the first available, safe opportunity, he informed the family of only what he really knew at the time: though he was not entirely sure, the patient had experienced what appeared to be a significant reaction and he told them exactly what he had just done in response and what his short-term plans were for the patient's care. This information was delivered with empathy, but in a highly factual, completely nondefensive manner. He used the informed consent discussion as a reference point for his conversation. He promised full disclosure, but only after seeing to the patient's medical needs and only after having a chance to gather more information.
- He called Risk Management, reported to them what he knew and what he had told the patient's family. Risk Management documented the information carefully in their system and dispatched a risk manager to the clinic to start the process of gathering information. In this case, the attending and the risk manager agreed that they would meet the family together, and Risk Management offered to serve as a resource for their questions and provide needed information.
- Several meetings occurred between the risk manager, the physicians caring for the patient, and the family between the first notification of the complication and the patient's death. Once checked for accuracy, information was freely shared and always placed in context and in language the family could understand.

The family later reflected on the care with which the pre- and postprocedure conversations had occurred. Although they could not recite every one of the risks the cardiologist had previously discussed, they remember being left with the impression that this catheterization was not as simple as they first thought. They remember

thinking that regardless of how careful, skilled, and experienced the cardiologist, there were serious risks that he could not control. They remembered the patience with which the cardiologist reviewed what he was going to do and why. They clearly knew they were part of a teaching effort, but later they remembered most the interest the attending seemed to show in their grasp of what he was going to do. Importantly, they never questioned the credibility of the cardiologist when he later told them that the investigation concluded that their husband and father did indeed have that rare anaphylactic reaction to dye. They did not doubt the factual information given to them about the sequence of events, believing that the staff moved with deliberate skill and speed. And perhaps most important, they never doubted that the cardiologist really cared about their loved one, notwithstanding the fact that this physician had met the patient only at one brief clinic visit before the catheterization and that the physician was deeply affected by the death of his patient. Table 3-1 is a list of tips for a successful disclosure.

TABLE 3-1 **Tips for Successful Disclosure**

- ALWAYS take care of patient first.
- Gather all facts needed for presentation of information.
- Presume goodwill on behalf of all parties.
- Approach the disclosure with honesty.
- Confidentiality of patient information is primary.
- Decisions are patient-centered.
- Input from family is invited, welcomed, and valued.
- Patient's primary caregivers are valued and welcomed.
- Recommendations, not decisions are the goals.
- Pay attention to patient preferences and cultural considerations.
- Do not speculate on causes or reasons for the adverse outcome—communicate what is known and plan to follow up as more information becomes available.
- Do not disclose in heat of the moment unless necessary and keep it fact-based. Opinions can always wait and almost always change with information.
- Commit to answering questions.
- Seek assistance: Call Risk Management or Department Head.

Impulsive Disclosure and Its Associated Costs

In early December, Brian W. underwent coronary artery bypass surgery for paroxysmal atrial fibrillation that was refractory to medical management. Postoperative episodes of atrial fibrillation were managed by Cardiology and he was discharged home on Christmas Eve. Four days later, the patient presented to the emergency department with shortness of breath, palpitations, atrial fibrillation, digoxin toxicity, and left pleural effusion. Reasoning that the patient seemed hemodynamically stable 2 weeks post op, the Emergency Medicine physician elected to contact Cardiology, who noted, "given patient's recent CABG, we felt that a post op surgical etiology was less likely." The patient was admitted to Cardiology. The patient decompensated over the ensuing hours and went into pulseless electrical activity (PEA) arrest at 2:32 AM. Echocardiogram done at 4:30 AM was reviewed at 7:00 AM and was thought to show possible tamponade. The surgeon was called and arrived at 7:30 AM. Versions of events according to the patient's wife, the cardiology fellow, and the surgeon follow:

PATIENT'S WIFE: "Dr. _____ was extremely upset and yelled at the doctors with Brian. He told them they didn't know what they were doing. He demanded to know why he wasn't called when Brian was admitted. He was furious and told me repeatedly that this should never have happened, that had he been called, he would have had Brian in the OR in no time. He said that an echo should have been done as soon as Brian came through the emergency room and he didn't know what the heck they were thinking. I told him I can't believe he wasn't notified when Brian got here. What kind of place are you running, anyway?"

CARDIOLOGY FELLOW: "He (the surgeon) was really out of line, right in front of the patient and his wife, yelling that he should have known about this patient when he arrived. That was not even my decision. I certainly couldn't reason with him and I can only imagine what the patient and his wife thought. I just knew I was going to be sued after that."

SURGEON: "No, I didn't yell at anyone. Mrs. W. asked me if I knew Brian was in the hospital and I told

them 'no'—what was I going to do, lie? Yes, I told them I should have known and had I known, I would have had him in the OR a lot sooner and with a better result. I don't know what they were thinking—why in the world did they admit this patient to Cardiology?"

The surgeon was right about one thing: at the time he erupted in front of the family, he didn't know what the emergency department physician had been thinking when the patient was admitted to Cardiology and not Cardiac Surgery. Had the surgeon taken the time to find out before he unloaded his criticism, many problems might have been avoided. The emergency physician actually had considered the issue thoroughly: He thought about these factors: (1) the patient was 2 weeks out from surgery and stable even on anticoagulants; (2) the patient had atrial fibrillation before and after surgery, so atrial fibrillation alone was no reason to suspect the leak; (3) the surgeon typically leaves the pericardium open, so tamponade as the mechanism for atrial fibrillation was very low on his differential; and (4) the patient was hemodynamically stable in the emergency department. Against this backdrop, even the surgeon later agreed that it was perfectly reasonable to admit the patient to Cardiology, but having expressed himself before he discovered the facts, it was impossible to undo the damage of his uninformed, impulsive remarks.

Ideally, the surgeon should have told the family, "I promise to get answers for you, but first, we need to attend to Brian's immediate medical needs. Once he's stable and I have a chance to get more information, we will talk. I have many of the same questions." After getting more facts, the surgeon would not have been so dogmatic on the decision to admit to Cardiology—a critical issue if the family decides to pursue a malpractice claim.

■ CONNECTING TO QUALITY WITH LESSONS LEARNED

One of the most important aspects of acknowledging an adverse outcome and at times an error is the opportunity of learning from those events. It is impossible to learn from a mistake and improve upon practices without first recognizing the error or problem. Interventional cardiologists should have a process in place to connect their lessons learned with quality improvement aims. Problems identified as "systems issues" need to be addressed, corrected, and disseminated institution-wide.

Recall that one of the factors that drives patients or families to sue is the hope that what happened to them will not happen to another (12). It is powerful to be able to tell a patient and family that their loss has not been utterly in vain. Of course, there are some for which the amount of compensation is paramount, but the number of people who find value in future quality improvements is grossly underappreciated.

Connecting to quality improvement after an error (negligent or not) has been made helps prevent the reduction of future adverse events. It allows for complications and trends to be studied so that problems can be predicted and prevented. This fosters the best risk management strategy: preventing the bad outcomes in the first place.

Examination of the intersection of law and medicine can be illuminating for both sides. Although many physicians see the duty to provide informed consent as a legal technicality imposed on them by operation of law, it is healthy to revisit the purpose of law in our society. Frederic Bastiat, the 19th-century author, economist, and statesman, described it this way in his treatise, *The Law* (12):

> We must remember that law is force, and that, consequently, the proper functions of the law cannot lawfully extend beyond the proper functions of force.
>
> When law and force keep a person within the bounds of justice, they impose nothing but a mere negation. They oblige him only to abstain from harming others. They violate neither his personality, his liberty, nor his property. They safeguard all of these. They are defensive; they defend equally the rights of all.

Patients under a physician's care are entirely vulnerable. Informed consent, at a minimum, protects a patient's inarguable right to determine who is permitted to touch them, to what extent, and under what circumstances. Rather than bridle at the obligation, or diminish it by reducing it to the act of obtaining a signature on a form, physicians should remember that in our

society, the purpose of the law is not so much to impose an obligation as it is to protect those who cannot protect themselves.

■ PEARLS

- View the informed consent process as a tool to manage risk. Use it as an opportunity to set reasonable expectations for the patient to minimize surprise when complications occur.
- Informed consent is not completing a consent form. It is the agreement that arises from the conversation between the physician and the patient during which the patient is educated sufficiently to make an informed decision about medical treatment.
- In general, adequate informed consent discussions should include a description of the proposed procedure and alternatives, including material risks and benefits of each in language a layman can understand and in sufficient detail to create a reasonably educated patient.
- The person intending to perform the procedure should secure the consent in a noncoercive way when the patient is fully competent and with time to change his or her mind.
- Document informed consent in both a well-written, up-to-date standardized consent form and a contemporary clinic note in the patient's chart.
- Whether to mention an off-label use of devices or medications in the informed consent conversation should be considered in every case. Disclosure of the off-label use is recommended if there is any question about whether to discuss the off-label use in advance.
- Well-executed and well-documented informed consent beforehand sets the stage for difficult disclosure conversations that may be required later. It allows the caregiver and the risk manager to build on the discussion of potential risks and complications established before the problem occurred.
- Disclosure of adverse outcomes is the ethical thing to do for all involved, makes practical sense, is a necessary precursor to learning from mistakes, and makes sense from a claims management perspective, but should never be done without help.
- Disclosure of an adverse outcome is a process, not a single event, and should not only be

handled in a way that is attentive to the patient and family's needs but also in a way that is prudent and deliberate.

- Take advantage of the opportunity to learn from an adverse event. Connect those lessons learned with quality improvement aims.

References

1. Vincent C, Young M, Phillips A. (2003). Why do people sue doctors? A study of patients and relatives taking legal action. *Lancet.* 1994;343:1609–1613.
2. *Mohr v Williams,* 104 NW 12 (Minn 1905).
3. *Schloendorff v The Society of the New York Hospital,* 211 NY 125, 105 NE 92, 93 (1914).
4. *Canterbury v Spence,* 464 F2d 772 (DC Cir 1972).
5. Robinson G, Merav A. Informed consent: recall by patients tested postoperatively. *Ann Thorac Surg.* 1976;22(3):209–212.
6. National Quality Forum Consensus Committee. *Safe Practices for Better Healthcare—2009 Update: A Consensus Report.* Washington, DC: National Quality Forum; 2009.
7. Boothman R, Blackwell A, Campbell D, et al. A better approach to medical malpractice claims? The University of Michigan approach. *J Health Life Sci L.* 2009;2(2):125–136.
8. Hickson G, Clayton EW, Githens P, Sloan F. Factors that prompted families to file medical malpractice claims following prenatal injuries. *JAMA.* 1992;267:1359–1361.
9. Federal Food, Drug and Cosmetic Act, Sec. 906. 21 USC sec. 396. Practice of Medicine.
10. http://www.fda.gov/ScienceResearch/Special Topics/RunningClinicalTrials/Guidances InformationSheetsandNotices/ucm116355.htm. Accessed June 18, 2010.
11. Kalra J, Massey KL, Mulla A. Disclosure of medical error: policies and practice. *JAMA.* 1992;267:1359–1363.
12. Bastiat F. *The Law.* Irvington-on-Hudson, NY: Foundation for Economic Education; 1996. Originally published in 1850.

4 Training and Facility Environment

ERON STURM AND JOHN W. HIRSHFELD JR

PREREQUISITES FOR SAFETY IN INVASIVE CARDIOVASCULAR PROCEDURES

Safety and effectiveness in invasive cardiovascular procedures require both appropriately knowledgeable and skilled physician operators and a working environment that fosters safety. Thus, both physician operator education and training and cardiac catheterization laboratory facility and operational procedures must be optimized to provide the best possible patient outcomes.

A skilled, knowledgeable operator constitutes a patient's best protection against complications of an interventional cardiovascular procedure. The operator affects the risk of a complication in multiple domains. Complication risk begins with appropriate case selection. It is also influenced by the skill with which the operator conducts a procedure, by the judgment used to make strategic intraprocedural decisions, and by the operator's ability to assess outcome, recognize complications promptly, and manage them appropriately.

The operation of the cardiac catheterization laboratory facility as a system is also vital to optimal patient safety and outcomes. Both the laboratory's physical equipment complement and its operational procedures are essential to safe and effective procedure conduct. It is axiomatic that the laboratory must be appropriately designed architecturally and have high-quality radiologic imaging, monitoring, and life support equipment that is maintained in perfect working order. In addition, the laboratory must have highly trained, skilled, clinical personnel and operate according to well-designed rigorous protocols that ensure reliable systematic quality execution of procedures and prompt appropriate responses to complications and other emergencies.

GOALS OF PHYSICIAN OPERATOR TRAINING IN INTERVENTIONAL CARDIOLOGY

The ideal interventional cardiologist is a skilled knowledgeable operator who selects cases appropriately, performs procedures skillfully, assesses results accurately, and manages undesirable outcomes appropriately. A well-designed training program should foster its trainees' acquisition of the knowledge and skills required to optimize procedure outcome while minimizing risk.

There are four basic domains of physician operator quality:

1. *Case selection:* Appropriate case selection requires application of cognitive knowledge and judgement. A procedure's appropriateness, as judged from the patient's baseline characteristics, is determined by the interaction of its likelihood of success, its attendant risk, and the potential benefit to the patient of a successful outcome. A skilled knowledgeable operator balances these considerations appropriately in making the decision to undertake the procedure.
2. *Procedure execution:* Quality procedure execution begins by selecting the optimal procedure strategy. This includes identifying the optimal devices and techniques for the patient's particular characteristics. Quality procedure execution also requires that the operator possess the necessary technical skill to execute the procedure effectively.

3. *Outcome assessment:* It is important to be able to assess a procedure's outcome with respect to both judging success and recognizing complications. Should a complication develop, the operator should be able to recognize it and manage it. In addition, the operator should be able to furnish appropriate aftercare for successful uncomplicated procedures to ensure the optimal durability of the procedure's result.

4. *Radiation safety and protection:* The physician operator should understand the X-ray imaging system's operation and the basic principles of radiation physics and X-ray fluorographic imaging in order to achieve optimal imaging while minimizing patient radiation exposure.

ORIGIN AND EVOLUTION OF TRAINING AND CERTIFICATION IN INTERVENTIONAL CARDIOLOGY

Evolution of Interventional Cardiology as a Discipline

The first coronary angioplasty procedure was performed by Andreas Gruentzig in 1977 (1). In the several years that followed, physicians skilled in diagnostic catheterization extended their skills to the nascent discipline of interventional cardiology through attendance at demonstration courses, organized initially by Gruentzig and subsequently by others and through communication within tightly knit groups who shared experiences and information. The discipline rapidly matured as equipment was refined and procedure indications were clarified. By the mid-1980s, many accredited general cardiovascular training programs were offering an additional year of training in invasive diagnostic and interventional cardiovascular procedures.

Development of Interventional Cardiology Training Programs and Certification

By the early 1990s, interventional cardiovascular procedures had become commonplace and it was becoming generally accepted that dedicated specialized training was needed to prepare a physician to perform interventional cardiovascular procedures at a state-of-the-art level. At this point, the American College of Cardiology (ACC) and the American Board of Internal Medicine (ABIM) approached the American Board of Medical Specialties (ABMS) with a proposal that a separate certification process be developed for interventional cardiology. The underlying rationale that the discipline should be separately recognized and certified was that the field had its own large specialized cognitive knowledge base that is not held by general cardiovascular specialists. This principle is derived from the attributes of an interventional cardiologist listed earlier in this chapter. It is self-evident that the technical skill dimension of interventional cardiology is a comparatively small component of the overall attribute complement required to be a quality interventionalist. Thus, the field of interventional cardiology, although a semi-surgical discipline, is actually dominated by its cognitive knowledge base. The recognition of this concept led to the acceptance of interventional cardiology as a separately certifiable discipline within cardiovascular medicine and the recognition that standards and criteria for training and experience in interventional cardiology were needed.

This acceptance led to parallel initiatives by ABIM to develop a certifying examination and by the American Council of Graduate Medical Education (ACGME) to develop standards and criteria for interventional cardiology training programs. The ABIM interventional cardiology examination was administered for the first time in 1999. The ACGME training standards are linked to the ABIM certifying process in that eligibility to sit for the ABIM now requires that the candidate have completed training in a residency review committee–approved training program that meets the standards and criteria adopted by the ACGME.

PROGRAMMATIC REQUIREMENTS FOR TRAINING IN INTERVENTIONAL CARDIOLOGY

The ACGME has specified detailed programmatic requirements that training programs must satisfy in order to achieve accreditation (2). This document specifies requirements for program structure, resources, conduct, faculty, and faculty responsibilities.

The ABIM stipulates that candidates for certification in interventional cardiology must have completed the required 1 year of training in an ACGME-accredited program (3). During that year trainees must perform a minimum of 250 cardiac interventional procedures.

The definition of "perform" is precise: "To receive credit for performance of a therapeutic interventional cardiac procedure in the training pathway, a fellow must meet the following criteria:

- Participate in procedural planning, including indications for the procedure and the selection of appropriate procedures or instruments.
- Perform critical technical manipulations of the case. (Regardless of how many manipulations are performed in any one 'case,' each case may count as only one procedure.)
- Be substantially involved in postprocedural management of the case.
- Be supervised by the faculty member responsible for the procedure. (Only one fellow can receive credit for each case even if others were present.)"

The examination covers the entire cognitive knowledge base of interventional cardiology. The specifics are listed in the examination blueprint published by ABIM (4).

The content areas covered and their relative proportions on the exam are as follows (4):

Case selection and management: 25%
Procedural techniques: 25%
Basic science: 15%
Pharmacology: 15%
Imaging: 15%
Miscellaneous: 5%

■ ELEMENTS OF THE TRAINING CURRICULUM

Cognitive Knowledge Base

Interventional cardiology is fundamentally a cognitive discipline. The mastery of the cognitive knowledge base detailed in the earlier section is closely tied to the ability to appropriately perform the technical aspects of the interventional cardiovascular procedures. For example, the fundamental understanding of the coronary anatomy and the three-dimensional relationship of coronary ostia in the sinuses of Valsalva are essential to appropriate catheter selection, procedural success, and avoidance of unnecessary procedural complications or delays (5).

The basic cognitive knowledge base expected of the cardiology trainee in the cardiac catheterization laboratory is based on their level of training. The most recently published update was published in 2008 as the ACC COCATS Task Force 3 statement on training in diagnostic and interventional cardiac catheterization (6). It details the cognitive knowledge base that cardiovascular medicine trainees should acquire in cardiac catheterization. It is organized into three levels of training.

The level 1 trainee, whose experience with cardiovascular procedures will be confined to critical care–level procedures, will not be trained to perform diagnostic or interventional cardiovascular procedures. This level of training, which should be achieved by all cardiovascular specialists, includes basic coronary anatomy and coronary artery physiology and interpretation of diagnostic coronary angiograms. In addition, the level I trainee should be able to understand and interpret complex cardiac hemodynamics in various cardiac conditions. The level 1 trainee should also understand the indications and contraindications for interventional cardiovascular procedures and be able to manage the various procedural complications from cardiac catheterization procedures. The level 1 trainee should also understand the basic principles of X-ray imaging and radiation safety and the indications for and complications of the drugs commonly used during invasive cardiovascular procedures.

Level 2 training prepares the trainee to perform diagnostic but not interventional cardiovascular procedures. Level 2 training includes further understanding of the basic operations of the hemodynamic recording equipment in the cardiac catheterization laboratory. In addition, the level 2 trainee should understand advanced invasive techniques of fractional flow and coronary flow reserve and understand the basics of peripheral vascular anatomy as it pertains to peripheral vascular disease and complications in the cardiac catheterization laboratory. The level 2 trainee should also have more advanced knowledge of the X-ray imaging system and the radiation physics and biology in order to both optimize image quality and minimize patient radiation exposure.

Level 3 training is a dedicated year of training to perform interventional cardiovascular procedures. In addition to mastering the cognitive knowledge base expected of the level 1 and level 2 trainee, the level 3 trainee should acquire the core cognitive knowledge and technical skill needed to perform balloon angioplasty, intracoronary stent placement, atherectomy techniques, intravascular ultrasound, transseptal catheterization, and measurement of fractional flow reserve. The level 3 trainee should also seek to gain as much knowledge as possible regarding the management of complications of interventional cardiovascular procedures including coronary perforation, no coronary reflow, coronary artery dissection, and stent thrombosis.

Technical Skills

The technical skill set required in interventional cardiology is derived from the cognitive knowledge base detailed in the previous section. The ACC COCATS Task Force 3 statement published in 2008 specifies a minimum procedural experience that is felt to be required to develop adequate technical skill. The level 3 requirements for the trainee in interventional cardiology include experience with greater than 550 cumulative invasive procedures including a minimum of 250 interventional procedures. The statement makes a point that more procedures is not always better and recommends a maximum of 600 interventional procedures, with 400 procedures considered optimal (5,6). The trainee clearly benefits from a diverse case selection, including experience with different vascular access sites, catheter designs and techniques, and the management of various complications.

The core procedural capabilities that should be offered in a contemporary comprehensive interventional cardiology training program for level 3 trainees are detailed in the 1999 ACC training statement on the structure of an optimal interventional cardiology training program and in the 2008 ACC COCATS Task Force 3 statement on training in diagnostic and interventional cardiology (5,6). These include the following techniques:

1. Conventional balloon angioplasty and percutaneous coronary stent placement

in various types of lesions including type A, B, C lesions in both native vessels and surgical bypass vessels. Experience with various techniques of bifurcation stenting, left main coronary artery stenting, and management of PCI-related complications.
2. Primary angioplasty for ST-elevation myocardial infarction.
3. Training in atherectomy techniques and the use of distal protection devices.
4. Intravascular ultrasound and measurement of fractional flow reserve.
5. Exposure to various types of mechanical circulatory support including the placement and management of intra-aortic balloon pumps, as well as more novel types of percutaneous mechanical circulatory support devices, if available.

The skill set and expertise of the interventional cardiology faculty and practice patterns at the training institution should include:

1. Cardiac balloon valvuloplasty
2. Endomyocardial biopsy in both native and transplanted hearts
3. Transcatheter closure of congenital defects with exposure to intracardiac and transesophageal echo imaging to guide percutaneous structural procedures
4. Transcatheter percutaneous valvular procedures with exposure to intracardiac and transesophageal echo imaging to assist with percutaneous structural procedures
5. Peripheral vascular angiography for both diagnostic and interventional indications
6. Alcohol septal ablation for hypertrophic obstructive cardiomyopathy

■ TRAINING ENVIRONMENT
Needs of the Trainee

In addition to the above cognitive knowledge base and procedural conduct experience, the interventional cardiology trainee benefits from a training environment that helps to prepare the trainee to practice interventional cardiology in today's dynamic practice environment. Modern interventional cardiology is only one of a number of techniques used to manage all types of heart disease including coronary artery disease, valvular disease, congenital disease, and primary myocardial/pericardial disease. Thus, the interventional training environment at a major academic medical center should achieve collaboration with other departments within cardiology, cardiothoracic surgery, and radiology that may be complementary in the education of the interventional cardiology trainee. In particular, a detailed understanding of the multiple cardiac imaging modalities is becoming increasingly important for the interventional cardiologist as the practice of percutaneous valve placement and structural heart disease expands, as well as for the potential future ability to noninvasively image the "vulnerable" coronary plaque. For example, the use of and the interpretation of intracardiac echo or transesophageal echo are now considered essential for percutaneous transeptal procedures and more novel percutaneous valve procedures. The use of and the interpretation of cardiovascular magnetic resonance (CMR) and computed tomography angiography are becoming standard in the preprocedural assessment of the complicated cardiovascular patient. Thus, complementary training in these imaging techniques will soon be an indispensable skill for the interventional cardiology trainee.

Faculty–Trainee Relationships

The interventional cardiology trainee benefits from a training environment where he or she is exposed to various skilled and experienced operators. The minimal faculty requirements have been outlined by both the ACGME and in the recent 2008 ACC COCATS Task Force statement on the training environment in diagnostic and interventional cardiology. The 2008 ACC COCATS Task Force 3 statement (5,6) states that an optimal program in interventional cardiology should have a minimum of three key faculty members, one of whom is program director, and each of whom maintains a minimum procedural volume of 150 annual diagnostic cases. To maximize the exposure for the trainee, it is important that institutions with adequate patient volume should include faculty with various skills in advanced interventional cardiovascular techniques such as septal ablation for hypertrophic obstructive cardiomyopathy, balloon valvuloplasty, percutaneous valve interventions, peripheral vascular interventions, and patent foramen ovale and atrial septal defect

closure. The number of faculty should be kept at a level to attain a key faculty (defined as those that devote at least 20 h/wk to the program)-to-trainee ratio of 0.5 trainees per faculty member (5). Having a large and/or diverse faculty provides the trainee with exposure to various procedural techniques, mentoring opportunities, and practice patterns.

Trainee Responsibilities

The trainee's participation in a particular procedure will vary depending on his or her experience level and the complexity of the procedure. As detailed in the 2008 ACC COCATS Task Force 3 statement (6), the trainee should have responsibility at every level of the procedure including the preprocedural evaluation of the patient, performance of the procedure itself under the direct supervision of a program faculty member, participation in the analysis of the angiographic and/or hemodynamic data obtained during the procedure, and involvement in the postprocedural management of the patient and any procedure-related complications.

1. Preprocedural evaluation: to review the patient's medical record and obtain a history and physical examination in order to assess appropriateness of the procedure and evaluate for specific risk factors of the procedure for the particular patient. In addition, the trainee should be able to obtain informed consent and address any patient concerns or alternatives to the procedure when appropriate.
2. Performance of the procedure under the direct supervision of a program faculty member: level 3 interventional cardiology trainees should assume progressive responsibility for the performance of interventional procedures as they acquire the appropriate skills and should be the primary operator on the majority of cases as dictated by their level of experience.
3. Participate in the analysis of the angiographic and/or hemodynamic data obtained during the procedure.
4. Involvement in the postprocedural management including completion of a postprocedural note and availability to respond to any adverse reactions or procedure-related complications.

In addition, under the direct supervision of the supervising faculty, the level 3 trainee has the responsibility to supervise advanced level 1 and level 2 trainees in the performance and mastery of diagnostic catheterization. The trainee also has a responsibility to participate in clinical research during the first 3 years of cardiology fellowship training or during the dedicated fourth year of interventional cardiology training. This may include participation in an ongoing clinical trial and/or institutional specific research in various facets of interventional cardiology.

■ TRAINING CONDUCT

Training in interventional cardiology may be divided into two domains, cognitive knowledge base training and procedure conduct training. Both domains are conducted concurrently and the training experiences are complementary.

Cognitive Training

Cognitive training includes the knowledge base underlying case selection, procedure conduct strategy assessment of outcome and management of complications. There is also an interaction with technical experiences as much of what might be considered technical skill is actually derived from cognitive knowledge.

Case Reviews

A training program needs a large case review experience. This is best conducted in conference at which the trainees and program faculty review selected cases to examine the case selection considerations, the procedure conduct strategy, and the procedure's short-term outcome. These reviews should be conducted in a spirit of open inquiry to examine the rationales behind the various decisions surrounding the procedure as well as alternative approaches including both case selection and procedure conduct strategy.

Such case reviews are necessarily focused on short-term outcomes and do not provide experience in long-term outcomes. However, training focused solely on short-term outcomes (how was the patient at the end of the procedure) is inadequate. As long-term outcome is a core underpinning of case selection, it is important that trainees be exposed whenever possible to long-term outcomes or interventional proce-

dures. Thus, interventional cardiology conferences should take pains to include presentation of long-term follow-up outcomes whenever they are available.

Morbidity and Mortality Review

Morbidity and mortality review is an important subset of case reviews. Often the most important lessons are learned from procedures that do not achieve optimal outcomes. Consequently, a training program should have a structured series of morbidity and mortality case reviews. These reviews should be comprehensive in that all complicated cases should be reviewed in a spirit of open inquiry in order that the entire group can derive lessons from the cases that will make them more sophisticated and successful operators.

Cognitive Seminars

Interventional cardiology has a large cognitive knowledge base that needs to be transmitted to trainees in a systematic manner. This includes, technical aspects of equipment—theory and operation, radiation safety, protection and biology, basic cardiovascular physiology and pharmacology, and the large clinical trial knowledge base. Review of this knowledge base is best accomplished through a structured series of seminars during which this knowledge base is presented and discussed. The topic selection for these seminars can be derived from multiple sources including the ABIM blueprint for the interventional cardiology certifying examination and professional society web sites.

Procedure Training

Direct hand-on procedure training is considered to be the core of the interventional cardiology training experience. It is important to keep in mind that the trainee's procedure-based experience is both technical and cognitive. It is also an important axiom that the trainee's experience requires more than just procedure execution experience.

Preprocedural Evaluation

Procedure-based training begins with the case selection—the decision that the case is appropriate for interventional treatment. It extends to planning the procedure strategy and the actual execution of the procedure. This includes device selection and plans for adjunctive therapy. This component of the trainee's experience is particularly important. If the trainee's experience is confined to scrubbing in as the procedure begins and assisting with procedure execution, a great deal of the procedure's educational value has been missed.

Procedure Conduct

During procedure execution, the trainee should personally perform (under the direct scrubbed supervision of the faculty trainer) as much of the procedure as his or her capabilities permit. The faculty trainer's responsibility is to coach the trainee in procedure execution. This places a responsibility on the trainer to be able to explain verbally how a procedure should be executed and how to solve technical problems. An important facet of this process is to review the procedure afterward to ensure that the trainee fully understood rationale and mechanisms for particular maneuvers and appropriately assessed the procedure's outcome. This postprocedure evaluation is particularly important in the event of a less than optimal outcome.

Postprocedure Management

The trainee should be actively involved in postprocedure management. This includes participation in management of the vascular access sites, assessing the patient's short-term clinical response to the procedure, participating in plans for postdischarge care and evaluation.

■ FACILITY OPERATING PRACTICES TO OPTIMIZE PATIENT SAFETY

Interventional cardiovascular procedure quality and safety, although, obviously, critically depends on physician operator knowledge and skill, is also strongly influenced by the facility environment in which the procedure is performed. The facility, both its physical equipment complement and its clinical staff, plays a vital role in providing the platform that supports the physician operator in conducting an interventional cardiovascular procedure.

Physical Environment

The physical environment includes the architectural design of the facility, its equipment complement, and its relationship to other hospital facilities needed to support interventional cardiovascular procedures.

Architectural Layout

The architectural layout of the procedure room and its support space are integral to effective operation of a cardiac catheterization laboratory. The procedure room must be of adequate size and its fixed equipment and utilities must be appropriately located. The control room should be a physically separate area isolated from radiation exposure with good audio communication to the procedure room. Some of these parameters, such as minimal procedure room size and the requirement for a separate control room, are now specified by many state department of health codes. As a general principal, a procedure room should have a minimum of 500 square feet of floor space (more if the room has biplane or other complex radiographic equipment). There should be a separate X-ray equipment room for the X-ray system's supporting electronics so that they do not occupy space in the procedure room. Particular attention should be paid to lighting control and design. The positioning of other equipment such as monitor booms, portable radiation shields, and operating lights also requires careful attention to detail. These should all be ceiling-mounted in order to minimize floor clutter and to simplify cleaning.

Equipment

The core of any interventional cardiovascular facility is its radiologic equipment. Currently available equipment from major manufacturers provides excellent radiologic images.

Relationship to Other Hospital Facilities

The procedure room's architectural relationship to other procedure rooms as well as support facilities in the cardiac catheterization suite and other hospital support services such as operating rooms and intensive care units are important architectural considerations. Appropriate consideration of these issues enables the design of a cardiac catheterization suite that functions smoothly and effectively, particularly when responding to emergency situations or moving critically ill patients from one facility to another.

Clinical Staff Capabilities and Training

The clinical staff of the laboratory facility (registered nurses (RN) and registered cardiovascular technicians (RCVT) qualified) are integral to the safe operation of the laboratory. They are integral partners of the physician staff. Their roles include providing patient assessments, monitoring patients during procedures, providing pharmacologic and respiratory treatment as necessary, and implementing responses to emergencies. Ideal staff RNs have prior critical care experience but can certainly develop the necessary knowledge and skills on the job with appropriate training and mentoring. The same is true for non-RN RCVT staff who, in general, have all the responsibilities for patient management and care other than to administer medications. It is axiomatic that the response to an emergency occurring during a procedure can only be as successful as the ability of the clinical staff's knowledge and skills allows.

Operating Protocols

Interventional cardiovascular procedures are complex processes that include many sequential steps and require numerous ancillary activities. Inadvertent omission of a step can be catastrophic (a classic example is failure to administer anticoagulation before beginning the procedure). In many respects, the process of performing an interventional cardiovascular procedure has much in common with the process of flying an airplane. The Federal Aviation Administration has learned over many years of experience that it is important to systematize the airplane flight procedures. This has led to rigidly prescribed procedures including checklists that are completed prior to takeoffs and landings. The exemplary safety record of United States commercial aviation testifies to the efficacy of these practices, particularly when compared to United States highway safety record. The safety of interventional cardiovascular procedures can be enhanced substantially if the cardiac catheterization laboratory facility puts in place procedures and protocols that minimize the risk of medical errors. These include the standard medical error reduction tactics such as "timeouts" and site of surgery verification. They extend to procedure conduct protocols that specify sequential steps to be followed during a procedure. In addition, they include suite organizational protocols intended to minimize the risk of drug identification and dosing errors, device selection errors, equipment calibration, and maintenance protocols and inventory monitoring. Successful achievement of systematic practice in each of these areas is an important underpinning of procedural safety.

References

1. Gruentzig AR, Senning A, Siegenthaler WE. Non-operative dilatation of coronary-artery stenosis: percutaneous transluminal coronary angioplasty. *N Engl J Med.* 1979;301:61–68.

2. Accreditation Council of Graduate Medical Education. *ACGME program requirements for graduate medical education in interventional cardiology.* http://www.acgme.org/acWebsite/downloads/RRC_progReq/152pr707_ims.pdf. Approved September 28, 2004. Revised July 1, 2009. Accessed July 7, 2010.

3. American Board of Internal Medicine. *Interventional cardiology policies.* http://www.abim.org/certification/ policies/imss/icard.aspx. Accessed July 7, 2010.

4. American Board of Internal Medicine. *Interventional cardiology: certification examination blueprint.* http://www.abim.org/pdf/blueprint/icard_cert.pdf. Accessed July 7, 2010.

5. Hirshfeld JW Jr, Banas JS Jr, Brundage BH, et al. American College of Cardiology training statement on recommendations for the structure of an optimal adult interventional cardiology training program: a report of the American College of Cardiology Task Force on clinical expert consensus documents. *J Am Coll Cardiol.* 1999; 34:2141–2147.

6. Jacobs AK, Babb JD, Hirshfeld JW Jr, Holmes DR Jr. Task Force 3: training in diagnostic and interventional cardiac catheterization endorsed by the Society for Cardiovascular Angiography and Interventions. *J Am Coll Cardiol.* 2008;51:355–361.

5

When Should a Procedure Not Be Performed?

P. MICHAEL GROSSMAN AND MAURO MOSCUCCI

■ RISK VERSUS BENEFIT OF INVASIVE CARDIOVASCULAR PROCEDURES

There is often perceived pressure to pursue an aggressive treatment strategy for severe cardiovascular disease. However, the decision to perform an invasive cardiovascular procedure is based upon a careful balance of the risk of the procedure weighed against the anticipated benefit to the patient. Before proceeding, the details of the planned procedure and its anticipated risks must be discussed with the patient and family. In addition to the specific procedure that is planned, the discussion should include a prediction of the benefits that are hoped for, the attendant risks and their probabilities, and how the risks and benefits compare with any potential alternative treatment strategies.

The risks and potential complications of a percutaneous cardiovascular procedure are detailed in this book. It is imperative that all individuals performing these procedures be familiar with the potential complications of the procedures that they perform. Furthermore, prompt recognition of complications, immediate corrective treatment, or referral for corrective treatment, where appropriate, is imperative. If a significant major complication does occur, the patient and family should be informed as soon as the procedure has been completed. The discussion should not only describe the nature of the complication but should indicate what long-term consequences are expected, and outline the corrective plan of action. These discussions should be frank but not place blame. The catheterizing physician should also visit the patient daily during the hospitalization after the complication, in order to offer input to the patient's care, and to avoid the feeling of abandonment on the part of the physician and the family. Communication, both before the procedure and after a complication has occurred, is the responsibility of the interventional physician and will limit the desire for retribution (i.e., a malpractice suit).

■ CONTRAINDICATIONS TO CARDIOVASCULAR PROCEDURES

In general, there is no absolute contraindication to the performance of a cardiovascular procedure. However, there are several correctable conditions that can increase the risk of specific complications, and which therefore represent relative contraindications to the performance of elective or semi-elective procedures. In addition, a relative contraindication in an emergency setting might become a strong contraindication in an elective setting. For example, uncontrolled hypertension can increase the risk of myocardial ischemia and heart failure during coronary angiography, and the risk of bleeding during vascular access or following arterial sheaths removal. Thus, uncontrolled hypertension is an indication to postpone the procedure until adequate blood pressure control has been achieved. Likewise, while severe renal dysfunction is not necessarily a contraindication to the performance of a procedure, worsening renal function either unexplained or following contrast administration can

TABLE 5-1	Relative Contraindications to Cardiac Catheterization and Angiography
Condition	**Increased Risk**
Hyperkalemia, hypokalemia, or digitalis toxicity	Arrhythmias
Uncontrolled hypertension	Bleeding, hemorrhagic stroke following anticoagulation, heart failure and myocardial ischemia during angiography
Febrile illness	Infection
Ongoing anticoagulation with warfarin (INR > 1.5 commonly used as a cutoff)	Bleeding
Severe thrombocytopenia. The general consensus is that a platelet count of 40,000/mL to 50,000/mL is sufficient to perform major invasive procedures with safety, in the absence of associated coagulation abnormalities (1)	Bleeding
History of severe allergy to contrast media	Life-threatening anaphylactoid reactions
Decompensated heart failure	Pulmonary edema following contrast administration. Inability to lay flat during the procedure
Severe renal insufficiency and/or anuria, unless dialysis is planned to remove fluid and as renal replacement therapy	Volume overload and pulmonary edema, nephropathy requiring dialysis
Worsening renal function: unexplained or following radiocontrast administration	Acute renal failure requiring dialysis
Active bleeding including gastrointestinal bleeding	Major bleeding secondary to administration of antiplatelets and antithrombotic agents

(Adapted and expanded from Donald S. Baim. *Cardiac Catheterization, Angiography, and Intervention.* 7th ed. Philadelphia, PA: Lippincott Williams & Wilkins; 2006:7.)

be considered a strong contraindication to an elective or semi-elective procedure requiring contrast administration. Table 5-1 includes a list of relative contraindications and corresponding complications. The risk/benefit ratio of the procedure, the clinical context, and the urgency or emergency of the procedure will be additional factors that must be included in the equation when deciding whether to postpone or to perform the procedure. Furthermore, what might be a relative contraindication to a therapeutic procedure requiring anticoagulation and resulting in implantation of a device might not be an issue in the setting of a purely diagnostic procedure.

■ FUTILE CARDIOVASCULAR INTERVENTIONS

Medical futility is described as proposed therapy that should not be performed because available data have shown that it will not improve the patient's medical condition. Medical futility remains ethically controversial for several reasons. Some health care providers claim that a treatment is futile without knowing the relevant outcome data. There is, unfortunately, no consensus as to the statistical threshold for a treatment to be considered futile. Many medical ethicists advise against the term "Futile care," especially with patients and families. Care is never futile, but some medical procedures, for example, invasive cardiovascular procedures, sometimes are (2,3).

The term "futile interventions" refers to interventions that are unlikely to produce any significant benefit for the patient. Two kinds of medical futilities are often distinguished: *quantitative futility*, where the likelihood that an intervention will benefit the patient is exceedingly poor (e.g., less than 1 in 20 or more conservatively, less than 1 in 100, chance of providing benefit), and *qualitative futility*, where the quality of benefit an intervention will produce is exceedingly poor (2).

The goal of medicine is to help the sick. The interventionist is not obliged to offer procedures that do not benefit a patient. Futile cardiovascular interventions are ill advised because they may increase a patient's pain and discomfort in the final days and weeks of life, give false hope to patients and their families, and because they can expend finite medical resources (4).

Who decides when a cardiovascular intervention is futile? The ethical authority to render futility judgments rests with the medical profession as a whole, not with individual physicians at the bedside. Thus, futility determinations in specific cases should conform to more general professional standards of care. The interventionist, therefore, must be aware of those professional standards, and effectively apply and communicate those in difficult clinical situations.

■ CARDIOVASCULAR INTERVENTIONS TO BE AVOIDED

Of course, the only guaranteed means to avoid the complication of a procedure is to not perform that procedure. The catheterization procedure must be performed for appropriate indications, where the risk/benefit balance is in favor of invasive treatment. The American College of Cardiology and American Heart Association have developed guidelines for the use of invasive, catheter-based procedures for the management of cardiovascular disease (5–8). These guidelines are updated frequently, as technology and scientific advancements warrant. These guidelines are intended to complement, not replace sound medical judgment and knowledge. The guidelines provide a foundation of knowledge and guidance, which in clinical practice should give the performing physician pause when considering the appropriateness of a catheter-based procedure. According to the guidelines, "Class III" indications are conditions for which there is evidence and/or general agreement that a procedure/treatment is not useful/effective and in some cases may be harmful.

The following are clinical conditions in which an invasive approach to the management of cardiovascular disease is not indicated (5–8).

Asymptomatic or Mildly Symptomatic (CCS I or II Angina) Patients

Percutaneous coronary intervention (PCI) is not recommended when these clinical conditions are present:

- Only a small area of viable myocardium at risk
- No objective evidence of ischemia
- Lesions that have a low likelihood of successful dilatation
- Mild symptoms that are unlikely to be due to myocardial ischemia
- Factors associated with increased risk of morbidity or mortality
- Insignificant disease (less than 50% coronary stenosis)

Patients With More Severe Angina Symptoms (CCS Class III Angina)

PCI is not recommended when these clinical conditions are present:

- CCS class III angina with single- or multivessel coronary artery disease (CAD), no evidence of myocardial injury or ischemia on objective testing, and no trial of medical therapy, or who have one of the following:
- Only a small area of myocardium at risk
- All lesions or the culprit lesion to be dilated with morphology that conveys a low likelihood of success
- A high risk of procedure-related morbidity or mortality
- Insignificant disease (less than 50% coronary stenosis)

Patients With Unstable Angina or Non-ST Segment Myocardial Infarction

PCI (or coronary artery bypass grafting [CABG]) is not recommended when these clinical conditions are present:

- One- or two-vessel CAD without significant proximal left anterior descending CAD with no current symptoms or symptoms that are unlikely to be due to myocardial ischemia and who have no ischemia on noninvasive testing
- In the absence of high-risk features associated with unstable angina/non-ST segment myocardial infarction (UA/NSTEMI), PCI is not recommended for patients with UA/NSTEMI who have single- or multivessel CAD and no

trial of medical therapy, or who have one or more of the following:

- Only a small area of myocardium at risk
- All lesions or the culprit lesion to be dilated with morphology that conveys a low likelihood of success
- A high risk of procedure-related morbidity or mortality
- Insignificant disease (less than 50% coronary stenosis)
- Significant left main CAD and candidacy for CABG
- A PCI strategy in stable patients with persistently occluded infarct-related coronary arteries after STEMI/NSTEMI is not indicated

Patients With ST Segment Myocardial Infarction

PCI is not recommended when these clinical conditions are present:

- Elective PCI should not be performed in a non–infarct-related artery at the time of primary PCI of the infarct-related artery in patients without hemodynamic compromise.
- Primary PCI should not be performed in asymptomatic patients more than 12 hours after the onset of STEMI who are hemodynamically and electrically stable.
- A planned reperfusion strategy using full-dose fibrinolytic therapy followed by immediate PCI may be harmful.
- A strategy of coronary angiography with intent to perform PCI (or emergency CABG) is not recommended in patients who have received fibrinolytic therapy if further invasive management is contraindicated or the patient or designee does not wish further invasive care.
- PCI of a totally occluded infarct artery greater than 24 hours after STEMI is not recommended in asymptomatic patients with one- or two-vessel disease if they are hemodynamically and electrically stable and do not have the evidence of severe ischemia.

Patients With a History of Coronary Artery Bypass Surgery (CABG)

PCI is not recommended in patients with prior CABG for chronic total vein graft occlusions.

- PCI is not recommended in patients who have multiple target lesions with prior CABG and

who have multivessel disease, failure of multiple saphenous vein grafts (SVGs), and impaired LV function unless repeat CABG poses excessive risk due to severe comorbid conditions.

Patients With Claudication

Endovascular treatment is not indicated:

- If there is no significant pressure gradient across a stenosis despite flow augmentation with vasodilators (8)
- Primary stent placement is not recommended in the femoral, popliteal, or tibial arteries (8)
- Endovascular intervention is not indicated as prophylactic therapy in an asymptomatic patient with lower extremity PAD (8)

Patients With Chronic Limb Ischemia (CLI)

Percutaneous (or surgical) revascularization is not indicated in patients with severe decrements in limb perfusion (e.g., ankle-brachial index (ABI) less than 0.4) in the absence of clinical symptoms of CLI (8).

Note

It is important to underscore that these class III indications provide a framework for guidance to practicing physicians, and that as technology evolves and more data become available through clinical trials and registries analysis, it is likely that some of those indications might change.

■ WHEN TO AVOID PROCEDURES IN HIGH-RISK PATIENTS

The decision to perform an invasive cardiovascular procedure in a high-risk patient is challenging not only because of the technical issues and higher likelihood of morbidity or mortality, but because there is often little medical evidence to guide the practitioner in decision making with the patient and family. Randomized trials comparing management strategies in high-risk patient populations are, therefore, exceedingly valuable.

In 2009, the Percutaneous Coronary Intervention versus Coronary-Artery Bypass Grafting for Severe Coronary Artery Disease (SYNTAX) Trial was published (9). This was the largest randomized trial to compare PCI with drug-eluting

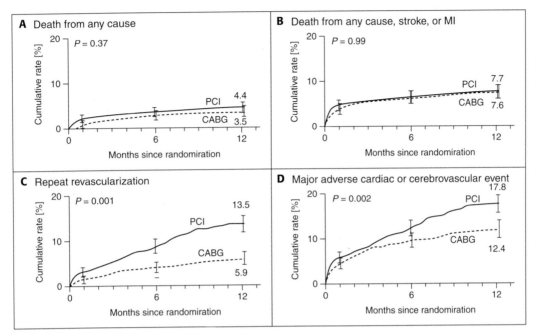

FIGURE 5-1. Rates of outcomes among the study patients, according to treatment group. Kaplan–Meier curves are shown for the percutaneous coronary intervention (PCI) group and the coronary artery bypass grafting (CABG) group for death from any cause (**A**); death, stroke, or myocardial infarction (MI) (**B**); repeat revascularization (**C**); and the composite primary end point of major adverse cardiac or cerebrovascular events (**D**). The two groups had similar rates of death from any cause (relative risk with PCI vs. CABG, 1.24; 95% confidence interval [CI], 0.78 to 1.98) and rates of death from any cause, stroke, or MI (relative risk with PCI vs. CABG, 1.00; 95% CI, 0.72 to 1.38). In contrast, the rate of repeat revascularization was significantly increased with PCI (relative risk, 2.29; 95% CI, 1.67 to 3.14), as was the overall rate of major adverse cardiac or cerebrovascular events (relative risk, 1.44; 95% CI, 1.15 to 1.81). The "I" bars indicate 1.5 SE. Relative risks were calculated from the binary rates. *P*-values were calculated with the use of the chi-square test (Reprinted from Serruys PW, Morice MC, Kappetein AP, et al. Percutaneous coronary intervention versus coronary-artery bypass grafting for severe coronary artery disease. *N Engl J Med.* 2009;360:961–972, with permission. © 2009 Massachusetts Medical Society.)

stents to CABG in patients with left main or three-vessel CAD. Rates of major adverse cardiac or cerebrovascular events at 12 months were significantly higher in the PCI group (17.8% vs. 12.4% for CABG; *P* = 0.002), in large part because of an increased rate of repeat revascularization (13.5% vs. 5.9%; *P* < 0.001); as a result, the criterion for noninferiority was not met. At 12 months, the rates of death and myocardial infarction were similar between the two groups; stroke was significantly more likely to occur with CABG (2.2% vs. 0.6% with PCI; *P* = 0.003). While overall, CABG was superior to PCI with DES based upon lower rates of the combined end point of major adverse cardiac or cerebrovascular events at 1 year (Fig. 5-1) (9).

In the SYNTAX Trial, a SYNTAX score was calculated; the SYNTAX score reflects a compre-

hensive anatomic assessment, with higher scores indicating more complex coronary disease; a low score was defined as ≤22, an intermediate score as 23 to 32, and a high score as ≥33 (the SYNTAX score calculator is available online at no charge at www.syntaxscore.com). In patients with a high SYNTAX score, not only was the overall rate of major adverse cardiac or cerebrovascular events significantly increased, but also the rate of the composite components of death, stroke, and myocardial infarction was slightly raised (11.9% vs. 7.6% in the CABG group; *P* = 0.08) (Fig. 5-2) (9). This finding suggests that a percutaneous approach should be avoided in patients with high SYNTAX scores. Similar findings were reported in three-vessel disease patients in the older ARTS II registry (10) and in more contemporary registries of patients with left main CAD (11).

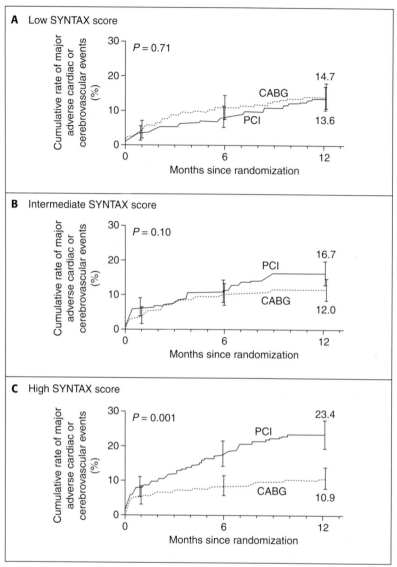

FIGURE 5-2. Rates of major adverse cardiac or cerebrovascular events among the study patients, according to treatment group and SYNTAX score category. Kaplan–Meier curves are shown for the percutaneous coronary intervention (PCI) group and the coronary artery bypass grafting (CABG) group for major adverse cardiac or cerebrovascular events at 12 months. The 12-month event rates were similar between the two treatment groups for patients with low SYNTAX scores (0 to 22) (**A**) or intermediate SYNTAX scores (23 to 32) (**B**). Among patients with high SYNTAX scores (≥33, indicating the most complex disease) (**C**) those in the PCI group had a significantly higher event rate at 12 months than those in the CABG group. SYNTAX scores were calculated at the core laboratory. The "I" bars indicate 1.5 SE. P-values were calculated with the use of the chi-square test (Reprinted from Serruys PW, Morice MC, Kappetein AP, et al. Percutaneous coronary intervention versus coronary-artery bypass grafting for severe coronary artery disease. *N Engl J Med.* 2009;360:961–972, with permission. © 2009 Massachusetts Medical Society.)

Although the purpose of training and reviewing texts such as this is to learn from the experience and mistakes of others, there is no substitute for operator experience when performing technically challenging procedures. Furthermore, the expertise and training of catheterization laboratory personnel, equipment, and availability of support (e.g., cardiovascular surgery backup on site) all contribute to an environment where potentially catastrophic complications may be avoided altogether or managed efficiently and effectively. In fact, outcomes related to percutaneous coronary interventions have been demonstrated to be superior at higher volume medical centers (12,17). Numerous studies have demonstrated an inverse relationship between physician operator volume and major adverse cardiac events (13–17). Furthermore, high-volume operators tend to have better outcomes than low-volume operators in both low- and high-risk patients (14).

In general, the guidelines do not support low-volume operators perform elective PCI at low-volume institutions (5), nor for elective PCI to be performed at institutions without on-site cardiac surgery. Yet, as new data are becoming available from centers that perform PCI without cardiac surgery on site, and as technology continues to evolve, it is possible that we will see a change in the guidelines surrounding operator volume and low-volume centers. However, the concept of "practice makes it perfect" and of the related "learning curve" will likely continue to be a mainstay, particularly with high-risk complex procedures or novel procedures.

■ CONCLUSIONS

The decision to perform an invasive cardiovascular intervention should be based upon the risk weighed against the perceived benefit. It is the responsibility of the interventionist to be aware of the appropriate indications for a procedure, to fully assess the clinical situation, to critically assess the competence and limitations of the medical team asked to perform the intervention, and to communicate the potential risks, benefits, and alternatives to the patient and family. Furthermore, the most successful invasive proceduralists learn from their own experiences and those of others, are able to avoid complications, and possess the grace under pressure to overcome difficulties.

References

1. Schiffer A, Anderson KC, Bennett CL, et al. Platelet transfusion for patients with cancer: clinical practice guidelines of the American Society of Clinical Oncology. *J Clin Oncol.* 2001;19:1519–1538.
2. Schneiderman LJ, Jecker NS, Jonsen AR. Medical futility: its meaning and ethical implications. *Ann Intern Med.* 1990;112:949–954.
3. Bernat JL. Medical futility: definition, determination, and disputes in critical care. *Neurocrit Care.* 2005;2:198–205.
4. Schneiderman LJ, Jecker NS, Jonsen AR. Medical futility: response to critiques. *Ann Intern Med.* 1996;125:669–674.
5. Smith SC Jr, Feldman TE, Hirshfeld JW Jr, et al. ACC/AHA/SCAI 2005 Guideline Update for Percutaneous Coronary Intervention—Summary Article: A Report of the American College of Cardiology/American Heart Association Task Force on Practice Guidelines (ACC/AHA/SCAI Writing Committee to Update the 2001 Guidelines for Percutaneous Coronary Intervention). *J Am Coll Cardiol.* 2006;47:216–235.
6. King SB III, Smith SC Jr, Hirshfeld JW Jr, et al. 2007 Focused Update of the ACC/AHA/SCAI 2005 Guideline Update for Percutaneous Coronary Intervention: a report of the American College of Cardiology/American Heart Association Task Force on Practice Guidelines: 2007 Writing Group to Review New Evidence and Update the ACC/AHA/SCAI 2005 Guideline Update for Percutaneous Coronary Intervention, Writing on Behalf of the 2005 Writing Committee. *Circulation.* 2008;117:261–295.
7. Kushner FG, Hand M, Smith SC Jr, et al. 2009 focused updates: ACC/AHA guidelines for the management of patients with ST-elevation myocardial infarction (updating the 2004 guideline and 2007 focused update) and ACC/AHA/SCAI guidelines on percutaneous coronary intervention (updating the 2005 guideline and 2007 focused update): a report of the American College of Cardiology Foundation/American Heart Association Task Force on Practice Guidelines. *J Am Coll Cardiol.* 2009;54:2205–2241.
8. Hirsch AT, Haskal ZJ, Hertzer NR, et al. ACC/AHA 2005 guidelines for the management of patients with peripheral arterial disease (lower extremity, renal, mesenteric, and abdominal aortic): executive summary a collaborative report from the American Association for Vascular Surgery/Society for Vascular Surgery, Society for Cardiovascular Angiography and Interventions, Society for Vascular Medicine and Biology, Society of Interventional Radiology, and the ACC/AHA Task Force on Practice Guidelines (Writing Committee to Develop Guidelines for the Management of Patients With Peripheral Arterial Disease) endorsed by the American Association of Cardiovascular and Pulmonary Rehabilitation;

National Heart, Lung, and Blood Institute; Society for Vascular Nursing; TransAtlantic Inter-Society Consensus; and Vascular Disease Foundation. *J Am Coll Cardiol.* 2006;47:1239–1312.

9. Serruys PW, Morice MC, Kappetein AP, et al. Percutaneous coronary intervention versus coronary-artery bypass grafting for severe coronary artery disease. *N Engl J Med.* 2009;360:961–972.

10. Valgimigli M, Serruys PW, Tsuchida K, et al. Cyphering the complexity of coronary artery disease using the syntax score to predict clinical outcome in patients with three-vessel lumen obstruction undergoing percutaneous coronary intervention. *Am J Cardiol.* 2007;99:1072–1081.

11. Capodanno D, Capranzano P, Di Salvo ME, et al. Usefulness of SYNTAX score to select patients with left main coronary artery disease to be treated with coronary artery bypass graft. *JACC Cardiovasc Interv.* 2009;2:731–738.

12. Brown DL. Analysis of the institutional volume-outcome relations for balloon angioplasty and stenting in the stent era in California. *Am Heart J.* 2003;146:1071–1076.

13. Hannan EL, Racz M, Ryan TJ, et al. Coronary angioplasty volume-outcome relationships for hospitals and cardiologists. *JAMA.* 1997;277:892–898.

14. Moscucci M, Share D, Smith D, et al. Relationship between operator volume and adverse outcome in contemporary percutaneous coronary intervention practice: an analysis of a quality-controlled multi-center percutaneous coronary intervention clinical database. *J Am Coll Cardiol.* 2005;46:625–632.

15. Ellis SG, Weintraub W, Holmes D, et al. Relation of operator volume and experience to procedural outcome of percutaneous coronary revascularization at hospitals with high interventional volumes. *Circulation.* 1997;95:2479–2484.

16. Shook TL, Sun GW, Burstein S, et al. Comparison of percutaneous transluminal coronary angioplasty outcome and hospital costs for low-volume and high-volume operators. *Am J Cardiol.* 1996;77:331–336.

17. Hannan EL, Wu C, Walford G, et al. Volume-outcome relationships for percutaneous coronary interventions in the stent era. *Circulation.* 2005;112(8):1171–1179.

6 Adjunctive Pharmacology

YURI B. PRIDE, MAURO MOSCUCCI, AND C. MICHAEL GIBSON

Technologic advancements in percutaneous coronary intervention (PCI) have been mirrored closely by the development of pharmacologic agents aimed at maintaining both short- and long-term vessel and intracoronary stent patency. Further advancements in the inhibition of both platelet and coagulation activation have decreased the incidence of ischemic outcomes among patients undergoing PCI but have come at the cost of higher rates of hemorrhagic events, which may independently portend a worse prognosis. As such, the current era of pharmacologic agents used prior to and during coronary intervention must balance the potential benefit of decreasing ischemic outcomes with the risk of bleeding events.

In this chapter, we will review the available antiplatelet and antithrombotic agents used in the management of patients undergoing PCI, including a brief review of the clinically relevant pharmacologic properties of the drugs as well as the evidence supporting their clinical application.

■ ANTIPLATELET AGENTS

Aspirin

Acetylated salicylic acid, or aspirin, is the cornerstone of antiplatelet therapy among patients undergoing PCI for elective indications and for those with acute coronary syndrome (ACS)(1). Aspirin exerts its antiplatelet activity via irreversible inhibition of cyclooxygenase, which catalyzes the production of thromboxane, a potent vasoconstrictor that also enhances platelet aggregation within platelets and the production of prostacyclin, a vasodilator and inhibitor of platelet activation, in endothelial cells (2).

Because endothelial cells have nuclei, they have the ability to produce more active cyclooxygenase. This, coupled with the short serum half-life of aspirin, sways the overall activity of aspirin toward its antiplatelet effect.

Aspirin first demonstrated efficacy in the management of patients with acute myocardial infarction (MI) in the ISIS-2 trial, in which the use of 160 mg of aspirin daily for 1 month led to a 2.4% absolute reduction in cardiovascular death (1). As aspirin has become the standard of care among patients with ACS, its role in the management of patients undergoing PCI is ubiquitous, and it has never been, nor will it likely ever be, studied in a randomized trial.

Current Guidelines for the Use of Aspirin

The American College of Cardiology (ACC)/American Heart Association (AHA) and European Society of Cardiology (ESC) guidelines for the management of patients with STEMI (3–6) and NSTEMI (7,8) recommend the administration of aspirin (162 to 325 mg) as soon as possible among patients presenting with symptoms suggestive of ACS (Table 6-1). Among patients undergoing PCI for stable coronary disease, the ACC/AHA/Society for Coronary Angiography and Intervention (SCAI) and ESC guidelines (5,9–11) recommend the administration of aspirin (300 to 325 mg among aspirin-naïve patients and 75 to 325 mg among aspirin-experienced patients) at least 2 hours prior to PCI and preferably 24 hours prior.

■ ADP-RECEPTOR ANTAGONISTS

Ticlopidine, clopidogrel, and prasugrel are the three commercially available ADP-receptor

TABLE 6-1	Guideline Recommendations for the Administration of Aspirin

Clinical Presentation	ACC/AHA or ACC/AHA/SCAI	ESC
STEMI undergoing primary PCI	Aspirin should be administered to STEMI patients as soon as possible after hospital presentation and continued indefinitely in patients not known to be intolerant of that medication.	Aspirin should be given to all patients with STEMI as soon as possible after the diagnosis is deemed probable.
NSTEACS undergoing an early invasive strategy	Aspirin should be administered to NSTEACS patients as soon as possible after hospital presentation and continued indefinitely in patients not known to be intolerant of that medication.	Aspirin is recommended for all patients presenting with NSTEACS without contraindication.
Elective PCI	Patients already taking daily chronic aspirin therapy should take 75–325 mg of aspirin before the PCI procedure is performed. Patients not already taking daily chronic aspirin therapy should be given 300–325 mg of aspirin at least 2 h and preferably 24 h before the PCI procedure is performed.	Aspirin should be given to all patients undergoing elective PCI.

ACC, American College of Cardiology; AHA, American Heart Association; ESC, European Society of Cardiology; NSTEACS, non-ST-segment elevation acute coronary syndrome; PCI, percutaneous coronary intervention; SCAI, Society for Coronary Angiography and Intervention; STEMI, ST-segment elevation myocardial infarction.
(Adapted from the ACC/AHA, ACC/AHA/SCAI, and ESC guidelines for the management of STEMI, NSTEACS, and elective PCI (3–11).)

antagonists (12,13). They are thienopyridine derivatives and act as irreversible inhibitors of the P2Y12 receptor (14). They differ not in their mechanism of action, but most significantly in their metabolism and side-effect profile. More novel non-thienopyridine ADP-receptor antagonists have been developed and studied in large-scale clinical trials but are not currently approved for use (15).

Ticlopidine

Ticlopidine was the first available ADP-receptor antagonist, and it greatly altered the landscape of pharmacologic management of patients undergoing coronary stent implantation (16). Although coronary stents improved the incidence of in-stent restenosis and abrupt vessel closure (17,18), they were initially hampered by higher-than-acceptable rates of acute and subacute stent thrombosis. Therapeutic anticoagulation with unfractionated heparin (UFH) bridged to oral vitamin K antagonists was therefore used. Unfortunately, this anticoagulation strategy was

associated with high rates of adverse hemorrhagic outcomes and increased length of stay among patients undergoing PCI with stent implantation.

The introduction of ticlopidine, which not only reduced bleeding complications but also significantly reduced the incidence of subacute stent thrombosis and shortened hospital stay substantially (19–21), obviated the need for therapeutic anticoagulation following stent implantation. A loading dose of 500 mg is generally given, followed by 250 mg twice daily. In the pivotal trial comparing aspirin in combination with UFH bridged to phenprocoumon (a vitamin K antagonist derivative of coumarin) with a goal international normalized ratio (INR) of 3.5 to 4.5 or ticlopidine 250 mg twice daily in the management of patients undergoing stent implantation for failed balloon angioplasty, ticlopidine was associated with a 75% reduction in the composite of death, MI, or target vessel revascularization (TVR) and substantial reductions in stent thrombosis (20). Moreover, there was a marked reduction in hemorrhagic events, even though with a relatively high target INR by current standards.

A larger study of patients undergoing routine stent implantation demonstrated a significant reduction in the incidence of the composite of death, TVR, angiographic evidence of thrombosis or recurrent MI favoring the combination of aspirin and ticlopidine over aspirin and warfarin with a target INR of 2.0 to 2.5 (21). With this lower target INR, however, there was no significant difference in the incidence of hemorrhagic events.

Ticlopidine, however, is associated with a not insignificant incidence of thrombotic thrombocytopenic purpura (TTP), and it was soon essentially replaced by clopidogrel (22).

Clopidogrel

Clopidogrel, in addition to having the ease of once-daily dosing, was not associated with a high incidence of TTP, and was found to be equivalent to ticlopidine in terms of a reduction in ischemic outcomes following stent implantation (23). Clopidogrel has therefore dominated the interventional landscape since its introduction, and it has been associated with a reduction in ischemic outcomes among patients undergoing stent implantation for both stable CAD as well as following ACS (24).

Clopidogrel is a prodrug that requires metabolism via the cytochrome P450 system to its active metabolite (25). Although clopidogrel has also been associated with TTP, the incidence is much lower (26). Clopidogrel has been evaluated in studies across the spectrum of ACS and among patients undergoing PCI for stable coronary artery disease. A loading dose of 300 mg or 600 mg is usually administered given its need for metabolism to its active form. Administration of such a loading dose prior to PCI has been associated with improved outcomes. In a post hoc analysis of the Clopidogrel for the Reduction of Events During Observation (CREDO) study, the administration of a loading dose of 300 mg of clopidogrel prior to PCI was associated with improved outcomes as long as it was administered at least 15 hours prior to intervention (27). Among patients with ACS who require urgent intervention, this is frequently not practical, and doses as high as 600 mg may provide more rapid platelet inhibition in this subset of patients (28).

Prasugrel

Prasugrel is the most recent addition to the thienopyridine family of drugs and has been shown to provide more rapid, sustained, and greater platelet inhibition than clopidogrel (Fig. 6-1) (29). Prasugrel, which was approved for use in the United States in 2009, has demonstrated efficacy among patients with ACS undergoing PCI (30). Although both clopidogrel and prasugrel are prodrugs that require metabolism to their active forms, clopidogrel has a highly variable antiplatelet response because of its metabolism via the cytochrome P450 system. Prasugrel metabolism does not include a "dead-end pathway" and it leads to more rapid, consistent, and effective platelet inhibition than clopidogrel (31,32). Prasugrel has not been evaluated in the setting of PCI for stable CAD.

In patients with ACS undergoing PCI, prasugrel has been shown to reduce adverse cardiovascular events (a composite of cardiovascular death, nonfatal MI, or nonfatal stroke) at the cost of a modest increase in hemorrhagic events (30). In a post hoc analysis, this benefit was not seen among patients with a history of stroke or transient ischemic attack, those who weighed less than 60 kg, and those aged 75 years or older. Therefore, prasugrel is currently not recommended for patients older than 75 years and for patients weighing less than 60 kg.

Ticagrelor

Ticagrelor is a non-thienopyridine, oral, reversible direct-acting inhibitor of the P2Y12 receptor (33). Like prasugrel, it provides faster, greater, and more consistent P2Y12 inhibition than clopidogrel. However, because ticagrelor is a reversible inhibitor, its antiplatelet effect dissipates more rapidly than the thienopyridines, which are irreversible inhibitors. Ticagrelor has been studied in a large clinical trial that enrolled patients presenting with high-risk ACS, the Study of Platelet Inhibition and Patient Outcomes (PLATO), in which more than 18,000 patients were randomized to ticagrelor or clopidogrel (34). Ticagrelor was administered as a 180-mg loading dose, followed by 90 mg twice daily thereafter. At 12 months, ticagrelor led to a significant 16% reduction in the composite of death from vascular causes, MI, or stroke (9.8%

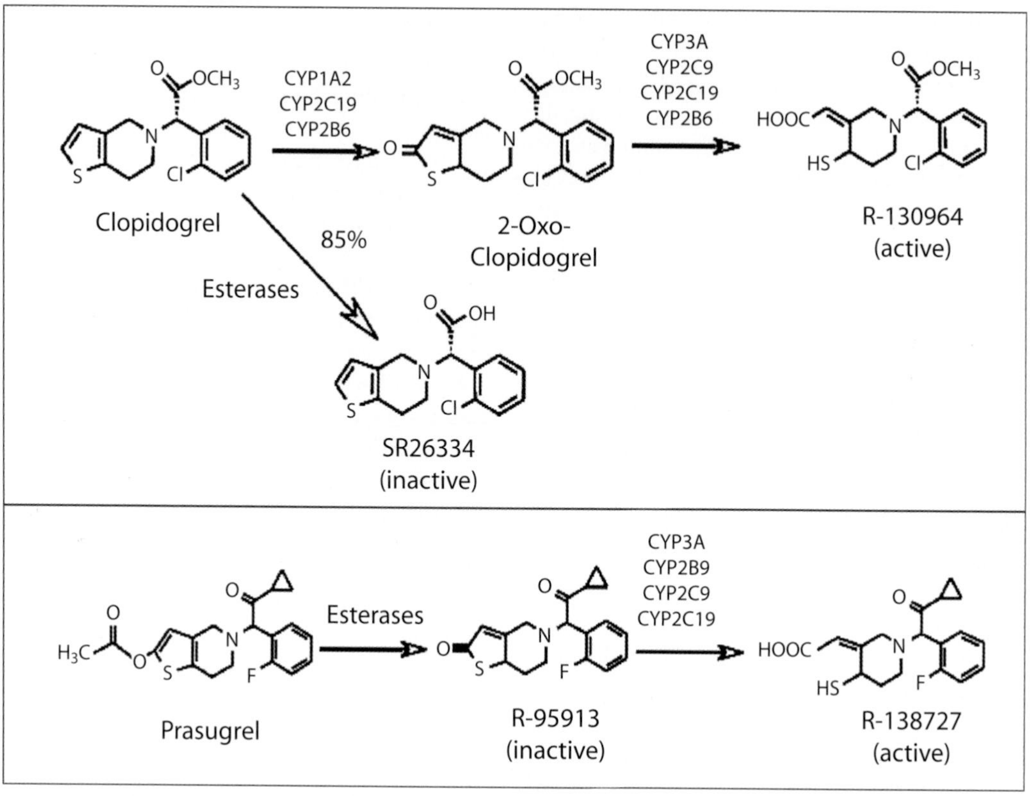

FIGURE 6-1. Metabolic pathways of clopidogrel and prasugrel. Both clopidogrel and prasugrel require activation to an active metabolite. Although the metabolic pathway of clopidogrel includes a "dead-end" pathway toward an inactive metabolite, the metabolic pathway of prasugrel does not include such "dead-end" pathway. (From Mega JL, Close SL, Wiviott SD, et al. Cytochrome P450 genetic polymorphisms and the response to prasugrel: relationship to pharmacokinetic, pharmacodynamic, and clinical outcomes. *Circulation.* 2009;119:2553–2560.)

vs. 11.7%) and a significant reduction in all-cause mortality (4.5% vs. 5.9%) without a significant difference in major bleeding (11.6% vs. 11.2%).

Ticagrelor has not specifically been studied among patients undergoing PCI. However, in the subgroup of patients undergoing invasive management in PLATO, there was also a significant reduction in the composite of vascular mortality, MI, or stroke favoring ticagrelor (35). Moreover, patients randomized to ticagrelor had a significant reduction in stent thrombosis.

Cangrelor

Cangrelor is an intravenous non-thienopyridine ADP-receptor antagonist that has a plasma half-life of 3 to 6 minutes and is therefore rapidly reversible (36). Platelet function normalizes within 30 to 60 minutes of discontinuation of

the infusion. It would therefore seem to be an attractive agent among patients undergoing PCI, as it has rapid onset and offset of action. Two large-scale randomized clinical trials, however, failed to demonstrate a significant benefit of cangrelor, when compared with clopidogrel, among patients undergoing PCI for ACS (37,38).

Genetic Polymorphism and Response to ADP Receptor Blockers

Both clopidogrel and prasugrel are metabolized to active metabolites by the cytochrome P450. As shown in Figure 6-1, the metabolism of clopidogrel includes an active pathway toward an active metabolite and a "dead-end" pathway toward an inactive metabolite. In contrast, the metabolism of prasugrel does not include the "dead-end" pathway. In addition, while the metabolism of clopidogrel depends predominantly on the CYP2C19 enzymatic pathway, prasugrel is rapidly de-esterified after oral administration, and the active metabolite is formed from the conversion of the intermediate mainly through the CYP3A and CYP2B enzymatic pathways. It has recently been shown that there are "reduced function" alleles of the CYP2C19 gene that result in a reduction in the metabolism of clopidogrel to the active metabolite. The same alleles do not result in a reduction in the metabolism of prasugrel. Importantly, it has also been shown that "reduced function" alleles of CYP2C19 are associated with worse clinical outcomes among patients receiving clopidogrel (Fig. 6-2), while they appear to have no effect on clinical outcomes among patients treated with prasugrel (Fig. 6-3). These novel discoveries have con-

tributed to a growing enthusiasm in pharmacogenomic and genetic polymorphism and to the realization that we might be able to reliably determine response to pharmacologic interventions through genetic testing.

Current Guidelines for the Use of ADP-Receptor Antagonists

Only the thienopyridine ADP-receptor antagonists are mentioned in current guidelines for the management of ACS in patients with stable coronary disease undergoing PCI, as neither ticagrelor nor cangrelor are approved for use (Table 6-2).

In STEMI patients undergoing primary PCI, the most recent ACC/AHA guideline updates in 2009 recommended a loading dose of a thienopyridine be given as soon as possible,

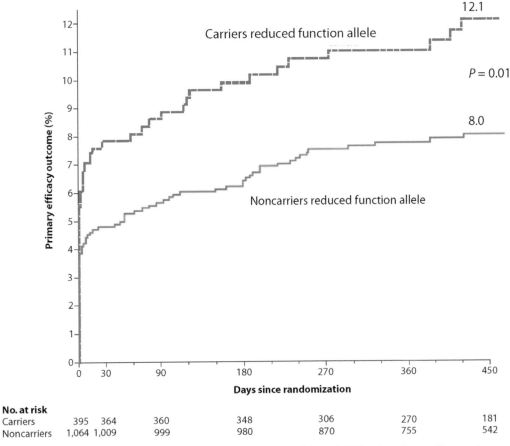

No. at risk

Carriers	395	364	360	348	306	270	181
Noncarriers	1,064	1,009	999	980	870	755	542

FIGURE 6-2. Relationship between *CYP2C19* reduced function allele and risk for the primary efficacy outcome of death from cardiovascular causes, myocardial infarction, or stroke in patients receiving clopidogrel in the TRITON-TIMI 38 clinical trial. (From Mega JL, Close SL, Wiviott SD, et al. Cytochrome P450 genetic polymorphisms and the response to prasugrel: relationship to pharmacokinetic, pharmacodynamic, and clinical outcomes. *Circulation*. 2009;119:2553–2560.)

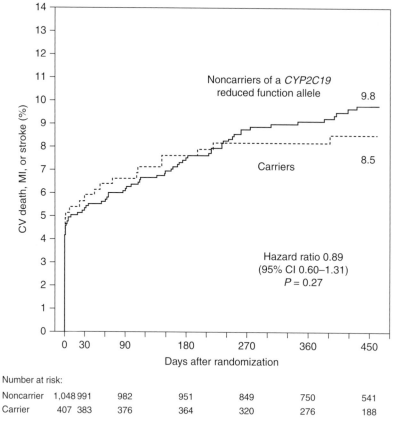

FIGURE 6-3. Relationship between *CYP2C19* reduced function allele and risk for the primary efficacy outcome of death from cardiovascular causes, myocardial infarction, or stroke in patients receiving prasugrel in the TRI-TON-TIMI 38 clinical trial. (From Mega JL, Close SL, Wiviott SD, et al. Cytochrome P450 genetic polymorphisms and the response to prasugrel: relationship to pharmacokinetic, pharmacodynamic, and clinical outcomes. *Circulation.* 2009;119:2553–2560.)

either 300 or 600 mg of clopidogrel or 60 mg of prasugrel (5). The most recent ESC guidelines, which were published in 2008, recommend administration of 300 to 600 mg of clopidogrel as soon as possible (6).

The 2007 ACC/AHA guidelines for the management of patients with unstable angina and NSTEMI recommend a loading dose of clopidogrel or a glycoprotein (Gp) IIb/IIIa inhibitor be used among patients undergoing an initially invasive strategy (8). In addition, they suggest that it is reasonable to administer both clopidogrel and a Gp IIb/IIIa inhibitor in patients undergoing an initially invasive strategy, although if bivalirudin is chosen as an initial antithrombin (AT), routine Gp IIb/IIIa use can be omitted. The ESC guidelines, published in 2007, recommend a 300-mg loading dose of clopidogrel be administered to all

patients and that a 600-mg loading dose may be used among patients undergoing an initially invasive strategy (7).

The 2005 ACC/AHA/SCAI guidelines for patients undergoing routine PCI recommend a loading dose of 300 mg of clopidogrel be administered at least 6 hours prior to the procedure (9). The 2005 ESC guidelines recommend 300 mg of clopidogrel be administered at least 6 hours prior to PCI or 600 mg of clopidogrel at least 2 hours prior to PCI (10).

■ GLYCOPROTEIN IIb/IIIa INHIBITORS

Gp IIb/IIIa inhibitors are intravenous agents that inhibit the final common pathway of platelet aggregation, which is mediated via platelet

TABLE 6-2	**Guideline Recommendations for the Administration of ADP-receptor Antagonists**	
Clinical Presentation	**ACC/AHA or ACC/AHA/SCAI**	**ESC**
STEMI undergoing primary PCI	A loading dose of thienopyridine is recommended for STEMI patients for whom PCI is planned. Regimens should be one of the following: 1. At least 300–600 mg of clopidogrel should be given as early as possible before or at the time of primary or nonprimary PCI. 2. Prasugrel 60 mg should be given as soon as possible for primary PCI. In STEMI patients with a prior history of stroke and transient ischemic attack for whom primary PCI is planned, prasugrel is not recommended as part of a dual-antiplatelet therapy regimen.	Clopidogrel should be given as soon as possible to all patients with STEMI undergoing PCI. It is started with a loading dose of at least 300 mg, but a 600-mg loading dose achieves a more rapid and stronger inhibition of platelet aggregation.
NSTEACS undergoing an early invasive strategy	Antiplatelet therapy in addition to aspirin should be initiated before diagnostic angiography (upstream) with either clopidogrel (loading dose followed by daily maintenance dose) or an intravenous Gp IIb/IIIa inhibitor. It is reasonable to initiate antiplatelet therapy with both clopidogrel (loading dose followed by daily maintenance dose) and an intravenous Gp IIb/IIIa inhibitor.	For all patients, an immediate 300-mg loading dose of clopidogrel is recommended. A loading dose of 600 mg of clopidogrel may be used to achieve more rapid inhibition of platelet function.
Elective PCI	A loading dose of clopidogrel should be administered before PCI is performed. An oral loading dose of 300 mg, administered at least 6 h before the procedure, has the best established evidence of efficacy. When a loading dose of clopidogrel is administered, a regimen of greater than 300 mg is reasonable to achieve higher levels of antiplatelet activity more rapidly, but the efficacy and safety compared with a 300-mg loading dose are less established.	Clopidogrel, at a dose of 300 mg, should be administered to all patients at least 6 h prior to undergoing elective PCI.

ACC, American College of Cardiology; AHA, American Heart Association; ESC, European Society of Cardiology; Gp, glycoprotein; NSTEACS, non-ST-segment elevation acute coronary syndrome; PCI, percutaneous coronary intervention; SCAI, Society for Coronary Angiography and Intervention; STEMI, ST-segment elevation myocardial infarction. (Adapted from the ACC/AHA, ACC/AHA/SCAI, and ESC guidelines for the management of STEMI, NSTEACS, and elective PCI (3–11).)

interaction with fibrinogen. The three commercially available agents are eptifibatide, a small peptide, tirofiban, a small molecule inhibitor, and abciximab, a monoclonal antibody.

Use of up-front Gp IIb/IIIa inhibitors in the setting of primary PCI for STEMI in the modern era of aggressive clopidogrel preloading has been shown to improve epicardial patency prior to PCI, myocardial perfusion, and ST-segment resolution as compared with provisional use in the cardiac catheterization laboratory (39–42). Ongoing Tirofiban in Myocardial Infarction Evaluation (ON-TIME) 2 trial, in which patients were randomized to tirofiban administered in the prehospital setting or provisionally in the cardiac catheterization laboratory, demonstrated a significant improvement in mean ST-segment resolution 60 minutes following primary PCI (40). In addition, the use of tirofiban was associated with a significant reduction in the composite of death, recurrent MI, urgent TVR, or blinded bailout use of tirofiban, although the composite outcome was predominately driven by a reduction in the use of bailout tirofiban. There was no significant difference in hemorrhagic outcomes.

In a smaller study, STEMI patients undergoing primary PCI were randomized to three arms: early tirofiban, tirofiban in the cardiac catheterization laboratory, or provisional tirofiban (39). Patients randomized to the early tirofiban group had higher rates of a patent infarct-related artery on initial angiography and had improved myocardial perfusion following primary PCI.

Eptifibatide has also been studied in a small randomized trial of early administration versus administration following initial angiography (41). Early administration led to a significant improvement in pre-PCI coronary flow and myocardial perfusion and no significant difference in adverse cardiovascular or hemorrhagic outcomes, although routine use of high-dose clopidogrel was not mandated. Likewise, early administration of abciximab improved coronary patency among STEMI patients treated with primary PCI, but no thienopyridine loading dose was administered (42).

The use of Gp IIb/IIIa inhibitors among patients with NSTEMI and unstable angina has likely been altered by more frequent use and higher dosing of clopidogrel preloading. Early

studies of Gp IIb/IIIa inhibitors suggested a small but significant reduction in the composite of death and MI.

The administration of abciximab was studied among over 2,000 high-risk patients with non-ST-segment elevation ACS (NSTEACS) (elevated cardiac biomarkers or ST-segment deviation) who received a 600-mg loading dose of clopidogrel at least 2 hours prior to PCI (43). Abciximab or placebo was administered after the decision to perform PCI but prior to wire passage. The administration of abciximab led to a significant reduction in the composite of death, MI, or urgent TVR within 30 days (8.9% versus 11.9%, $P = 0.03$) compared with placebo. This difference was driven by a significant reduction in events in the subgroup of patients with elevated troponin, and there was no significant difference in outcomes among patients without elevated cardiac biomarkers. There was no significant difference between the groups in the rates of major or minor hemorrhage or the need for blood transfusion.

However, a more recent large clinical trial including patients presenting with high-risk NSTEACS (2 or more of ST-segment deviation, elevated cardiac biomarkers, or age > 60 years) failed to show a meaningful clinical benefit of early administration of eptifibatide (44).

The Early Glycoprotein IIb/IIIa Inhibition in Non-ST-Segment Elevation Acute Coronary Syndrome (EARLY ACS) trial randomized 9,492 such patients to administration of eptifibatide as soon as the diagnosis was made versus provisional administration in the cardiac catheterization laboratory prior to PCI. All patients received aspirin and antithrombotic therapy. Loading doses of clopidogrel were not mandated, but nearly three-quarters of patients received early clopidogrel. Early use of eptifibatide had no significant impact on the primary outcome, a composite of death, MI, recurrent ischemia requiring urgent revascularization, or a thrombotic complication during PCI that required bolus therapy opposite to the initial study-group assignment at 96 hours. There was a trend toward a reduction in the composite of death or MI favoring the early eptifibatide group, but there was also a significantly higher incidence of bleeding and red-cell transfusion in the early eptifibatide group.

Current Guidelines for the Use of Gp IIb/IIIa Inhibitors

The 2009 ACC/AHA guidelines for the management of STEMI suggest that it is reasonable to start the treatment with a Gp IIb/IIIa inhibitor (abciximab has the most compelling evidence, but tirofiban and eptifibatide can also be considered) at the time of primary PCI (Table 6-3) (5). The safety and efficacy of Gp IIb/IIIa inhibitors prior to arrival in the cardiac catheterization laboratory is uncertain; the 2008 ESC guidelines give similar recommendations for STEMI patients undergoing primary PCI (6).

The ACC/AHA guidelines recommend initiation of a Gp IIb/IIIa inhibitor (or high loading dose clopidogrel) in patients with NSTEACS undergoing an early invasive strategy (8). In addition, the guidelines suggest that it is reasonable to administer a Gp IIb/IIIa inhibitor to patients undergoing an initial conservative strategy who have recurrent chest discomfort and to patients undergoing an initially invasive strategy who have already received clopidogrel. The 2007 ESC guidelines recommend initiation of eptifibatide or tirofiban for initial early treatment in addition to oral antiplatelet agents for intermediate- to high-risk NSTEACS patients. Patients who receive initial treatment with eptifibatide or tirofiban prior to angiography should be maintained on the same drug during and after PCI (7).

The 2005 ACC/AHA/SCAI guidelines suggest that it is reasonable to administer a Gp IIb/IIIa inhibitor to patients undergoing elective PCI with stent implantation (9), whereas the 2005 ESC guidelines suggest that Gp IIb/IIIa inhibitors should be considered on a case-by-case basis for elective PCI (10).

■ ANTITHROMBOTIC AGENTS

Unfractionated Heparin

UFH was discovered almost 90 years ago and is the prototype of its derivatives (45). It is a natural product that can be isolated from beef lung or porcine intestinal mucosa. It consists of highly sulfated polysaccharide chains with a mean of about 45 saccharide units. Only one-third of the heparin chains possess a unique pentasaccharide sequence that exhibits high affinity for AT, and it is this fraction that is responsible for most of the anticoagulant activity of heparin.

In clinical trials comparing the association of heparin plus aspirin versus aspirin alone in NSTEACS, a trend toward benefit was observed in favor of the heparin–aspirin combination, but at the cost of an increase in bleeding (46).

UFH is the most commonly used anticoagulant during PCI. Randomized trials have shown UFH to reduce ischemic complications (47,48). UFH in a dose of 60 to 100 IU/kg and a target activated clotting time (ACT) between 250 and 350 seconds are recommended. A target of 200 seconds is advocated for UFH dosing in conjunction with a Gp IIb/IIIa inhibitors (49,50). After completion of PCI, UFH is not indicated, as continued treatment does not reduce ischemic complications and is associated with a higher risk of bleeding (51).

Low-Molecular-Weight Heparins

Based on early experience with low-molecular-weight heparins (LMWHs) (52,53), two pivotal trials examined the efficacy and safety of enoxaparin in patients presenting with ACS. The Efficacy and Safety of Subcutaneous Enoxaparin in Non-Q-Wave Coronary Events (ESSENCE) randomized more than 3,000 patients to enoxaparin or UFH for at least 48 hours (54). At 14 days, the incidence of death, MI, or recurrent angina was significantly lower in patients randomized to enoxaparin than those receiving UFH, and the outcomes remained significantly different at 30 days. Although there was no significant difference in major bleeding, the incidence of any bleeding event was significantly higher in the enoxaparin group, primarily driven by an increase in injection-site ecchymosis. The TIMI 11B trial, which randomized nearly 4,000 patients to either UFH or enoxaparin, again demonstrated a statistically significant difference in ischemic outcomes favoring enoxaparin with no difference in major bleeding (55).

The Superior Yield of the New Strategy of Enoxaparin, Revascularization and Glycoprotein IIb/IIIa Inhibitors (SYNERGY) trial randomized more than 10,000 patients presenting with NSTEACS and high risk features undergoing an early invasive strategy to enoxaparin versus UFH (56). More than half received a Gp IIb/IIIa inhibitor and two-thirds received

TABLE 6-3	Guideline Recommendations for the Administration of Glycoprotein IIb/IIIa Receptor Antagonists	
Clinical Presentation	ACC/AHA or ACC/AHA/SCAI	ESC
STEMI undergoing primary PCI	It is reasonable to start treatment with Gp IIb/IIIa (abciximab has a higher level of evidence than tirofiban or eptifibatide) at the time of primary PCI (with or without stenting) in selected patients with STEMI. The usefulness of Gp IIb/IIIa receptor antagonists (as part of a preparatory pharmacologic strategy for patients with STEMI before their arrival in the cardiac catheterization laboratory for angiography and PCI) is uncertain.	The weight of evidence is in favor of efficacy of abciximab. The efficacy of tirofiban and eptifibatide is less well established.
NSTEACS undergoing an early invasive strategy	Antiplatelet therapy in addition to aspirin should be initiated before diagnostic angiography (upstream) with either clopidogrel (loading dose followed by daily maintenance dose) or a Gp IIb/IIIa inhibitor. Abciximab as the choice for upstream Gp IIb/IIIa therapy is indicated only if there is no appreciable delay to angiography and PCI is likely to be performed; otherwise, eptifibatide or tirofiban is the preferred choice of Gp IIb/IIIa inhibitor. It is reasonable to initiate antiplatelet therapy with both clopidogrel (loading dose followed by daily maintenance dose) and a Gp IIb/IIIa inhibitor. Abciximab as the choice for upstream Gp IIb/IIIa therapy is indicated only if there is no appreciable delay to angiography and PCI is likely to be performed; otherwise, IV eptifibatide or tirofiban is the preferred choice of GP IIb/IIIa inhibitor. Abciximab should not be administered to patients in whom PCI is not planned.	In patients at intermediate to high risk, particularly patients with elevated troponins, ST-segment depression, or diabetes, either eptifibatide or tirofiban for initial early treatment is recommended in addition to oral antiplatelet agents. Patients who receive initial treatment with eptifibatide or tirofiban prior to angiography should be maintained on the same drug during and after PCI. In high-risk patients not pretreated with Gp IIb/IIIa inhibitors and proceeding to PCI, abciximab is recommended immediately following angiography. When anatomy is known and PCI planned to be performed within 24 h with Gp IIb/IIIa inhibitors, most secure evidence is for abciximab.
Elective PCI	In patients undergoing elective PCI with stent placement, it is reasonable to administer a Gp IIb/IIIa inhibitor. If clopidogrel is given at the time of procedure, supplementation with Gp IIb/IIIa receptor antagonists can be beneficial to facilitate earlier platelet inhibition than with clopidogrel alone.	Gp IIb/IIIa inhibitors are reasonable for use in elective PCI with complex lesions, threatening/actual vessel closure, visible thrombus, no/slow reflow.

ACC, American College of Cardiology; AHA, American Heart Association; ESC, European Society of Cardiology; Gp, glycoprotein; NSTEACS, non-ST-segment elevation acute coronary syndrome; PCI, percutaneous coronary intervention; SCAI, Society for Coronary Angiography and Intervention; STEMI, ST-segment elevation myocardial infarction.
(Adapted from the ACC/AHA, ACC/AHA/SCAI and ESC guidelines for the management of STEMI, NSTEACS and elective PCI (3–11).)

TABLE 6-4 Dosing of Enoxaparin in the Cardiac Cauterization Laboratory According to Time of Last SQ Dose and Number of SQ Doses

Time of Last SQ Dose of Enoxaparin or Number of SQ Doses	Additional Dosing
<8 h and at least ≥ 3 SQ doses administered	No additional dosing
8–12 h	LMWH—additional intravenous bolus of 0.3 mg/kg
>12 h	Standard full dose anticoagulation
<3 consecutive SQ doses	LMWH—additional intravenous bolus of 0.3 mg/kg

clopidogrel or ticlopidine. There was no significant difference in the incidence of death or non-fatal MI by 30 days between patients who received enoxaparin or UFH. In addition, the rates of acute complications, including abrupt closure, threatened abrupt closure, unsuccessful PCI, and emergency CABG surgery were not significantly different between the groups. There was, however, a significantly higher incidence of major bleeding in the enoxaparin group, and particularly among patients in whom anticoagulation was switched from UFH to LMWH and vice versa. The lack of a readily available monitoring system for LMWH makes its use in the cardiac catheterization laboratory less appealing. Current guidelines recommend dosing of LMWH in the cardiac catheterization laboratory, which is strictly dependent on the time of the last SQ administration. No additional anticoagulation should be given if the last subcutaneous dose of enoxaparin was given ≤8 hours prior to PCI. An additional intravenous bolus of 0.3 mg/kg is recommended if the last dose was given between 8 and 12 hours prior to PCI, whereas standard full anticoagulation should be used if the last dose was given >12 hours prior to PCI (Table 6-4). Timing of arterial sheath removal also varies according to the dose and route of LMWH administration (Table 6-5).

Fondaparinux

A synthetic analogue of the AT-binding pentasaccharide sequence found in UFH and LMWH, fondaparinux binds AT and enhances its reactivity with factor Xa (57).

The Organization to Assess Strategies for Ischemic Syndromes (OASIS)-5 trial randomized 20,078 patients with NSTEACS (2 or more

of age > 60 years, elevated cardiac biomarkers or ischemic ECG changes) to fondaparinux or enoxaparin for a mean of 6 days (58). Fondaparinux was not inferior to enoxaparin in terms of the composite of death, MI, or refractory ischemia at 9 days, and major bleeds were halved with fondaparinux compared with enoxaparin with lower rates of bleeding complications at the access site among the approximately two-thirds of patients who underwent coronary angiography. Alarmingly, however, there was a higher incidence of catheter thrombosis in patients receiving fondaparinux.

The OASIS-6 trial evaluated the effect of fondaparinux, given for up to 8 days, compared with standard adjuvant anticoagulant treatment in 12,092 patients with STEMI (59). The trial had a complicated design with two strata. In the subgroup of patients undergoing primary PCI, there was again a significantly higher rate of guiding catheter thrombosis and more coronary complications with fondaparinux.

Bivalirudin

Direct thrombin inhibitors (DTIs) are derivatives of hirudin, a polypeptide first isolated from the salivary glands of the medicinal

TABLE 6-5 Timing of Arterial Sheath Removal in Patients Receiving Enoxaparin

Route of Administration of LMWH	Timing of Arterial Sheath Removal
Subcutaneous	8 h after the last dose
Intravenous	4 to 6 h after the last dose

leech, *Hirudo medicinalis* (60). They are bivalent molecules that are capable of binding the active site and fibrin-binding site of thrombin. Rather than catalyzing the production of endogenous thrombin inhibitors, DTIs bind directly to thrombin and inhibit its interaction with substrate, thereby preventing fibrin formation, thrombin-mediated activation of the coagulation cascade, and thrombin-induced platelet aggregation (61). While indirect thrombin inhibitors such as UFH and LMWH lead to the inactivation of only circulating thrombin, because of their mechanism of action, DTIs are capable of inactivating clot-bound thrombin as well. Importantly, in comparison with heparin derivatives (and even fondaparinux), heparin-induced thrombocytopenia has not been reported in patients receiving bivalirudin, the only DTI approved for use among patients undergoing PCI.

The Randomized Evaluation in Percutaneous Coronary Intervention Linking Angiomax to Reduced Clinical Events (REPLACE)-2 trial randomized over 6,000 patients undergoing urgent or elective PCI to UFH plus planned Gp IIb/IIIa blockade or bivalirudin plus provisional Gp IIb/IIIa blockade (62). Bivalirudin was not inferior in terms of the composite primary outcome of the 30-day incidence of death, MI, urgent repeat revascularization, and in-hospital major bleeding. However, in-hospital major bleeding was significantly less common among patients receiving bivalirudin.

The Acute Catheterization and Urgent Intervention Triage Strategy (ACUITY) trial randomized almost 13,819 patients with NSTEACS and planned early invasive strategy to three arms: UFH or enoxaparin plus Gp IIb/IIIa blockade, bivalirudin plus Gp IIb/IIIa blockade, or bivalirudin monotherapy with provisional Gp IIb/IIIa blockade at the discretion of the treating physician (63). There were three primary 30-day end points: (1) a composite ischemia end point (death from any cause, MI, or unplanned revascularization), (2) major bleeding, and (3) a composite of the ischemia end point plus major bleeding. There was no significant difference in any of the three primary end points among patients who received a heparin product plus Gp IIb/IIIa blockade compared with those who received bivalirudin plus Gp IIb/IIIa blockade. Compared with those who

received a heparin product plus Gp IIb/IIIa blockade, bivalirudin alone was associated with a noninferior rate of ischemic outcomes but significantly reduced major bleeding and the composite ischemic and hemorrhagic outcome. A subsequent subgroup analysis of patients who underwent PCI in the ACUITY trial (nearly 8,000 patients) reported similar findings (64).

Finally, bivalirudin was studied among patients presenting with STEMI undergoing primary PCI in the Harmonizing Outcomes with Revascularization and Stents in Acute Myocardial Infarction (HORIZONS-AMI) study, in which more than 3,500 patients were randomized to receive bivalirudin or UFH plus a Gp IIb/IIIa inhibitor (65). Patients randomized to bivalirudin had a significantly lower incidence of the composite of death, reinfarction, TVR for ischemia, stroke, or major bleeding when compared with UFH plus a Gp IIb/IIIa inhibitor. This was driven by a significant reduction in major bleeding favoring bivalirudin monotherapy. Stent thrombosis was significantly more common among patients randomized to bivalirudin in the first 24 hours, but the difference in rates of stent thrombosis were not significantly different at 30 days. Most striking, perhaps, was the finding that bivalirudin monotherapy was associated with a significant reduction in cardiovascular mortality and death from all causes.

Current Guidelines for the Use of Antithrombotic Agents

The 2009 ACC/AHA STEMI guidelines recommend UFH or bivalirudin as parenteral anticoagulant therapy in the cardiac catheterization laboratory whether or not UFH was initially administered in the emergency department (Table 6-6) (5). In addition, bivalirudin is a reasonable option among patients with a high risk of bleeding. In the 2008 ESC STEMI guidelines, UFH is recommended, bivalirudin is a reasonable alternative and fondaparinux may be considered as long as an initial dose of UFH was administered (6).

The 2007 ACC/AHA guidelines for the management of unstable angina and NSTEMI recommend anticoagulation therapy be initiated as soon as possible after presentation (8). For patients in whom an invasive strategy is selected, enoxaparin and UFH have the highest level of

TABLE 6-6 **Guideline Recommendations for the Administration of Antithrombotic Therapy**

Clinical Presentation	ACC/AHA or ACC/AHA/SCAI	ESC
STEMI undergoing primary PCI	For patients who have been treated with aspirin and a thienopyridine, recommended supportive anticoagulant regimens include the following: 1. For prior treatment with UFH, additional boluses of UFH should be administered as needed to maintain therapeutic activated clotting time levels, taking into account whether Gp IIb/IIIa receptor antagonists have been administered. 2. Bivalirudin is useful as a supportive measure for primary PCI with or without prior treatment with UFH.	UFH is standard anticoagulant therapy during PCI. The weight of evidence favors the use of bivalirudin. Fondaparinux should not be used.
NSTEACS undergoing an early invasive strategy	Recommended regimens include enoxaparin and UFH, which have the highest level of evidence, and bivalirudin, which has some evidence for use.	Anticoagulation is recommended for all patients in addition to antiplatelet therapy. In an urgent invasive strategy, UFH, enoxaparin or bivalirudin (I-B) should be immediately started.
Elective PCI	UFH should be administered to patients undergoing PCI. It is reasonable to use bivalirudin as an alternative to UFH and Gp IIb/IIIa antagonists in low-risk patients undergoing elective PCI.	UFH is recommended among patients undergoing elective PCI with monitoring of the ACT.

ACC, American College of Cardiology; AHA, American Heart Association; ESC, European Society of Cardiology; Gp, glycoprotein; NSTEACS, non-ST-segment elevation acute coronary syndrome; PCI, percutaneous coronary intervention; SCAI, Society for Coronary Angiography and Intervention; STEMI, ST-segment elevation myocardial infarction; UFH, unfractionated heparin.
(Adapted from the ACC/AHA, ACC/AHA/SCAI, and ESC guidelines for the management of STEMI, NSTEACS, and elective PCI (3–11).)

evidence, but fondaparinux and bivalirudin may also be considered. The 2008 ESC guidelines give similar recommendations (7).

Among patients undergoing elective PCI, the 2005 ACC/AHA/SCAI guidelines recommend UFH be administered; bivalirudin is considered as a reasonable alternative (9). The 2005 ESC guidelines recommend UFH be used (10).

■ REVERSAL OF ANTITHROMBOTIC THERAPY

In case of life-threatening bleeding, the interventionalist will be faced with the need of reversing antithrombotic therapy. Except for UFH and protamine, there is no perfect "antidote" for other antithrombotic agents. Table 6-7 summarizes suggested interventions in an attempt to reverse or blunt the anticoagulant effect of antiplatelet and antithrombotic agents.

■ ADJUNCTIVE PHARMACOTHERAPY OTHER THAN ANTITHROMBOTIC AND ANTIPLATELET THERAPY

While the field of adjunctive pharmacotherapy in interventional cardiology has been traditionally focused on the prevention of thrombotic complications, the past decade

| TABLE 6-7 | Suggested Pharmacologic Interventions to Reverse or Blunt the Effect of Antiplatelet and Antithrombotic Agents |

Antiplatelet or Antithrombotic Agent	Reversal Agent
Aspirin	• Desmopressin (DDAVP) 0.3 mcg/kg. DDAVP is a synthetic analogue 8-arginine vasopressin. It promotes the release of von Willebrand factor and factor VIII from endothelial cells, and it has been used in coagulation disorders such as von Willebrand disease, mild hemophilia A (factor VIII deficiency), and thrombocytopenia. The increase is evident within 30 min, and it is maximal at a dose of 0.3 mcg/kg. DDAVP shortens the prolonged activated partial thromboplastin time and bleeding time, probably as a result from the increases in factor VIII and vWF. It can be used with uremic induced platelet dysfunction. Although it has no effect on platelet count or aggregation, it has been shown to increase platelet adhesion to the vessel wall. In contrast to vasopressin, DDAVP has little effect on blood pressure and is therefore relatively safe in the setting of acute administration • Platelet transfusion
Thienopyridines	• DDAVP can shorten the prolonged bleeding time of individual taking thienopyridines • Platelet transfusion
GP IIb/IIIa receptor blockers	• Platelet transfusion (efficacy uncertain) • DDAVP • Fresh frozen plasma (15 ml/kg body weight) • Cryoprecipitate
Heparin	• Protamine. Recommend dosing is 10 mg/1,000 units of UFH or 1 mcg/100 units of UFH
LMWH	• Protamine. Recommend dosing is 1 mg for each mg of LMWH
Bivalirudin	• DDAVP 0.3 mcg/kg. It can shorten the prolonged bleeding time of rabbits treated with hirudin • Cryoprecipitate (10 units) • Fresh frozen plasma (15 ml/kg body weight)

(From Mannucci PM. Desmopressin (DDAVP) in the treatment of bleeding disorders: the first 20 years. *Blood.* 1997;90:2515–2521; Crowther MA, Warkentin TE. Bleeding risk and the management of bleeding complications in patients undergoing anticoagulant therapy: focus on new anticoagulant agents. *Blood.* 2008;111:4871–4879.)

has been characterized by new development in the use of adjunctive pharmacotherapy in the prevention or reversal of other complications. Chapters 13 and 17 address specifically the use of adjunctive pharmacotherapy in the prevention of contrast nephropathy and other contrast reactions, and in the prevention and management of no reflow. The reader is referred to those chapters for an in-depth review.

■ CONCLUSION

The interventional landscape has advanced significantly in the past three decades, and not merely because of innovative percutaneous techniques. PCI has been made safer, easier, and more efficacious because of major advances in pharmacologic strategies to prevent angioplasty and stent complications. Appropriate and judicious use of these powerful pharmacologic agents will be required in order to further advance our ability to treat stable and unstable coronary disease.

References

1. Randomised trial of intravenous streptokinase, oral aspirin, both, or neither among 17,187 cases of suspected acute myocardial infarction: ISIS-2. ISIS-2 (Second International Study of Infarct Survival) Collaborative Group. *Lancet.* 1988; 2(8607):349–360.

2. Awtry EH, Loscalzo J. Aspirin. *Circulation.* 2000; 101(10):1206–1218.

3. Antman EM, Anbe DT, Armstrong PW, et al. ACC/AHA guidelines for the management of patients with ST-elevation myocardial infarction: a report of the American College of Cardiology/ American Heart Association Task Force on Practice Guidelines (Committee to Revise the 1999 Guidelines for the Management of Patients with Acute Myocardial Infarction). *Circulation.* 2004; 110(9):e82–e292.

4. Antman EM, Hand M, Armstrong PW, et al. 2007 Focused Update of the ACC/AHA 2004 Guidelines for the Management of Patients With ST-Elevation Myocardial Infarction: a report of the American College of Cardiology/American Heart Association Task Force on Practice Guidelines: developed in collaboration With the Canadian Cardiovascular Society endorsed by the American Academy of Family Physicians: 2007 Writing Group to Review New Evidence and Update the ACC/AHA 2004 Guidelines for the Management of Patients With ST-Elevation Myocardial Infarction, Writing on Behalf of the 2004 Writing Committee. *Circulation.* 2008;117(2): 296–329.

5. Kushner FG, Hand M, Smith SC Jr, et al. 2009 Focused Updates: ACC/AHA Guidelines for the Management of Patients With ST-Elevation Myocardial Infarction (updating the 2004 Guideline and 2007 Focused Update) and ACC/AHA/ SCAI Guidelines on Percutaneous Coronary Intervention (updating the 2005 Guideline and 2007 Focused Update): a report of the American College of Cardiology Foundation/American Heart Association Task Force on Practice Guidelines. *Circulation.* 2009;120(22):2271–2306.

6. Van de Werf F, Bax J, Betriu A, et al. Management of acute myocardial infarction in patients pre-senting with persistent ST-segment elevation: the Task Force on the Management of ST-Segment Elevation Acute Myocardial Infarction of the European Society of Cardiology. *Eur Heart J.* 2008;29(23):2909–2945.

7. Bassand JP, Hamm CW, Ardissino D, et al. Guidelines for the diagnosis and treatment of non-ST-segment elevation acute coronary syndromes. *Eur Heart J.* 2007;28(13):1598–1660.

8. Anderson JL, Adams CD, Antman EM, et al. ACC/AHA 2007 guidelines for the management of patients with unstable angina/non ST-elevation myocardial infarction: a report of the American College of Cardiology/American Heart Association Task Force on Practice Guidelines (Writing Committee to Revise the 2002 Guidelines for the Management of Patients With Unstable Angina/Non ST-Elevation Myocardial Infarction): developed in collaboration with the American College of Emergency Physicians, the Society for Cardiovascular Angiography and Interventions, and the Society of Thoracic Surgeons: endorsed by the American Association of Cardiovascular and Pulmonary Rehabilitation and the Society for Academic Emergency Medicine. *Circulation.* 2007;116(7):e148–e304.

9. Smith SC Jr, Feldman TE, Hirshfeld JW Jr, et al. ACC/AHA/SCAI 2005 Guideline Update for Percutaneous Coronary Intervention—summary article: a report of the American College of Cardiology/American Heart Association Task Force on Practice Guidelines (ACC/AHA/SCAI Writing Committee to Update the 2001 Guidelines for Percutaneous Coronary Intervention). *Circulation.* 2006;113(1):156–175.

10. Silber S, Albertsson P, Aviles FF, et al. Guidelines for percutaneous coronary interventions. The Task Force for Percutaneous Coronary Interventions of the European Society of Cardiology. *Eur Heart J.* 2005;26(8):804–847.

11. King SB III, Smith SC Jr, Hirshfeld JW Jr, et al. 2007 Focused Update of the ACC/AHA/SCAI 2005 Guideline Update for Percutaneous Coronary Intervention: a report of the American College of Cardiology/American Heart Association Task Force on Practice Guidelines: 2007 Writing Group to Review New Evidence and Update the ACC/AHA/SCAI 2005 Guideline Update for Percutaneous Coronary Intervention, Writing on Behalf of the 2005 Writing Committee. *Circulation.* 2008;117(2):261–295.

12. Savi P, Herbert JM. Clopidogrel and ticlopidine: P2Y12 adenosine diphosphate-receptor antagonists for the prevention of atherothrombosis. *Semin Thromb Hemost.* 2005;31(2):174–183.

13. Toth PP. The potential role of prasugrel in secondary prevention of ischemic events in patients with acute coronary syndromes. *Postgrad Med.* 2009;121(1):59–72.

14. Hashemzadeh M, Goldsberry S, Furukawa M, et al. ADP receptor-blocker thienopyridines: chemical structures, mode of action and clinical use. A review. *J Invasive Cardiol.* 2009;21(8):406–412.

15. Angiolillo DJ, Guzman LA. Clinical overview of promising nonthienopyridine antiplatelet agents. *Am Heart J.* 2008;156(2 suppl):S23–S28.

16. Bruno JJ. The mechanisms of action of ticlopidine. *Thromb Res Suppl.* 1983;4:59–67.

17. Fischman DL, Leon MB, Baim DS, et al. A randomized comparison of coronary-stent placement and balloon angioplasty in the treatment of coronary artery disease. Stent Restenosis Study Investigators. *N Engl J Med.* 1994;331(8):496–501.

18. Serruys PW, de Jaegere P, Kiemeneij F, et al. A comparison of balloon-expandable-stent implantation with balloon angioplasty in patients with coronary artery disease. Benestent Study Group. *N Engl J Med.* 1994;331(8):489–495.

19. Bertrand ME, Legrand V, Boland J, et al. Randomized multicenter comparison of conventional anticoagulation versus antiplatelet therapy in unplanned and elective coronary stenting. The full anticoagulation versus aspirin and ticlopidine (fantastic) study. *Circulation.* 1998;98(16):1597–1603.

20. Schomig A, Neumann FJ, Kastrati A, et al. A randomized comparison of antiplatelet and anticoagulant therapy after the placement of coronary-artery stents. *N Engl J Med.* 1996;334(17):1084–1089.

21. Leon MB, Baim DS, Popma JJ, et al. A clinical trial comparing three antithrombotic-drug regimens after coronary-artery stenting. Stent Anticoagulation Restenosis Study Investigators. *N Engl J Med.* 1998;339(23):1665–1671.

22. Chen DK, Kim JS, Sutton DM. Thrombotic thrombocytopenic purpura associated with ticlopidine use: a report of 3 cases and review of the literature. *Arch Intern Med.* 1999;159(3):311–314.

23. Bennett CL, Weinberg PD, Rozenberg-Ben-Dror K, et al. Thrombotic thrombocytopenic purpura associated with ticlopidine. A review of 60 cases. *Ann Intern Med.* 1998;128(7):541–544.

24. Yusuf S, Zhao F, Mehta SR, et al. Effects of clopidogrel in addition to aspirin in patients with acute coronary syndromes without ST-segment elevation. *N Engl J Med.* 2001;345(7):494–502.

25. Farid NA, Kurihara A, Wrighton SA. Metabolism and disposition of the thienopyridine antiplatelet drugs ticlopidine, clopidogrel, and prasugrel in humans. *J Clin Pharmacol.* 2010;50(2):126–142.

26. Oo TH. Clopidogrel-associated thrombotic thrombocytopenic purpura presenting with coronary artery thrombosis. *Am J Hematol.* 2006;81(11):890–891.

27. Steinhubl SR, Berger PB, Brennan DM, et al. Optimal timing for the initiation of pretreatment with 300 mg clopidogrel before percutaneous coronary intervention. *J Am Coll Cardiol.* 2006;47(5):939–943.

28. Cuisset T, Frere C, Quilici J, et al. Benefit of a 600-mg loading dose of clopidogrel on platelet reactivity and clinical outcomes in patients with non-ST-segment elevation acute coronary syndrome undergoing coronary stenting. *J Am Coll Cardiol.* 2006;48:1339–1345.

29. Wiviott SD, Trenk D, Frelinger AL, et al. Prasugrel compared with high loading- and maintenance-dose clopidogrel in patients with planned percutaneous coronary intervention: the Prasugrel in Comparison to Clopidogrel for Inhibition of Platelet Activation and Aggregation-Thrombolysis in Myocardial Infarction 44 trial. *Circulation.* 2007;116(25):2923–2932.

30. Wiviott SD, Braunwald E, McCabe CH, et al. Prasugrel versus clopidogrel in patients with acute coronary syndromes. *N Engl J Med.* 2007;357(20):2001–2015.

31. Brandt JT, Payne CD, Wiviott SD, et al. A comparison of prasugrel and clopidogrel loading doses on platelet function: magnitude of platelet inhibition is related to active metabolite formation. *Am Heart J.* 2007;153(1):66.e9–66.e16.

32. Jernberg T, Payne CD, Winters KJ, et al. Prasugrel achieves greater inhibition of platelet aggregation and a lower rate of non-responders compared with clopidogrel in aspirin-treated patients with stable coronary artery disease. *Eur Heart J.* 2006;27(10):1166–1173.

33. Capodanno D, Dharmashankar K, Angiolillo DJ. Mechanism of action and clinical development of ticagrelor, a novel platelet ADP P2Y(12) receptor antagonist. *Expert Rev Cardiovasc Ther.* 2010;8(2):151–158.

34. Wallentin L, Becker RC, Budaj A, et al. Ticagrelor versus clopidogrel in patients with acute coronary syndromes. *N Engl J Med.* 2009;361(11):1045–1057.

35. Cannon CP, Harrington RA, James S, et al. Comparison of ticagrelor with clopidogrel in patients with a planned invasive strategy for acute coronary syndromes (PLATO): a randomised double-blind study. *Lancet.* 2010;375(9711):283–293.

36. Storey RF, Wilcox RG, Heptinstall S. Comparison of the pharmacodynamic effects of the platelet ADP receptor antagonists clopidogrel and AR-C69931MX in patients with ischaemic heart disease. *Platelets.* 2002;13(7):407–413.

37. Bhatt DL, Lincoff AM, Gibson CM, et al. Intravenous platelet blockade with cangrelor during PCI. *N Engl J Med.* 2009;361(24):2330–2341.

38. Harrington RA, Stone GW, McNulty S, et al. Platelet inhibition with cangrelor in patients undergoing PCI. *N Engl J Med.* 2009;361(24):2318–2329.

39. Shen J, Zhang Q, Zhang RY, et al. Clinical benefits of adjunctive tirofiban therapy in patients with acute ST-segment elevation myocardial infarction undergoing primary percutaneous coronary intervention. *Coron Artery Dis.* 2008;19(4):271–277.

40. Van't Hof AW, Ten Berg J, Heestermans T, et al. Prehospital initiation of tirofiban in patients with ST-elevation myocardial infarction undergoing primary angioplasty (On-TIME 2): a multicentre, double-blind, randomised controlled trial. *Lancet.* 2008;372(9638):537–546.

41. Gibson CM, Kirtane AJ, Murphy SA, et al. Early initiation of eptifibatide in the emergency department before primary percutaneous coronary intervention for ST-segment elevation myocardial infarction: results of the Time to Integrilin Therapy in Acute Myocardial Infarction (TITAN)-TIMI 34 trial. *Am Heart J.* 2006;152(4):668–675.

42. Montalescot G, Barragan P, Wittenberg O, et al. Platelet glycoprotein IIb/IIIa inhibition with coronary stenting for acute myocardial infarction. *N Engl J Med.* 2001;344(25):1895–1903.

43. Kastrati A, Mehilli J, Neumann FJ, et al. Abciximab in patients with acute coronary syndromes undergoing percutaneous coronary intervention after clopidogrel pretreatment: the ISAR-REACT 2 randomized trial. *JAMA.* 2006;295(13):1531–1538.

44. Giugliano RP, White JA, Bode C, et al. Early versus delayed, provisional eptifibatide in acute coronary syndromes. *N Engl J Med.* 2009;360(21):2176–2190.

45. De Caterina R, Husted S, Wallentin L, et al. Anticoagulants in heart disease: current status and perspectives. *Eur Heart J.* 2007;28(7):880–913.

46. Collins R, MacMahon S, Flather M, et al. Clinical effects of anticoagulant therapy in suspected acute myocardial infarction: systematic overview of randomised trials. *BMJ.* 1996;313(7058):652–659.

47. Boccara A, Benamer H, Juliard JM, et al. A randomized trial of a fixed high dose vs a weight-adjusted low dose of intravenous heparin during coronary angioplasty. *Eur Heart J.* 1997;18(4):631–635.

48. Koch KT, Piek JJ, de Winter RJ, et al. Early ambulation after coronary angioplasty and stenting with six French guiding catheters and low-dose heparin. *Am J Cardiol.* 1997;80(8):1084–1086.

49. Avendano A, Ferguson JJ. Comparison of Hemochron and HemoTec activated coagulation time target values during percutaneous transluminal coronary angioplasty. *J Am Coll Cardiol.* 1994;23(4):907–910.

50. Kereiakes DJ, Lincoff AM, Miller DP, et al. Abciximab therapy and unplanned coronary stent deployment: favorable effects on stent use, clinical outcomes, and bleeding complications. EPILOG Trial Investigators. *Circulation.* 1998;97(9):857–864.

51. Friedman HZ, Cragg DR, Glazier SM, et al. Randomized prospective evaluation of prolonged versus abbreviated intravenous heparin therapy after coronary angioplasty. *J Am Coll Cardiol.* 1994;24(5):1214–1219.

52. Low-molecular-weight heparin during instability in coronary artery disease, Fragmin during Instability in Coronary Artery Disease (FRISC) study group. *Lancet.* 1996;347(9001):561–568.

53. Gurfinkel EP, Manos EJ, Mejail RI, et al. Low molecular weight heparin versus regular heparin or aspirin in the treatment of unstable angina and silent ischemia. *J Am Coll Cardiol.* 1995;26(2):313–318.

54. Cohen M, Demers C, Gurfinkel EP, et al. A comparison of low-molecular-weight heparin with unfractionated heparin for unstable coronary artery disease. Efficacy and Safety of Subcutaneous Enoxaparin in Non-Q-Wave Coronary Events Study Group. *N Engl J Med.* 1997;337(7):447–452.

55. Antman EM, McCabe CH, Gurfinkel EP, et al. Enoxaparin prevents death and cardiac ischemic

events in unstable angina/non-Q-wave myocardial infarction. Results of the thrombolysis in myocardial infarction (TIMI) 11B trial. *Circulation.* 1999;100(15):1593–1601.

56. Ferguson JJ, Califf RM, Antman EM, et al. Enoxaparin vs unfractionated heparin in high-risk patients with non-ST-segment elevation acute coronary syndromes managed with an intended early invasive strategy: primary results of the SYNERGY randomized trial. *JAMA.* 2004;292(1):45–54.

57. Boneu B, Necciari J, Cariou R, et al. Pharmacokinetics and tolerance of the natural pentasaccharide (SR90107/Org31540) with high affinity to antithrombin III in man. *Thromb Haemost.* 1995;74(6):1468–1473.

58. Yusuf S, Mehta SR, Chrolavicius S, et al. Comparison of fondaparinux and enoxaparin in acute coronary syndromes. *N Engl J Med.* 2006;354(14):1464–1476.

59. Yusuf S, Mehta SR, Chrolavicius S, et al. Effects of fondaparinux on mortality and reinfarction in patients with acute ST-segment elevation myocardial infarction: the OASIS-6 randomized trial. *JAMA.* 2006;295(13):1519–1530.

60. Nowak G, Schror K. Hirudin—the long and stony way from an anticoagulant peptide in the saliva of medicinal leech to a recombinant drug and beyond. A historical piece. *Thromb Haemost.* 2007;98(1):116–119.

61. White CM. Thrombin-directed inhibitors: pharmacology and clinical use. *Am Heart J.* 2005; 149(1 suppl):S54–S60.

62. Lincoff AM, Bittl JA, Harrington RA, et al. Bivalirudin and provisional glycoprotein IIb/IIIa blockade compared with heparin and planned glycoprotein IIb/IIIa blockade during percutaneous coronary intervention: REPLACE-2 randomized trial. *JAMA.* 2003;289 (7): 853–863.

63. Stone GW, McLaurin BT, Cox DA, et al. Bivalirudin for patients with acute coronary syndromes. *N Engl J Med.* 2006;355(21): 2203–2216.

64. Stone GW, White HD, Ohman EM, et al. Bivalirudin in patients with acute coronary syndromes undergoing percutaneous coronary intervention: a subgroup analysis from the Acute Catheterization and Urgent Intervention Triage strategy (ACUITY) trial. *Lancet.* 2007;369(9565): 907–919.

65. Stone GW, Witzenbichler B, Guagliumi G, et al. Bivalirudin during primary PCI in acute myocardial infarction. *N Engl J Med.* 2008;358(21): 2218–2230.

7

Moderate Sedation in Diagnostic and Therapeutic Cardiovascular Procedures

CHRISTINA M. MATADIAL AND RICARDO MARTINEZ-RUIZ

onscious sedation, more accurately termed "sedation/analgesia" or "moderate sedation," describes a state in which patients are able to tolerate unpleasant procedures while maintaining adequate cardiorespiratory function as well as the ability to respond purposefully to verbal commands and tactile stimulation. Moderate sedation does not refer to medications given for postoperative pain relief, premedication, or pain control during labor and delivery. The ability to independently maintain a patent airway is an important distinguishing feature of moderate sedation. Deep sedation, which involves the use of medications to induce a controlled state of depressed consciousness or unconsciousness, may also cause partial or complete loss of protective reflexes including the ability to independently and continuously maintain a patent airway. The deeply sedated patient may not be easily aroused and may not purposefully respond to verbal commands or physical stimulation (1). Only anesthesia providers may administer deep sedation. It should be recognized that sedation is a continuum. A patient may progress from one degree of sedation to another depending on his or her underlying medical status, the medication(s) administered, and the dosage and route of administration. It is important, therefore, that the monitoring and staffing requirements be based on the patient's acuity and the potential response of the patient to the procedure. Progress from one level of sedation to another requires appropriate changes in monitoring and observation of the patient.

The responsibilities of those care providers, physicians or nurses, administering moderate sedation is to prepare and monitor the patient before, during, and after the procedure. Informed consent, including options and risks, for both the procedure and the level of sedation must be obtained prior to the procedure and prior to the patient's sedative medication. For outpatient procedures, before sedating the patient, discharge and follow-up instructions may need to be given to the patient and/or the person responsible for transporting the patient postsedation (2).

In the 1980s, anesthesiology's role in sedation was to intersperse requests for help with sedation among surgical cases, especially in patients with multiple, significant comorbidities in whom sedation was anticipated to be difficult. The anesthesiologist's first priority is always the operating suite. Hence, there was more likely to be time for sedation cases in low-volume hospitals, but as facility volumes (mostly surgical) increased, anesthesiologists became increasingly absorbed by the demands of surgery. As the demand for anesthesia providers became greater than the supply, the use of nonanesthesia providers grew and spread to more sites within and soon beyond the hospital. With the introduction of midazolam in the mid-1980s, moderate sedation grew in demand. Compared with diazepam, midazolam enjoyed a far steeper dose–response curve, much greater potency, and faster onset. Unfortunately, these advantages resulted in more than 80 early deaths when used by proceduralists accustomed to rapid bolus administration in darkened rooms with little or no patient monitoring. Those deaths and a growing awareness that sedation by nonanesthesia personnel, particularly in combination with narcotic drugs, posed substantial morbidity and mortality risks, prompted the Joint Commission on Accreditation of Healthcare Organizations (JCAHO) in the early 1990s to promulgate explicit sedation standards. The Commission required processes inherent in monitored anesthesia care (MAC) (e.g., presedation assessment, intraprocedure patient monitoring, discharge criteria), as well as monitoring and evaluation of sedation practices throughout the hospital by the anesthesia department (3).

■ TERMINOLOGY

Many organizations have defined different levels of sedation. These definitions are consistent among the organizations and are clearly outlined by the American Society of Anesthesiologists (ASA).

Minimal sedation (anxiolysis) is a drug-induced state during which patients respond normally to verbal commands. Although cognitive function and coordination may be impaired, ventilatory and cardiovascular functions are unaffected.

Moderate sedation (conscious sedation) is a drug-induced depression of consciousness during which patients respond purposefully to verbal commands. *NOTE: Reflex withdrawal from a painful stimulus is not considered a purposeful response, either alone or accompanied by light tactile stimulation.* No interventions are required to maintain a patient airway, and spontaneous ventilation is adequate. Cardiovascular function is usually maintained.

Deep sedation is a drug-induced depression of consciousness during which patients cannot be easily aroused, but respond purposefully after repeated or painful stimulation. The ability to independently maintain ventilatory function may be impaired. Patients may require assistance in maintaining a patent airway and spontaneous ventilation may be inadequate. Cardiovascular function is usually maintained.

General anesthesia is a drug-induced loss of consciousness during which patients are not arousable, even by painful stimulation. The ability to independently maintain ventilatory function is often impaired. Patients often require assistance in maintaining a patent airway, and positive pressure ventilation may be required because of depressed spontaneous ventilation or drug-induced depression of neuromuscular function. Cardiovascular function may be impaired. Because sedation is a continuum, it is not always possible to predict how an individual patient will respond. Hence, practitioners intending to produce a given level of sedation should be able to rescue patients whose level of sedation becomes deeper than initially intended. Individuals administering moderate sedation/analgesia (conscious sedation) should be able to rescue patients who enter a state of deep sedation/analgesia, whereas those administering deep sedation should be able to rescue patients who enter a state of general anesthesia (4).

Moderate sedation is part of a spectrum of drug-induced alteration in consciousness. This spectrum can range from minimal sedation (anxiolysis) through general anesthesia (Table 7-1).

■ CARDIOLOGY PROCEDURES REQUIRING MODERATE SEDATION

The cardiac catheterization laboratory (CCL) has evolved into a multimodal interventional suite in which patients undergo various diagnostic and therapeutic procedures. Cardiologists, surgeons, and interventional radiologists continue to develop protocols for procedures performed in the CCL, and patient needs are ever-changing because of the increased complexity of procedures. As the complexity of procedures increases, the monitoring and sedation requirements increase as well.

Procedures performed in the CCL may include, but are not limited to, diagnostic angiography, percutaneous coronary interventions,

TABLE 7-1   **Range of Sedation**

Category	Minimal Sedation (Anxiolysis)	Moderate Sedation/Analgesia ("Conscious Sedation")	Deep Sedation/Analgesia	General Anesthesia
Responsiveness	Normal response to verbal stimulation	Purposeful response to verbal or tactile stimulation	Purposeful response following repeated or painful stimulation	Unarousable even with painful stimulus
Airway	Unaffected	No intervention required	Intervention may be required	Intervention often required
Spontaneous ventilation	Unaffected	Adequate	May be inadequate	Frequently inadequate
Cardiovascular function	Unaffected	Usually maintained	Usually maintained	May be impaired

(From Practice guidelines for sedation and analgesia by non-anesthesiologists: an updated report by the American Society of Anesthesiologists Task Force on Sedation and Analgesia by Non-Anesthesiologists. *Anesthesiology.* 2002;96(4):1004–1017.)

valvuloplasty, percutaneous valve replacement and repair, electrophysiology mapping studies, and radiofrequency ablations of arrhythmias. Endovascular repair of both thoracic aortic aneurysms and abdominal aortic aneurysms (AAAs), transcatheter closure of atrial septal defects, implantation of pacing and defibrillator devices and even the placement of percutaneous ventricular assist devices (pVAD) are also performed in the CCL.

Sedation for Pediatric Procedures

Similar to adult procedures, interventional procedures in infants and children may be lengthy, and the potential exists for hemodynamic instability and significant blood loss. The scope and practice of pediatric cardiac catheterization have continued to expand as well, and now include a multitude of interventional procedures. Because noninvasive imaging with echocardiography and/or magnetic resonance scanning is frequently used for anatomic diagnosis, cardiac catheterization is reserved for smaller, more critically ill patients with complex congenital heart disease who may require interventional procedures and diagnostic imaging prior to surgical intervention.

Some procedures, such as device closure of an atrial septal defect, may be accomplished with deep sedation and spontaneous ventilation in children. However, general anesthesia with endotracheal intubation is commonly performed in infants and children undergoing procedures such as balloon valvuloplasty, coiling of aortopulmonary collaterals, dilation or stenting of pulmonary arteries, balloon dilatation of coarctation of the aorta, and device closure of a ventricular septal defect.

Up to 25% of children with congenital heart disease have syndromes or other anomalies that may affect their anesthesia care and require optimization prior to a procedure. Interventional cardiology procedures may involve considerable physiologic perturbation, and the cardiovascular status of the pediatric patient, as well as the extent of the procedure should be considered carefully before proceeding with any anesthetic technique (5).

■ PRINCIPLES OF SEDATION

As diagnostic and interventional catheterizations are performed on patients with higher number of comorbidities and with increasingly complex pathology, skillful physiologic monitoring becomes critical in maintaining stable hemodynamics and in managing rapidly any complications that may occur during the procedure. Proper application of sedation to obtain the required depth of sedation requires thorough consideration of the optimal anesthetic technique and familiarity with multiple aspects of sedation, including patient and procedure factors, the pharmacology of the medications in use, and the ability to recognize and manage issues arising from the wide variability in these factors.

Dose Titration

A key principle in the administration of sedative agents is that drugs must be titrated in incremental doses to a desired sedative effect. Although certain patient characteristics may help predict the dosage required to achieve adequate sedation to complete the procedure (e.g., patient's age, comorbidities, body mass, race, previous responses to sedation, and current use of oral narcotics or benzodiazepines), it is impossible to predict accurately the exact dose that will be successful in a given patient. This is because the pharmacologic response of individual patients to specific agents is variable. Therefore, the practicing provider attempting to achieve moderate sedation must deliver an initial bolus selected through a process of clinical estimation and then titrate the drug by incremental dosing to the desired effect. The general process is to start with a low dose; assess the response of the patient's sedation level, ventilatory function, and cardiovascular status; and proceed gradually with titration. Knowledge of pharmacokinetic properties of the agents used is critical. However, it is reasonable to expect that for any given sedative or analgesic, the range of individual responses is three- to fivefold. For this reason, training in any regimen directed toward moderate sedation should include a period of observation of an expert performing the administration of sedation, followed by a period of supervised administration in which a mentor supervises the trainee in selecting doses and performing patient assessment.

Synergistic Effects

Another important general principle of targeting moderate sedation is that combinations of drugs in different classes typically have synergistic effects rather than just additive effects. Therefore, administration of even a small amount of narcotics can substantially reduce the amount of either benzodiazepines or propofol required to perform endoscopy. Understanding the impact of the synergistic effects on appropriate dosage selection is a critical aspect of the training process for administration of moderate sedation.

Time to Onset of Action

A final general principle that nonanesthesiologists must understand is that each sedative agent has unique properties with regard to the length of time between intravenous (IV) injection, onset of sedative action, and the peak effect of the drug. If additional boluses of agent are given before earlier boluses have been allowed to peak, then sedative effects may accumulate rapidly and push patients to deeper than desired levels of sedation. Therefore, each agent must be allowed an appropriate length of time to reach its peak effect before injecting additional boluses of the drug, both during the initial titration process and during the maintenance phase of sedation. For example, midazolam has a longer interval to peak effect (8 to 12 minutes) than diazepam (2 to 5 minutes). Combined with its increased potency relative to diazepam, this effect contributed to the deaths of 73 persons reported to the Food and Drug Administration (FDA) and attributed to midazolam in the first 4 years after its introduction.

■ PRESEDATION CONSIDERATIONS

Patients presenting for moderate sedation should undergo a focused physical examination, including vital signs, auscultation of the heart and lungs, and evaluation of the airway (see "airway assessment"). Preprocedure laboratory testing should be guided by the patient's underlying medical condition and the likelihood that the results will affect the management of sedation. These evaluations should be confirmed immediately before sedation is initiated (6).

Clinicians administering moderate sedation should be familiar with the patient's medical history and how it might alter the patient's response to hypnotic agents. Things to be on the lookout for include the following:

- Abnormalities of the major organ systems
- Previous adverse experience with anesthesia
- Drug allergies, current medications, and potential drug interactions
- Time and nature of last oral intake

- History of tobacco, alcohol, or substance use or abuse
- Factors predictive of airway difficulties

Airway Assessment for Sedation

How easy or difficult it will be to intubate a patient depends on these important points. Do they have a short neck and small mouth? Are they obese, and to what extent can they open their mouth? Is there any soft tissue swelling at the back of the mouth or any limitations in neck flexion or extension (rheumatoid arthritis or ankylosing spondylitis). Some airway abnormalities may increase the likelihood of airway obstruction during spontaneous ventilation.

Many factors should be taken into account when assessing an airway (Table 7-2), including history and physical examination (including airway assessment).

TABLE 7-2	Approach to Airway Assessment Procedures for Sedation and Analgesia

History
Previous problems with anesthesia or sedation
Stridor, snoring, or sleep apnea
Advanced rheumatoid arthritis
Chromosomal abnormality (e.g., trisomy 21)

Physical examination

Habitus
Significant obesity (especially involving the neck and facial structures)

Head and neck
Short neck, limited neck extension, decreased hyoid–mental distance (≤3 cm in an adult), neck mass, cervical spine disease or trauma, tracheal deviation, dysmorphic facial features (e.g., Pierre–Robin syndrome)

Mouth
Small opening (<3 cm in an adult); edentulous; protruding incisors; loose or capped teeth; dental appliances; high, arched palate; macroglossia; tonsillar hypertrophy; nonvisible uvula

Jaw
Micrognathia, retrognathia, trismus, significant malocclusion

(Adapted from Practice guidelines for sedation and analgesia by non-anesthesiologists: an updated report by the American Society of Anesthesiologists Task Force on Sedation and Analgesia by Non-Anesthesiologists. *Anesthesiology.* 2002;96(4):1004–1017.)

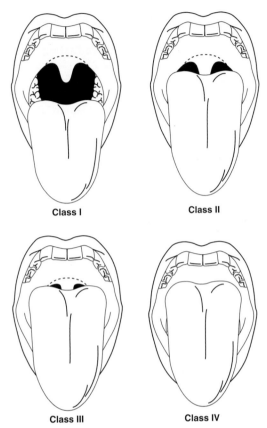

FIGURE 7-1. Mallampati classification. Class I: can see soft palate, anterior and posterior tonsillar pillars, and uvula. Class II: cannot see tonsillar pillars. Class III: only uvula base can be seen. Class IV: cannot see uvula at all. (From Blackbourne LH. *Advanced Surgical Recall.* 2nd ed. Baltimore, MD: Lippincott Williams & Wilkins, 2004.)

The Mallampati scoring system uses a simple visual scale to grade each patient based on the visual vertical distance between the tongue and soft palate or uvula at the back of the pharynx (Fig. 7-1). Grade I shows a large vertical distance between the uvula and the base of the tongue, and you could imagine that this patient is a lot easier to intubate than a patient with a grade IV score (7).

Fasting Guidelines for Moderate Sedation

Although the goals of moderate sedation are anxiolysis and analgesia with preservation of laryngeal and pharyngeal reflexes, the possibility of entering into deep sedation is always present. For this reason, the fasting guidelines for deep sedation and anesthesia should also apply to patients undergoing moderate sedation (Table 7-3).

TABLE 7-3	Summary of American Society of Anesthesiologists Preprocedure Fasting Guidelines

Ingested Material	Minimum Fasting Period[a] (h)
Clear liquids[b]	2
Breast milk	4
Infant formula	6
Nonhuman milk[c]	6
Light meal[d]	6

These recommendations apply to healthy patients who are undergoing elective procedures. They are not intended for women in labor. Following the Guidelines does not guarantee complete gastric emptying has occurred.
[a]The fasting periods apply to all ages.
[b]Examples of clear liquids include water, fruit juices without pulp, carbonated beverages, clear tea, and black coffee.
[c]Since nonhuman milk is similar to solids in gastric emptying time, the amount ingested must be considered when determining an appropriate fasting period.
[d]A light meal typically consists of toast and clear liquids. Meals that include fried or fatty foods or meat may prolong gastric emptying time. Both the amount and type of foods ingested must be considered when determining an appropriate fasting period.[8]
(From Practice guidelines for sedation and analgesia by non-anesthesiologists: an updated report by the American Society of Anesthesiologists Task Force on Sedation and Analgesia by Non-Anesthesiologists. *Anesthesiology.* 2002;96(4):1004–1017.)

It is important to note that some conditions will result in a full stomach, or risk of aspiration, despite adequate preprocedure fasting guidelines. These conditions include pregnancy, acute abdominal pathology (peritonitis, bowel obstruction), severe gastrointestinal reflux, hiatal hernia, morbid obesity (BMI > 40), esophageal dysmotility, previous esophageal surgery, long-standing diabetes mellitus, increased intracranial pressure, and multiple trauma. Such patients are not good candidates for sedation and should be managed by an anesthesia provider with possible endotracheal intubation for the procedure.

Presedation Assessment and Plan

Because sedation carries risks, administration of sedation is part of a planned process. A sedation plan is developed to meet each patient's needs identified through a presedation assessment. A presedation assessment is required prior to administration of sedation. The presedation assessment must be documented in the patient's medical record. This assessment must be reviewed with respect to the patient's condition immediately **prior to** administration of sedation by the practitioner directing the sedation. A presedation assessment includes but is not limited to the following:

1. Physical status assessment (review of systems, vital signs, airway, cardiopulmonary reserve), past and present drug history including drug allergies
2. Previous adverse experience with sedation and analgesia as well as with regional and general anesthesia
3. Results of relevant diagnostic studies
4. Verification of patient NPO status
5. Assignment of physical status classification using ASA Physical Status Classification (Table 7-4) (9)
6. Informed consent—should clearly document that moderate sedation is planned

Candidates for sedation shall be in good general medical health and have adequate ventilatory reserve. For patients who have significant medical problems (e.g., severe systemic disease, morbid obesity, sleep apnea, upper or lower structural airway abnormalities), consideration shall be given for consultation with an anesthesiologist or an attending physician specializing in the primary disease process affecting the patient.

Immediately prior to moderate sedation, baseline values of blood pressure, heart rate, respiratory rate, oxygen saturation, and responses to verbal stimuli or level of consciousness shall be recorded.

IV moderate sedation requires continuous IV access until the patient has recovered. This can be accomplished with an indwelling catheter with or without IV fluid administration. In patients receiving moderate sedation by non-IV routes or whose IV access has become nonfunctional, the practitioner directing the moderate sedation shall determine the advisability of establishing or reestablishing IV access. In all circumstances, an individual capable of establishing IV access should be readily available.

| TABLE 7-4 | American Society of Anesthesiologists Physical Status Classification System |

Class[a]	Description
ASA 1	A normal healthy patient
ASA 2	A patient with mild systemic disease
ASA 3	A patient with severe systemic disease
ASA 4	A patient with severe systemic disease that is a constant threat to life
ASA 5	A moribund patient who is not expected to survive without the operation
ASA 6	A declared brain-dead patient whose organs are being removed for donor purposes

[a]The addition of the letter E to the ASA status denotes an emergency procedure.
(Adapted from Practice guidelines for sedation and analgesia by non-anesthesiologists: an updated report by the American Society of Anesthesiologists Task Force on Sedation and Analgesia by Non-Anesthesiologists. *Anesthesiology.* 2002;96(4):1004–1017.)

■ MONITORING

A monitoring individual must be present to continuously assess patient's well-being and facilitate patient's safety and comfort, and maintain, support, and record vital signs of the patient at appropriate intervals (see the following text). This individual shall not be the technical assistant and have no other responsibilities that will leave the patient unattended or compromise continuous monitoring.

Heart rate, blood pressure, oxygen saturation, and electrocardiogram should be monitored continuously. Capnography, although not a standard of care and not always readily available, can be used as a way to further assess the effectiveness of the patient's respiratory efforts while sedated, especially in situations in which access to the head and airway are limited, and when the patient is placed in a position other than supine.

The following items must be monitored and recorded at 5-minute intervals or more frequently, if indicated, on a time-based record:

1. Blood pressure, heart rate, respiratory rate, and oxygen saturation
2. Responses to verbal stimuli or level of consciousness
3. Medications and dosages

■ PHARMACOLOGY

No one drug fits the needs of all sedation cases.

The choice of sedative should take into consideration certain variables, such as pain threshold of the procedure, the need for amnesia, and the need for altered level of consciousness.

Phenothiazine and Buterophenone Sedatives

These sedatives include chlorpromazine, prochlorperazine, and droperidol. These drugs have good sedative properties, as well as muscle relaxant, antiemetic, and antiarrhythmogenic effects. They have no analgesic activity, but when administered with other anesthetics can potentiate their effect. Droperidol is not widely used anymore because of recent FDA warnings regarding prolonged QT interval associated with its use. Cases of QT prolongation and/or torsade de pointes have been reported in patients receiving Droperidol at doses at or below recommended doses. Some cases have occurred in patients with no known risk factors for QT prolongation and some cases have been fatal (10). Disadvantages of these sedatives are that they are α-adrenergic blockers and cause peripheral vasodilation, which can lead to hypothermia. Chlorpromazine decreases seizure threshold, and it is relatively contraindicated in CNS lesions. Because these sedatives lack analgesic activity, it is important to realize that any painful stimulation of the patient may cause reflex movement and withdrawal from the painful source.

Benzodiazepines

The benzodiazepines include diazepam, midazolam, and alprazolam. These drugs are antianxiety and anticonvulsant drugs with good muscle relaxant activity. They have minimal cardiovascular and respiratory effects. The primary use of these drugs in moderate sedation is in combination with other drugs, such as opiates.

Opiates

The opiates, sometimes referred to as "narcotics," are a large class of drugs that exert their effects on opiate receptors in the central nervous system. Depending on the type of opiate receptors the drug binds, and depending on the type of action on the receptor, the effects of narcotics can be primarily analgesic, or a mixture of analgesia and euphoria with sedation. Opiates generally are cardiostable; however, there can be significant respiratory depression, as well as other side effects such as nausea and vomiting, delayed gastric emptying, hypotension, and bradycardia.

Antihistamines

Diphenhydramine is the commonly used antihistamine in most centers. It is an H_1-receptor antagonist with anticholinergic and sedative effects. It is also used as an antiemetic. It has synergistic effects when used with opioids and benzodiazepines.

Other Agents Used in Sedation

Although mentioned here in this chapter, the drugs listed in the following text are commonly used to achieve a deeper level of sedation, titrated by an anesthesia provider with knowledge and expertise in managing untoward side effects of the medications.

Propofol

Propofol is used as an alternative to standard benzodiazepine and opioid-based regimens for various reasons. Advantages of propofol over traditional agents include ultra-short onset of action of approximately 30 to 60 seconds (through rapid redistribution throughout the entire body) with peak effect in 1 to 3 minutes, short half-life, minimal risk of nausea, and short recovery time. For example, among patients who had previously received a combination of midazolam and meperidine for colonoscopy, 85% preferred propofol sedation.

However, some characteristics of propofol can make it difficult to use for moderate sedation. As the drug has no analgesic effects, patients may experience agitation, confusion, and withdrawal from painful stimuli when under moderate sedation. Because propofol has a relative narrow therapeutic range, it must be titrated carefully to achieve moderate sedation without inadvertently inducing deeper levels of sedation. Patients can quickly slip from moderate to deep sedation risking life-threatening respiratory depression. Unlike opioids and benzodiazepines, propofol cannot be quickly reversed pharmacologically. There is no antagonist for propofol, so patients experiencing overdose will need assistance with ventilation until spontaneous ventilation resumes. Propofol can also cause a drop in blood pressure and heart rate. Additionally, propofol is vulnerable to microbial contamination and once drawn up should be used within a few hours.

Nurse-administered propofol sedation (NAPS) involves the administration of propofol by a registered nurse (RN) under the supervision of a medical practitioner. The nurse's sole responsibility during the procedure is for the administration of propofol through physician-ordered titration and patient monitoring. The goal is to anticipate the portions of the endoscopy that may be more painful or stimulating, and administer propofol to achieve a deeper level of sedation while monitoring for airway obstruction, as well as respiratory rate and other vital signs. With NAPS, propofol is used as a monotherapy for moderate sedation. NAPS was the initial model for nonanesthesiologist-administered propofol (11).

The use of propofol by nonanesthesiologists is off-label. The current dispensing literature notes that for general anesthesia or MAC sedation, propofol should be administered only by persons trained in the administration of general anesthesia and not involved in the conduct of the surgical/diagnostic procedure.

The American Association of Nurse Anesthetists and American Society of Anesthesiology (AANA–ASA) issued a Joint Statement

Regarding Propofol Administration on April 14, 2004 (12) (See http://www.aana.com/news.aspx?id=761):

> Because sedation is a continuum, it is not always possible to predict how an individual patient will respond. Due to the potential for rapid, profound changes in sedative/anesthetic depth and the lack of antagonistic medications, agents such as propofol require special attention. Whenever propofol is used for sedation/anesthesia, it should be administered only by persons trained in the administration of general anesthesia, who are not simultaneously involved in these surgical or diagnostic procedures. This restriction is concordant with specific language in the propofol package insert, and failure to follow these recommendations could put patients at increased risk of significant injury or death. Similar concerns apply when other IV induction agents are used for sedation, such as thiopental, methohexital, or etomidate.

The ASA maintains that propofol is a drug meant only for use in a medical setting by professionals trained in the provision of general anesthesia.

Dexmedetomidine

Dexmedetomidine HCl, an imidazole compound, is the pharmacologically active S-enantiomer of medetomidine. The agent's sedative, anxiolytic, and analgesic effects are produced through specific and selective activation of postsynaptic α_2-adrenoreceptors. It is approximately eight times more selective for the α_2-adrenergic receptor than clonidine and is 1,620 times more potent as an α_2-adrenergic receptor agonist than as an α_1-adrenergic receptor agonist.

The recommended dexmedetomidine dose is an IV infusion bolus of 1 mcg/kg over a 10-minute period, followed by a continuous IV infusion of 0.2 to 0.7 mcg/kg per hour. The maintenance dose should be titrated until the sedation goal is reached. It is not necessary to discontinue dexmedetomidine before, during, or after extubation. Doses up to 2.5 mcg/kg per hour for up to 7 days, with no rebound effect on withdrawal and no compromise in hemodynamic stability have been used in clinical trials. Dexmedetomidine is as effective as propofol and midazolam for producing and maintaining

adequate short-term sedation of critically ill, mechanically ventilated patients. The benefits of dexmedetomidine over currently available sedative agents include its lack of respiratory depression and its ability to decrease the need for opioid analgesics (13).

Although a review of the literature produced anecdotal information regarding the efficacy and safety of dexmedetomidine in moderate sedation cases, its use as a mainstream drug for noncritical care or nonoperative settings remains yet to be established.

Fospropofol

Fospropofol is an IV, sedative-hypnotic agent indicated for sedation in adult patients undergoing diagnostic or therapeutic procedures. The primary action of fospropofol is to produce sedation or general anesthesia. Fospropofol is a water-soluble prodrug that is rapidly hydrolyzed in patients and derives its sedative and anesthetic actions by releasing propofol into the blood and tissues. The primary anesthetic action of the active metabolite propofol is thought to be produced by positive modulation of the inhibitory function of the neurotransmitter gama-aminobutyric acid (GABA) through GABA-A receptors.

Although fospropofol is not primarily marketed to produce general anesthesia, it shares many of the properties and side effects of its primary metabolite propofol, which is a general anesthetic. These properties include respiratory and cardiovascular depression, and rapid loss of consciousness. Individual responses to propofol vary considerably because of wide differences in its concentration–response curve in different individuals. Because of this variability in its active product, the response to the administration of fospropofol can be unpredictable in that a small dose might produce a minimal effect, but a repeated dose could suddenly produce a profound anesthetic effect. Obviously, this would be particularly dangerous in the uncontrolled environment (14).

In 2008, the ASA submitted formal comments and testified before the FDA's Anesthetic and Life Support Drugs Advisory Committee (ALSDAC) requesting that the labeling for fospropofol disodium injection 35 mg/mL (fospropofol) include a similar warning to that which is included on the label for propofol.

Because fospropofol is a prodrug and it is metabolized in the blood stream into propofol, for patient safety reasons the ASA believes that the drug should be administered only by persons trained in the administration of general anesthesia and not involved in the conduct of the surgical/diagnostic procedure (15).

■ RISKS AND COMPLICATIONS

Cardiopulmonary events related to sedation and analgesia are the most frequent causes of procedure-related morbidity and mortality. These complications range in severity from transient, minor oxygen desaturation to life-threatening events such as apnea, shock/hypotension, and myocardial infarction. Severe oxygen desaturation is rare, but some level of desaturation is estimated to occur in up to 70% of patients.

Respiratory Depression

The patient's level of consciousness, pulmonary ventilation, oxygenation, and hemodynamics should be monitored continuously during moderate or deep sedation (see section on monitoring). Lack of response to verbal stimulation is often the first sign of impending respiratory depression. In addition to clinical observation, however, pulse oximetry and capnography are valuable adjuncts for detecting early signs of respiratory depression.

Cardiac Arrhythmias and Hemodynamic Instability

Rare cases of ventricular tachycardia and cardiac arrest due to ventricular fibrillation have been reported. Continuous ECG monitoring is recommended for patients who are undergoing deep sedation or have existing cardiac or pulmonary disease.

Sedation can cause both hypertension and hypotension. Pain can cause blood pressure to rise. Benzodiazepines used alone generally cause a mild drop in blood pressure. However, sedation with a benzodiazepine–opioid combination can lead to a more profound drop as can the administration of propofol. Monitoring heart rate and blood pressure every 5 minutes throughout sedation is recommended. Blood pressure should be determined before sedation/analgesia is established when possible (16).

Paradoxical Reactions

A state of excitement can occur in some patients as a reaction to sedation with benzodiazepines, which can prevent the performance of an endoscopic procedure. These so-called paradoxical reactions can include excessive talkativeness, movement, and emotional release. Certain factors predispose a patient to having a paradoxical reaction; however, these reactions are relatively uncommon, occurring in less than 1% of cases (17).

Predisposing patient characteristics for paradoxical reactions include the following:

- Young and advanced age
- Genetic predisposition
- Alcoholism or drug abuse
- Psychiatric and/or personality disorders

Other Non–Sedation-Related Risks

The use of fluoroscopy and X-radiation are prominent in the CCL; therefore, it is imperative that all personnel strictly adhere to the following three radiation safety principles: maximize distance from the radiation source, minimize exposure times, and always use proper shielding with leaded glass, acrylic, gowns, gloves, thyroid collars, and stands. Dosimeters must be worn at all times to help track cumulative exposure, and practitioners should keep all radiation doses "as low as reasonably achievable" (the ALARA principle), a concept fully supported by the radiation safety program at the Centers for Disease Control and Prevention.

Patients with pacing devices and implantable cardioverter-defibrillator devices (ICDs) should be observed carefully in the CCL. When using electrocautery, exit pads should be placed in positions that direct electrical current away from pacing and ICD leads; otherwise suppression of pacing and inappropriate triggering of ICDs may occur. Because of the negative effects of electromagnetic interference, a transdermal magnet should be available at all times to convert pacemakers into asynchronous mode and also to suppress antitachycardiac therapies on ICDs. When specifically working on a pacing device, the practitioner must be aware of the presence of unipolar leads; if the generator loses physical contact with the patient on a unipolar lead setup, the device will be unable to pace because of an open circuit, and immediate means for backup pacing must be readily available to avoid hemodynamic compromise.

There is always the potential for a catastrophe, such as acute blood loss during the stenting of a tortuous AAA due to perforation or rupture of the aneurysm. The presence of a rapid transfusion device and experienced colleagues and assistants are imperative, including access to laboratory, anesthesia providers for advanced airway management, and surgical colleagues in the event that the CCL is converted into an operating suite, and the need for frequent blood sampling and rapid transfusion is immediate.

■ RESCUE TECHNIQUES

The risk for complications while providing moderate and deep sedation is greatest when caring for patients already medically compromised. In most cases, significant untoward events can generally be prevented by careful preoperative assessment, along with attentive intraoperative monitoring and support. Nevertheless, we must be prepared to manage untoward events should they arise.

■ RESPIRATORY COMPLICATIONS

Assessment of Respiration

The management of any medical emergency should commence with a primary assessment, with emphasis on the airway, breathing, and circulation (ABCs) taught during all courses of basic life support. Although it is common and appropriate for the procedure team to assess these parameters simultaneously, airway patency must be given initial priority. The airway should be assessed for obstruction. The head should be tilted back while the chin is lifted, and the mouth and throat examined for any foreign material. In the unconscious patient, it may be necessary to perform a "jaw-thrust" maneuver in addition to the head-tilt, chin-lift procedure. Once the airway is in an optimal position, attention can be placed on ventilation. Asking a sedated but conscious patient to take a slow, deep breath at regular intervals may be enough to restore normal oxygen saturation. If the patient is unconscious, the monitoring operator should "look, listen, and feel" for ventilatory effort and airflow. A useful maneuver may be to place one hand over the face and nostrils and

feel for breathing, or over the diaphragm, since during quiet breathing the chest does not always raise noticeably. If breathing is still in question, a stethoscope can be used to auscultate the apices of the lungs for breath sounds. The carotid pulse can be palpated either during or following this assessment.

While airway patency and breathing are being assessed by the practitioner, other portions of primary assessment can be performed simultaneously by additional team members.

Oxygen Supplementation

The equipment required to provide supplemental oxygen includes a 100% oxygen source, a regulator, tubing, and either a nasal cannula or mask and suction system. Every office and procedure area should be equipped with at least a portable E-cylinder of oxygen. These E-cylinders should be replaced when their content falls below 1,000 psi to ensure appropriate O_2 supply.

The nasal cannula is suitable for administering supplemental oxygen to conscious patients who may less well tolerate a mask. Flow rates of 4 L/min may be adequate supplementation for most situations in which the patient is breathing.

The nonrebreather mask with a reservoir may be appropriate to deliver higher oxygen concentrations to unconscious, breathing patients. When using any mask, the flow rate should be at least 6 L/min. Provided the mask has a reservoir, this flow rate will deliver an oxygen concentration of 60%, and each additional L/min will increase FIO_2 by approximately 5%.

Advanced Airway Intervention

The apneic patient is usually unconsciousness and will require positive pressure ventilation. Bag-valve-mask (BVM) devices with reservoirs can provide 90% to 95% oxygen concentrations, but their proper use requires considerable skill on the part of the operator. Proper head position, effective mask seal, and bag compression are essential skills that must be developed if they are to be used effectively. If ventilation remains difficult, airway adjuncts are indicated.

Oropharyngeal and nasopharyngeal airways are adjuncts that improve airway patency by keeping the mouth open and preventing the base of the tongue from sagging against the posterior pharyngeal wall. Some styles of airway are hollow and facilitate the insertion of a suction catheter to clear the pharynx of secretions.

When attempting to ventilate an apneic patient, a reasonable stepped approach is to attempt ventilation with a BVM alone, followed, if necessary, by insertion of an oropharyngeal airway. If this proves inadequate, one must consider advanced airway adjuncts such as tracheal intubation or insertion of a laryngeal mask airway (LMA). Tracheal intubation is the gold standard of airway adjuncts. However, its use is limited to those having advanced anesthesia training such as oral and maxillofacial surgeons, dentists, and anesthesiologists. If intubation is unsuccessful or if the provider is not trained in this procedure, an LMA has gained status as the "second-best" airway adjunct because it is reasonably effective and technically less difficult to insert. The LMA is an airway adjunct that fits over the top of the larynx. The apex of the mask is inserted in the mouth, advanced toward the uvula, and continued through the natural bend of the oropharynx until it comes to rest over the pyriform fossa at the glottis. At this point, the cuff around the mask is inflated with enough air to create a relatively airtight seal. However, training in the insertion of the LMA on simulation mannequins or live patients is still necessary to be able to accomplish it successfully in an actual emergency (18).

Management of Respiratory Depression

In general, the use of sedation has a positive influence on patients undergoing procedures. By reducing fear and anxiety, there is less stress on the cardiovascular system, and vasovagal reactions are less likely to occur. When compared with local anesthesia alone, the two most significant negative variables introduced by moderate sedation, as well as deep sedation and general anesthesia, are the added risks for either respiratory depression, that is, hypoventilation, or airway obstruction.

Respiratory depression may present as a decrease in depth and/or rate of ventilation and is attributed to depression of respiratory control centers, which normally trigger breathing as carbon dioxide levels in the blood rise slightly above the normal threshold. All sedatives, opioids, and potent general anesthesia inhalation agents have the potential to depress central hypercapnic and/or peripheral hypoxemic drives, but this risk is minimal with moderate sedation, provided one uses conventional doses and monitors the patient appropriately. Nevertheless, one must be thoroughly skilled in managing respiratory depression in the event it should occur.

Like any complication, management of respiratory depression should commence with standard airway support as noted earlier.

Pharmacologic reversal of the sedative agents is indicated whenever a sedation provider is faced with an unconscious patient, since airway complications such as laryngospasm, airway obstruction, aspiration, etc., may result in apnea or failure to respond adequately to oxygen supplementation and attempts at positive pressure ventilation (Table 7-5).

Among the drug classes used for moderate sedation, opioids are the most powerful respiratory depressants. If an opioid has been included in the regimen, naloxone (Narcan) should be the first reversal drug administered. Depending on

TABLE 7-5	Reversal Agents for Moderate Sedation	
Cause of Respiratory Depression	Agent	Action/Administration/Dose
Opioids	Naloxone	Opioid receptor antagonist IV: 0.1–0.4 mg q2–3min
Benzodiazepines	Flumazenil	Benzodiazepine receptor antagonist IV: 0.2 mg q3–4min IM/SLI: 0.2 mg q4–5min Maximum _ 1 mg

(Adapted from Karch AM, ed. 2009 *Lippincott's Nursing Drug Guide*. Philadelphia, PA: Lippincott Williams & Wilkins; 2009 (19).)

the perceived urgency of the emergency treatment, it can be titrated intravenously in 0.1- to 0.4-mg increments every 3 to 5 minutes or 0.4 mg injected sublingually or intramuscularly (IM) every 5 minutes. Careful titration in no more than 0.1-mg increments is advised for any patient susceptible to cardiac irritability or hypertension. Generally, the maximum recommended dose is 0.8 mg, followed by a search for other causes if the response is inadequate. Naloxone should not be administered to a patient with a current history of opioid dependence, unless the event is life-threatening and other interventions have been futile.

Although less likely to cause respiratory depression when used alone compared with narcotics, benzodiazepines can be reversed using the specific antagonist, flumazenil (Romazicon). Depending on the perceived urgency of the emergency treatment, it can be titrated in 0.2- to 1-mg increments intravenously every 2 to 3 minutes. Although minimal research is available on the speed and efficacy of intramuscular or sublingual injections (SLI) of flumazenil in patients with benzodiazepine overdose, it may be injected via those routes if IV access is not readily available. Flumazenil should not be administered to patients having a history of dependence on benzodiazepines, a seizure disorder managed by a benzodiazepine, or evidence of tricyclic antidepressant overdose.

Management of Airway Obstruction

Laryngospasm

Airway obstruction must be distinguished from respiratory depression. Although obstruction may result in hypoventilation, the patient's actual drive to ventilate (breathe) may or may not be obtunded. Upper airway obstruction may be attributed to anatomic structures or foreign material, both of which are addressed during the initial "airway patency" portion of the primary assessment. When these procedures fail to establish patency, pathologic causes of obstruction must be considered, namely laryngospasm or laryngeal edema. These events can be distinguished visually by those trained in direct laryngoscopy, but otherwise the distinction is made empirically. Laryngospasm is a reflex closure or spasm of the glottis muscles including vocal cords. In the conscious or moderately sedated

patient, it is very transient and self-limiting in a patient with otherwise normal reflexes and anatomy. It also occurs during deep sedation or light planes of general anesthesia, but the obtunded patient may not be able to clear the irritating material, and therefore, the laryngospasm can be prolonged. It occurs frequently in children and in adults who are smokers. Most often the patient is unconscious and the head, neck, and upper torso exhibit a "bucking" or "rocking" movement as the patient's central mechanisms make attempts to ventilate against the obstruction. Rather than the upper abdomen and the chest rising simultaneously during attempts to breathe, these movements will alternate due to laryngospasm or any other type of airway obstruction. In most cases, the spasm will relax following sustained pressure using a BVM, but hypoxemia may result if the obstruction does not resolve quickly, particularly if supplemental oxygen was not being used prior to the spasm. The airway should be suctioned followed by a forceful jaw thrust to open the airway, and the BVM should then be placed with enough force to establish a tight mask seal. Gentle continuous pressure from the bag should be applied until ventilations are successful. Pharmacologic reversal of sedative agents should be considered whenever a practitioner is faced with an unconscious patient or when airway complications such as laryngospasm are diagnosed or even suspected. Once the patient has regained consciousness, the laryngeal spasm should resolve following vigorous coughing. In the event that the cords fail to relax or severe hypoxemia develops, additional pharmacologic intervention requires the use of neuromuscular blockers, such as IV succinylcholine. Generally, a very small dose (0.1 to 0.2 mg/kg) is all that is required and should only supplement the continued application of positive pressure using a BVM. A full intubating dose of succinylcholine (1 to 2 mg/kg) should be considered if direct laryngoscopy and/or tracheal intubation are anticipated. Succinylcholine is ideally administered by an anesthesia provider, or someone trained in the use of advanced airway devices.

Laryngeal Edema

Laryngeal edema is among the constellation of events associated with major allergic (anaphylactoid) reactions. The swelling of laryngeal mucosa, as well as neighboring pharyngeal mucosa and tongue, may accompany anaphylactoid reactions and will generally present as stridor or high-pitched "croaking" sounds during ventilation. The conscious patient will complain of throat tightness or tongue swelling. Management may require administration of epinephrine, which "decongests" the mucosa via vasoconstriction. It may be administered by several routes and doses listed among the other emergency drugs summarized in Table 7-5. The most conventional dose is 0.3 to 0.5 mg Subcutaneous/Intramuscular (IM). IV titration of 0.1-mg increments is reserved for more severe episodes.

Additional agents for allergic or anaphylactic reactions include antihistamines and corticosteroids. Steroids are not used for initial acute treatment because of limited efficacy and delayed onset, for example, several hours. Minor allergic reactions may manifest cutaneously such as pruritus or rash and are not life-threatening. They are attributed to histamine release and can be managed with an antihistamine such as diphenhydramine.

Bronchospasm

Bronchospasm may result from a type I anaphylactic allergic reaction or an anaphylactoid reaction, independently or in combination with laryngeal edema, or as a consequence of the hyperreactive airway typical in patients with asthma. Regardless of the cause for bronchospasm, the patient will exhibit dyspnea and wheezing attributed to obstruction in the chest, not the throat or mouth. Bronchial smooth muscle is under autonomic nervous control and requires β_2 sympathomimetics for relaxation. Following primary assessment, including oxygen supplementation, a selective β_2-agonist such as albuterol should be administered by a metered inhaler. This is preferred over epinephrine because it is less likely to produce cardiovascular side effects attributed to stimulation of cardiac β_1 receptors. In severe or refractory episodes, including status asthmaticus, parenteral epinephrine can be administered (Table 7-6).

■ CARDIOVASCULAR COMPLICATIONS

Moderate sedation and lighter levels of deep sedation usually have minimal influence on cardiovascular function. However, excessive drug dosages, including local anesthetics alone or with vasoconstrictors, and consequences of interventions, such as inadequate anesthesia, may trigger cardiovascular changes.

Vasovagal Reaction

Vasovagal reaction is a common medical complication during interventional procedures. In some cases, vagal influences are severe enough to induce transient periods of asystole. Regardless of the cause or severity, vasovagal events will generally subside during the time primary measures for assessment and airway support are instituted. Subsequently, attention must be directed toward abnormalities in blood pressure and heart rate that may or may not require pharmacologic intervention. If suspected vasovagal syncope does not spontaneously resolve quickly, and it does not respond to the administration of atropine, other much more serious conditions such as complete heart block, stroke, myocardial ischemia, and drug overdose should be considered and appropriate emergency procedures should commence.

Hypotension

The blood pressure required to perfuse tissues adequately varies from patient to patient and is influenced by their medical status and posture at the time of assessment. Numerical values that change significantly from baseline should alert the clinician, but evaluation of tissue perfusion is the most significant component of cardiovascular assessment. Color changes in the skin and mucosa and the rate of capillary refill subsequent to squeezing of the nail beds can be used as a guide for assessing perfusion of peripheral tissues prior to blood pressure measurement. The adequacy of blood perfusion within the central nervous system can be estimated by the conscious patient's response to verbal and painful stimuli, or by the papillary reflex of the unconscious or heavily sedated patient. If perfusion is considered inadequate, the practitioner may elect to increase blood pressure.

In general, a systolic pressure of 90 mm Hg should sustain mean arterial pressure sufficient to perfuse tissues in the supine patient. However, if systolic and/or diastolic pressures drop 15 to 20 mm Hg below baseline, tissue perfusion

TABLE 7-6 Emergency Drugs for Moderate Sedation

Indication	Agent	Action/Administration/Dosage
Laryngospasm	Succinylcholine	(20 mg/mL) Nicotinic receptor agonist; depolarization neuromuscular block IV: 0.1–0.2 mg/kg (5 to 20 mg)
Bronchospasm	Albuterol (metered inhaler) Epinephrine (1:1,000/1 mg/mL) (1:10,000/0.1 mg/mL)	Selective β$_2$-receptor agonist 2–3 inhalations q1–2min 3 if needed α- and β-receptor agonist IM/Subcutaneous: 0.3–0.5 mg SLI: 0.2 mg IV: 0.1 mg q3–5min based on vital signs and ECG
Laryngeal edema or anaphylaxis	Epinephrine (1:1,000/1 mg/mL) (1:10,000/0.1 mg/mL)	α- and β-receptor agonist IM/Subcutaneous: 0.3–0.5 mg SLI: 0.2 mg IV: 0.1 mg q3–5min based on vital signs and ECG
Bradycardia/hypotension	Atropine (0.4, 0.5, and 1.0 mg/mL) Ephedrine (50 mg/mL)	Cholinergic (muscarinic) receptor antagonist IV, IM/SLI: 0.5 mg q4–5min up to 2 mg if needed Releases norepinephrine; α-/β-receptor agonist IV: dilute; 1 mL in 5 mL (10 mg/mL); then 5–10 mg q5min up to 50 mg IM/SLI: (undiluted) 25 mg q5min up to 50 mg if needed
Hypotension	*Phenylephrine (10 mg/mL)	Selective α-agonist IV: (double-dilute); 1 mL in 10 mL (1 mg/mL) Then discard 9 mL and dilute remaining 1 mL in 10 mL (0.1 mg/mL); administer 0.1 mg increments q3min to 0.5 mg
Hypertension	Nitroglycerin (0.4-mg tablet) Labetalol (5 mg/mL) Morphine 2.5 mg	Venodilator topical sublingual: 1 tablet q5min α- and β-receptor antagonist IV: 10 mg q5min–0.5 mg/kg bolus if needed for desired effect. Repeat as needed Opioid receptor agonist IV: 2.5 mg q3–5min to 10 mg

(Adapted from Karch AM, ed. *2009 Lippincott's Nursing Drug Guide*. Philadelphia, PA: Lippincott Williams & Wilkins; 2009 (19).)

could be compromised and therefore should be assessed. Stroke volume and systolic pressure can be elevated in two manners:

- Improve venous return by repositioning the patient (Trendelenburg position), administering IV fluid boluses, or administering drugs that provide venoconstriction to increase venous pressure and preload (see Table 7-5).

- Increase myocardial contractility (inotropy) using drugs that activate β$_1$ receptors on myocardial cells, providing a positive inotropic influence. If a hypotensive patient exhibits syncopal signs and symptoms, continuation of the procedure should be delayed until a full primary assessment is completed. A 250 to 500 mL of physiologic solution, such as saline or Ringer's lactate, should be administered rapidly unless congestive heart failure with pulmonary edema is suspected. Generally, this will increase preload sufficiently to improve stroke volume and raise systolic pressure.

Hypotension encountered during cardiology procedures is usually attributed to either vasovagal episodes or the use of sedatives and analgesics that depress sympathetic outflow to the cardiovascular system. In either case, ephedrine specifically counters these influences indirectly by stimulating norepinephrine release from sympathetic nerve endings. Ephedrine can be administered intravenously in 5- to 10-mg increments every 3 to 5 minutes, or 25 mg of ephedrine can be administered by intramuscular injection. Exceeding a total dose of 50 mg is not recommended.

Sometimes, hypotension may be accompanied by tachycardia, so the cardiotonic effects of ephedrine may be undesirable. This situation occurs most often when hypotension is the result of hypovolemia or dehydration.

Phenylephrine is an α-adrenergic agonist that is useful for treating hypotension when tachycardia is present or when any increase in heart rate should be avoided, such as for a patient with significant coronary artery disease. Phenylephrine produces venoconstriction, improving preload and systolic pressure, and produces arterial constriction, which increases diastolic pressure. The elevation in mean arterial pressure may trigger a baroreceptor-mediated reduction in heart rate. Phenylephrine is typically administered intravenously in 0.1-mg increments or by continuous IV infusion. The use of phenylephrine is best reserved for those with training in deep sedation and general anesthesia.

Hypertension

Sudden elevations in blood pressure are not uncommon in cardiology procedures, regardless of whether sedation is being provided. What establishes a significant elevation has not been well defined, but "hypertensive crisis" is the conventional term for sudden elevations in diastolic pressure >120 mm Hg. It should be noted that this term does not take into account the patient's baseline pressure. In patients with chronic hypertension, autoregulation of cerebral blood flow is reset to a higher level, and abruptly lowering pressure can lead to cerebral ischemia. This is particularly true for geriatric patients, where the risk of cardiovascular and cerebrovascular disease is greater. Considerations for drugs to reduce blood pressure may include β-blockers such as esmolol or labetalol, which are available for IV use. Unlike other IV vasodilators such as hydralazine, the β-blocking activity prevents reflex tachycardia. Careful titration is the key to avoid overshoot of the desired blood pressure end point. β-Blockers should be used with caution in patients with asthma because the antagonist action on bronchial β_2 receptors may induce bronchospasm. In these cases, the use of selective β_1-blockers such as esmolol is a safer option. Esmolol can be administered intravenously in increments of 10 mg up to 0.5 mg/kg. Because of its very short duration of action, additional doses every 10 minutes may be needed to maintain the effect. Neither labetalol nor esmolol should be administered without continuous ECG monitoring and continual blood pressure assessment.

Tachycardias

Transient episodes of tachycardia are triggered most often by pain, stress, and vasopressors included in local anesthetic solutions to which epinephrine has been added. However, tachycardia can also be a reflex response to hypoxia or hypotension, and these should be considered during patient assessment before treatment. A selective β_1-receptor antagonist such as esmolol can be titrated intravenously in the above dose range to gradually decrease sympathetic stimulation. Esmolol has a short duration so that in case the heart rate drops too precipitously, it should recover within a few minutes (20).

It is important to remember that in the CCL, many of the diagnostic and electrophysiology studies performed under sedation trigger rate and rhythm abnormalities. Therefore, prior to performing any pharmacologic intervention, close communication with the interventional team is required.

Management of Paradoxical Reactions

When a paradoxical reaction occurs, additional doses of benzodiazepines and opioids usually worsen the problem. Flumazenil, a benzodiazepine antagonist, has been shown to be effective in managing these reactions with a minimum of side effects (17).

Emergency Equipment for Sedation

Given the known cardiovascular and respiratory adverse effects of sedative drugs, when administering sedation, emergency equipment to manage adverse events should always be available. Table 7-7 includes a list of essential equipment recommended by the American Society of Anesthesiologists Practice Guidelines (6).

TABLE 7-7	Emergency Equipment for Sedation

Intravenous equipment
  Gloves
  Tourniquet
  Alcohol wipes
  Sterile gauze pads
  Intravenous catheters
  Intravenous tubing
  Intravenous fluid
  Assorted needles for drug aspiration and
    intramuscular injection
  Variety of sizes of syringes
  Tape

Basic airway management equipment
  Source of compressed oxygen (tank with regulator
    or pipeline supply with flowmeter)
  Source of suction
  Suction catheters
  Yankauer-type suction
  Face masks
  Self-inflating breathing bag-valve set
  Oral and nasal airways
  Lubricant

Advanced airway management equipment (for practitioners with intubation skills)
  Laryngeal mask airways
  Laryngoscope handles
  Laryngoscope blades
  Endotracheal tubes
    Cuffed 6.0, 7.0, 8.0 mm ID
  Stylet (appropriately sized for endotracheal tubes)
  Rigid videolaryngoscope

(Adapted from Practice guidelines for sedation and analgesia by non-anesthesiologists: an updated report by the American Society of Anesthesiologists Task Force on Sedation and Analgesia by Non-Anesthesiologists. *Anesthesiology*. 2002;96(4):1004–1017.)

TRAINING AND CREDENTIALS REQUIRED FOR SEDATION

The literature does not make specific recommendations regarding training requirements for personnel supervising, administering, and monitoring moderate sedation. It is recommended that the knowledge of the pharmacology of the drugs used during the sedation process be required, as well as knowledge of basic airway management and basic life support.

At least one individual capable of establishing a patent airway and positive pressure ventilation, as well as a means for summoning additional assistance, should be present whenever sedation–analgesia is administered. It is recommended that an individual with advanced life support skills be immediately available (within 5 minutes) for moderate sedation and within the procedure room for deep sedation (6).

RED FLAGS FOR ANESTHESIA CONSULTATION

There are several areas that raise "red flags" for anesthesia consultation, which can be summarized according to the categories shown in Table 7-8. The conditions listed in the table can be used as a reference for maintaining safe procedural conditions. The final decision on consultation should be with the primary provider performing the procedure, however.

Obstructive sleep apnea (OSA), a common breathing disorder, is a risk factor deserving of special mention. Polysomnographic recordings of sleep stages, respiration, and oxygenation reveal characteristics of OSA. Complete cessation of airflow for more than 10 seconds (apnea) or airflow reduction more than 50% (hypopnea) despite continuing breathing efforts results in hypoxemia and hypercapnia. This obstructive apnea or hypopnea is caused by complete or partial closure of the pharyngeal airway. The apnea or hypopnea is usually terminated in association with cortical arousal and opening of the pharyngeal airway.

Breathing is reestablished with loud snoring, normalizing of oxygenation, and often overshooting ventilation. OSA patients repeat the obstructive apnea or hypopnea, resulting in blood gas oscillation and sleep fragmentation.

TABLE 7-8 **Red Flags for Anesthesia Consultation**

Airway assessment
History
- History of snoring or obstructive sleep apnea
- Advanced rheumatoid arthritis with cervical spine involvement
- Previous problems with anesthesia and sedation or intubation

Physical examination
- Significant obesity especially involving the neck and facial structures
- Dysmorphic facial features (e.g., trisomy 21, Pierre–Robin syndrome)
- Short neck, limited neck extension, neck masses, cervical spine trauma or immobilization, tracheal deviation, decreased hyomental distance <3 cm in an adult)
- Trismus, significant malocclusion, retrognathia, micrognathia, unstable mandibular fracture

Assessment of aspiration risk
- History of frequent gastroesophageal reflux with or without hiatal hernia
- Gastroparesis in patients with diabetes mellitus
- Decreased airway reflexes, including gag and cough
- Recent vomiting or concurrent nausea
- Ingestion of full liquids or food within 6 hours of the procedure
- Bowel obstruction

Assessment of central nervous system or mental status
- Extremes of age (<1 or >70 years of age)
- Intoxication (drugs or alcohol)
- Delirium
- Psychosis
- Demonstrated inability to cooperate
- Mentally challenged

Other comorbidities of concern
- Chronic lung disease, including oxygen dependence
- Severe renal disease
- Neuromuscular diseases (myotonias, muscular dystrophies, Guillain–Barré, etc.)
- Elevated intracranial pressure
- Patients on multiple sedatives or antipsychotics

Recent growing evidence indicates that OSA is an independent risk factor for the development of hypertension, cardiovascular morbidity and mortality and sudden death. Daytime somnolence, a common clinical symptom in OSA patients, can result in increased risk of motor vehicle accident. Perioperative pharyngeal obstruction in OSA patients is thus a major concern when subjecting these patients to an altered state of consciousness. Accordingly, practitioners planning sedation should consider OSA as a risk factor for perioperative pharyngeal obstruction regardless of daytime sleepiness symptom. A high Mallampati score and large neck circumference are associated with difficult tracheal intubation within obese persons, suggesting potential involvement of anatomic imbalance in difficult tracheal intubation (21).

■ RECOVERY AND DISCHARGE CRITERIA AFTER SEDATION AND ANALGESIA

Each patient-care facility in which sedation–analgesia is administered should develop recovery and discharge criteria that are suitable for its specific patients and procedures. Some of the basic principles that might be incorporated in these criteria are listed in the following text.

General Principles

1. Medical supervision of recovery and discharge after moderate or deep sedation is the responsibility of the operating practitioner or of a licensed physician.
2. The recovery area should be equipped with, or have direct access to, appropriate monitoring and resuscitation equipment.
3. Patients receiving moderate or deep sedation should be monitored until appropriate discharge criteria are satisfied. The duration and frequency of monitoring should be individualized depending on the level of sedation achieved, the overall condition of the patient, and the nature of the intervention for which sedation/analgesia was administered.
4. Oxygenation should be monitored until patients are no longer at risk for respiratory depression.
5. Level of consciousness, vital signs, and oxygenation (when indicated) should be recorded at regular intervals.
6. A nurse or other individual trained to monitor patients and recognize complications should be in attendance until discharge criteria are fulfilled.

7. An individual capable of managing complications (e.g., establishing a patent airway and providing positive pressure ventilation) should be immediately available until discharge criteria are fulfilled.

Guidelines for Discharge

1. Patients should be alert and oriented; infants and patients whose mental status was initially abnormal should have returned to their baseline status. Practitioners and parents must be aware that pediatric patients are at risk for airway obstruction should the head fall forward while the child is secured in a car seat.
2. Vital signs should be stable and within acceptable limits.
3. Use of scoring systems may assist in the documentation of fitness for discharge.
4. Sufficient time (up to 2 hours) should have elapsed after the last administration of reversal agents (naloxone, flumazenil) to ensure that patients do not become resedated after reversal effects have worn off.
5. Outpatients should be discharged in the presence of a responsible adult who will accompany them home and be able to report any postprocedure complications.
6. Outpatients and their escorts should be provided with written instructions regarding postprocedure diet, medications, activities, and a phone number to be called in case of emergency.

Discharge Criteria

The primary provider may discharge the patient by written order or the RN may discharge the patient based on established criteria if so ordered by the provider.

Medical staff approved criteria are as follows for RN discharge using the Modified Aldrete Scoring System (Table 7-9) (21):

1. Completion of Modified Aldrete Scoring System as shown below.
2. Additionally, the patient must
   a. Demonstrate intact motor/sensory function, for example, enough motor strength to change, position in bed and sufficient sensory function to prevent

TABLE 7-9 **Modified Aldrete Scoring System**

Parameter	Score
Activity	
Able to move four extremities	2
Able to move two extremities	1
Able to move no extremities	0
Respiration	
Deep breath, cough freely	2
Dyspnea or limited breathing	1
Apneic	0
BP ± 20% preanesthesia level	2
BP ± 20–50% preanesthesia level	1
BP ± 50% preanesthesia level	0
Consciousness	
Fully awake	2
Arouse on calling	1
Not responding	0
Oxygenation	
Able to maintain O_2 saturation >92% (or preprocedural level) on room air	2
Requires O_2 inhalation to maintain saturation >90%	1
O_2 saturation <90% even with O_2	0

(Adapted from Ahmad S, Yilmaz M, Marcus R-J, et al. Impact of bispectral index monitoring on fast tracking of gynecologic patients undergoing laparoscopic surgery. *Anesthesiology.* 2003;98:849–852.)

possible injury, or consistent with preprocedure examination.
   b. Demonstrate the level of pain, nausea, or vomiting at acceptable level, for example, most minimal.
   c. Level of pain and minimal level of nausea.
   d. No evidence of procedural complications/other issues.
3. Notation that discharge criteria are met.

■ KEY POINTS

Any patient receiving a reversal agent must be observed for 1 to 2 hours after the last dose of reversal agent. Any patient who does not meet the above discharge criteria and who exhibits any untoward reaction, including but not limited to respiratory insufficiency, hypoxemia, hypotension/hypertension, bradycardia/

tachycardia, adverse reactions such as rash and use of reversal agent, must be evaluated by the practitioner performing the procedure.

If the patient is being transferred to another area, verbal report must be given to the nurse caring for the patient. Additionally, the name of the nurse, where the patient was transported, how the patient was transported, and the time the patient was transported must be noted as appropriate on the moderate sedation record.

■ CONCLUSION

Moderate sedation administration is growing in popularity. Recent statistics indicate that it is used in hospitals and physician offices for an estimated 200 million procedures each year in the United States. Thus, there is a need to increase the effectiveness of training for non-anesthesiologists who administer moderate sedation. The JCAHO and the ASA have created guidelines for safe administration of moderate sedation. Specifically, JCAHO requires that practitioners who administer sedation be trained in the safe use of sedative agents and in the rescue of patients who inadvertently slip into a deeper-than-expected level of sedation. With the advent of shorter-acting, less-potent respiratory depressant medications, an increase in the demand for moderate sedation for specific diagnostic and interventional procedures can be expected. Universal guidelines regarding training, credentialing, and patient selection do not yet exist. It will be up to the practitioner to exercise appropriate caution and common sense in patient selection and pharmacologic manipulation, to maintain their patients in the golden zone of the sedation continuum.

References

1. Becker E, Haas DA. Management of complications during moderate and deep sedation: respiratory and cardiovascular considerations. *Anesth Prog.* 2007;54:59–69.

2. Odom-Forren J, Watson D. *Practical Guide to Moderate Sedation/Analgesia.* St Louis, MO: Mosby; 2005.

3. Orkin F, Duncan P. Substrate for healthcare reform: anesthesia's low-lying fruit. *Anesthesiology.* 2009;111:734–740.

4. Joint Commission on the Accreditation of Healthcare Organizations. *Comprehensive Accreditation Manual for Hospitals.* Oakbrook Terrace, IL: JCAHO; 2004.

5. Coté CJ, Lerman J, Todres ID. *A Practice of Anesthesia for Infants and Children.* 3rd ed. Philadelphia, PA: Saunders; 2008.

6. Practice guidelines for sedation and analgesia by non-anesthesiologists: an updated report by the American Society of Anesthesiologists Task Force on Sedation and Analgesia by Non-Anesthesiologists. *Anesthesiology.* 2002;96:1004–1017.

7. Blackbourne LH. *Advanced Surgical Recall.* 2nd ed. Baltimore, MD: Lippincott Williams & Wilkins, 2004.

8. American Society of Anesthesiology. Practice guidelines for preoperative fasting and the use of pharmacological agents to reduce the risk of pulmonary aspiration: application to healthy patients undergoing elective procedures. *Anesthesiology.* 1999;90:896–905.

9. ASA Physical Status Classification System. American Society of Anesthesiologists website. www.asahq.org/clinical/physicalstatus.htm. Accessed October 28, 2009.

10. Droperidol. Drugs.com website. www.drugs.com/pro/droperidol.html. Revised May 2006. Accessed October 23, 2009.

11. Chen SC, Rex DK. Review article: registered nurse-administered propofol sedation for endoscopy. *Aliment Pharmacol Ther.* 2004;19:147–155.

12. AANA-ASA Joint Statement Regarding Propofol Administration, April 14, 2004. Available at: http://www.aana.com/news.aspx?id=761 (Accessed July 12, 2010).

13. Abramov D, Nogid B, Nogid A. The role of dexmedetomidine (Precedex®) in the sedation of critically ill patients. *P&T J.* 2005;30:158–161.

14. Schedules of controlled substances: placement of fospropofol into schedule IV. *ASA Newsletter,* October 6, 2009. Docket No. DEA–327. www.asahq.org/publications.

15. ASA comments at FDA hearing on fospropofol. American Society of Anesthesiologists website. Posted May 8, 2008. www.asahq.org/news/asanews050808.htm; accessed November 4, 2009.

16. Bell G, et al. Cardio-pulmonary and sedation-related complications. British Society of Gas-

troenterology Guidelines in Gastroenterology, November 2006. (Available at: www.health. uce.ac.uk/webmodules/GM607Z/Handouts/ complications.pdf. Access Date July 13, 2010)

17. Mancuso C, Tanzi MG, Gabay M. Paradoxical reactions to benzodiazepines: literature review and treatment options. *Pharmacotherapy*. 2004; 24(9):1177–1185.

18. Cairo JM, Pilbean SP. *Mosby's Respiratory Care Equipment*. 7th ed. Philadelphia, PA: Mosby; 2004: 62–88.

19. Karch AM, ed. 2009 *Lippincott's Nursing Drug Guide*. Philadelphia, PA: Lippincott Williams & Wilkins; 2009.

20. Hazinski MF, Chameides L, Hemphill R, eds. 2005 American Heart Association Guidelines for cardiopulmonary resuscitation and emergency cardiovascular care. *Circulation*. 2005;112(suppl): IV1–IV196.

21. Isono S. Obstructive sleep apnea of obese adults: pathophysiology and perioperative airway management. *Anesthesiology*. 2009;110:908–921.

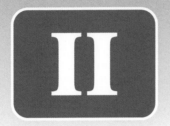

SECTION

II

Systemic and Local Complications of Invasive Procedures in General

8

Predicting and Avoiding Death, Emergency Surgery, and Other Complications of Percutaneous Coronary Intervention

STEPHEN G. ELLIS

At the dawn of the age of intervention, untreatable coronary dissection led to the need for emergency bypass surgery in 4% to 8% of patients, and this was the principal cause of periprocedural death, as patients presenting with acute myocardial infarction (AMI) were largely avoided. In the "Middle Ages" of intervention, increased use of atheroablative devices shifted the cause of unwanted emergency bypass surgery to a near-even mixture of perforation and dissection. At the same time, increased application of percutaneous coronary intervention (PCI) for patients with AMI offset reduced the risk of dissection-related mortality. Today, with the near-uniform use of coronary stents and more aggressive treatment of patients with resuscitated sudden cardiac death and major myocardial infarction, untreatable dissection and perforation are rare with good technique, and brain death and pump failure have become the most common reasons for untoward outcomes with PCI (1). Overall in-hospital PCI-related mortality and bypass surgery rates are presently approximately 1.5% and 0.5%, respectively, but depend greatly on case mix. With this gradually changing scenario of use and outcomes with PCI, old risk-triaging strategies need to be reassessed, while at the

same time lessons learned regarding technique must not be forgotten.

■ MODELS FOR PREDICTING RISK OF PCI

Over the years, several models to predict outcome with PCI have been developed with the aim to provide risk-adjusted comparisons across operators and institutions, and in an attempt to predict individual patient's prognosis. These models should be assessed based upon their ability to discriminate the risk (c statistic), their calibration (2), and their relevance to the contemporary era. In general, models for mortality have had much better c statistics (>0.85) than models for MACE (0.60 to 0.75). Perhaps the most widely used mortality model is that emanating from the very large ACC-NCDR database (3). This model, containing 16 relatively easy-to-evaluate parameters, was both developed and validated in large numbers of patients from multiple institutions and found to have excellent discrimination (c statistic = 0.89). Calibration was also excellent, except possibly among highest-risk individuals (the highest single risk group had 37% predicted mortality; the descriptive manuscript provides inadequate information to assess calibration among the most

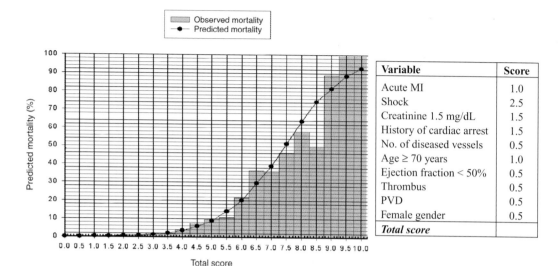

Variable	Score
Acute MI	1.0
Shock	2.5
Creatinine 1.5 mg/dL	1.5
History of cardiac arrest	1.5
No. of diseased vessels	0.5
Age ≥ 70 years	1.0
Ejection fraction < 50%	0.5
Thrombus	0.5
PVD	0.5
Female gender	0.5
Total score	

FIGURE 8-1. Michigan risk model for death after PCI and bedside risk prediction tool. For the estimation of risk, calculate the total score by adding individual scores if the comorbidity is present. For number of diseased vessels, add 0.5 for each major epicardial vessel that has >70% stenosis. Identify total score on the horizontal axis of the plot and corresponding probability on the vertical axis. Scores ≤2.5 are associated with a risk of death <0.8%, whereas scores >7 are associated with a risk of death >40%. (Adapted from Moscucci M, Share D, Kline-Rogers E, et al. Simple bedside additive tool for prediction of in-hospital mortality after percutaneous coronary interventions. *Circulation.* 2001;104:263–268.)

high-risk patients). The ramifications of this limitation are particularly acute in this era of score-carding, as these are exactly the individuals for whom the interventionalist would most like to predict the outcome and to have an adequate risk adjustment tool.

Similarly to the ACC model, the Michigan mortality model, which was developed for bedside use in the prediction of individual patient's prognosis, had excellent discrimination (4). This model had also good calibration across different patients' risk groups (Fig. 8-1).

Another widely used risk adjustment calculator is that from the Mayo Clinic, which uses eight simple risk factors (age, creatinine, ejection fraction, preprocedural shock, myocardial infarction within 24 hours, congestive heart failure, gender, and the presence or absence of peripheral arterial disease) (5,6) to predict both mortality and MACE (Figs. 8-2 and 8-3). In validation testing, this model had a *c* statistic of 0.88 for mortality. Only 1.5% of patients had mortality estimated at >10% and the confidence limits about the point estimate for this group were rather wide. The *c* statistic for MACE was 0.74.

Another recently developed prognostic tool is the SYNTAX score (http://www.Syntaxscore.

com), which has been validated to correlate with 1-year MACE in three-vessel and left main intervention (Fig. 8-4). It is available at http://www. Syntaxscore.com.

Aside from their ability in scorecarding, it is uncertain how these tools should be used in clinical practice. One might presume that operator technique and experience are at least as important as some of the other key risk factors in determining the outcome. Surgical results also vary considerably from institution to institution. It is not at all unreasonable however, to at least ask that for all but the most simple (≤3 focal/simple lesions) patients with three-vessel coronary artery disease (CAD) undergoing elective procedures have a quick SYNTAX score calculated. Ad hoc elective PCI, unless detailed options have been previously discussed or there are extenuating comorbidities, should not be performed in the highest-risk tercile patients.

The utility of these models in helping the clinician choose which patients to avoid in the high-risk elective or emergency setting is debatable. Most of the mortality risk is in the highest-risk decile (typically >6% to 10% risk, compared with <2% risk in all other deciles), but the discriminatory capacity within this decile is modest

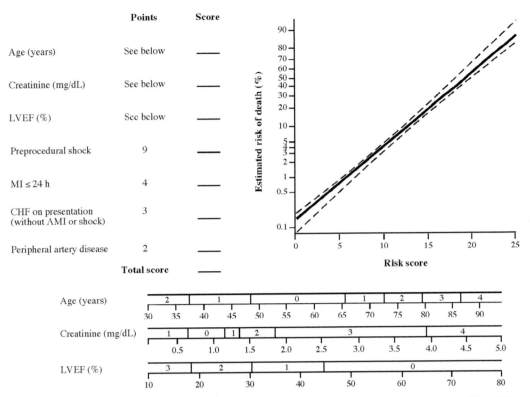

FIGURE 8-2. Mayo Clinic risk model for death after PCI. (From Singh M, Gersh BJ, Li S, et al. Mayo Clinic Risk Score for percutaneous coronary intervention predicts in-hospital mortality in patients undergoing coronary artery bypass graft surgery. *Circulation.* 2008;117:356–362.)

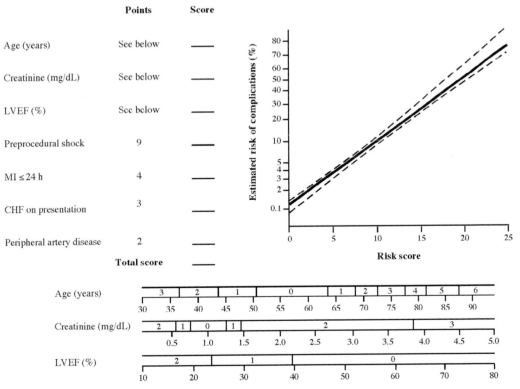

FIGURE 8-3. Mayo Clinic model for risk of complications after PCI. (From Singh M, Gersh BJ, Li S, et al. Mayo Clinic Risk Score for percutaneous coronary intervention predicts in-hospital mortality in patients undergoing coronary artery bypass graft surgery. *Circulation.* 2008;117:356–362.)

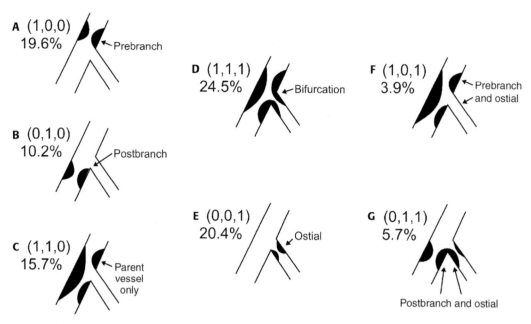

FIGURE 8-4. Distribution of bifurcation types using Medina classification in SYNTAX ($n = 380$ lesions). (From Morice MC. Results from SYNTAX left main cohort: impact of SYNTAX score and bifurcation techniques on outcome. Presented at the American Heart Association Annual Meeting; November 14–18, 2009; Orlando, FL.)

at best (c statistics 0.70 to 0.75). No model yet developed can provide the clinician with a clear definition of mortality risk >50%. Shock or salvage procedures in patients over 80 years are at the highest risk, but that risk is typically underestimated by these models. Ultimately decisions to proceed in high-risk patients depend on patient, family and societal expectations, and the willingness of the interventionalist and the system within which they work to assume the reporting risk of treating such patients.

■ AVOIDING COMPLICATIONS— CRITICAL ISSUES AND TECHNIQUES

To a large extent, fatal outcomes are determined by patient selection and technique, whereas the risk of emergency bypass surgery and the occurrence of very large myocardial infarctions principally relate to laps in technique. The latter can largely be divided into "clumsiness" and more commonly "failure to anticipate."

Patient Selection

Although it is in some ways trivial to state that one must always consider the balance of benefit

and risk, to neglect this judgment turns the physician into a technician. Given recent trial results (COURAGE (7), FAME (8)), under almost all circumstances the patient must be symptomatic and the lesion to be treated should be ischemia and symptom-causing to proceed. Lesions under consideration should be well seen in two complementary views, with supplementary perfusion imaging, FFR, or intravascular ultrasound (IVUS) as necessary. Perfusion to all parts of the myocardium must be accounted for so as not to miss anomalies or bypass graphs. In general, the extremely complex lesions should be attempted only in patients for whom the hemodynamic consequences of vessel closure are modest, or the patient with no other reasonable treatment options. Selection of which patients recently resuscitated from sudden cardiac death with unclear neurologic status to intervene upon is an especially challenging task, the outcome of which may depend principally on societal expectations regarding near futility and reporting. Availability and outcomes with post arrest cooling protocols also need to be considered (9,10). At present, we are hesitant to perform emergency PCI on patients known to have suffered cardiac arrest for more than 10 minutes before CPR is initiated (these exact times are often difficult to obtain), but we do offer systemic cooling for patients with downtimes <30 minutes and Glasgow coma score ≤8 if cooling can be initiated within 6 hours of arrest.

Adjunctive Medication

Based upon contemporary trial results (11) for all procedures except those involving chronic total occlusions (CTOs) or other anatomy at risk of perforation, patients should receive aspirin, clopidogrel or prasugrel (especially preferred in ACS patients), bivalirudin, and a statin reload. Because of the inability to immediately reverse bivalirudin in the event of a perforation, heparin is preferred in patients for whom that risk is higher than usual (e.g., CTOs, rotational atherectomy use in conjunction with highly eccentric or angulated lesions). Glycoprotein IIb/IIIa inhibitors still appear to have a role in the emergency treatment of ACS patients when the antiplatelet effect of thienopyridines has yet to take place (30 to 45 minutes for a 60-mg loading dose of prasugrel, 2 to 3 hours for 600-mg loading dose of clopidogrel).

Guide Catheters

There remain two general approaches to guide catheter use—active (with 5- or 6-F catheters) and passive (with 7- or 8-F catheters). The former can be safely used if one remembers two general dictums—avoid deep vessel intubation in the presence of even modest amounts of protruding proximal plaque or the fragile internal mammary artery, and always bring the guide forward over a device providing some support, preferably a guidewire and a balloon. The latter group is especially helpful when one is concerned about ostial trauma such as treatment of ostial unprotected left main or right coronary stenoses, or small in situ internal mammary arteries. Large-diameter catheters are, of course, required when one may need to deliver bulky devices (e.g., SKS for LMT requiring ≥3.0-mm stents). Both require shape choice to provide coaxiality of approach. Actively used catheters should also be chosen to have relatively straight distal aspects for safe deep intubation (e.g., Judkins right 4), whereas passively used catheters also require shape for sufficient support either through inherent stiffness or pressure off an opposing coronary sinus or wall (e.g., Amplatz

left series). Operators in our laboratory generally use XB or EBU shape guide catheters as the first choice to cannulate the left main and ARI or AR2, or Judkins right guide catheter for the right coronary artery.

Other than relating to proximal vessel dissection due to intentionally or inadvertently using active technique with guide catheters better suited for passive technique (use particular care that the guide catheter does not "dive in" when withdrawing somewhat bulky devices), the principal impact of guide catheter choice on complications is the avoidance of guide catheters with insufficient support to deliver the needed device (most commonly a stent) to the lesion always consider worst-case scenario. Calcified and tortuous vessels (the combination is particularly a challenge), as well as those prone to perforation (e.g., elderly females with tortuous vessels (12)) require particular attention. Choice of guide catheter size also, of course, has ramifications to assess site choice—generally the radial artery is of sufficient size to accommodate 6-F catheters in women and 7-F catheters in men.

Guide Wires

There are a number of excellent workhorse guide wires today. Specialty wires should be used judiciously—for example, hydrophilic wires for extreme tortuosity or subtotally occluded vessels with microchannels, stiff wires to deliver bulky devices, and CTO specialty wires for their intended usage. In all cases, the tip should be actively rotated as the wire is advanced and the operator attentive to tactile and visual resistance. Hydrophilic and stiff wires are particularly prone to advance through softer portions of the lesion outside from the lumen, with less feedback to the operator that a dissection is imminent. Generally, if such a wire is required to deliver a balloon distally, once the lesion has been crossed the wire should be exchanged for a workhorse wire. Hydrophilic wires are particularly prone to distal migration and vessel perforation with poor technique. When advancing any device, but particularly a stiff or bulky device, one must learn to keep an eye not only on the guide catheter and device but also on the distal wire. Hydrophilic wires also tend to move forward (or backward) when the inexperienced operator is removing a balloon or similar device. A particularly important but basic adage is that, as long as the operator has the guidewire secure beyond the lesion with a guide catheter of sufficient support, they have control and can manage almost any dissection or perforation related complication (excepting wire tip perforations).

Balloons and Stents

Except for predilatation when one is simply trying to make a channel large enough to deliver the primary treatment device, balloons and stents should be sized 1.1:1 to the "normal" adjacent vessel. With DES, as possible, one should stent from normal to normal vessel. Ballooning outside of the area to be stented should be assiduously avoided (STELLR) (13). The problem is often knowing what is "normal." Use of IVUS in the presence of diffuse disease or an apparently rapidly tapering vessel is often very helpful. That said, one must consider the effects of vessel remodeling, which often maximally occurs at the site of the stenosis. Sizing to 0.5 mm less than the media-to-media dimension is often appropriate, although it is difficult to make hard

and fast rules. Sizing larger runs the risk of a perforation. One must also consider the balloon compliance that may vary considerably between devices, and also the fact that the expanded stent size in the body is almost never that which is listed on the compliance chart outside the body (average stent MLD is 75% of expected at 15 atm) (14). Depending on the compliance of the delivery balloon (with stents currently available in the United States such as Cypher, Taxus, Xience V/Promus, Endeavor), often postdilatation with a noncompliant balloon is prudent to avoid the unwanted "dog boning" effect (risking an edge tear) of a compliant balloon delivering a stent. Most contemporary stents should be postdilated to 16 to 20 atm. One further caution—if because of the presence of fluoroscopic calcium or other issues, one is not certain that the stent can be fully expanded, test dilatation at low pressure should be undertaken before the stent is delivered. If a standard balloon will not inflate fully, a scoring device or rotational atherectomy (caution with tortuosity or extremely eccentric lesions due to the risk of perforation) should be used to pretreat the lesion. A poorly expanded stent is a setup for stent thrombosis.

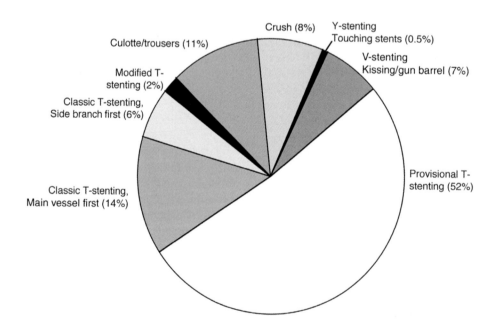

89% of provisional T-stenting lesions used only 1 stent; 9% used 2 stents

FIGURE 8-5. Techniques utilized for distal left main stenting in SYNTAX ($n = 211$ lesions treated). (From Morice MC. Results from SYNTAX left main cohort: impact of SYNTAX score and bifurcation techniques on outcome. Presented at the American Heart Association Annual Meeting; November 14–18, 2009; Orlando, FL.)

Side Branch Management

Before even proceeding to treat side branch narrowings, it is important to recall that angiography often overestimates their severity (15).

Once the need to treat has been established, the message from the multiple small randomized trials attempting to ascertain best technique for side branch management is that single stent use with provisional side branch stenting is generally superior to other approaches (16). Although true in most cases, the heterogeneity of side branch anatomy makes generalization difficult. The Medina classification is an attempt to categorize lesions among this heterogeneity. Many experienced interventionalists continue to see merit in routine side branch stenting for large side branches (>2.5 mm) where there is significant ostial disease (Medina 1, 1, 0; 0, 1, 1 or 1, 1, 1). In this case, a mini crush, Culotte or "V-stenting" with minimal stent overlap may be preferred. In the first two, it is very important to perform a final "kiss" (sequential high-pressure inflations in each stent, followed by simultaneous low-pressure inflation). Proximal oversizing can be avoided by recalling that the diameter of the parent vessel = diameter of two daughter vessels × 0.67 (17). T-stenting may also be applied in the relatively rare instance when the side branch angle is 80 to 100 degrees (otherwise a gap will invariably be left at the side branch ostium). Distribution of lesion types, approaches, and results for the distal LMT bifurcation subset of SYNTAX are shown in Figures 8-4, 8-5, and 8-6. With provisional stenting, the risk of side branch loss may be minimized by prewiring the side branch before delivering the main branch stent. Care must be taken to leave only a short wire segment in the side branch when the main branch stent is delivered, and to avoid this technique although if the vessel is highly calcified or if the side branch wire must traverse a long segment of the main branch stent (both increasing the risk of the wire becoming trapped).

Avoiding Stent Thrombosis

Acute and subacute stent thrombosis is rare but most likely to occur in the setting of AMI, gross stent undersizing, or extreme hypercoagulable

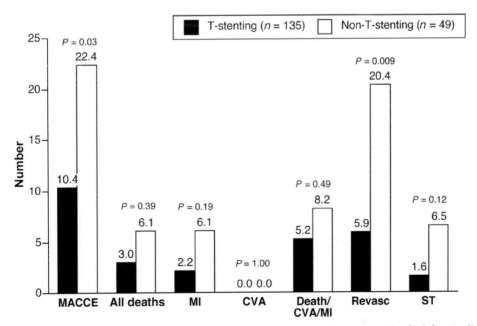

FIGURE 8-6. Nonrandomized comparison of outcomes after T-stenting and non-T-stenting for left main distal lesions in SYNTAX. (From Morice MC. Results from SYNTAX left main cohort: impact of SYNTAX score and bifurcation techniques on outcome. Presented at the American Heart Association Annual Meeting; November 14–18, 2009; Orlando, FL.)

states (e.g., HITS). Protection in these settings involves intracoronary nitroglycerin use to minimize spasm and misjudgment of vessel size (not always effective in the thrombus-laden myocardial infarction–associated vessel), IVUS when there is doubt about vessel size or stent apposition, prasugrel instead of clopidogrel loading in high-risk ACS states, and attention to clues that the patient may be especially hypercoagulable.

Special Issues With CTOs

The wiring technique when approaching CTOs (unintended or often near deliberate perivascular advancing of a wire, with high risk of wire perforation), as well as other issues related to traversing collaterals mandates attention to several other adages otherwise unnecessary for the interventionalist. First, anticoagulants that cannot be readily reversed (bivalirudin, glycoprotein IIb/IIIa antagonists) must be avoided until the wire has been successfully placed and there is no question about the presence of a perforation. Second, before aggressively ballooning and stenting, one must attempt to ascertain the degree to which the wire may have exited the true lumen. Certainly in most instances intravascular but extraluminal wire placement without perforation will allow successful completion of the procedure. However, there have been more than a handful of significant perforations while ballooning or stenting in this situation. Optimal strategy is not well defined. Based upon our own experience, however, I would advocate dilating any questionable channel with a 1.5-mm balloon, followed by IVUS. If there appears to be very little tissue between the channel and the pericardium, one should consider halting the procedure or recrossing the lesion with another guidewire. If the choice is made to proceed, one needs be very careful not to oversize the stents that are placed and generally deliver them at a lower-than-usual pressure. Third, septals should only be dilated with ≤1.5-mm balloons at very low pressure (2 to 3 atm). Septal perforation or closure is rarely catastrophic but has been reported to cause ventricular septal rupture. Fourth, if the technique involves externalization of a 300-cm guide wire, one must "protect" both the septals and the lesion itself with a balloon or other device to prevent "slicing" the vessel. Lastly, one should not attempt to traverse epi-cardial collaterals for fear of perforation without devices especially intended for this use (e.g., Corsair device).

■ TREATING COMPLICATIONS: CRITICAL TECHNIQUES

Coronary Dissection

Perhaps the most important aspect of managing coronary dissections is the realization that they may occur with any lesion (or with guide catheter trauma). Proximal or mid RCA lesions in relatively nondiseased vessels are notorious for occasionally "unraveling" distally. That said, longer lesions, vessel calcification, and angulation still are risk factors for dissection, and degenerated SVG or thrombus containing lesions are risk factors for embolization/"slow flow." When selecting equipment, one should always anticipate the potential utilization of more bulky devices (e.g., longer stents) than necessarily required to treat the lesion per se. Once a dissection is identified, it is mandatory to assess its length in at least two angiographic views and secure its length by passage of a stable guide wire. With a good guide catheter and guidewire, one can treat almost any dissection. One should then proceed to place stents distal to proximal, extending 3 to 5 mm in both directions beyond its evident length. Major side branches can then be rescued although one needs to resist the temptation to be "too cute." One must accept loss of minor side branches. Use of IVUS to assess complete expansion of long or multiply placed stents is often advisable. Coronary dissection is further discussed in Chapter 15.

Coronary Perforation

Coronary perforation is a rare (approximately 0.5%) complication that can be fatal, particularly if the operator is not prepared to deal with its consequences. Risk factors have been well described—older females, tortuous, angulated or calcified lesions, use of very high pressure or ablative devices (11). Rotational atherectomy is particularly hazardous with eccentric lesions on bends when wire bias tends to draw the device to the outer curvature and when the lesion is on the inner curvature of the vessel. If at all possible, rotablation should be avoided in this instance. If no other choice is available, one should use a 1.25-mm burr. Also, in general in the DES era when rotational atherectomy is simply used to open a channel or modify vessel compliance, burr to artery ratios should be kept to <0.6. All interventional laboratories should have a coronary perforation kit and a pericardiocentesis kit readily available. The former should include various covered stents and coils. Generally, perforation is evident (and sometimes very obvious) on routine angiography. One should be aware, however, that about 10% of perforations present as delayed cardiac tamponade. We have found that the 1 to 3 grading scheme for perforation suggested more than a decade ago (12) with some modification is still useful, although treatment algorithms have changed.

Class 1: Perforations

These are sometimes difficult to distinguish from dissections. Generally prolonged balloon inflation (approximately 5 minutes) and/or stent implantation, without change in anticoagulation, is sufficient for treatment. One should be aware, however, of the risk of delayed tamponade.

Class 2: Perforations

These are often caused by balloon or stent over-expansion, or by distal wire migration. Sometimes they occur with ablative device use. The former can usually be treated by immediate prolonged balloon inflation, followed by careful observation. Sometimes, the delivery balloon itself is sufficient to occlude flow, but often a balloon 0.5 mm larger than the target vessel with inflation at low pressure is required. Partial reversal of antithrombin agents (if possible) and discontinuation of GP IIb/IIIa inhibitors should be routine. Transthoracic echocardiography should be performed to establish a baseline and rule out unexpected pericardial fluid. Distal wire migration-associated perforation may require placement of a coil (e.g., Terumo Embolization Microcoil, Terumo, Somerset, NJ) to achieve intravascular hemostasis. Continued leakage via collaterals should be considered. Class 2 perforations are more hazardous in the presence of glycoprotein IIb/IIIa antagonists. Abciximab should be reversed with platelets for all but the simplest perforations (see the following text).

Class 3: Perforations

These are most frequently caused by ablative devices but can also occur with high-pressure balloon/stent implantation. Treatment requires immediate local tamponade with balloon inflation, readiness for pericardiocentesis (transthoracic echocardiography called for but utilized carefully so as not to delay other necessary procedures) and reversal of anticoagulation and placement of covered stent (or an emergency trip to the operating room). We have found the "dueling guide catheter" approach to place the covered stent in this instance useful. A second 8-F guide catheter with wire and covered stent is placed in the appropriate coronary ostia (while the other guide catheter is backed out with leak-occluding balloon in place) and the wire advanced with the occluding balloon still in place. That balloon is transiently deflated and the second guide wire advanced across the lesion. Then, quickly, the occluding balloon is deflated and withdrawn while the covered stent is advanced and inflated.

Class 2–3: Contained Perforations

Perforations with egress into the myocardium or in the presence of a scarred/previously opened pericardium (prior cardiac surgery) are usually much more benign in presentation. The former can often simply be observed. The latter should be treated as per classification, however, as their hemodynamic effect is not always predictable. Coronary perforation is further discussed in details in Chapter 16.

■ "SLOW REFLOW"

Slow reflow is not a cause for, nor should be treated with, emergency bypass surgery. It can, however, cause death due to infarction and pump failure. Management of slow reflow is considered in Chapter 17.

■ DEVICE RETRIEVAL

Rarely stents, balloons, and guidewires (or other device fragments) are dislodged or fractured and need to be retrieved. This appears to occur in approximately 0.3% of intended stents (18). Data on the incidence of balloon or guide wire loss are more difficult to obtain.

Stents appear to be dislodged principally under two circumstances—when, because of proximal calcification or a severe lesion, the operator attempts to force the stent distally and the stent is stripped off proximally to the balloon; and when the operator encounters difficulty delivering the stent and attempts to pull it back into a misaligned guide catheter, thereby completely stripping the stent off the delivery system altogether (except for the wire). The most important technical point to remember is to keep the guide wire across the dislodged stent.

The simplest approach in both cases, when it works, is simply to advance a small-diameter balloon so that its tip protrudes slightly beyond the stent, inflate at approximate 2 atm, and drag the stent back out of the guide catheter. Under certain circumstances, it may be better to expand the stent where it sits. This also is rather simple to achieve, as long as one has not lost the guidewire position.

If neither of these approaches is suitable, one is left with the option of trying to actually retrieve the stent with a retrieval device or crush the stent out-of-the-way. A partially expanded stent cannot be left in the coronary arteries (those embolized into peripheral arteries seem to have infrequent clinical consequences—possibly because of brisk flow). Perhaps the simplest retrieval technique is the two-wire technique. This is easiest when the initial guide wire remains in place through the stent. A second guide wire is advanced through the struts of the lost stent, and then the guide wires are rotated in opposite directions to entwine their distal ends. The wires are then pulled back removing the stent. A variety of loop snares are also available. These are generally easy to use if the original guide wire remains in place and if the 2- to 4-mm snare can be advanced distally over the stent. These devices are bulky, however. Care must be taken that the stent is not pushed distally. The snare is simply advanced beyond the stent, narrowed, and retrieved. If the original guidewire position has been lost, another guide wire may be advanced alongside the stent in the snare advanced over this guide wire. In this case, the snare must be positioned around the stent before the latter is lassoed. Other retrieval devices are available (vascular retrieval device, biliary stone forceps, biopsy forceps, retained-fragment retriever), although they are too bulky to be useful unless the stent itself protrudes from the coronary ostia.

Guidewires themselves are most often trapped when a stent is expanded over them or when they are forcefully advanced distally in a diffusely diseased coronary artery. If they cannot be removed with moderate traction, it is generally best to advance an OTW balloon over the wire as near as possible to the wire tip and then remove both the balloon and the wire simultaneously. Sometimes considerable force is required.

■ DO NOT PANIC

Major complications are nowadays so infrequent that few of us have frequent exposure to them. Keep your cool, collect your thoughts, and prioritize. Summon help. It is useful to delegate pharmacologic management of the code or near-code situation to a colleague while you attend to the technical challenges (or vice versa). Above all, be prepared. Do not attempt high-risk elective PCI in the evening or on weekends, when experienced physician and nursing help might not be available. With ready access to experienced hands, devices (e.g., Impella 2.5, TandemHeart), surgical support and tools to treat perforations, and with recalling to keep the guidewire across the lesion, virtually all complications can be successfully managed. That said, all laboratories should critically review all of their major complications and benchmark their results against those of high-quality laboratories.

■ WHEN YOU THINK YOU ARE DONE

Especially when you have finished an especially challenging procedure, there is a tendency to say "whew" and not be as meticulous as you should be with the aspects of the final procedure. Wire out completion angiography in two views focusing on the lesion itself, all aspects of the anatomy traversed by the guide catheter and areas in the vicinity of the distal guide wire tip should be mandatory. Lastly, although access site angiography should be routinely performed prior to initiating intervention, if it has not been done at the point of the completion of the procedure, it should be done then. Hypotension due to a retroperitoneal hemorrhage can lead to thrombotic closure of even a perfectly treated coronary stenosis. Other issues relating to access site management are discussed in Chapter 14.

References

1. Resnic F, Welt F. The public health hazards of risk avoidance associated with public reporting of risk-adjusted outcomes in coronary intervention. *J Am Coll Cardiol.* 2009;53:825–830.

2. McGeechan K, Macaskill P, Irwig L, et al. Assessing new biomarkers and predictive models for use in clinical practice. *Arch Intern Med.* 2008; 168(21):2304–2310.

3. Shaw RE, Anderson V, Brindis RG, et al. Updated Risk Adjustment Mortality Model using the complete 1.1 dataset from the American College of Cardiology National Cardiovascular Data Registry. *J Invasive Cardiol.* 2003;15:578.

4. Moscucci M, Share D, Kline-Rogers E, et al. Simple bedside additive tool for prediction of in-hospital mortality after percutaneous coronary interventions. *Circulation.* 2001;104:263–268.

5. Singh M, Rihal CS, Lennon RJ, et al. Bedside estimation of risk from percutaneous coronary intervention: the new Mayo Clinic risk scores. *Mayo Clin Proc.* 2007;82:701–708.

6. Singh M, Peterson ED, Milford-Beland S, et al. Validation of the Mayo Clinic risk score for in-hospital mortality after percutaneous coronary interventions using the national cardiovascular data registry. *Circ Cardiovasc Interv.* 2008;1:36–44.

7. Boden WE, O'Rourke RA, Teo KK, et al. Optimal medical therapy with or without PCI for stable coronary disease. *N Engl J Med.* 2007;356(15): 1503–1516.

8. Tonino PAL, De Bruyne B, Pijls NHJ, et al. Fractional flow vs angiography for guiding percutaneous coronary intervention. *N Engl J Med.* 2009: 360(3):213–224.

9. The Hypothermia after Cardiac Arrest Study Group. Mild therapeutic hypothermia to improve the neurologic outcome after cardiac arrest. *N Engl J Med.* 2002;346(8):549–556.

10. Bernard SA, Gray TW, Buist MD, et al. Treatment of comatose survivors of out-of-hospital cardiac arrest with induced hypothermia. *N Engl J Med.* 2002;346(8):557–563.

11. Stone GW, McLaurin BT, Cox DA, et al, for the ACUITY Investigators. Bivalirudin for patients with acute coronary syndromes. *N Engl J Med.* 2006;355(21):2203–2216.

12. Ellis SG, Ajluni, Arnold ZA, et al. Increased coronary perforation in the new device era. Incidence, classification, management, and outcome. *Circulation.* 1994;90:2725–2730.

13. Costa MA, Angiolillo DJ, Tannenbaum K, et al. Impact of stent deployment procedural factors on long-term effectiveness and safety of sirolimus-eluting stents (final results of the Multicenter Prospective STLLR Trial). *Am J Cardiol.* 2008;101(12):1704–1711.

14. Costa JR, Mintz GS, Carlier SG, et al. Bifurcation coronary lesions treated with the "crush" technique: an intravascular ultrasound analysis. *Am J Cardiol.* 2005;96(1):74–78.

15. Koo BK, Kang HJ, Youn TJ, et al. Physiologic assessment of jailed side branch lesions using fractional flow reserve. *J Am Coll Cardiol.* 2005;45:633–637.

16. Steigen TK, Maeng M, Wiseth R, et al. Randomized study on simple versus complex stenting of coronary bifurcation lesions: the Nordic Bifurcation Study. *Circulation.* 2006;114: 1955–1961.

17. Finet G. Fluid dynamics and rheology in bifurcation lesions. Presentation at 13th Annual Angioplasty Summit, TCT Asia Pacific; 2008.

18. Eggebrecht H, Haude M, von Birgelsen C, et al. Nonsurgical retrieval of embolized coronary stents. *Catheter Cardiovasc Interv.* 2000;51(4):432–440.

Stroke and Neurovascular Rescue

SUDHIR KATHURIA, DHEERAJ GANDHI, AND
LEWIS B. MORGENSTERN

O ver the past several decades, cardiac catheterization has undergone tremendous advancement and is frequently used as a definitive means for the diagnostic evaluation of various cardiac diseases. It is also playing an increasingly important therapeutic role, with percutaneous cardiac interventions now being routinely performed as an alternative to medical and surgical treatment. Cardiac catheterization is generally regarded safe with rates of serious complication at less than 1% for most types of procedures (1). Among the possible complications, stroke is perhaps one of the most devastating complications and has been reported in 0.11% to 0.38% of patients undergoing these procedures (2). Although the fraction of patients experiencing stroke from these procedures is relatively low, with more than 2 million cardiac catheterization procedures performed annually in the United States, it adds up to significantly large numbers (3).

Acute ischemic and acute hemorrhagic strokes are the two main subtypes of strokes. Acute ischemic stroke is generally caused by a blood clot (or occasionally other material including calcium from cardiac valves) obstructing the blood flow to the brain, whereas acute hemorrhagic stroke is due to the rupture of blood vessels leading to intraparenchymal or subarachnoid hemorrhage. In the general population, the majority of strokes are of ischemic type with hemorrhagic strokes constituting only 10% to 20% of these cases (4). However, the relative incidence of acute hemorrhagic subtype is more frequent in the setting of stroke arising as a complication of percutaneous coronary interventions and ranges from 22% to 46.5% perhaps due to the use of antiplatelet, antithrombotic,

and thrombolytic agents during these procedures (2,5,6).

There are a number of possible causes of acute ischemic stroke during cardiac catheterization, but thromboembolic phenomenon accounts for a vast majority (7–9). Mechanical force from the catheters, guidewires, and adjunctive mechanical devices can result in fragmentation of atherosclerotic plaques in vessels leading to embolic stroke. Keeley and Grines reported plaque dislodgement from the aortic arch in more than 50% of percutaneous revascularization procedures based on prospective evaluation of 1,000 consecutive patients. The patients in this study were undergoing percutaneous interventions using large-lumen guiding catheters (8 and 9 F). After the guiding catheter was advanced over a 0.035-in wire into the descending aorta and around the aortic arch, the wire was removed from this catheter and blood was allowed to exit the back of the catheter for at least three cardiac cycles. The blood and any suspended fragments were collected on a sterile towel. The operator examined this material for the presence and relative quantity of atheromatous material. Catheter shapes and debris scores were recorded for all 1,000 procedures (10). Other possible sources of embolism include clot formation due to prolonged procedures, air embolism, and arterial dissection related to guidewire manipulation (11–13). Certain types of procedures such as electrophysiologic ablation are associated with even higher rates of stroke likely due to procedure-related denuded endothelium along with additional release of tissue factors and other thrombogenic substances. In addition, ablation procedures often require larger catheters that may potentially be more traumatic, and prolonged catheter manipulation in left-sided cardiac chambers (14,15).

There is a paucity of data regarding outcomes of percutaneous cardiac intervention–related acute ischemic stroke. However, one study reported a very high hospital mortality rate of 47.6% among 21 acute ischemic stroke patients resulting from 9,662 consecutive cardiac procedures (2). This rate is much higher compared with 3% to 9% in hospital mortality rate in acute ischemic stroke patients from the general population (16,17). This increased mortality from stroke in the setting of percutaneous cardiac interventions is attributed to certain patient characteristics seen more commonly in this patient population such as older age, advanced atherosclerosis, noninsulin-dependent diabetes mellitus, and periprocedural complications that often require the use of an intra-aortic balloon pump (16,17).

Most of the experience, evidence, and literature currently available is based upon stroke in general population. Many of the comments and suggestions in the following sections are based on this general experience. The reader is suggested to utilize commonly accepted acute ischemic and acute hemorrhagic stroke guidelines (4,18). Specific issues related to stroke in the setting of cardiac endovascular procedures are also discussed and suggestions have been made accordingly.

■ PERIPROCEDURAL MONITORING AND EARLY IDENTIFICATION OF STROKE

The potential morbidity and mortality from periprocedural strokes can be limited by its timely recognition, prompt evaluation as well as institution of appropriate therapy. The entire team involved in cardiac interventional procedures should be aware of this potential complication and ideally formulate a plan of action to deal with an acute stroke victim in the catheterization lab. Every patient should be informed and counseled about the risk of stroke from percutaneous cardiac procedures. Ideally, these procedures should be performed at centers where multidisciplinary team support from neurology, neurosurgery, and neuroendovascular specialist is available at all times.

Preprocedure Monitoring

A well-documented baseline neurologic examination before the start of the procedure is necessary. A focused neurologic examination should include the patient's mental status, memory, orientation, language, visual fields, lower cranial nerve function, motor power, gait, and gross coordination. Any known or suspected neurologic deficit should be carefully evaluated and documented before starting the procedure. This will allow prompt and correct detection of any change in neurologic deficit arising as a complication from the procedure.

Intraprocedure and Postprocedure Monitoring

Identification of the onset of stroke can be extremely challenging during cardiovascular procedures. This is due to lack of awareness, administration of sedative medications, and restricted access to the patient due to the presence of sterile patient field. The majority of diagnostic procedures can be conducted using mild sedation alone, and any unnecessary heavy sedation should be avoided. The physician and the nurse in charge should actively monitor for any signs of potential stroke during the procedure.

Intraprocedure clinical neurologic evaluation can be extremely limited during cases performed under deep sedation or general anesthesia. In situations that may place the patient at high risk, certain neuromonitoring techniques can potentially be used to evaluate any changes in the neurologic status; however, none of these techniques have been demonstrated to improve outcome in stroke complications, and we certainly cannot recommend these procedures for routine cardiac catheterization procedures. The ideal technique should provide continuous, real-time information about the cerebral function and flow hemodynamics. The functional information can be obtained by electroencephalography (EEG) and somatosensory evoked potentials (SSEPs). EEG tracing can detect cerebral ischemia by measuring slowing of frequencies or reduced amplitude produced by neuronal dysfunction. These changes tend to be more generalized in global ischemia and regional in focal ischemia. The depth of ischemia is associated with severity of EEG changes. SSEP, on the other hand, detects cerebral ischemia by delay in the arrival or reduction in amplitude of evoked responses. Hemodynamic information can be obtained using transcranial Doppler ultrasonography (TCD) and near-infrared spectroscopy (NIRS) during endovascular procedures. TCD can detect hemodynamic compromise by measuring changes in mean flow velocities in the concerned vessel. In addition, it can detect cerebral microemboli by changes in intensity of received signals after they are reflected by gaseous or particulate matter in the insonated cerebral artery. On the other hand, NIRS technique uses light optical spectroscopy to evaluate the brain oxygen saturation. A reduction in this saturation is believed to reflect the occurrence of cerebral ischemia (19–24). These evolving neuromonitoring techniques are not perfect but can be utilized in complex and high-risk procedures under general anesthesia. Further research is needed to see whether they improve outcome and are cost-effective.

A thorough neurologic examination after the completion of the procedure should be performed with special attention toward any change in neurologic status from the baseline examination conducted before the procedure. Continued observation and vigilance for signs and symptoms of stroke are warranted in the postoperative and recovery units.

■ EVALUATION OF ACUTE STROKE VICTIM IN THE CATHETERIZATION LAB

Prompt diagnosis and evaluation of the ischemic stroke patient are vital as the brain tissue becomes increasingly less salvageable as time progresses (25). Ideally, every hospital should have an acute stroke care plan that utilizes all essential resources including emergency medicine physicians, stroke neurologists, nursing staff, radiologists, neuroendovascular specialists, anesthesiologists, and pharmacists to expedite the evaluation and initiation of proper treatment of acute stroke patients (26). Whenever there is concern or frank signs of acute stroke, it is crucial to promptly inform and mobilize the stroke team. Many hospitals now have 24-hour coverage through active stroke

beeper and a well-established stroke team with members from neurology, emergency radiology, and interventional neuroradiology (27).

As with any critically ill patient, assessment of the airway, breathing, and circulation (ABCs) and providing life support to unstable patients is essential. This should start simultaneously with mobilization of the stroke team. An intravenous (IV) line should be established, if it is not already in place, for administration of drugs as well as for resuscitation. If a stroke is recognized during the procedure and an arterial sheath is in place, it should preferably be retained, sutured, and secured. An established arterial sheath may be useful in case endovascular stroke treatment may be necessary and can save valuable time.

If possible and safe to do so, the interventional team should consider stopping the anticoagulant or antiplatelet agents administered during the endovascular procedure. This is in case the stroke is hemorrhagic which is not known until a noncontrast head CT is performed (see the following text). Anticoagulant reversal should not be performed until after the head CT confirms a hemorrhage since making an ischemic stroke patient more prone to coagulate is not advocated.

Physical Examination

Because the time to start treatment is critical, the physical examination should be strategic and not exhaustive. A focused neurologic examination to assess level of consciousness, mental status, localizing focal signs, and evaluation of stroke severity is performed. The National Institute of Health Stroke Scale (NIHSS) is a preferred neurologic examination that is based upon level of consciousness, motor and sensory function, speech, and language. This helps in localizing the stroke lesion, quantification of the deficit, and helps in decision making about the appropriate treatment (28).

Imaging

The primary goals of imaging in acute stroke patients are to distinguish hemorrhagic stroke from ischemic stroke, presence of early complications, and further evaluation of the ischemic stroke patient for reperfusion therapy. There are limited published data in the context of stroke during cardiac interventions. This section is intended to be a guide to select appropriate neuroimaging techniques based on the author's experience and available literature on stroke in the general population.

Urgent noncontrast CT scan should always be obtained and be the next step after strategic physical examination. This test is rapid, easily available, and serves as an accurate tool for stroke triage (29). A CT should ideally be obtained in matter of minutes and should take precedence over any routine diagnostic study on the first available CT scanner (Fig. 9-1). The major utility of CT is to identify or exclude acute intracranial hemorrhage and its complications. It can also help exclude other conditions that may occasionally mimic stroke such as tumors and other space-occupying lesions. In some cases, CT can be helpful in demonstrating early ischemic changes during the first few hours of stroke, especially in cases of major vessel occlusion. A thrombus in the main stem of middle cerebral artery (MCA) can demonstrate intravascular linear high density as the so-called "Hyperdense MCA sign." Other early CT signs of acute ischemia include subtle hypodensities involving the gray matter structures, such as the basal ganglia, producing loss of margins and distinction of the lentiform nucleus. Sulcal effacement resulting from cytotoxic edema along insular cerebral cortex produces so-called "loss of the insular ribbon sign" (30).

If the clinical evaluation and initial noncontrast CT study are suggestive of acute ischemic stroke, the decision making regarding an attempt at thrombolysis involves the assessment of patient's status, duration from the onset of symptoms, severity of clinical stroke, and presence of any contraindication to thrombolytic therapy. If the clinical deficits are very mild (NIHSS < 4 or considered nondisabling) or improving spontaneously, acute thrombolytic therapy is generally not indicated. Similarly, the presence of contraindications to thrombolytic therapy, established advanced ischemic changes or hemorrhage on CT, and recognition of symptoms beyond the generally accepted 6- to 8-hour treatment window would generally contraindicate thrombolysis as well. Such patients generally benefit from a prompt admission to a dedicated stroke unit or neurologic intensive care unit where they can be managed and evaluated further. Stroke units have indeed been shown to be the most important factor in stroke outcome.

In contrast, if the head CT does not reveal any contraindications, many centers would proceed directly to intra-arterial (IA) thrombolysis. However, another approach is to perform further imaging evaluation to identify the site of arterial occlusion and quantify the presence of salvageable brain tissue (penumbra). The potential advantage of this approach is to use the anatomic and physiologic information that can be so readily obtained by using advanced imaging techniques of CT angiography (CTA) and CT perfusion (CTP) or MR, MR angiography and MR perfusion. However, this approach has a disadvantage of adding a slight delay to the thrombolysis procedure.

As stated earlier, the critical variables in further assessment of the patient at this stage are location of the intracranial occlusion and the status of vascular collaterals supplying the ischemic brain. The choice of imaging study (CT angiogram/CT perfusion or MR/MR angiogram/MR perfusion) or omitting this in favor of more expeditious transfer to neurovascular laboratory depends upon the availability of resources, expertise, and local experience with one modality or the other. Each imaging modality provides specific advantages in specific situations, but again these imaging strategies do not currently have class I evidence supporting their link to improved stroke outcomes. Diffusion-weighted imaging (DWI) sequence of MR is the most sensitive imaging technique available in detecting brain parenchyma likely to reflect completely infarcted brain. It is a preferred modality in patients having posterior fossa ischemia, or small deep white matter cortical lesions. On the other hand, CT is the preferred modality in patients with pacemakers, unstable patients, and those with other contraindications for MR. CTA can be easily obtained in these patients and has a higher spatial resolution than MR angiography (31).

At our institution (DG, SK), we perform a very rapid stroke protocol MR imaging that includes whole-brain DWI, fast fluid attenuation inversion recovery (FLAIR), susceptibility weighted imaging (SWI), MR angiogram, and MR perfusion data to evaluate at-risk brain. This abbreviated MR stroke protocol can be

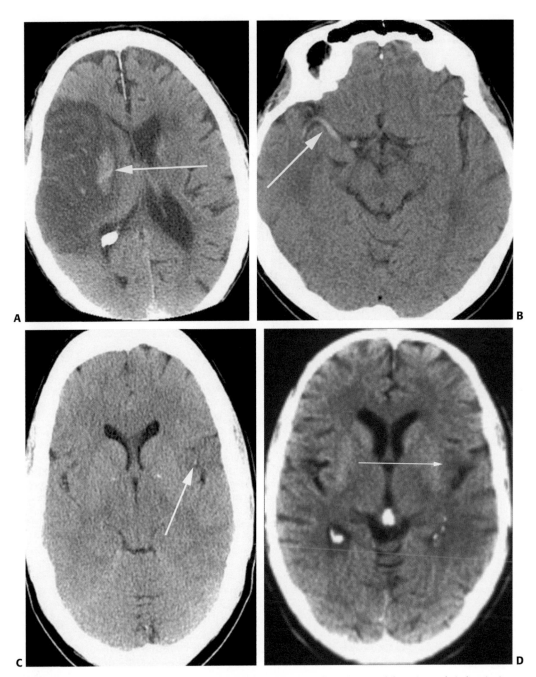

FIGURE 9-1. Role of initial noncontrast CT in evaluating acute stroke patients and detecting early ischemic signs as seen in images obtained from different acute stroke patients. (**A**) Patient with acute right MCA stroke on clinical evaluation. Noncontrast CT reveals a large area of low density associated with edema and sulcal effacement in the right MCA territory. High-density focus in the medial aspect (*arrow*) represents acute hemorrhage. The findings of large area of established ischemic changes as well as presence of hemorrhage should be recognized as these contraindicate any attempt at revascularization. (**B**) Hyperdense MCA sign on right side (*arrow*) representing an acute embolus within the middle cerebral artery. No acute hemorrhage was seen. This patient was treated with intra-arterial thrombolysis. (**C**) MCA dot sign (*arrow*) on the left side representing thrombus in the distal part of MCA. Subtle hypodensity seen in the adjacent brain parenchyma is suggestive of early ischemic change in the brain. (**D**) Insular ribbon sign seen as a subtle hypodensity along the insular cortex and an additional early indicator of MCA stroke.

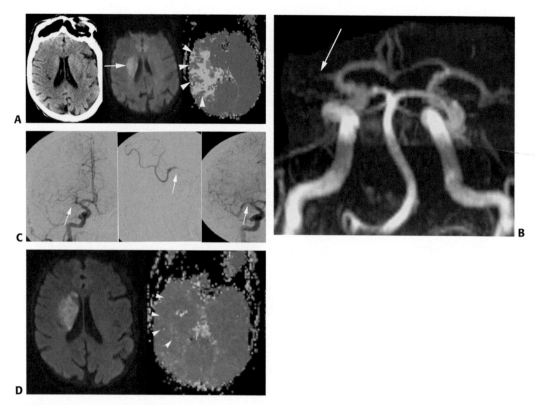

FIGURE 9-2. Example of abbreviated stroke protocol performed at our institution. Within 12 to 15 minutes, a comprehensive stroke assessment is possible with this technique and aids considerably in appropriate decision making. (**A**) Noncontrast CT image in this patient with left hemiplegia and aphasia shows no acute hemorrhage or other contraindication for thrombolysis. Diffusion-weighted imaging (DWI) in the middle shows an area of bright signal (*arrow*) suggestive of restricted diffusion that is consistent with an acute infarct. Colored mean transit time (MTT) image on the right shows a larger area (*arrowheads*) of increased MTT (relative to the DWI image) suggestive of penumbra or salvageable brain. (**B**) MR angiogram image obtained at the same time demonstrates the site of occlusion (*arrow*) in M1 segment of right MCA. (**C**) With the knowledge that there is no hemorrhage, large area of salvageable brain and right MCA occlusion, intra-arterial thrombolysis was offered to the family. DSA image on the left confirms the same site of occlusion (*arrow*) as seen on MRA, the image in the middle shows contrast injection through the microcatheter during the intra-arterial thrombolysis showing distal portion of MCA that was not seen earlier, and the image on the right shows successful recanalization with complete opening at the previous occlusion site (*arrow*). (**D**) Follow-up MRI shows no significant increase in DWI high signal area with resolution of abnormal area seen on MTT before thrombolysis (*arrowheads*). (See color insert.)

completed within 12 to 15 minutes. It provides valuable information about the site of arterial occlusion and the extent of infarcted tissue on diffusion-weighted sequences. Additionally, MR can help identify and quantify penumbra (salvageable, at-risk brain) by evaluating mismatch between diffusion and perfusion sequences (Fig. 9-2). Unstable patients and those with contraindications to MR imaging can just as easily be evaluated with a combination CTA/CTP study. The CTA can identify the site of arterial occlusion and CTP can help identify the tissue level perfusion. The areas of ischemic tissue

(infarct and penumbra) demonstrate increased mean transit time (MTT) and reduced cerebral blood flow (CBF) on the perfusion maps (REF). Areas of decreased cerebral blood volume (CBV) on perfusion studies are consistent with areas of established infarction. Subtraction of areas of decreased CBV (infarcted tissue) from areas of MTT/CBF abnormalities (ischemic tissue) reveals tissue at risk (penumbra) that may be salvaged with timely intervention (Figs. 9-3 and 9-4).

As stated earlier, much controversy and debate exists about using comprehensive stroke

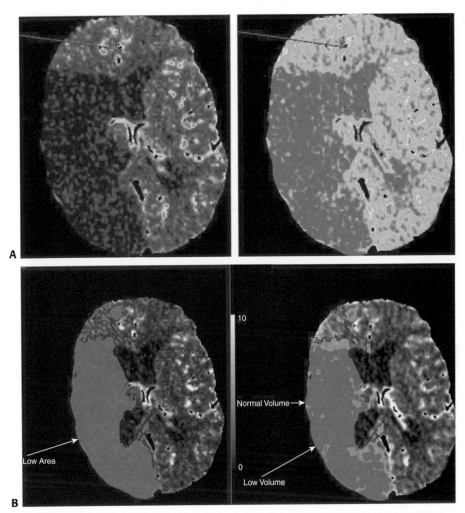

FIGURE 9-3. This 80-year-old patient developed signs of right hemispheric stroke and she was status post an aortic intervention. The NIHSS was 24. CT scan was completely unremarkable. Because of the recent procedure and medical instability, a CTA and CT perfusion was performed. (**A**) CBF perfusion map image on the left shows large abnormal area with decreased cerebral blood flow with matched defect of cerebral blood volume as seen on CBV perfusion map image on the right. (**B**) Lack of penumbra as shown by now commercially available penumbra maps that are constructed from CBF and CBV perfusion maps images shown here. In this patient, there does not appear to be any significant salvageable penumbra. An attempt at revascularization is not indicated and would only result in further injury by reperfusing already infarcted brain.

imaging including CT or MR perfusion data in this setting. The only class I evidence that is available to support improved stroke outcome is to give IV recombinant tissue plasminogen activator (rt-PA) therapy within 4.5 hours for which only noncontrast CT is sufficient. However, most of patients in the setting of cardiac vascular interventions have contraindications to IV rt-PA therapy due to the use of anticoagulant drugs. Some experts (including the senior author LM) favor proceeding directly with digital subtraction angiography after obtaining bare

minimum noncontrast CT imaging in favor of saving time and good neurologic exam. These choices are open to debate at this time and future longitudinal studies will likely answer this question.

■ STROKE MANAGEMENT
Goal

Stroke is the third most common cause of death in industrialized nations and the single most common reason for permanent disability (32).

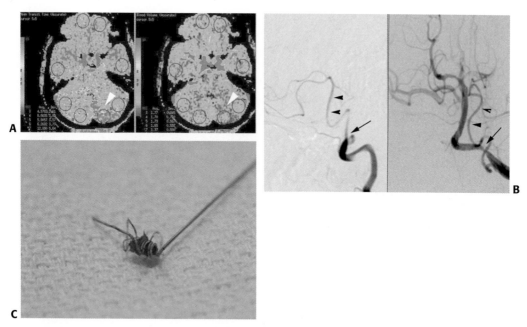

FIGURE 9-4. Successful clot retrieval using MERCI device, 8 hours after the onset of symptoms in a patient with basilar artery occlusion and very poor initial neurologic exam. (**A**) Perfusion images obtained 7 hours after the onset of symptoms show penumbra or mismatch in cerebellar hemispheres between MTT map image on the left and CBV map image on the right (*arrowhead*). (**B**) DSA image on the left shows the site of complete occlusion (*arrow*) in the left vertebral artery distal to the origin of the left posterior inferior cerebellar artery (*black arrowheads*), with nonvisualization of the basilar artery. Image on the right is after clot removal using MERCI device showing recanalization with underlying focal area of stenosis (*arrow*) at the previous site of occlusion. (**C**) MERCI retriever device with clot engaged in distal coiled nitinol loops. This patient made a dramatic recovery. He had mild neurologic deficits the day following the procedure and went on to make a full clinical recovery in the subsequent 3 months. (See color insert.)

This creates a massive financial and personal burden on our society. The estimated direct and indirect cost of stroke for 2008 has been shown to be approximately 65.5 billion dollars (33). Thus, the treatment of stroke is targeted not only at complete functional recovery by timely intervention but also at salvaging at-risk brain and limiting the brain damage to as little as possible. Minimizing the brain damage by saving at-risk brain can provide an opportunity to lead an independent life, and it can make a huge difference in the lives of patients, their family members, and on society as a whole.

The prompt initiation of treatment for acute stroke has been established as the standard of care and includes both well-established medical therapies and constantly evolving newer endovascular techniques. The role and place of the important techniques will be discussed in general followed by their application in the unique setting of stroke during cardiac catheterization. It is important to note that rescuing ischemic neurons is very different from rescuing ischemic cardiac muscle. Any hemorrhage is unfavorable and damaging to the brain. A strategy of opening the occlusion at all costs can be deadly. Prudence in patient selection and knowing when to stop in the battle to open the vessel are critically important.

IV Thrombolysis

The only FDA-approved thrombolytic agent for the treatment of acute ischemic stroke is IV rt-PA. We do not recommend the use of any other thrombolytic agent because of the lack of any substantial safety and efficacy data. IV rt-PA thrombolysis was the first treatment for acute stroke shown to effectively treat the direct underlying cause of vascular occlusion. The time limit for this treatment is within 4.5 hours of the onset of stroke, and it is based on the results of the National Institute of Neurological Disorder and Stroke (NINDS), rt-PA Stroke Study Group trial, and the ECASS-III data (34,35).

This treatment has the advantage of being rapidly available, and it does not require any special equipments. Even though IV thrombolysis was initially a matter of controversy, over time it has been recommended and endorsed as a class 1A level of evidence by major national guideline development organizations (18,36). Nonetheless IV thrombolysis, despite its promise, also suffers from many limitations (37). The recanalization rates of IV rt-PA for proximal arterial occlusion are quite low; only 10% for internal carotid artery (ICA) occlusion and 30% for proximal MCA occlusion (38), and the time constraints for thrombolysis (4.5 hours) are too restrictive for more widespread use (39).

Although IV rt-PA should be considered for any patient with stroke onset within 4.5 hours, it is generally not a useful option for patients with recent cardiac endovascular procedures. This is due to the frequent use of anticoagulants and antiplatelet agents in this patient population, which represents a contraindication to the use of IV rt-PA.

IA Thrombolysis

The ability to provide rapid local delivery of thrombolytics with a greater concentration at the site of occlusion while lowering overall systemic dose led to the concept of IA thrombolysis.

The efficacy and safety of IA r-pro-UK-based thrombolysis were established in two randomized multicenter controlled trials, PROACT I and II (40). IA thrombolysis in patients with MCA occlusion has shown to be more effective in opening the occluded artery even with a longer 6-hour window from symptom onset, and it was at least as effective as IV thrombolysis in improving outcomes. Recanalization rates for major cerebrovascular occlusions such as proximal MCA, ICA, and intracranial carotid artery "T" occlusion are generally far superior (70% vs. 34%) compared with the IV approach (41). However, the risk of intracranial hemorrhage within 24 hours of stroke onset is also higher in the thrombolysis group than in control group (10% vs. 2%). Head-to-head comparisons of IV versus IA thrombolysis are ongoing. Until then, it should be recognized that the level of evidence supporting IV rt-PA is superior to the level of evidence supporting IA rt-PA. It is the special circumstance of the pericardiac catheterization that lends one to consider IA before IV rt-PA. Those factors include the fact that most patients have already received antiplatelet or antithrombotic treatment, which is an absolute contraindication to IV rt-PA, but only a relative contraindication to IA rt-PA, and convenience of having the arterial sheath in place.

IAT has the potential to improve outcome of patients with acute ischemic stroke (see Fig. 9-2). However, it is a high-risk treatment and should only be administered by neurointerventionalists (generally neuroradiologists, neurosurgeons, and neurologists) who have not only received specific training in catheter-based treatment but also understand neuroanatomy and cerebrovascular diseases. Evidence from phase IV studies on IV administration has shown that, unless the protocols for treatment are strictly adhered to, outcomes can be worse.

Combined IA and IV Thrombolysis

This approach is based upon combining the advantage of rapid, easy use of IV rt-PA along with direct local titrated dose and higher rates of recanalization of IAT, promising to improve the speed and frequency of recanalization. In addition, thrombolysis can also be used along with mechanical devices to obtain superior recanalization results, but with additional bleeding concerns.

A large multicenter randomized IMS III trial is currently underway with hope to further optimize the results of endovascular thrombolytic treatment. It promises to provide the safety and efficacy data, not only for combined IA and IV thrombolytic therapy, but also for additional use of mechanical devices in clot removal.

■ ENDOVASCULAR MECHANICAL APPROACHES

Mechanical means of clot removal are rapidly gaining popularity and have several advantages over IV and IA thrombolytic therapy. Mechanical removal can be used as the only method or in combination with thrombolytic therapy. By reducing or avoiding the use of thrombolytics, the risk of hemorrhage is likely reduced. Moreover, the mechanical approach allows a much wider window of treatment, as far as 8 hours after symptom onset. When used in conjunction with thrombolytics, it increases the speed of their action by exposing a larger surface area of the fragmented clot to the drug (37). However, there are no randomized, controlled trials demonstrating the safety and efficacy of these devices yet. More studies are needed, and while we employ these devices routinely for patient care, we feel obligated to inform patients and their families regarding the limited published data about their use.

Mechanical devices may be the best or sometimes the only option for many patients who have contraindications to thrombolytic therapy, including the use of anticoagulants or glycoprotein IIb–IIIa inhibitors, recent surgery, bleeding disorders, or when patients are already beyond the therapeutic time window for IV and IA thrombolysis (42–44). However, the mechanical approach at times can be technically challenging especially in navigation of these devices through extremely tortuous vessels. In untrained hands, devices can cause excessive trauma to the vasculature causing vasospasm, vessel dissection, or perforation. Mechanical retrieval devices can sometimes migrate the clot into more proximal larger vessel and potentially cause a larger stroke. However, the various distinct advantages of mechanical stroke treatment discussed earlier still make the use of this strategy very attractive.

Thrombus Disruption Technique

This technique is most commonly used in conjunction with thrombolytic therapy. Generally, the tip of the microwire is used to break the thrombus with great caution not to injure the wall of vessel. Passing the distal end of the microwire few times through the thrombus makes a small channel and increases the surface area of the clot exposed to the thrombolytic agent. Other means that can be used to break the thrombus include snares, percutaneous transluminal angioplasty, and low-pressure balloon angioplasty.

The MicroLysUS infusion catheter has an inbuilt piezoelectric sonography element at its distal tip that creates ultrasonic vibration to facilitate thrombolysis. It involves the separation of fibrin strands using noncavitating sonography, along with an increase in fluid permeation by acoustic streaming and thus exposing larger surface area of thrombus to the thrombolytic drug. This approach results in faster clot disso-

lution with less fragmentation of the thrombus (45). However, we favor the use of alternative mechanical devices (MERCI, PENUMBRA) as discussed in the following text.

Mechanical Embolectomy Using the MERCI Device

The Merci retriever (Concentric Medical) was the first mechanical stroke device to be approved by the FDA in 2004 to restore blood flow by removing thrombus from occluded vessels in patients experiencing ischemic stroke. Patients who are otherwise ineligible for treatment with IV rt-PA or who fail IV rt-PA therapy may qualify for this treatment.

The Merci retriever device consists of a flexible nitinol wire with multiple helical loops at its distal end that are meant to engage the thrombus for retrieval. This is advanced through a microcatheter and a larger 8- or 9-F balloon guiding catheter. Once the thrombus is engaged in the loops, the guiding catheter balloon is inflated to temporarily reduce or stop the antegrade flow to help retrieving the clot. Since the initial approval in 2004, this device has undergone several modifications to improve the recanalization success rate. First-generation devices (X5 and X6) had tapering helical-shaped nitinol wire loops at its distal end. In the second-generation devices (L4, L5, and L6), some additional arcading filaments were attached to a nontapering helical nitinol coil with 90-degree angle to the proximal wire. In the next-generation devices, variable pitch was introduced in the loops in linear fashion with attached filaments (37).

The international multicenter Multi MERCI trial was conducted in patients who had either contraindications to IV rt-PA, or in whom IV rt-PA failed to recanalize the arterial occlusions. Successful recanalization was achieved in 55% of cases by retriever alone and in 68% of cases with adjunctive therapy. The Merci device can be especially useful and more effective in large-vessel occlusions (Fig. 9-4) with a safety profile similar to previously discussed stroke interventions (42,43,46).

Mechanical Embolectomy Using Penumbra System

The Penumbra system is a new addition to mechanical devices by which a thrombus can be

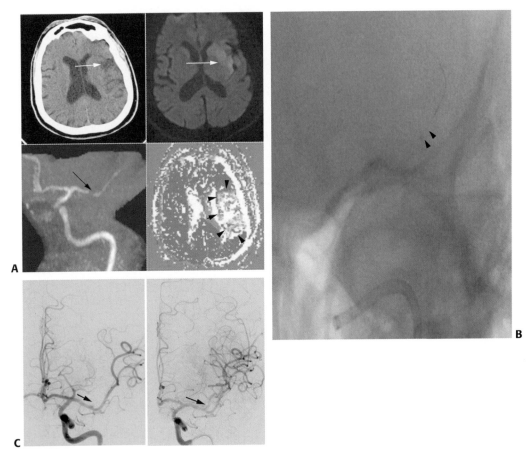

FIGURE 9-5. Usefulness of penumbra device for mechanical thrombolysis. This patient developed acute hemiplegia following endovascular cardiac intervention. Given the recent use of heavy anticoagulation during cardiac procedure, mechanical thrombolysis was offered. (**A**) Noncontrast CT image in upper left corner shows subtle hypodensity (*arrow*) with no hemorrhage. There is penumbra present with obvious mismatch between upper right DWI image (*arrow*) and lower right perfusion map (*arrowheads*). MR angiogram in lower left corner shows nonvisualization of upper division of MCA with occlusion at its origin (*black arrow*). (**B**) Unsubtracted angiogram image showing the placement of penumbra mechanical device at occlusion site (*arrowheads*). (**C**) Digital subtraction images before and after successful recanalization of superior division of MCA using Penumbra mechanical device (*arrow*). Subsequent MR imaging (not shown) revealed resolution of mismatch between DWI and PWI images. (See color insert.)

removed from large intracranial vessels (Fig. 9-5). The device disrupts the thrombus by mechanical force and removes it by extraction and aspiration. The system is composed of three main components: a reperfusion catheter, a separator, and a thrombus removal ring. First, the catheter is placed just proximal to the clot and then connected to an aspiration pump that generates vacuum force of −20 in of Hg to remove the clot. Any residual thrombus portion can be engaged and removed directly by using the thrombus removal ring (47). It is a promising system and contrary to the MERCI device works from the proximal portion to the distal portion of the thrombus.

In a prospective international multicenter trial (Penumbra Stroke Trial) conducted in the United States and Europe, complete or partial recanalization was achieved in 81.6% of occluded vessels. Similar results were also found in a retrospective review of 139 patients who were treated with this device at seven international centers, thus reflecting a favorable efficacy profile in real-world setting (48). However, there are no randomized studies or studies comparing mechanical with lytic therapy.

■ STROKE UNIT MONITORING

The postprocedure stroke patient should be monitored with the aim to minimize preventable complications and to improve the overall functional independence. However, the presence of underlying cardiac diseases can make it challenging to properly balance the different needs of recovering brain and at-risk heart. Proper maintenance of important physiologic parameters such as oxygenation, blood pressure, temperature, and glycemic status is extremely important. Any possible effect on these parameters should be considered while using postprocedure medications. The extent of monitoring required depends upon the severity, the cause of stroke, and the overall condition of the patient. Serial clinical monitoring every 4 hours may be appropriate for a stable recovering patient, whereas continuous monitoring may be needed for a patient who has suffered an intracranial bleeding and who is prone to various complications. As with any acute disease process, maintenance of airways for adequate oxygenation is crucial. Stroke patients with brainstem involvement and reduced consciousness often require endotracheal intubation to protect their airways and provide adequate oxygenation. The oxygen saturation must be maintained at greater than or equal to 95% (18).

Poststroke patients may develop hypotension or more commonly hypertension. Potential causes of hypotension include aortic dissection, dehydration, blood loss, sepsis, and decreased cardiac output (18). Whenever hypotension is noted, the underlying cause should be sought and immediate treatment should be started. However, vasopressors should be avoided if possible, as they can potentially cause myocardial infarction, pulmonary edema, and systemic end organ ischemia. Recommendation for patients undergoing reperfusion therapy is to maintain systolic blood pressure (SBP) of less than 180 mm Hg and diastolic blood pressure (DBP) of less than 105 mm Hg (18).

Fever, hypoxia, and glucose dysregulation are very toxic to ischemic neurons. Efforts to avoid these perturbations are warranted. Hyperglycemia is seen in up to one-third of patients with acute ischemic stroke (49) and is associated with increased brain edema after stroke and increased risk of hemorrhagic transformation

(50). Hypoglycemia, on the other hand, can mimic the symptoms of ischemic stroke and its correction should lead to rapid resolution of associated neurologic deficits.

■ CONCLUSION

Although acute stroke is one of the most feared complications of cardiac catheterization, there are treatment options that can reduce the damage. Importantly, the management of stroke patients should include a team approach involving stroke neurology and neurointerventional experts. Judicious use of rt-PA in carefully selected patients by IV or IA routes, consideration for a mechanical approach, and close monitoring in a stroke unit with aggressive prevention of complications, metabolic optimization, and early rehabilitation are crucial parts of stroke recovery.

References

1. Segal AS, Abernethy WB, Palacios IF, et al. Stroke as a complication of cardiac catheterization: risk factors and clinical features. *Neurology.* 2001;56: 975–977.
2. Fuchs S, Stabile E, Kinnaird TD, et al. Stroke complicating percutaneous coronary interventions: incidence, predictors, and prognostic implications. *Circulation.* 2002;106:86–91.
3. National Center for Health Statistics. *1999 National Hospital Discharge Survey: Annual Summary with Detailed Diagnosis and Procedure Data.* DHHS Publication (PHS) 2001–1722. Washington, DC: US Department of Health and Human Services; September 2001, No. 151.
4. Broderick J, Connolly S, Feldmann E, et al. Guidelines for the management of spontaneous intracerebral hemorrhage in adults: 2007 update. A guideline from the American Heart Association/American Stroke Association Stroke Council High Blood Pressure Research Council; Quality of Care and Outcomes in Research Interdisciplinary Working Group. *Stroke.* 2007;38:2001–2023.
5. Weintraub WS, Mahoney EM, Ghazzal ZM, et al. Trends in outcome and costs of coronary intervention in the 1990s. *Am J Cardiol.* 2001;88:497–503.
6. Akkerhuis KM, Deckers JW, Lincoff AM, et al. Risk of stroke associated with abciximab among patients undergoing percutaneous coronary intervention. *JAMA.* 2001;286:78–82.

7. Hand PJ, Wardlaw JM, Rivers CS, et al. MR diffusion weighted imaging and outcome prediction after ischemic stroke. *Neurology.* 2006;66:1159–1163.

8. Hedberg M, Boivie P, Edstrom C, et al. Cerebrovascular accidents after cardiac surgery: an analysis of CT scans in relation to clinical symptoms. *Scand Cardiovasc J.* 2005;39:299–305.

9. Hogue CW Jr, Murphy SF, Schechtman KB, et al. Risk factors for early or delayed stroke after cardiac surgery. *Circulation.* 1999;100:642–647.

10. Keeley EC, Grines CL. Scraping of aortic debris by coronary guiding catheters: a prospective evaluation of 1000 cases. *J Am Coll Cardiol.* 1998; 32:1861–1865.

11. Qureshi AI, Luft AR, Sharma M, et al. Prevention and treatment of thromboembolic and ischemic complications associated with endovascular procedures, part 1: pathophysiological and pharmacological features. *Neurosurgery.* 2000;46:1344–1359.

12. Wijman CA, Kase CS, Jacobs AK, et al. Cerebral air embolism as a cause of stroke during cardiac catheterization. *Neurology.* 1998;51:318–319.

13. Hinkle DA, Raizen DM, McGarvey ML, et al. Cerebral air embolism complicating cardiac ablation procedures. *Neurology.* 2001;56:792–794.

14. Zhou L, Keane D, Reed G. Thromboembolic complications of cardiac radiofrequency catheter ablation: a review of the reported incidence, pathogenesis and current research directions. *J Cardivasc Electrophysiol.* 1999;10:611–620.

15. Kok LC, Mangrum JM, Haines DE, et al. Cerebrovascular complication associated with pulmonary vein ablation. *J Cardiovasc Electrophysiol.* 2002;13:764–767.

16. Heuschmann PU, Kolominsky-Rabas PL, Misselwitz B, et al. Predictors of in-hospital mortality and attributable risks of death after ischemic stroke: the German Stroke Registers Study Group. *Arch Intern Med.* 2004;164:1761–1768.

17. Reed SD, Cramer SC, Blough DK, et al. Treatment with tissue plasminogen activator and inpatient mortality rates for patients with ischemic stroke treated in community hospitals. *Stroke.* 2001;32: 1832–1840.

18. Adams HP Jr, del Zeppo G, Alberts MJ, et al. Guidelines for the early management of adults with ischemic stroke: a guideline from the American Heart Association/American Stroke Association Stroke Council, Clinical Cardiology Council, Cardiovascular Radiology and Intervention Council, and the Atherosclerotic Peripheral Vascular Disease and Quality of Care Outcomes in Research Interdisciplinary Working Groups. *Stroke.* 2007;38:1655–1711.

19. Haupt WF, Horsch S. Evoked potentials in carotid surgery: a review of 994 cases. *Neurology.* 1992; 42:835–838.

20. Sloan MA, Alexandrov AV, Tegeler CH, et al. Assessment: transcranial Doppler ultrasonography. Report of the Therapeutic and Technology Assessment Subcommittee of the American Academy of Neurology. *Neurology.* 2004;62:1468–1481.

21. Razumovsky AY, Gugino LD, Owen JH. Advanced neurological monitoring for cardiothoracic and vascular surgery. *Semin Cerebrovascular Dis Stroke.* 2005;5:141–154.

22. Arnold M, Sturzenegger M, Schaffler L, et al. Continuous intraoperative monitoring of middle cerebral artery blood flow velocities and electroencephalography during carotid endarterectomy. *Stroke.* 1997;28:1345–1350.

23. Dinkel M, Schweiger H, Georlitz P. Monitoring during carotid surgery: somatosensory evoked potentials versus carotid stump pressure. *J Neruosurg Anesthesiol.* 1992;4:167–175.

24. Halsley JH, McDowell HA, Gelman S. Transcranial Doppler and rCBF compared in carotid endarterectomy. *Stroke.* 1986;17:1206–1208.

25. Albers GW, Amarenco P, Easton JD, et al. Antithrombotic and thrombolytic therapy for ischemic stroke: the seventh ACCP conference on antithrombotic and thrombolytic therapy. *Chest.* 2004;126:483S–512S.

26. Gorelick AR, Gorelick PB, Sloan EP. Emergency department evaluation and management of stroke: acute assessment, stroke teams and carepathways. *Neurol Clin.* 2008;26:923–942.

27. Hamidon BB, Dewey HM: Impact of acute stroke team emergency calls on in-hospital delays in acute stroke care. *J Clin Neurosci.* 2007;14:831–834.

28. Cohen SN. *Management of Ischemic Stroke.* New York, NY: McGraw-Hill; 2000.

29. Wintermark M, Rowley H, Lev M. Acute stroke triage to intravenous thrombolysis and other therapies with advanced CT or MR imaging: pro CT. *Radiology.* 2009;251:619–926.

30. Nakano S, Iseda T, Yoneyama T, et al. Early CT signs in patients with acute middle cerebral artery occlusion: incidence of contrast staining and hemorrhagic transformations after intra-arterial

reperfusion therapy. *Clin Radiol.* 2006;61:156–162.

31. Bash S, Villablanca JP, Jahan R, et al. Intracranial vascular stenosis and occlusive disease: evaluation with CT angiography, MR angiography, and digital subtraction angiography. *AJNR Am J Neuroradiol.* 2005;26:1012–1021.

32. Stroke: 1989—recommendations on stroke prevention, diagnosis, and therapy: report of the WHO Task Force and Other Cerebrovascular Disorders. *Stroke.* 1989;20:1407–1431.

33. Rosamond W, Flegal K, Furie K, et al. Heart disease and stroke statistics: 2008 update—a report from the American Heart Association Statistics Committee and Stroke Statistics Subcommittee. *Circulation.* 2008;117:e25–e146.

34. Tissue plasminogen activator for acute ischemic stroke: The National Institute of Neurological Disorders and Stroke rtPA Stroke Study Group. *N Engl J Med.* 1995;333:1581–1587.

35. Hacke W, Kaste M, Bluhmki E, et al. Thrombolysis with alteplase 3 to 4.5 hours after acute ischemic stroke. *N Engl J Med.* 2008;359:1317–1329.

36. Sacco RL, Adams R, Albers G, et al. Guidelines for prevention of stroke in patients with ischemic stroke or transient ischemic attack: a statement for healthcare professionals from the American Heart Association/American Stroke Association Council on Stroke. *Stroke.* 2006;37:577–617.

37. Nogueira RG, Schwamm LH, Hirsch JA. Endovascular approaches to acute stroke, part 1: drugs, devices, and data. *Am J Neuroradiol.* 2009;30:649–661.

38. Wolpert SM, Bruckmann H, Greenlee R, et al. Neuroradiologic evaluation of patients with acute stroke treated with recombinant tissue plasminogen activator: the rtPA Acute Stroke Study Group. *AJNR Am J Neuroradiol.* 1993;14:3–13.

39. Rosamond W, Flegal K, Friday G, et al. Heart disease and stroke statistics—2007 update: a report from the American Heart Association Statistics Committee and Stroke Statistics Subcommittee. *Circulation.* 2007;115:e172.

40. Furlan A, Higashida R, Wechsler L, et al. Intra-arterial prourokinase for acute ischemic stroke. The PROACT II study: a randomized controlled trial. Prolyse in Acute Cerebral Thromboembolism. *JAMA.* 1999;282(21):2003–2011.

41. Von Kummer R, Holle R, Rosin L, et al. Does arterial recanalization improve outcome in carotid territory stroke? *Stroke.* 1995;26:581–587.

42. Nogueira RG, Smith WS. Safety and efficacy of endovascular thrombectomy in patients with abnormal hemostasis: pooled analysis of the MERCI and Multi MERCI trials. *Stroke.* 2009;40:516–522.

43. Smith WS, Sung G, Starkman S, et al. Safety and efficacy of mechanical embolectomy in acute ischemic stroke: results of the MERCI trial. *Stroke.* 2005;36:1432–1438.

44. Smith WS, Sung G, Saver J, et al. Mechanical thrombectomy for acute ischemic stroke: final results of the Multi MERCI trial. *Stroke.* 2008;39:1205–1212.

45. Tomsick T, Broderick J, Carrozella J, et al. Revascularization results in the Interventional Management of Stroke II trial. *AJNR Am J Neuroradiol.* 2008;29:582–587.

46. Gobin YP, Starkman S, Duckwiler GR, et al. MERCI 1: a phase 1 study of Mechanical Embolus Removal in Cerebral Ischemia. *Stroke.* 2004;35:2848–2854.

47. Bose A, Henkes H, Alfke K, et al. The Penumbra System: a mechanical device for the treatment of acute stroke due to thromboembolism. *AJNR Am J Roentgenol.* 2008;29:1409–1413.

48. Tarr R, Alfke K, Stingele R, et al. Initial postmarket experience of the Penumbra System: revascularization of large vessel occlusion in acute ischemic stroke in the United States and Europe. *Stroke.* 2009;40:46.

49. Scott JF, Robinson GM, French JM, et al. Prevalence of admission hyperglycemia across clinical subtypes of acute stroke. *Lancet.* 1999;353:376–377.

50. Lindsberg PJ, Roine RO. Hyperglycemia in acute stroke. *Stroke.* 2004;35:363–364.

10 Periprocedural Myocardial Infarction

ASHEQUL M. ISLAM AND AARON D. KUGELMASS

Myocardial infarction (MI) resulting from percutaneous coronary intervention (PCI) has been an acknowledged complication since the introduction of balloon angioplasty. Although the incidence of abrupt closure has been almost negated by the introduction of stents and adjunct therapies, clinically significant periprocedural MI remains an important complication. Controversy has centered on the importance of periprocedural cardiac enzyme leaks. Despite this debate, periprocedural MI remains a critical component of any determination of major adverse cardiovascular events (MACE). Periprocedural MI is pertinent to the evaluation and introduction of new interventional devices as well as standardized outcome registries of routine clinical interventional cardiology practice. This chapter reviews the definition of periprocedural MI, its incidence, and the debate around its prognostic significance. The pathophysiologic mechanisms of PCI-related infarction are reviewed, as is the efficacy of therapeutic approaches to reduce this complication. Recommendations for the management of patients with periprocedural infarction follow.

DEFINITION OF MI

The term "myocardial infarction" defines myocardial cell necrosis due to ischemia secondary to perfusion imbalance between supply and demand. Traditionally, MI was defined in studies of disease prevalence by the World Health Organization (WHO) by symptoms, EKG abnormalities, and enzyme elevation. However, with the availability of highly sensitive biomarkers, very small or even silent MIs are now detected. Elevations of biomarkers above the 99th percentile upper limit of normal after PCI, assuming a normal baseline troponin value, are indicative of postprocedural myocardial necrosis. There is currently no specific scientific basis for defining a biomarker threshold for the diagnosis of periprocedural MI. Pending further data, and by arbitrary convention, it is suggested to designate increases more than three times the 99th percentile upper limit of normal as PCI-related MI (1).

Any elevation in cardiac enzymes after PCI is a result of cell death secondary to myocardial ischemia and should be identified as MI according to the new criteria (2). Periprocedural MI is classified as type 4a by the ACC and ESC consensus panel (2). Pathologically, infarctions are typically classified by size: microscopic (focal necrosis), small (less than 10% of the left ventricular [LV] myocardium), moderate (10% to 30% of the LV myocardium), and large (more than 30% of the LV myocardium), and by location.

Myocardial cell injury occurring after angioplasty may be a one-time event as opposed to often repetitive nature of spontaneously occurring myocardial ischemia and injury. However, it is likely that patients who develop a coronary microembolism and periprocedural infarcts have atherosclerotic lesions that are unstable, and hence, represent a subgroup at risk for future events.

INFARCTION TYPE AND INCIDENCE

Q Wave (ST-Segment Elevation MI)

Large, clinically significant MI was a common and serious complication in the early percutaneous transluminal coronary angioplasty (PTCA) experience. The initial NHLBI angioplasty registry (1977 through 1981) reported a 4.4% incidence of MI (3). Additionally, 6% of patients required emergent coronary artery bypass graft (CABG). These figures improved over the subsequent 5 years. The second NHLBI registry enrolled patients from 14 centers between 1985 and 1986 (4). The success rate improved to 90% with reduction of emergency CABG rates from 5.8% to 3.5%, and a reduction of mortality rate for patients with single-vessel coronary artery disease from 0.85% to 0.2%. However, the periprocedural MI rate remained constant (4.3%), even though in a more complex patient cohort.

Among patients with abrupt closure that proceeded to bypass surgery within 90 minutes, up to 50% sustained a Q-wave MI. Thus, the "true" rate of Q-wave MI related to PTCA significantly exceeded 6% when patients requiring emergent CABG are also considered. In a large study of all elective cases of PTCA for stable or unstable angina between 1980 and 1986 at Emory University Hospital, there were 316 patients undergoing CABG after failed PTCA. Of those, 202 patients had surgery emergently and the rest electively (5). There was significantly higher in-hospital Q-wave MI in emergent CABG group compared with the elective CABG group (27% vs. 4%). With the introduction of the coronary perfusion balloon and maintenance of distal coronary perfusion, there was less injury to myocardial tissue in patients sent for emergency CABG and the risk of Q-wave MI decreased to approximately 10% (6). However, by the late 1980s to early 1990s, the incidence of periprocedural Q-wave MI still exceeded 1.5%, and emergent surgery in 3%. The introduction of stents in 1993 reduced the complication rates even more with major adverse cardiac event in 3% (death 1%, emergency CABG 0.7%, and Q-wave and large non–Q-wave MI 1.3%) (7). Currently, the incidence of PCI-related Q-wave and large non–Q-wave infarctions approximates 1% (8).

Contemporary large periprocedural infarcts, as will be discussed in greater detail, are often due to clinically detectable procedural complications such as severe coronary dissection not treatable with a stent resulting in abrupt vessel closure. In the absence of a stent, the presence of complex dissection is associated with five times more abrupt closure during coronary balloon angioplasty (9). Other factors include large side branch occlusion, disruption of collateral flow, distal embolization, protracted "slow flow" or "no reflow" phenomenon, and stent thrombosis.

Non–ST-Segment Elevation MI

When creatine phosphokinase (CPK) is routinely measured following PCI, there is often elevation of this (and other) cardiac marker in the absence of clinical or angiographic suggestion of a complication or myocardial necrosis. Depending on the threshold, the incidence of periprocedural CPK elevation can range from 10% to 35% (10) (Table 10-1). Likewise, numerous studies have demonstrated elevation of troponin T and I isoforms. Some series have reported periprocedural elevations of this more sensitive marker of myonecrosis in more than 50% of patients undergoing PCI (11).

Large non–ST-segment elevation infarctions, as will be discussed in greater detail, are most often the result of abrupt closure, side branch occlusion, transient flow diminution, and macroscopic embolization. In contrast, small biomarker releases, often clinically and angiographically silent, are more frequent. These are postulated to be the result of microemboli from disrupted atherosclerotic plaques and thrombus during percutaneous interventions. While initial discussion focused on whether small biomarker release resulted from cellular ischemia without actual infarction, magnetic resonance imaging has demonstrated irreversible myocardial necrosis in patients with only mild or borderline elevations of either CPK-MB or troponin with and without angiographic evidence of vessel occlusion and an absence of EKG changes or wall motion abnormalities (25,26) (Fig. 10-1). Selvanayagam et al. showed that there was a strong correlation between the rise in troponin I measurements at 24 hours and mean mass of new myocardial hyperenhancement, both at 24 hours and a median of 8 months after PCI (Fig. 10-2). The magnitude of this injury correlates directly with the extent of troponin elevation.

■ PROGNOSTIC SIGNIFICANCE

It has been broadly accepted that Q wave and large, clinically apparent non–Q-wave MIs following PCI were associated with poor long-term

TABLE 10-1   **Incidence of CPK-MB Release Following PCI**

Author	Year	n	>1× ULN (%)	≥3× ULN (%)	≥5× ULN (%)	≥8× ULN (%)
Klein et al. (12)	1991	272	15.3	—	—	—
Kugelmass et al. (13)	1994	565	11.5	—	2.3	—
Tardiff et al. (14)	1999	2,341	24.0	13.8	3.7	—
Kini et al. (15)	1999	1,675	18.7	5.9	2.4	—
Saucedo et al. (16)	2000	900	35.0	—	8.5	—
Mehran et al. (17)	2000	2,256	25.8	—	12.9	0
Stone et al. (18)	2001	7,147	37.3	17.9	11.8	7.7
Ellis et al. (19)	2002	8,409	17.2	—	3.6	—
Brener et al. (20)	2002	3,478	24.2	9.8	5.3	—
Jeremias et al. (21)	2004	5,850	21.3	8.7	—	2.6
Pasceri et al. (22)	2004	153	35.0	—	—	—
Briguori et al. (23)	2004	451	—	16.4	15.6	—
Lindsey et al. (24)	2009	5,961	—	7.2	3.7	—

ULN, upper limit of normal.

outcomes. In a study of over 7,000 patients by Stone et al., the development of Q waves following PCI was associated with a 38% 2-year mortality with a hazard ratio of 9.9 (18). Although there has been unanimity around the significance of large periprocedural infarctions, there has been significant debate over the clinical significance of smaller infarctions. This has been especially true of clinically and angiographically "silent" enzyme releases. Specifically, there has been little

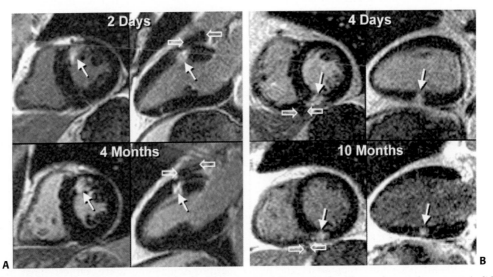

FIGURE 10-1. Contrast-enhanced MRI views of two patients demonstrating discrete hyperenhancement (*solid arrows*) immediately adjacent to the stent (*open arrows*), both early and late after PCI. (**A**) Patient 7 had a stent in the proximal left anterior descending artery. (**B**) Patient 2 had a stent in the mid-posterior descending artery. Both patients had minor side branch occlusion. (From Ricciardi MJ, Wu E, Davidson CJ, et al. Visualization of discrete microinfarction after percutaneous coronary intervention associated with mild creatine kinase-MB elevation. *Circulation.* 2001;103:2780–2783.)

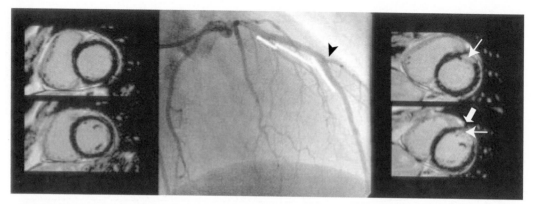

FIGURE 10-2. Two basal short-axis images (**left**) in a patient before left anterior descending coronary artery (LAD) PCI showing no delayed hyperenhancement. Contrast-enhanced images in the same image plane after PCI (**right**) reveal new anterolateral wall hyperenhancement (*long arrows*) adjacent to LAD stent (*short arrow*). Center shows post-PCI angiogram with position of three stents highlighted and good flow in LAD and second diagonal branch (likely affected territory; *black arrowhead*). (From Selvanayagam JB, Porto I, Channon K, et al. Troponin elevation after percutaneous coronary intervention directly represents the extent of irreversible myocardial injury: insights from cardiovascular magnetic resonance imaging. *Circulation.* 2005;111:1027–1032.)

agreement over what threshold of CPK-MB release should be considered "large" or of prognostic significance.

In numerous studies, periprocedural myocardial biomarker release has been associated with increased risk-adjusted mortality (13,14,18,27–35). However, the threshold above which myocardial enzyme elevation is associated with adverse long-term clinical outcomes is still controversial. Most studies have examined CPK-MB as the marker for periprocedural MI. At one end of the spectrum, numerous studies have suggested that any degree of CPK-MB elevation is associated with increased mortality (14,27,29–32,35). In a meta-analysis of seven studies with 23,230 PCI patients, significantly increased mortality was observed with elevated CPK-MB level (32). Mean follow-up was 6 to 34 months. Compared with subjects with normal CPK-MB, there was a dose–response relationship with relative risks for death being 1.5 (95% CI, 1.2 to 1.8) with one- to three-fold CPK-MB elevations, 1.8 (95% CI, 1.4 to 2.4) with three- to five-fold CPK-MB elevations, and 3.1 (95% CI, 2.3 to 4.2) with over five-fold CPK-MB elevations ($P <$ 0.001 for all). Simoon et al. also showed any elevation of CPK-MB has a dose–response relationship with mortality at 6 months in a meta-analysis of EPIC, CAPTURE, and EPILOG trials (35).

It is also controversial whether periprocedural MI and spontaneous MI have similar clinical implications. Akkerhuis et al. demonstrated in their analysis of patients with unstable angina and non–ST-elevation MI that there is a gradual increase in 6-month mortality with increasing level of CPK-MB, which occurred spontaneously or after PCI (29). Although the absolute mortality rates were lower after procedure-related infarcts compared with spontaneous infarcts, the relative increase in 6-month mortality with each increase in peak CPK-MB level was similar for PCI-related myocardial necrosis and spontaneous myocardial necrosis. These authors concluded that any periprocedural CPK-MB release carried the same long-term prognostic significance as a "spontaneous" infarction.

Abdelmeguid et al. examined 4,664 consecutive patients at Cleveland Clinic with successful PTCA or directional atherectomy (27). In this study, elevation of total CPK level twice normal and higher was associated with increased cardiac mortality at 36 ± 22 months compared with a group with CPK level equal to or less than twice normal level. Other studies (13,15,16,33) reported a threshold of five times above normal CPK-MB elevation as a predictor of increased cardiovascular mortality. Others have found only Q-wave MI or CPK-MB elevation $> 8\times$ normal predictive of increased late mortality (18,21). A recent (2009) analysis of the EVENT registry of contemporary "real-world" PCI, including the widespread use of drug-eluting stents, glycoprotein (Gp) IIb/IIIa inhibitors, thienopyridines, and statins, demonstrated that any periprocedural CPK-MB > 3× ULN was associated with increased 1-year mortality (36). However, when enzyme thresholds were employed, only patients with CPK-MB > 10× ULN had a significant increase in mortality (24). In one analysis of close to 6,000 pooled stent trial patients, lack of procedural success was the only predictor of late mortality, as even patients with Q waves and CPK-MB > 8× ULN who had successful stent procedures had no significant increased late risk (21).

There is greater agreement concerning the implications or periprocedural troponin elevation. As discussed, troponin I and T isoforms are frequently elevated following PCI. Minor elevations do not appear to impact long-term prognosis, whereas large elevations (>5× ULN) are associated with worsened outcomes (37).

To the extent that periprocedural MI confers or is associated with a late mortality risk, that risk appears to be greatest comparatively early following PCI. In an analysis of patients with periprocedural CPK-MB release, the increase in mortality abated by 4 months (19). Time-specific analysis of the EVENT registry demonstrated that the association of periprocedural MI was significant through 30 days but not days 31 to 365 (36).

As unclear as the "absolute" threshold for a significant periprocedural enzyme release is the causal relationship of periprocedural infarction and late mortality. Some authors have suggested that myonecrosis following PCI, even when comparatively small, establishes a nidus for arrhythmias, or in patients with compromised preprocedural reduced LV function, it begets further LV failure. Alternatively, others have suggested that these infarctions identify patients at increased risk of future ischemia-based events. Periprocedural enzyme elevation is associated with increased plaque burden in both the lesion and reference vessel, elevated preprocedural hsCRP, and reduced by pretreatment with statins (17,22,38). This suggests that periprocedural myonecrosis may be a marker of significant vulnerable plaque and a proinflammatory state, which, in turn, are the causal factors in increased late mortality in these patients.

■ RISK FACTORS FOR PERIPROCEDURAL MI

The propensity for atheromatous or thrombotic embolization, vessel occlusion, and/or protracted flow diminution predicts the likelihood of a patient developing periprocedural myonecrosis (Table 10-2). Plaque volume, both at the lesion and the reference vessel, as well as lesion length and lesion complexity are all associated with an increase in biomarker release (17,36,39–41). Lesions with friable plaque or adherent thrombus and an increased risk of distal embolization, as well as a proinflammatory state also predispose to periprocedural infarction. Patients with acute coronary syndromes, de novo as opposed to restenotic lesions, saphenous vein graft (SVG) targets, angiographic thrombus, and increased preprocedural hsCRP are all at increased risk (11,36,39,40,42,43). Of these, SVG lesions and in situ thrombus appear to confer the greatest hazard (11). Procedural technique also impacts infarction. Compared with balloon angioplasty, increased myonecrosis is observed after stenting or atherectomy, directional or rotational (11,16,18,39). Stent length, the number of stents deployed, and stent balloon inflation pressure are all variables associated with

TABLE 10-2 **Predictors of Periprocedural Myocardial Infarction**

Lesion specific
  Thrombus
  Saphenous vein graft
  Complex (type C)
  De novo
  Bifurcation
  Plaque volume
  Lesion length

Device specific
  Atherectomy
  Stent
  Stent length
  Number of stents
  Inflation pressure

Patient specific
  Acute coronary syndrome
  Multivessel PCI
  ↑ hsCRP

periprocedural infarction (11,16,36). Side branch occlusion, discussed further in the following text, is also an important factor in this process. As such, bifurcation PCI is also associated with an increased incidence of infarction (11,40).

Angiographic Findings

Mechanical, as well as physiologic, obstruction to blood flow during PCI is the fundamental cause of periprocedural MI. Frequently, these events are angiographically and/or clinically evident in the interventional suite. However, often periprocedural myonecrosis is angiographically and/or clinically silent. In a retrospective analysis of 251 consecutive PCI procedures, an adverse outcome was identified in only 53% of those with periprocedural myonecrosis on the basis of the angiogram (40). Thus, it is critical that the interventionalist should pay careful attention to clinical and angiographic events that may result in or herald infarction.

Abrupt vessel closure due to dissection, in situ thrombosis, and other factors was common in the early angioplasty and was associated with both MI and emergent CABG, as discussed previously (Table 10-3). Although complete, sustained vessel closure is rare in contemporary practice, it can still occur due to technical issues and results in large MI and emergent CABG. In a large pooled stent analysis, only MI associated with unsuccessful procedures predicted late mortality (21). More common, even in the stent era, is threatened or transient vessel closure (Fig. 10-3). These unanticipated interruptions of coronary flow, along with suboptimal angiographic outcomes such as

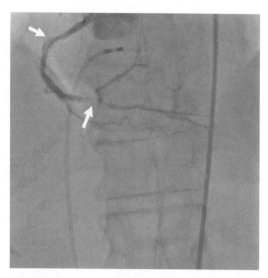

FIGURE 10-3. Spiral dissection of a right coronary artery after rotational atherectomy and angioplasty (*arrows*), which caused transient abrupt closure.

persistent dissections and filling defects are associated with both symptomatic and asymptomatic CPK-MB release (44). Stent thrombosis, the majority of which occurs within 2 days of implantation, is another etiology of vessel closure. Occurring in 1% to 2% of stent patients, angiographically confirmed stent thrombosis is associated with a 16% and 44% incidence of Q-wave and non–Q-wave MI, respectively (45). A more detailed consideration of dissection and vessel closure follows in Chapter 15.

Occlusion of large (2.1 mm or greater) side branches is a known risk of bifurcation stenting (Fig. 10-4). Occlusion of branch vessels (>1 mm) has been noted to occur in 3% to 20% of patients with myocardial injury (13,46). The occlusion of otherwise smaller, "angiographically invisible" branches also contributes to myocardial necrosis. A more detailed discussion of side branch occlusion, including strategies for prevention and management, is included in Chapter 15.

Embolization of atheromatous or thrombotic particulate material to the distal vessel bed is thought to constitute 50% to 75% of periprocedural MIs (11). These emboli can be either angiographically evident (Fig. 10-5) or "invisible." In addition to mechanical macrovascular obstruction, physiologic reductions in coronary flow can result in periprocedural infarction. Embolic occlusion of the microvasculature, myocardial edema, and vasoactive mediators are thought to

TABLE 10-3	**Angiographic Markers of Periprocedural Myocardial Infarction**

Abrupt closure
Transient closure
Dissection
Side branch occlusion
Distal embolization
"No reflow"
Stent thrombosis
Perforation

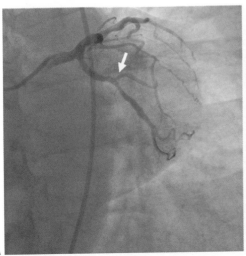
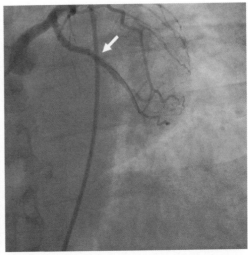

FIGURE 10-4. (A) A medium to large obtuse marginal branch (*arrow*) of the left circumflex artery following balloon angioplasty (predilation), but before stent implantation. **(B)** Circumflex artery after stent placement resulting in complete loss of obtuse marginal side branch (*arrow*).

be responsible for the "no reflow" phenomenon. Angiographically manifested by normal macrovascular appearance with diminished or absent flow, this is another etiology of periprocedural myocardial necrosis identified by the angiogram. It is more common in primary PCI, SVG intervention, and atherectomy. Both distal embolization and "no reflow" are further discussed in Chapter 17.

Periprocedural infarction often accompanies PCI-induced coronary artery perforation. Accepted treatments of perforation including protracted balloon inflation and vessel occlusion, coil-induced occlusion, and emergent CABG are all associated with MI (11).

◼ STRATEGIES FOR PREVENTION
Antiplatelet Agents

Platelet aggregation resulting in both vessel occlusion and subsequent platelet aggregate embolization is central in the pathogenesis of acute coronary syndromes. This same mechanism contributes to many of the ischemic complications of PCI, including periprocedural infarction. Pretreatment with aspirin prior to PCI remains a clinical standard today. Platelet Gp IIb/IIIa inhibitors potently prevent platelet aggregation by binding to platelet integrin. Numerous randomized controlled trials have shown that both abciximab and eptifibatide significantly reduce periprocedural myonecrosis in patients undergoing elective or urgent PCI (47–49). These studies demonstrated significant reductions (20% to 50%) in 30-day composite end points of death, urgent revascularization, and MI. The majority of this benefit resulted from an approximate 40% to 60% reduction in periprocedural MI. Many of these were clinically silent. The likely mechanisms for reducing periprocedural myonecrosis include reduced platelet-rich thrombus formation, macro and microscopic embolization during PCI, and reduced abrupt closure during PTCA without stenting.

High-dose clopidogrel pretreatment prior to PCI decreases periprocedural MI (50). Two hundred and fifty-five patients scheduled to undergo PCI for both stable angina and acute coronary syndrome were randomized to a 600-mg or 300-mg loading regimen of clopidogrel 4 to 8 hours before the procedure. The primary end point (30-day death, MI, and repeat revascularization) occurred in 4% of patients in the high loading dose versus 12% of those in the conventional loading dose group and was due entirely to the reduction in periprocedural MI. Upon multivariate analysis, the high loading regimen was associated with a 50% risk reduction of MI. An incremental benefit was observed in patients randomized to the 600-mg dose who were receiving statins, with an 80% risk reduction. In stable patients undergoing elective PCI, pretreatment with 600 mg of clopidogrel provides platelet inhibition sufficient to enable a safe

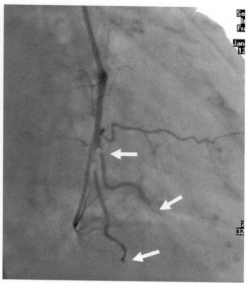

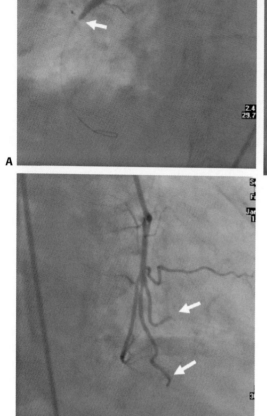

FIGURE 10-5. (A) A thrombotic occlusion (*arrow*) of proximal right coronary artery in a patient with acute myocardial infarction. **(B)** Following balloon angioplasty and aspiration thrombectomy, there is distal embolization in a side branch marked by intraluminal thrombus (*top arrow*) and acute vessel "cutoff" (*lower arrows*). **(C)** Following balloon angioplasty of side branch, distal embolization is still evident in the terminal branches (*arrows*).

procedure without the need of Gp IIb/IIIa inhibitors. Kastrati et al. showed that clopidogrel pretreatment using 600-mg loading dose offers a benefit in reducing MACE at 30 days similar to the benefit observed with pretreatment with the Gp IIb/IIIa inhibitor abciximab in patients undergoing elective PCI (51). The incidence of nonfatal MI was similar in those treated with high-dose clopidogrel and those treated with the Gp IIb/IIIa inhibitor (4%). Similar findings were found in troponin-negative patients undergoing PCI. In a 2,000-patient controlled trial of abciximab versus high-dose (600 mg) clopidogrel pretreatment among patients without an elevated troponin level, there was no difference in the incidence of primary end point. However, in

patients with positive preprocedural biomarkers, outcomes were significantly better in the glycoprotein IIb/IIIa inhibitor–treated group (52).

HMG CoA Reductase Inhibitors (Statins)

Statins have been ascribed the pleiotropic attribute of reducing vascular inflammation and providing plaque stabilization beyond their direct effect from lipid lowering. Given the role of plaque fragmentation and embolization, as well as inflammation in periprocedural myonecrosis, it should not be surprising that statin pretreatment reduces periprocedural MI. This benefit appears to be conferred on both statin-naïve and previously treated patients. In a study of 451 statin-naïve patients undergoing elective PCI, stains pretreatment 3 days prior to procedure significantly reduced the incidence of large periprocedural non–Q-wave MI (CPK-MB > 5× ULN) by nearly 50%. There were also significant decreases in the incidence of any CPK-MB or troponin release (23). In a similar study in stable angina patients who had not previously received the drugs, pretreatment with statins 7 days prior to PCI resulted in a significantly reduced incidence of myonecrosis as determined by both CPK-MB and troponin (22). High-dose atorvastatin reloading in patients on chronic therapy reduces periprocedural MI. In a study of 383 patients on chronic statin therapy with both stable angina and non—ST-segment elevation acute coronary syndromes undergoing PCI, preprocedural reloading with atorvastatin resulted in a near 50% reduction in periprocedural myonecrosis (53).

Other Pharmacologic Interventions

A variety of vasodilating agents, including calcium channel blockers have been utilized to reduce or reverse "no reflow." The efficacy of these agents for this indication remains equivocal. With regard to periprocedural MI, however, calcium channel blockers have been associated with an accelerated release of CPK after PCI compared with NTG, although a reduction in myonecrosis has not been demonstrated (54). There has been similar interest in the potential benefit of nicorandil. A meta-analysis of 17 studies employing this agent in PCI demonstrated no benefit of the agent relative to peak periprocedural CPK-MB release, despite overall improvements in TIMI flow scores and LV function (55).

The administration of β-blockers prior PCI has shown no benefit in preventing periprocedural enzyme elevation, although they remain an essential agent in aggressive secondary prevention. Preprocedural treatment with β-blockers did not reduce periprocedural biomarker release in a prospective trial (56).

Embolic Protection Devices

Devices designed to reduce the lodgment of atherothrombotic debris in small epicardial vessels and the microvasculature, embolic protection devices, represent an attractive strategy for preventing periprocedural infarctions that result from distal embolism. This approach has borne success in saphenous vein bypass graft stenting. In the SAFER trial of 800 SVG PCI, use of the balloon occlusion Guardwire device significantly reduced periprocedural non–Q-wave MI. This represented the primary basis for a 42% reduction in overall MACE (57). Other embolic protection devices have shown similar benefit since the initial report and are approved for SVG intervention (58–61). However, these devices have not proven clinically efficacious in the treatment of MI, although some surrogate end points have suggested potential reductions in microvascular embolism (58). A more detailed description of these devices is found in Chapter 17.

Thrombectomy

The physical extraction of thrombus, thrombectomy, during acute MI PCI could reduce distal thromboembolism. Although identifying myonecrosis attributable to the procedure in the midst of a spontaneous infarction is impossible, this benefit could be manifest by reduced incidence of angiographic embolism, as well as improved myocardial perfusion due to reductions in microvascular obstruction. Aspiration thrombectomy has been shown beneficial in acute MI setting with improved short- and long-term myocardial perfusion, as well as clinical outcomes (62). However, rheolytic thrombectomy has not been shown to reduce infarct size, improve TIMI flow grade, tissue myocardial perfusion, ST-segment resolution or 30-day mortality or MACE compared with traditional intervention (63).

■ DIAGNOSIS AND MANAGEMENT

Diagnosis of periprocedural MI is based on clinical, electrocardiographic, and biochemical determinations. Despite the prevalence of periprocedural myonecrosis and the recommendation of both the American and European Colleges of Cardiology, routine measurement of postprocedural cardiac enzymes remains uncommon. In a recent analysis of the ACC-NCDR PCI registry, nearly 65% of participating hospitals measured postprocedure CPK-MB in fewer than 20% of patients, whereas only 13% of hospitals determined them in >70% of patients (64). ACC/AHA/SCAI guidelines direct that CPK-MB should be obtained in patients with suspected ischemia, and in these patients a CPK-MB > 5× ULN is indicative of periprocedural MI (37). Thus, in patients in whom there is angiographic, clinical, or EKG suggestion of periprocedural ischemia, serial CPK-MB and EKGs should be obtained in order to both detect myocardial necrosis and direct individual management. Although routine enzyme determinations may be an ideal recommendation, they do not reflect current practice in the United States. Ongoing debate concerning the significance of isolated enzymatic determinations of myonecrosis, as well as the regulatory and financial implications of identifying "periprocedural MI" and other complications will likely prevent the widespread adoption of routine enzymatic determinations following PCI.

Patients with clinical and/or angiographic features of procedural infarction (vessel closure, large side branch occlusion, distal embolization) may require hemodynamic support with intra-aortic balloon pump or vasopressors. The use of "bailout" Gp IIb/IIIa inhibitors may be considered. Repeat angiography, and possible repeat revascularization, should be considered in patients with suspected acute/subacute stent thrombosis, large CPK-MB release, EKG changes, or hemodynamic compromise that ensue following PCI. Assessment of LV function is advisable in patients with large periprocedural CPK-MB release, new Q waves, or in those patients with smaller degrees of myocardial necrosis but with significant LV dysfunction at baseline. The incidence of in-hospital events in patients with small and medium CPK-MB elevations (<5× ULN) has been shown to be similar to those without myonecrosis (15). Thus, extending hospital observation solely because of an otherwise unsuspected small or moderate CPK-MB elevation is unlikely to result in clinical benefit. Current guidelines recommend additional in-hospital observation only in patients with CPK-MB > 5× ULN (37).

Optimal post-PCI care includes continued treatment with aspirin, thienopyridines, β-blockers, and HMG Co-A reductase inhibitors (statins) in accordance with current guidelines, in all patients. This certainly applies to the subset of PCI patients with periprocedural biomarker elevation. Use of renin–aldosterone pathway inhibitors (ACE inhibitors and ARBs) should be considered in patients with myonecrosis, especially those with diminished LV function.

■ CONCLUSION

MI has been a well-recognized complication since the inception of PTCA and was primarily attributable to vessel closure. The introduction of stents, potent platelet inhibitors, and other adjuncts has markedly reduced the incidence of large, clinically apparent periprocedural MI due to vessel closure. Periprocedural myonecrosis, as determined by CPK-MB and other markers, remains common and is most often attributable to atherothrombotic occlusion of side branch or distal vessels. Significant debate persists over the threshold at which this myonecrosis has prognostic implications. Adequate platelet inhibition, pretreatment with statins, and embolic protection devices appear to reduce the incidence of myonecrosis and periprocedural MI.

References

1. Thygesen K, Alpert JS, White HD, et al. Universal definition of myocardial infarction. *Circulation.* 2007;116(22):2634–2653.
2. Thygesen K, Alpert JS, White HD. Universal definition of myocardial infarction. *J Am Coll Cardiol.* 2007;50(22):2173–2195.
3. Kent KM, Bentivoglio LG, Block PC, et al. Long-term efficacy of percutaneous transluminal coronary angioplasty (PTCA): report from the National Heart, Lung, and Blood Institute PTCA Registry. *Am J Cardiol.* 1984;53(12): 27C–31C.
4. Detre K, Holubkov R, Kelsey S, et al. Percutaneous transluminal coronary angioplasty in 1985–1986 and 1977–1981. The National Heart, Lung, and Blood Institute Registry. *N Engl J Med.* 1988;318(5):265–270.
5. Talley JD, Jones EL, Weintraub WS, et al. Coronary artery bypass surgery after failed elective percutaneous transluminal coronary angioplasty. A status report. *Circulation.* 1989;79(6 Pt 2): I126–131.
6. Paik GY, Kuntz RE, Baim DS. Perfusion therapy to reduce myocardial ischemia en route to emergency coronary artery bypass grafting for failed percutaneous transluminal coronary angioplasty. *J Interv Cardiol.* 1995;8(3):319–327.
7. Detre K, Yeh W, Kelsey S, et al. Has improvement in PTCA intervention affected long-term prognosis? The NHLBI PTCA Registry experience. *Circulation.* 1995;91(12):2868–2875.

8. Baim D. *Grossman's Cardiac Catheterization, Angiography, and Intervention. 7th ed.* Philadelphia: Lippincott Williams & Wilkins; 2006.

9. Ellis SG, Roubin GS, King SB, et al. Angiographic and clinical predictors of acute closure after native vessel coronary angioplasty. *Circulation.* 1988;77(2):372–379.

10. Califf RM, Abdelmeguid AE, Kuntz RE, et al. Myonecrosis after revascularization procedures. *J Am Coll Cardiol.* 1998;31(2):241–251.

11. Herrmann J. Peri-procedural myocardial injury: 2005 update. *Eur Heart J.* 2005;26(23):2493–2519.

12. Klein LW, Kramer BL, Howard E, et al. Incidence and clinical significance of transient creatine kinase elevations and the diagnosis of non-Q wave myocardial infarction associated with coronary angioplasty. *J Am Coll Cardiol.* 1991;17(3):621–626.

13. Kugelmass AD, Cohen DJ, Moscucci M, et al. Elevation of the creatine kinase myocardial isoform following otherwise successful directional coronary atherectomy and stenting. *Am J Cardiol.* 1994;74(8):748–754.

14. Tardiff BE, Califf RM, Tcheng JE, et al. Clinical outcomes after detection of elevated cardiac enzymes in patients undergoing percutaneous intervention. IMPACT-II Investigators. Integrilin (eptifibatide) to Minimize Platelet Aggregation and Coronary Thrombosis-II. *J Am Coll Cardiol.* 1999;33(1):88–96.

15. Kini A, Marmur JD, Kini S, et al. Creatine kinase-MB elevation after coronary intervention correlates with diffuse atherosclerosis, and low-to-medium level elevation has a benign clinical course: implications for early discharge after coronary intervention. *J Am Coll Cardiol.* 1999;34(3):663–671.

16. Saucedo JF, Mehran R, Dangas G, et al. Long-term clinical events following creatine kinase–myocardial band isoenzyme elevation after successful coronary stenting. *J Am Coll Cardiol.* 2000;35(5):1134–1141.

17. Mehran R, Dangas G, Mintz GS, et al. Atherosclerotic plaque burden and CK-MB enzyme elevation after coronary interventions : intravascular ultrasound study of 2256 patients. *Circulation.* 2000;101(6):604–610.

18. Stone GW, Mehran R, Dangas G, et al. Differential impact on survival of electrocardiographic Q-wave versus enzymatic myocardial infarction after percutaneous intervention: a device-specific analysis of 7147 patients. *Circulation.* 2001;104(6):642–647.

19. Ellis SG, Chew D, Chan A, et al. Death following creatine kinase-MB elevation after coronary intervention: identification of an early risk period: importance of creatine kinase-MB level, completeness of revascularization, ventricular function, and probable benefit of statin therapy. *Circulation.* 2002;106(10):1205–1210.

20. Brener SJ, Ellis SG, Schneider J, et al. Frequency and long-term impact of myonecrosis after coronary stenting. *Eur Heart J.* 2002;23(11):869–876.

21. Jeremias A, Baim DS, Hoe KK, et al. Differential mortality risk of postprocedural creatine kinase-MB elevation following successful versus unsuccessful stent procedures. *J Am Coll Cardiol.* 2004;44(6):1210–1214.

22. Pasceri V, Patti G, Nusca A, et al. Randomized trial of atorvastatin for reduction of myocardial damage during coronary intervention: results from the ARMYDA (Atorvastatin for Reduction of Myocardial Damage during Angioplasty) study. *Circulation.* 2004;110(6):674–678.

23. Briguori C, Colombo A, Airoldi F, et al. Statin administration before percutaneous coronary intervention: impact on periprocedural myocardial infarction. *Eur Heart J.* 2004;25(20): 1822–1828.

24. Lindsey J. What is the Optimal Threshold for Defining a Periprocedural Myocardial Infarction? Prognostic Implications of Creatinine Kinase-MB Elevation After Percutaneous Coronary Interventions. *Am J Cardiol.* 2009;104(6): 36D.

25. Ricciardi MJ, Wu E, Davidson CJ, et al. Visualization of discrete microinfarction after percutaneous coronary intervention associated with mild creatine kinase-MB elevation. *Circulation.* 2001;103(23):2780–2783.

26. Selvanayagam JB, Porto I, Channon K, et al. Troponin elevation after percutaneous coronary intervention directly represents the extent of irreversible myocardial injury: insights from cardiovascular magnetic resonance imaging. *Circulation.* 2005;111(8):1027–1032.

27. Abdelmeguid AE, Ellis SG, Sapp SK, et al. Defining the appropriate threshold of creatine kinase elevation after percutaneous coronary interventions. *Am Heart J.* 1996;131(6):1097–1105.

28. Abdelmeguid AE, Topol EJ, Whitlow PL, et al. Significance of mild transient release of creatine kinase-MB fraction after percutaneous

coronary interventions. *Circulation.* 1996;94(7): 1528– 1536.

29. Akkerhuis KM, Alexander JH, Tardiff BE, et al. Minor myocardial damage and prognosis: are spontaneous and percutaneous coronary intervention-related events different? *Circulation.* 2002;105(5):554–556.

30. Andron M, Stables RH, Egred M, et al. Impact of periprocedural creatine kinase-MB isoenzyme release on long-term mortality in contemporary percutaneous coronary intervention. *J Invasive Cardiol.* 2008;20(3):108–112.

31. Harrington RA, Lincoff AM, Califf RM, et al. Characteristics and consequences of myocardial infarction after percutaneous coronary intervention: insights from the Coronary Angioplasty Versus Excisional Atherectomy Trial (CAVEAT). *J Am Coll Cardiol.* 1995;25(7):1693–1699.

32. Ioannidis, JP, Karvouni E, Katritsis DG. Mortality risk conferred by small elevations of creatine kinase-MB isoenzyme after percutaneous coronary intervention. *J Am Coll Cardiol.* 2003;42(8): 1406–1411.

33. Kini AS, Lee P, Marmur JD, et al. Correlation of postpercutaneous coronary intervention creatine kinase-MB and troponin I elevation in predicting mid-term mortality. *Am J Cardiol.* 2004;93(1): 18–23.

34. Kong TQ, Davidson CJ, Meyers SN, et al. Prognostic implication of creatine kinase elevation following elective coronary artery interventions. *JAMA.* 1997;277(6):461–466.

35. Simoons ML, van den Brand M, Lincoff M, et al. Minimal myocardial damage during coronary intervention is associated with impaired outcome. *Eur Heart J.* 1999;20(15):1112–1119.

36. Lindsey JB, Marso SP, Pencina M, et al. Prognostic impact of periprocedural bleeding and myocardial infarction after percutaneous coronary intervention in unselected patients: results from the EVENT (evaluation of drug-eluting stents and ischemic events) registry. *JACC Cardiovasc Interv.* 2009;2(11):1074–1082.

37. Smith SC, Jr., Feldman TE, Hirshfeld JW Jr, et al. ACC/AHA/SCAI 2005 guideline update for percutaneous coronary intervention: a report of the American College of Cardiology/American Heart Association Task Force on Practice Guidelines (ACC/AHA/SCAI Writing Committee to Update the 2001 Guidelines for Percutaneous Coronary Intervention). *J Am Coll Cardiol.* 2006; 47(1): e1–121.

38. Saadeddin SM, Habbab MA, Sobki SH, et al. Association of systemic inflammatory state with troponin I elevation after elective uncomplicated percutaneous coronary intervention. *Am J Cardiol.* 2002;89(8):981–983.

39. Bhatt DL, EJ. Topol, Does creatinine kinase-MB elevation after percutaneous coronary intervention predict outcomes in 2005? Periprocedural cardiac enzyme elevation predicts adverse outcomes. *Circulation.* 2005;112(6):906–915; discussion 923.

40. Blankenship JC, Islam MA, Wood GC, et al. Angiographic adverse events during percutaneous coronary intervention fail to predict creatine kinase-MB elevation. *Catheter Cardiovasc Interv.* 2004;63(1):31–41.

41. Holmes DR Jr, Berger PB. Troponisms, necrosettes, enzyme leaks, creatinine phosphokinase bumps, and infarctlets: what's behind this new lexicon and what does it add? *Circulation.* 2001;104(6):627–629.

42. Ellis SG, Guetta V, Miller D, et al. Relation between lesion characteristics and risk with percutaneous intervention in the stent and glycoprotein IIb/IIIa era: An analysis of results from 10,907 lesions and proposal for new classification scheme. *Circulation.* 1999;100(19):1971–1976.

43. Hong MK, Mehran R, Dangas G, et al. Creatine kinase-MB enzyme elevation following successful saphenous vein graft intervention is associated with late mortality. *Circulation.* 1999;100(24): 2400–2405.

44. Piana RN, Ahmed WH, Chaitman B, et al. Effect of transient abrupt vessel closure during otherwise successful angioplasty for unstable angina on clinical outcome at six months. Hirulog Angioplasty Study Investigators. *J Am Coll Cardiol.* 1999;33(1):73–78.

45. Cutlip DE, Baim DS, Ho KK, et al. Stent thrombosis in the modern era: a pooled analysis of multicenter coronary stent clinical trials. *Circulation.* 2001;103(15):1967–1971.

46. Arora RR, et al. Side branch occlusion during coronary angioplasty: incidence, angiographic characteristics, and outcome. *Cathet Cardiovasc Diagn.* 1989;18(4):210–212.

47. Use of a monoclonal antibody directed against the platelet glycoprotein IIb/IIIa receptor in high-risk coronary angioplasty. The EPIC Investigation. *N Engl J Med.* 1994;330(14):956–961.

48. EPISTENT Investigators. Randomised placebo-controlled and balloon-angioplasty-controlled

trial to assess safety of coronary stenting with use of platelet glycoprotein-IIb/IIIa blockade. *Lancet.* 1998;352(9122):87–92.

49. ESPRIT Investigators. Novel dosing regimen of eptifibatide in planned coronary stent implantation (ESPRIT): a randomised, placebo-controlled trial. *Lancet.* 2000;356(9247):2037–2044.

50. Patti G, Colonna G, Pasceri V, et al. Randomized trial of high loading dose of clopidogrel for reduction of periprocedural myocardial infarction in patients undergoing coronary intervention: results from the ARMYDA-2 (Antiplatelet therapy for Reduction of MYocardial Damage during Angioplasty) study. *Circulation.* 2005;111 (16):2099–2106.

51. Kastrati A, Mehilli J, Schuhlen H, et al. A clinical trial of abciximab in elective percutaneous coronary intervention after pretreatment with clopidogrel. *N Engl J Med.* 2004;350(3):232–238.

52. Kastrati A, Mehilli J, Neumann FJ, et al. Abciximab in patients with acute coronary syndromes undergoing percutaneous coronary intervention after clopidogrel pretreatment: the ISAR-REACT 2 randomized trial. *JAMA.* 2006;295(13): 1531–1538.

53. Di Sciascio G, Patti G, Pasceri V, et al. Efficacy of atorvastatin reload in patients on chronic statin therapy undergoing percutaneous coronary intervention: results of the ARMYDA-RECAPTURE (Atorvastatin for Reduction of Myocardial Damage During Angioplasty) Randomized Trial. *J Am Coll Cardiol.* 2009;54(6):558–565.

54. Matthews MA, Kunselman SJ, Gascho SA, et al. Differential release of cardiac enzymes after percutaneous coronary intervention. *Catheter Cardiovasc Interv.* 2005;65(1):19–24.

55. Iwakura K, Ito H, Okamura A, et al. Nicorandil treatment in patients with acute myocardial infarction: a meta-analysis. *Circ J.* 2009;73(5): 925–931.

56. Ellis SG, Brener SJ, Lincoff AM, et al. beta-blockers before percutaneous coronary intervention do not attenuate postprocedural creatine kinase isoenzyme rise. *Circulation.* 2001;104(22): 2685–2688.

57. Baim DS, Wahr D, George B, et al. Randomized trial of a distal embolic protection device during percutaneous intervention of saphenous vein aorto-coronary bypass grafts. *Circulation.* 2002; 105(11):1285–1290.

58. De Luca G, Suryapranata H, Stone GW, et al. Adjunctive mechanical devices to prevent distal embolization in patients undergoing mechanical revascularization for acute myocardial infarction: a meta-analysis of randomized trials. *Am Heart J.* 2007;153(3):343–353.

59. Halkin A, Masud AZ, Rogers C, et al. Six-month outcomes after percutaneous intervention for lesions in aortocoronary saphenous vein grafts using distal protection devices: results from the FIRE trial. *Am Heart J.* 2006;151(4):915 e1–7.

60. Kereiakes DJ, Turco MA, Breall J, et al. A novel filter-based distal embolic protection device for percutaneous intervention of saphenous vein graft lesions: results of the AMEthyst randomized controlled trial. *JACC Cardiovasc Interv.* 2008;1 (3):248–257.

61. Stone GW, Rogers C, Hermiller J, et al. Randomized comparison of distal protection with a filter-based catheter and a balloon occlusion and aspiration system during percutaneous intervention of diseased saphenous vein aorto-coronary bypass grafts. *Circulation.* 2003;108(5):548–553.

62. Svilaas T, Vlaar PJ, van der Horst IC, et al. Thrombus aspiration during primary percutaneous coronary intervention. *N Engl J Med.* 2008; 358(6):557–567.

63. Ali A, Cox D, Dib N, et al. Rheolytic thrombectomy with percutaneous coronary intervention for infarct size reduction in acute myocardial infarction: 30-day results from a multicenter randomized study. *J Am Coll Cardiol.* 2006;48(2): 244–252.

64. Wang TY, Peterson ED, Dai D, et al. Patterns of cardiac marker surveillance after elective percutaneous coronary intervention and implications for the use of periprocedural myocardial infarction as a quality metric: a report from the National Cardiovascular Data Registry (NCDR). *J Am Coll Cardiol.* 2008;51(21):2068–2074.

11 Cardiac Arrhythmias Complicating Interventional Procedures

ERIC D. GOOD AND HAKAN ORAL

■ ANATOMIC AND PHYSIOLOGIC CONSIDERATIONS

Basic information on the anatomy and physiology of the normal cardiac conduction system is important to better understand how electrophysiologic complications may develop and thereby minimize the risk of potential complications. The core components of normal cardiac rhythm are specialized cells within the sinoatrial (SA) node, the bundle of His, bundle branches, and Purkinje fibers, which initiate and propagate electrical excitation to the myocardium.

The SA node is located at the junction of the superior vena cava and high right atrium and consists of a central group of cells called the *compact zone*, responsible for impulse formation, and a more peripheral group of cells that form the border zone that serve to propagate impulses to the atrium. The region of the SA node is supplied by the sinus node artery, which arises as the second major branch off the right coronary artery (RCA) in 60% to 66% of the patients, as a branch of the left circumflex artery (LCX) in 27% to 40% of the patients, and as a dual supply (RCA and LCX) in approximately 6% (1–3).

Although individual atrial myocytes are capable of propagating impulses, there are three bundles of Purkinje-like fibers in the atria that form intra-atrial tracts that propagate impulses rapidly through the atria and toward the atrioventricular (AV) node. These are the anterior internodal bundle of Bachman, the middle internodal tract of Wenckebach, and the posterior internodal tract of Thorel. These tracts have a vascular supply derived predominantly from tributaries of the SA node artery. The tracts converge to the AV node, which consists of three regions: the transitional cell zone, the compact AV node, and the penetrating AV bundle, located in the anterior interventricular septum at the apex of the triangle of Koch (bounded by the base of the septal leaflet of the tricuspid valve, tendon of Todaro, a fibrous extension of the Eustachian valve, and the coronary sinus ostium). The distal end of the penetrating AV node continues in the membranous septum as the bundle of His (Fig. 11-1). Fluoroscopically, this region is most often located contiguous to the dome of a temporary pacing catheter as it enters the right ventricle from an inferior vena cava approach (Fig. 11-2). The region of the AV node is supplied by AV nodal artery, which arises from the distal RCA, just after the takeoff of the posterior descending artery in 80% to 87% of the patients, from the distal LCX in 8% to 11% of the patients, and as a dual supply (RCA and LCX) in 2% to 13% of the patients and courses very close to right atrial wall at the base of the triangle of Koch (Fig. 11-3) (1–3). Additional sources of arterial blood supply to the region of the AV node include contributions from the first septal perforator (off the left anterior descending artery), the descending septal artery, and anterior atrial branches, including Kugel anastomotic artery (connecting RCA and LCX) (2).

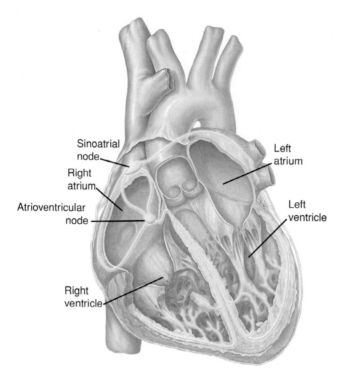

FIGURE 11-1. Anatomy of the intrinsic conduction system of the heart. (Asset provided by Anatomical Chart Co., 2008.)

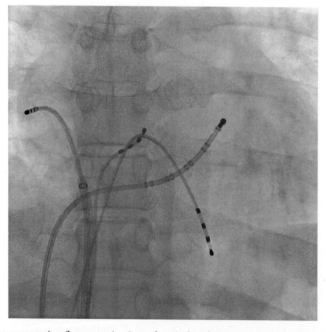

FIGURE 11-2. Anteroposterior fluoroscopic view of typical catheter positions during an electrophysiologic study. Note that HIS position usually resides at dome of the RV (right ventricle) catheter. Also shown are right atrial (RA) catheter, coronary sinus (CS) catheter, and HIS catheter (at "HIS position").

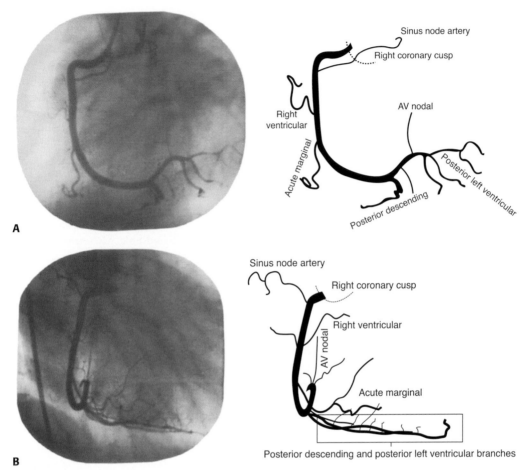

FIGURE 11-3. Blood supply to the sinoatrial node is from the sinus node artery (*open arrow*) and supply to the atrioventricular (AV) node is from the AV nodal artery (*closed arrow*). These typically arise as tributaries from the proximal and distal right coronary artery, respectively, but may arise from the distal left circumflex artery in some, and rarely from both. (**A**) Left anterior oblique projection. (**B**) Right anterior oblique projection. (From Pepine C, ed. *Diagnostic and Therapeutic Cardiac Catheterization.* 2nd ed. Philadelphia, PA: Lippincott Williams and Wilkins; 1994.)

The bundle of His begins to bifurcate on the left side, where the common bundle emerges from the central fibrous body, giving rise to the bundle branches immediately distal to the membranous septum. The left bundle branches off most immediately and cascades down the high, left ventricular septum just below the noncoronary cusp before fanning out into the left anterior and left posterior fascicles. The concept of a discrete left fascicle with a thin, anterosuperior and thick, posteroinferior, as opposed to indiscrete fiber radiations, is a debated but useful distinction. The right bundle branch is a direct continuation of the penetrating bundle along the superficial right, membranous interventricular septum. It does not give rise to branches as it

courses subendocardially in the middle and lower third of the ventricular septum, before reaching the apex. The left bundle receives dual arterial blood supply from septal perforators off the left axis deviation (supplying anterior and medial radiations) and from perforators of the posterior descending branch of the RCA. The right bundle receives similar dual blood supply (4).

Purkinje fibers connect the distal ends of the bundle branches to the endocardium of both ventricles by forming an intervening network. They are predominantly located subendocardially, tend to be concentrated at papillary muscle heads, and receive oxygen and other nutrients via diffusion from cavitary blood, independent of coronary artery occlusion. Perhaps for this reason, Purkinje fibers tend to be more resistant to ischemic insult than do surrounding myocardial fibers (4). These cells, therefore, often remain structurally intact amid the ischemic milieu in which they are embedded, such that they have been increasingly recognized as important triggers (early or delayed after depolarizations) of ventricular arrhythmias (VAs), including premature ventricular contractions (PVCs), ventricular tachycardia (VT), and ventricular fibrillation (VF).

■ DIAGNOSTIC VENTRICULOGRAPHY AND CORONARY ANGIOGRAPHY

Arrhythmias associated with diagnostic cardiac catheterizations are rare, estimated to complicate fewer than 5 in 1,000 procedures. VAs are the most commonly occurring arrhythmias during ventriculography. Single premature ventricular depolarizations, couplets, triplets, or even runs of VT are associated with mechanical stimulation of the ventricular myocardium by the guide wire, pigtail catheter, or other ventricular catheters. When these arrhythmias occur, the wire or catheter should be immediately withdrawn until ectopy ceases, since continued ventricular ectopy could induce sustained VT or VF. Only rarely will VAs be sustained with complete removal of the catheter or wire from the ventricle. In instances of sustained VT or VF, immediate cardioversion is required.

Optimal positioning of the ventriculography catheter in the midbasal ventricular cavity minimizes ventricular ectopy, avoids proarrhythmic catheter entanglement in the mitral chordal apparatus, and minimizes the chances for catheter–myocardial contact during power contrast infusion. Catheter design, including shape and number of side holes also may influence ventriculography-associated VAs. Caracciolo et al. (5) and Geggel et al. (6) demonstrated that a novel Halo catheter resulted in less movement and a reduced incidence of ventricular ectopy than did conventional 5F and 6F pigtail catheters without compromising the diagnostic quality of ventriculograms. Hirose et al. (7) showed that the 5F Jet Balance pigtail catheter, which has 52 side holes on the catheter and also an end hole, had significantly lower incidences of ventricular ectopy (21.8% vs. 42.9%, $P = 0.02$), VT (1.9%

vs. 14.3%, $P = 0.02$), and multiple ventricular ectopic beats (9.0% vs. 34.7%, $P = 0.001$), respectively, than 6F conventional pigtail catheters. The side holes of the Jet Balance catheter have an oval shape and are arranged symmetrically on the center of the shaft (Fig. 11-4).

Utilizing diagnostic coronary catheters for ventriculography (typically a multipurpose diagnostic coronary catheter) is a common practice by many experienced operators. While this technique saves procedure time by eliminating the need for additional catheter exchanges, it may be more likely to result in myocardial staining due to concentration of contrast flow through a single end hole. Myocardial staining, the deposition of contrast material in the endocardium, has been associated with increased risk of VAs with risk related to the size of the stain. While small areas of staining typically do not result in arrhythmic sequelae, large areas of staining may result in medically refractory ventricular tachyarrhythmias requiring immediate cardioversion (8).

Inadvertent injection of air or thrombus during either ventriculography or coronary angiography likely poses the greatest risk for arrhythmias, in particular VF. Attention to frequent flushing of catheters with heparinized saline solution, use of closed-system controller injection syringes, prophylactic systemic heparinization, and avoidance of apical positioning of the ventriculography catheter might minimize these risks. In rare instances, VF has been reported to result from use of an ungrounded power injector (8).

High-grade AV block (AVB) has also been described during contrast left ventriculography (9). This can occur due to mechanical impingent on the His–Purkinje system, particularly in patients with a preexisting right bundle branch block (RBBB). It may also occur as a result of persistent contrast staining of the high interventricular septum, 5 to 10 mm beneath the aortic valve (Fig. 11-5). It is in this region that the bundle of His gives rise to the left bundle branch, which promptly divides into the left anterior and posterior fascicles. In most instances, this block will resolve spontaneously given enough time, but it may require urgent insertion of a temporary pacing catheter. Permanent pacemaker placement is required in rare instances, usually in the presence of underlying AV conduction disease.

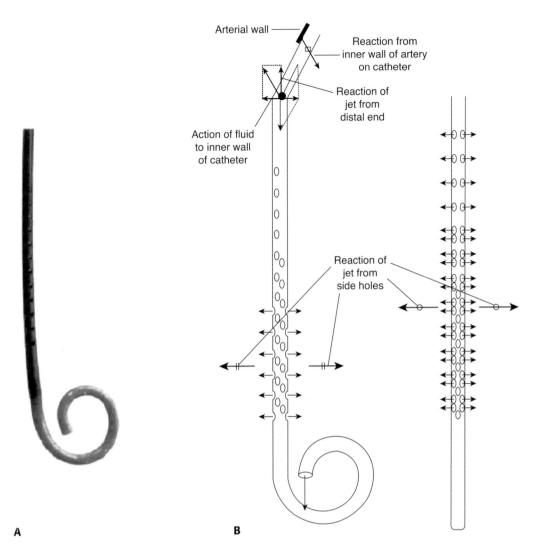

FIGURE 11-4. (**A**) Appearance of a 5 Fr Jet Balance pigtail catheter. It has 52 side holes on its catheter shaft and an end hole. The side hole has an oval shape, which size is 0.4 × 0.2mm. (**B**) Hydromechanics of the 5 Fr Jet Balance pigtail catheter. Side holes are arranged symmetrically on the center of the shaft, so reactions from side holes are canceled. Other action and reaction canceled each other. (From Hirose M, Shimada K, Sakanoue Y, et al. Usefulness of newly designed pigtail catheter with multiple side holes by reducing incidence of ventricular ectopy. Cathet Cardiovasc Interv. 1999;48:220–225.)

The left anterior fascicle is in very close proximity to the septal portion of the left ventricular outflow tract and is particularly susceptible to block from retrograde, mechanical catheter impingement. In patients with baseline normal conduction, developing left anterior fascicular block is usually of little consequence. In patients presenting with preexisting bifascicular block, that is, RBBB and left posterior fascicular block, however, complete AVB could ensue with rapid and deleterious hemodynamic sequelae. Therefore, it is important to assess the precatheterization electrocardiogram (ECG) for RBBB or bifascicular block to identify patients who might be best served by prophylactic temporary transvenous pacemaker placement.

Estimates of the incidence of VAs occurring during diagnostic, selective coronary angiography vary widely among studies, ranging from 0.4% to 5% (5–7). Several factors might influence somewhat disparate results, including type and size of diagnostic coronary catheter, acute ischemia, osmolarity and volume of contrast agent, and comorbid conditions. In a study of

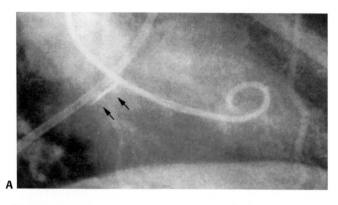

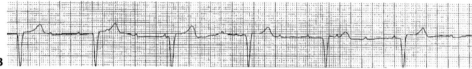

FIGURE 11-5. Ventriculogram after injection of contrast (**A**) (right anterior oblique 30 degrees) shows intramyocardial contrast staining just below aortic valve, which was associated with development of a third-degree atrioventricular block (**B**). (From Marine J, Smith TW, Monahan KM. High-grade atrioventricular block caused by His-Purkinje injury during contrast left ventriculography. *Circulation*. 2001;104:e77–e78.)

18,365 patients undergoing diagnostic coronary angiography, Chan et al. (10) found an incidence of pathologic VAs (sustained VT or VF) of only 0.131%. While some reports suggest that occurrences of VAs are related to the presence of underlying coronary disease, Bove et al. (11) found a wide variety of angiographic findings, ranging from normal coronaries to three-vessel coronary disease, in a study of 7,915 patients undergoing diagnostic coronary angiography for evaluation of chest pain.

Most VAs during catheterization relate to catheter manipulation (58%), ischemia (33%), or contrast medium (8%) (10). Injection of contrast into the RCA is more often associated with VAs than left main injections and more frequently observed with use of Judkins than Sones techniques (11). Factors increasing risks of VF during coronary injection include slow clearance of contrast from the coronary, use of high osmolar contrast, underlying electrolyte or acid–base imbalance, myocardial ischemia, and prolonged bradycardia.

Acute ECG changes that might be observed during coronary injection include T-wave tenting or inversions in the inferior limb leads (for left and right coronary injections, respectively); PR, QRS, and QT interval prolongation; and sinus slowing or asystole (8). These tend to

occur almost exclusively with use of high-osmolar contrast agents.

Vagally mediated slowing of the sinus rate may also result in prolonged periods of bradycardia that further delay the clearance of contrast from the coronary artery, thereby causing QRS widening and QT interval prolongation, which promote VAs. In addition, deep-seating of the RCA catheter in particular can mechanically occlude the takeoff of the sinus nodal artery, which is in proximity to the RCA ostium, and may result in ischemia and bradycardia-induced ventricular proarrhythmias. Rarely, catheter manipulation in the aortic arch itself can cause baroreceptor stimulation and a vasovagal response (12).

■ CORONARY INTERVENTIONS

VF is characterized by continuous, uncoordinated, and ineffective contraction of the ventricles, which results in life-threatening cessation of cardiac output (13). It is often the first manifestation of previously unknown structural heart disease, in particular, coronary artery disease, and is often associated with syncope, "seizures," and sudden death (14). The vast majority of survivors of VF arrests (>90%) are found to have impaired coronary flow and myocardial ischemia at angiography due to coronary atherosclerosis, coronary plaque rupture, cardiocoronary thromboembolism, coronary artery vasospasm, or cardiomyopathy (15).

While VT or VF in the clinical setting is usually a marker of underlying structural heart disease, especially coronary disease, its occurrence as a complication of coronary interventions is less well understood. VT or VF occurring at any time following fibrinolysis has consistently been shown to be a marker of poor in-hospital and long-term outcome (16–20), but the prognostic significance of VT or VF occurring after primary coronary interventions is less clear.

Investigators in the Primary Angioplasty in Myocardial Infarction study found a 4.3% incidence of periprocedural VT or VF among patients undergoing primary percutaneous coronary interventions (PCIs) but did not find a difference in in-hospital or 1-year mortality compared with those without VT or VF (21). Paccini et al. (22), on the other hand, found a similar incidence (5.2%) of VT or VF complicating PCI in a study of 9,000 patients presenting within 24 hours of symptom onset of an acute myocardial infarction (MI) but showed a significantly higher mortality (16.3% vs. 3.7%) for the cohort of patients with VT or VF.

More recently, in a post hoc, multicenter analysis of 5,745 patients with acute ST-elevation MIs (STEMIs) undergoing primary percutaneous transluminal coronary angioplasty, Mehta et al. (23) found a 5.7% incidence of VT or VF occurring mostly (90%) within 48 hours after cardiac catheterization (median time = 28 hours from catheterization). Mortality among patients with periprocedural VT or VF was significantly higher (23.2% vs. 3.6%) at 90 days when compared with those without VT or VF, and the excess mortality occurred mostly within the first 30 days. In addition, those with VT or VF had a worse acute clinical course that was more likely to be complicated by shock, congestive heart failure, or recurrent MIs.

Several clinical factors have been identified as risk factors for the development of periprocedural VT or VF among patients presenting for primary PCI. These include older age, higher heart rates and ST-segment deviations, lack of β-blockers in emergency department, RCA-associated infarct, lower blood pressures, lower creatinine clearance (chronic renal disease), less

postprocedure ST-segment resolution (<70%), and coronary flow restoration less than Thrombolysis in Myocardial Infarction (TIMI) grade 3. The lowest event rates for VT or VF occurred in those patients with complete postprocedure ST-segment resolution and restoration of TIMI 3 grade coronary flow (23). In addition, utilization of adjuvant therapies such intra-aortic balloon pumps, dialysis, blood transfusions, and use of antiarrhythmics were higher in patients with postprocedure VT or VF, and repeat catheterization was performed at a threefold higher rate.

Acute treatment of VT or VF often requires emergent use of cardioversion, which in most instances is sufficient as the sole treatment. Rarely, immediate recurrences require repeated cardioversions and initiation of antiarrhythmic therapy. In most instances, empiric initiation of amiodarone through an intravenous load and maintenance infusion is warranted. It should be recognized, however, that amiodarone increases defibrillation thresholds and may make subsequent external cardioversion more difficult. Cases of urgent interventions with radiofrequency catheter ablation of monomorphic VT and PVC-initiated VF have been described, but applicability is limited to centers able to commit the resources necessary to have dual coronary and electrophysiology interventional teams available on call for such cases. In rare instances, when VT or VF proves refractory to both cardioversions and medical interventions, emergent use of ventricular assist devices or initiation of cardiopulmonary bypass is required.

Monomorphic VT is a regular VT which most often (but not always) is associated with a wide QRS complex. It is important to distinguish VT from a supraventricular tachycardia (SVT) with aberrant ventricular conduction occurring during catheter interventions, since each would represent a different long-term risk of sudden death and certainly would require different treatment approaches. Sometimes it is quite difficult to differentiate VT from SVT with aberrancy. The presence of hemodynamic instability during a wide QRS tachycardia by no means excludes SVT as the rhythm. In the setting of hemodynamic instability, rapid cardioversion should be performed. ECG clues that suggest a wide-complex tachycardia is SVT with aberrancy include documentation of the same cycle length tachycardia at times with both broad and narrow QRS complexes (Fig. 11-4), initiation of the tachycardia by an atrial premature depolarization, and initiation of broad QRS morphology by a long-short sequence. ECG supporting the diagnosis of VT over SVT with aberrancy include evidence of AV dissociation (Fig. 11-5), concordance of QRS complexes in precordial leads (either all upright or inverted), and the presence of very broad QRS complexes. In general, QRS durations more than 160 ms during left bundle branch morphology or more than 140 ms during a right bundle branch morphology suggest VT. In addition, widening of the RS interval in the precordial more than 100 ms suggests VT. Further, VT is also more likely if there is deviation of axis that is atypical for bundle branch pattern (such as right-axis deviation in the presence of a baseline left bundle branch morphology). The "classic" axis deviation suggesting VT is the so-called northwest axis in the frontal plane.

The effect of vagal maneuvers may be utilized to help differentiate wide complex tachycardias, as well, providing the presence of relative hemodynamic stability. Such maneuvers can terminate SVTs or slow them with AVB but do not usually affect VT, unless it is related to bundle branch reentry. Administration of intravenous adenosine can be similarly helpful, but one must recognize that some idiopathic VTs are adenosine-sensitive and may terminate after administration of it.

■ ALCOHOL SEPTAL ABLATION

Alcohol septal ablation is an effective therapy in patients with medically refractory symptoms related to dynamic outflow tract obstruction in the setting of a hypertrophic cardiomyopathy. This technique involves delivery of absolute alcohol into the first septal perforator branch of the left anterior descending coronary artery to elicit a "controlled infarction" (and resultant thinning) of the hypertrophied, basal septum with a goal of decreasing the outflow gradient. QRS widening and PVCs are frequently observed during alcohol infusion but usually quickly resolve. High-grade AVB complicates the *acute* ablation procedure in about half of cases and may persist during convalescence as well. For this reason, a temporary transvenous pacer should be placed in the right ventricle prior to the procedure in patients who do not have preexisting pacemakers or defibrillators.

Historically, the initial incidence of AVB requiring permanent pacing was up to 40%, with a reported incidence in more recent and larger case series of 7% to 12% (24–26). Reapplication of additional amounts of alcohol in adjacent septal perforators increases the risk of permanent AVB. Fortunately, with the evolution of the ablation technique, lower doses and fewer instillations of alcohol, use of contrast echocardiography to guide instillation, and better awareness of the potential for conduction system complications, AVB has been reported in 4% to 12% of the patients in more recent studies (26–29).

Several authors have proposed utilizing a preprocedure scoring system to identify patients at highest risk of permanent AVB. Farber et al. (28) proposed a scoring system based on the collection of several baseline and peri-interventional variables within the first 48 hours after the procedure. In this model, patients were risk stratified into low-, intermediate-, and high-risk groups based on risk scores of less than 8, 8 to 12, and more than 12 points, respectively. Analysis of ECG and 48-hour Holter tracings for preprocedure rhythm and AV conduction disturbances revealed that isolated first-degree AVB, RBBB, or atrial fibrillation did not confer an increased risk for postintervention high-grade AVB, while preexisting left bundle branch block (LBBB) resulted in a need for permanent pacing in all cases. Furthermore, no significant differences between the three risk groups was found with respect to patient age, gender, left ventricular morphology, ethanol dose, or peak creatine kinase levels. Finally, on the basis of this model, one might expect 100%, 87%, and 13% of patients in the low-, intermediate-, and high-risk groups to have spontaneous AV conduction recovery 3 ± 2, 6 ± 3, and 9 ± 3 days following the procedure, which might provide the operator with preprocedure insight into the likelihood of a need for permanent pacing postprocedure.

The timing of the decision to place a permanent pacing device is somewhat controversial, with some authors recommending placement within 48 hours of persisting AVB and others suggesting a period of "watchful waiting" for the return of AV conduction (24,25,28–32). By incorporating risk stratification scheme outlined earlier, one might move to place a pacer in high-risk patients sooner, while waiting longer (up to a week) for spontaneous return of conduction in intermediate- or low-risk patients. In addition, patients with the presence of a preexisting LBBB who are left with postprocedural complete AVB should be considered more acutely for permanent pacemaker placement as this is an independent predictor of long-term need for pacing (33).

■ TRANSSEPTAL OCCLUDER DEVICES

Percutaneous transcatheter closure of patent foramen ovale (PFO) and secundum atrial septal defects (ASDs) is now a validated and increasingly utilized interventional procedure for the treatment of paradoxical and cryptogenic, thromboembolic strokes. Although contemporary occluder devices have demonstrated a good safety profile, less is known about their acute and chronic proarrhythmic potential. Premature atrial complexes, atrial fibrillation, atrial flutter, and atrial tachycardias are the arrhythmias most often encountered.

Baseline ECG abnormalities commonly observed in patients with ASD include rightward axis deviation, first-degree AVB, and incomplete RBBB pattern (34,35). Sinus (40%–70%) and AV node dysfunction (10%–45%) are common and thought to be related to prolongation of atrial refractoriness due to right atrial enlargement from volume overload (35). Premature atrial contractions are commonly observed following occluder device placement (70%), independent of the degree of residual shunt. There is a small risk of complete AVB.

A history of paroxysmal or persistent atrial fibrillation was encountered in approximately 6% of more than 1,000 patients presenting for placement of a septal occlusion device and was more commonly found in patients with ASDs than in those with PFOs (36). The annual incidence of new-onset atrial fibrillation was found in 4% of patients following ASD occlusion and 2.5% of PFO occlusion, while the annual incidence was 2.9% in the overall population over 2,454 years of cumulative follow-up. The majority of new-onset AF occurs soon after device placement, usually during the first month, and tends to be associated with the use of larger occluder devices in instances of PFO closure but not for ASD closure.

Recommendations for treatment of arrhythmias associated with ASD or PFO closure are largely anecdotal. Left atrial ablation prior to occluder device deployment is often performed preferentially when atrial fibrillation is documented, but the efficacy of this approach is uncertain.

Natale et al. (37) compared a series of 45 patients who had previously undergone ASD or PFO repairs with 45 age–, gender–, and AF-type–matched controls who did not have ASD or PFO closure. They demonstrated that percutaneous transseptal access and ablation in the left atrium was feasible, safe, and efficacious in such patients when guided by intracardiac echocardiography. Access to the left atrium was successful in 98% of ASD-/PFO-repaired patients, including those with occluder devices, without significant differences noted in the 3-month echo parameters as compared with the control group. Most ASD or PFO closure devices were noted to be situated in the antero-superior aspect of the interatrial septum, allowing an area in the posterioinferior area for transseptal puncture.

■ ENDOMYOCARDIAL BIOPSY

Nonsustained atrial and VAs are observed during instrumentation for endomyocardial biopsy (1.0%–1.5%) and are usually self-limited (38–41). Occasionally, sustained arrhythmias, usually SVTs, occur. In these instances, gentle manipulation of the bioptome against the atrial or ventricular myocardium to elicit a premature atrial or ventricular contraction is often all that is necessary to terminate the arrhythmia. In instances of persisting atrial fibrillation or atrial flutter, synchronized cardioversion may be required. Biopsy-related sustained VAs are exceedingly rare, and when they do occur, they usually relate to the myocardial substrate more than the procedure itself. For these, prompt cardioversion is necessary to avoid deleterious hemodynamic compromise.

Development of complete heart block may also be an infrequent complication of endomyocardial biopsy. In a study of 2,415 patients undergoing 3,048 endomyocardial allograft biopsy procedures via right femoral venous approach, Holtzmann et al. (39) found very rare instances of complete AVB requiring temporary pacing (0.2%) and even rarer instances where long-term pacing (0.04%) was required. For those requiring pacing, durations of temporary pacing ranged from 7 to 31 minutes, and the need for permanent pacing was associated with the presence of a preexisting LBBB. Pacing was more often required in patients with relatively smaller left ventricular diastolic dimensions (≤65 mm) than in those with significantly dilated left ventricles.

Other less serious conduction abnormalities can sometimes (0.6%–3.7%) complicate endomyocardial biopsy procedures (39–41). De novo RBBB is observed following approximately 1% of biopsy procedures but is transient in all but a third of cases (39). Avoiding mechanical trauma to or biopsy of the high anterior intervetricular septum may reduce the likelihood of developing RBBB. Mobitz-II AVB or temporary third-degree AVB occurs in approximately 0.3% of biopsy procedures and readily responds to administration of 0.5 to 1.0 mg of atropine (39).

■ PACEMAKER OR DEFIBRILLATOR COMPLICATIONS

Special considerations are required in patients presenting for cardiac interventional procedures who have a preexisting pacemaker or defibrillator.

It is essential for the prepared interventionalist to be familiar with the type of device, device manufacturer, number of leads, date of and reason for implant, and device settings to avoid the pitfalls of device-related procedural complications.

As a matter of practice, it may later prove useful to obtain and store orthogonal fluoroscopic views (typically anteroposterior and left anterior oblique 40-degree projection) of the device leads before obtaining access for any right-sided interventions to have a reference should device-related complications subsequently arise (Fig. 11-6). Care should be taken to avoid mechanically dislodging pacing or defibrillation leads with wire, catheter, or bioptome manipulation. This is of particular concern for atrial leads, which most often produce a free loop as they course anterior into the right atrial appendage. In general, right heart procedures (Swann–Gantz catheterization, endomyocardial biopsy, right ventriculography, etc.) should be avoided during the first 6 weeks following a new device implant so as to allow the leads to stabilize at their endocardial insertion.

In addition, familiarity with patient-specific device programming may be of particular importance to particular interventions. For example, patients who have received pacemakers for sinus node dysfunction may have devices or programming that provides only atrial-based

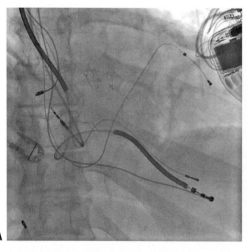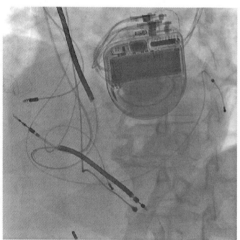

A   **B**

FIGURE 11-6. Fluoroscopic views of biventricular implantable cardioverter defibrillator in a patient with multiple prior devices/leads (**A**) right anterior oblique 10 degrees; (**B**) left anterior oblique 40 degrees). This "nest" of wires poses risks for dislodgement or damage with right-sided interventional procedures and may obscure coronary segments at angiography. Obtaining preprocedure fluoroscopic orthogonal views for later comparison might prove useful should complications occur.

pacing support. If complete AVB were to develop during the course of alcohol septal ablation, for example, atrial-based pacing support would be insufficient and the mere presence of a pacemaker might have provided a preprocedural false sense of security. Likewise, in patients with similar pacing indications but programmed to dual chamber pacing modes (e.g., DDD), it is common that inadequate programming of AV delays results in forced ventricular pacing even though intrinsic AV conduction is present (Fig. 11-7). In these instances, reprogramming to longer AV delays or changing the pacing mode to provide ventricular backup only (e.g., ventricular

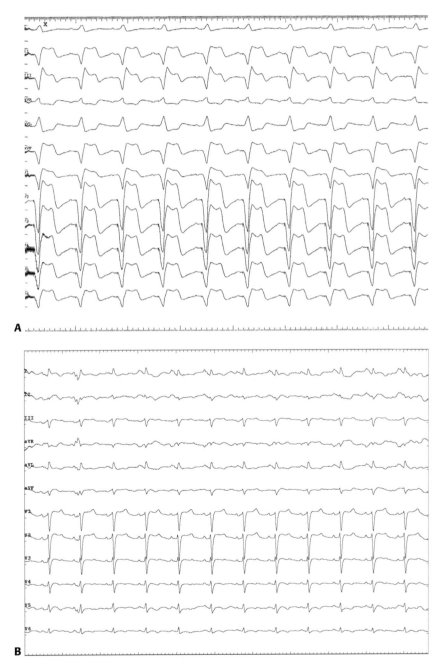

FIGURE 11-7. Atrioventricular (AV) sequential pacing (**A**) in a patient with inappropriate programmed AV delay such that intrinsic ventricular conduction (**B**) is preempted by ventricular pacing, masking the procedural complication of the complete AV block (*continued*)

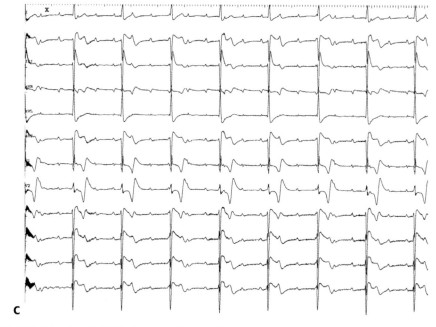

FIGURE 11-7. (*Continued*) (**C**) during alcohol septal ablation.

demand pacing (VVI) 40 bpm), could prove helpful in monitoring for procedural-related development of AV conduction disturbances or ST–T wave changes that would otherwise be "masked" by forced ventricular pacing. This may prove especially important in the cases of coronary interventions or alcohol septal ablations, where the presence of such changes might signal the operator to consider altering the manner of the intervention.

In some instances, forced pacing may prove a useful therapeutic tool. VT or VF that is "pause dependent," or initiated by "long–short" sequences is often suppressed by forced pacing

at rates of 90 bpm (Fig. 11-8). Patients with balloon pumps or ventricular assist devices may benefit from titration of pacing rates according to hemodynamic response, especially when devices are ECG-triggered.

In recent years, the use of specialized pacing modes designed to minimize ventricular pacing have become popular. Although they have vendor-specific proprietary names, functionally they are operating in the AAI(R) mode and switch to a DDD(R) mode upon loss of one beat of AV conduction, such that they are commonly ascribed to be in the AAI(R) ↔ DDD(R) mode. In this manner, they eliminate the AV delay

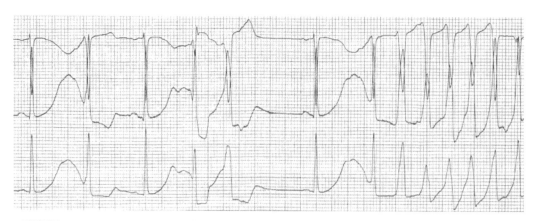

FIGURE 11-8. Polymorphic ventricular tachycardia induced by a long–short sequence resulted in multiple implantable cardioverter defibrillator shocks and later was suppressed by VVI pacing at 90 bpm.

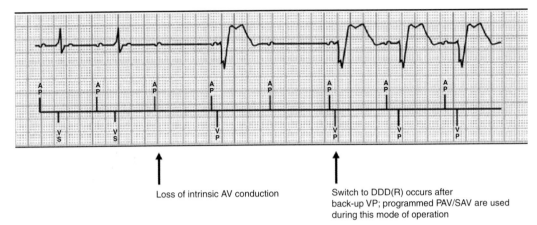

Loss of intrinsic AV conduction

Switch to DDD(R) occurs after
back-up VP; programmed PAV/SAV are used
during this mode of operation

FIGURE 11-9. AAI(R) (Atrial pacing, Atrial sensing, Inhibited, Rate adaptive) → DDD(R) (Dual pacing, Dual sensing, Dual triggering/inhibition, Rate adaptive) pacing mode. This mode is functionally operational as AAI(R) mode with monitoring for intrinsic atrioventricular (AV) conduction. If there is persistent loss of AV conduction (*arrow*), the mode will provide ventricular "backup" pacing and transition to DDD(R) mode. The device will continue to monitor for restoration of AV conduction and transition back to AAI(R) mode once it is restored.

"interlocks" of refractory periods that often confound the programming in patients with sinus node dysfunction (Fig. 11-9). It is important for the interventionalist to recognize that this unique programming mode can result in significantly long AV delays (sometimes up to 400 ms) under normal operating conditions and also allow a single dropped beat from AV conduction before switching modes.

■ CONCLUSION

It is important for the interventional cardiologist to have a basic understanding of the electrophysiology of the heart and potential arrhythmias that may develop during or after an intervention. Heightened awareness and preparedness for rather infrequent, however, important arrhythmogenic complications should result in outcomes and minimize often-preventable arrhythmogenic complications.

References

1. Patel S. Normal and anomalous anatomy of the coronary arteries. *Semin Roentgenol.* 2008;43(2): 100–112.

2. Saremi F, Abolhoda A, Ashikyan O, et al. Arterial supply to sinuatrial and atrioventricular nodes: imaging with multidetector CT. *Radiology.* 2008; 246(1):99–107.

3. Vieweg WV, Alpert JS, Hagan AD. Origin of the sinoatrial node and atrioventricular node arteries in right, mixed, and left inferior emphasis systems. *Cathet Cardiovasc Diagn.* 1975;1(4):361–373.

4. Waller BF, Gering LE, Branyas NA, Slack JD. Anatomy, histology, and pathology of the cardiac conduction system: part II. *Clin Cardiol.* 1993; 16(4):347–352.

5. Caracciolo EA, Kern MJ, Collis WC, et al. Improved left ventriculography with the new 5F helical-tip Halo catheter. *Am Heart J.* 1994; 128(4):724–732.

6. Geggel RL, Hijazi ZM. Reduced incidence of ventricular ectopy with a 4F Halo catheter during pediatric cardiac catheterization. *Cathet Cardiovasc Diagn.* 1998;43:55–57.

7. Hirose M, Shimada K, Sakanoue Y, et al. Usefulness of newly designed pigtail catheter with multiple side holes by reducing incidence of ventricular ectopy. *Cathet Cardiovasc Interv.* 1999;48:220–225.

8. Baim D, ed. *Cardiac Catheterization, Angiopraphy, and Intervention.* 7th Edition. Baltimore, MD: Lippincott Williams and Wilkins; 2006.

9. Marine J, Smith TW, Monahan KM. High-grade atrioventricular block caused by His-Purkinje injury during contrast left ventriculography. *Circulation.* 2001;104:e77–e78.

10. Chen J, Gao L, Yao M, Chen J. Ventricular arrhythmia onset during diagnostic coronary angiography with a 5F or 4F universal catheter. *Rev Esp Cardiol.* 2008;61(10):1092–1095.

11. Nishimura RA, Holmes DR Jr, McFarland TM, Smith HC, Bove AA. Ventricular arrhythmias during coronary angiography in patients with

angina pectoris or chest pain syndromes. *Am J Cardiol.* 1984;53:1496–1499.

12. Petch MC, Sutton R, Jefferson KE. Safety of coronary arteriography. *Br Heart J.* 1973;35:377–380.

13. Hayes D. Maue-Dickson W, Stanton D. *Dictionary of Cardiac Pacing Electrophysiology and Arrhythmias.* Miami Lakes, Florida: Peritus Corp; 1993.

14. Priori SG, Napolitano C, Grillo M. Concealed arrhythmogenic syndromes: the hidden substrate of idiopathic ventricular fibrillation? *Cardiovasc Res.* 2001;50(2):218–223.

15. Wever EF, Robles de Medina EO. Sudden death in patients without structural heart disease. *J Am Coll Cardiol.* 2004;43(7):1137–1144.

16. Gressin V, Louvard Y, Pezzano M, Lardoux H. Holter recording of ventricular arrhythmias during intravenous thrombolysis for acute myocardial infarction. *Am J Cardiol.* 1992;69(3):152–159.

17. Six AJ, Louwerenburg JH, Kingma JH, Robles de Medina EO, van Hemel NM. Predictive value of ventricular arrhythmias for patency of infarct-related coronary artery after thrombolytic therapy. *Br Heart J.* 1991;66(2):143–146.

18. Buckingham TA, Devine JE, Redd RM, Kennedy HL. Reperfusion arrhythmias during coronary reperfusion therapy in man: clinical and angiographic correlations. *Chest.* 1986;90(3):346–351.

19. Berger PB, Ruocco NA, Ryan TJ, Frederick MM, Podrid PJ. Incidence and significance of ventricular tachycardia and fibrillation in the absence of hypotension or heart failure in acute myocardial infarction treated with recombinant tissue-type plasminogen activator: results from the Thrombolysis in Myocardial Infarction (TIMI) phase II trial. *J Am Coll Cardiol.* 1993;22(7):1773–1779.

20. Newby KH, Thompson T, Stebbins A, et al; for the GUSTO Investigators. Sustained ventricular arrhythmias in patients receiving thrombolytic therapy: incidence and outcomes. *Circulation.* 1998;98(23):2567–2573.

21. Mehta RH, Harjai KJ, Grines L, et al; for the Primary Angioplasty in Myocardial Infarction (PAMI) Investigators. Sustained ventricular tachycardia or fibrillation in the cardiac catheterization laboratory among patients receiving primary percutaneous coronary intervention: incidence, predictors, and outcomes. *J Am Coll Cardiol.* 2004;43(10):1765–1772.

22. Piccini JP, Berger JS, Brown DL. Early sustained ventricular arrhythmias complicating acute myocardial infarction. *Am J Med.* 2008;121(9):797–804.

23. Mehta RH, Starr AZ, Lopes RD, et al; for the APEX AMI Investigators. Incidence of and outcomes associated with ventricular tachycardia or fibrillation in patients undergoing primary percutaneous coronary intervention. *JAMA.* 2009; 301(17):1779–1789.

24. Maron BJ. Role of alcohol septal ablation in treatment of obstructive hypertrophic cardiomyopathy. *Lancet* 2000;355:425–426.

25. Cheng TO. Conservative management of complete heart block complicating percutaneous transluminal septal myocardial ablation for patients with obstructive hypertrophic cardiomyopathy. *J Am Coll Cardiol.* 2004;94:982.

26. Talreja DR, Nishimura RA, Edwards WD, et al. Alcohol septal ablation versus surgical septal myectomy. *J Am Coll Cardiol.* 2004;44(12):2329–2332.

27. Faber L, Welge D, Fassbender D, et al. One-year follow-up of percutaneous septal ablation for symptomatic hypertrophic obstructive cardiomyopathy in 312 patients: predictors of hemodynamic and clinical response. *Clin Res Cardiol.* 2007;96(12):864–873.

28. Faber L, Welgea D, Fassbendera D, Schmidta HK, Horstkottea D, Seggewiss H. Percutaneous septal ablation for symptomatic hypertrophic obstructive cardiomyopathy: managing the risk of procedure-related AV conduction disturbances. *Int J Cardiol.* 2007;119(2):163–167.

29. Faber L, Seggewiss H, Gleichmann U. Percutaneous transluminal septal myocardial ablation in hypertrophic obstructive cardiomyopathy: results with respect to intra-procedural myocardial contrast echocardiography. *Circulation.* 1998; 98:2415–2421.

30. Lakkis NM, Nagueh SF, Kleiman NS, et al. Echocardiography-guided ethanol septal reduction for hypertrophic obstructive cardiomyopathy. *Circulation.* 1998;98:1750–1755.

31. Faber L, Meissner A, Ziemssen P, Seggewiss H. Percutaneous transluminal septal myocardial ablation for HOCM: long-term follow-up in the first series of 25 patients. *Heart.* 2000;83: 326–331.

32. Veselka J, Duchonová R, Procházková S, Páleníčková J, Sorajja P, Tesar D. Effects of varying ethanol dosing in percutaneous septal ablation for obstructive hypertrophic cardiomyopathy on early hemodynamic changes. *Am J Cardiol.* 2005;95:675–678.

33. Alam M, Dokainish H, Lakkis N. Alcohol septal ablation for hypertrophic obstructive cardiomy-

opathy: a systematic review of published studies. *J Interv Cardiol*. 2006;19(4):319–27.

34. Hill SL, Berul CI, Patel HT, et al. Early ECG abnormalities associated with transcatheter closure of atrial septal defects using the Amplatzer septal occluder. *J Interv Card Electrophysiol*. 2000; 4(3):469–474.

35. Shiku DJ, Stijns M, Lintermans JP, Vliers A. Influence of age on atrioventricular conduction intervals in children with and without atrial septal defect. *J Electrocardiol*. 1982;15:9–14.

36. Spies C, Khandelwal A, Timmermanns I, Schräder R. Incidence of atrial fibrillation following transcatheter closure of atrial septal defects in adults. *Am J Cardiol*. 2008;102:902–906.

37. Lakkireddy D, Rangisetty U, Prasad S, et al. Intracardiac echo-guided radiofrequency catheter ablation of atrial fibrillation in patients with atrial septal defect or patent foramen ovale repair: a feasibility, safety, and efficacy study. *J Cardiovasc Electrophysiol*. 2008;19(11):1137–1142.

38. Oldham N, Ott RA, Allen BA, Fopiano P, Dwyer M. Ventricular fibrillation complicating endomyocardial biopsy of a cardiac allograft. *Cathet Cardiovasc Diagn*. 1991;23(4):300–301.

39. Holzmann M, Nicko A, Kühl U, et al. Complication rate of right ventricular endomyocardial biopsy via the femoral approach: a retrospective and prospective study analyzing 3048 diagnostic procedures over an 11-year period. *Circulation*. 2008;118(17):1722–1728.

40. Deckers JW, Hare JM, Baughman KL. Complications of transvenous right ventricular endomyocardial biopsy in adult patients with cardio-myopathy: a seven-year survey of 546 consecutive diagnostic procedures in a tertiary referral center. *J Am Coll Cardiol*. 1992;19(1): 43–47.

41. Felker GM, Hu W, Hare JM, et al. The spectrum of dilated cardiomyopathy: the Johns Hopkins experience with 1,278 patients. *Medicine (Baltimore)*. 1999;78:270–283.

Infection

GIO J. BARACCO

The cardiac catheterization suite has become a place where increasingly more complex procedures are performed, including placement of many implantable devices. While most nonsurgical cardiac procedures still involve only percutaneous puncture and catheterization of an artery and/or vein, these procedures are now associated with the implantation of vascular stent grafts, atrial septal defect closure devices, and percutaneous heart valves. Vascular closure devices (VCDs) are being utilized with increasing frequency. In addition, the cardiovascular interventional suite is frequently used for the implantation and revision of pacemakers, implanted defibrillators, and other forms of cardiovascular implantable electronic devices (CIEDs). This involves performing clean surgical incisions, inserting a permanent implant, and closing the wounds by primary intention, blurring the differentiation between the interventional suite and an operating room. Given the increase in complexity and invasiveness of the procedures, it is not surprising that some of these patients will become infected. Infection occurs infrequently after cardiovascular procedures, but when it does, it becomes a potentially devastating complication, resulting in prolonged hospitalization, readmission, surgical procedures, or death. Infections associated with cardiovascular procedures are frequently underrecognized and underreported, much of it stemming from the fact that they occur several days after the procedure, thus not being counted as "complications from the procedure" (1).

Pacemakers and implanted defibrillators account for the bulk of infections associated to cardiovascular (CV) procedures. Cardiac stents may also become infected, although very infrequently. Arteritis at the puncture site of a cardiac catheterization procedure, especially when VCDs are used, and sepsis related to the infusion of contaminated products are very rare and seldom reported.

◼ INFECTIONS ASSOCIATED WITH CIEDs

Incidence

Over the past decade, the volume of implanted cardiac devices has soared, with newer and better devices being introduced to the market, new indications for their use, and improved accessibility. The incidence of infections, however, has increased at a much greater pace than the volume of device implantations. Voigt and colleagues (2) reported a population-based study, in which the volume of device implantations increased by 49% between 1996 and 2003, yet the number of infections increased 3.1-fold, 2.8-fold for pacemakers and 6-fold for implanted defibrillators. The same group published a follow-up study showing a 12% increment in the number of implanted devices between 2003 and 2006, with a corresponding increase in the number of infections, of 57%. Analysis of these data indicated that the increase in the incidence of infection between 1996 and 2006 is likely related to the selection of patients receiving CIEDs. While the age of the recipients did not change significantly during the 10-year study period, the proportion of patients with end-organ failures and diabetes mellitus increased over time. In addition, the proportion of white recipients of CIEDs decreased over time (3). Cabell and collaborators (4) confirmed this trend in a study of Medicare beneficiaries in which the rate of increase of cardiac device-associated infections (CDIs) between 1990 and 1999 was greater (124%) than the rate of increase in device implantations during the same period (42%).

The actual incidence of CDI varies according to the population studied and the methodology used. In a retrospective population-based study in Minnesota, Uslan (5) followed 1,524 patients with cardiac devices for a total of 7,578 device-years. The incidence rate of device infection was 1.9 per 1,000 device-years (5). Klug et al. (6) followed a cohort of 6,319 CIEDs implanted in 1 year and followed them for 1 year. The incidence of infection in his study was 0.68% (6).

The frequency of infection varies according to the type of device used and the type of infection under study. The probability of device infection is higher among patients with defibrillators compared with those with pacemakers (5). The incidence rate of pocket infection has been estimated at 1.37 per 1,000 device-years. The rate of CDI that include bloodstream infection or device endocarditis has been calculated at 1.14 per 1,000 device-years in Olmstead County, Minnesota (5). In a different study based on a cohort of 45 patients with pacemaker (PM) endocarditis in France, extrapolated to the total number of device implantations in that region in 1999, the incidence of infection was calculated at 550 cases of pacemaker endocarditis per million pacemakers implanted (7).

Pathogenesis

Implanted cardiovascular devices may become infected through one of several mechanisms. Early (within 1 year) infections are frequently related to contamination of the implant during the operative procedure. Later infections are occasionally caused by erosion of the implant through the skin and exposure of parts of it to the environment (8). Hematogenous seeding from a remote site of infection is also possible, but it is infrequent. The notable exception is bacteremia caused by *Staphylococcus aureus.* Up to 75% of patients who develop *S. aureus* bacteremia within 1 year of device implantation and about one-third of patients with *S. aureus* bacteremia after more than 1 year of device implantation have a cardiac device infection (9). Approximately 60% of these patients will show no signs or symptoms of CDI (9). Therefore, patients with staphylococcal bacteremia and no other source should be considered for removal of the device and leads, even if there are no local signs of infection (9). Gram-negative bacteremia, on the other hand, rarely results in an infection of a CIED (10). Factors that have been associated with an increased risk of infection related to CIEDs are listed in Table 12-1.

TABLE 12-1   **Risk Factors for Cardiac Implanted Electronic Device Infection**

Immunosuppression (renal dysfunction and corticosteroid use (11))
Oral anticoagulation use
Patient coexisting illnesses, including fever within 24 hours before implantation (6)
Periprocedural factors, including the failure to administer perioperative antimicrobial prophylaxis
Device revision/replacement
The amount of indwelling hardware, including the number of pacing leads (11)
Operator experience
The microbiology of bloodstream infections in patients with indwelling CIEDs
Abdominal placement (12)
Fever within 24 hours before implantation (6)
Use of temporary pacing before the implantation procedure (6)

CIED, cardiovascular implantable electronic device. (Adapted from Baddour L, Epstein A, Erickson C, et al. Update on cardiovascular implantable electronic device infections and their management: a scientific statement from the American Heart Association. *Circulation.* 2010;121:458–477.)

Clinical Presentation and Management

The initial presentation of patients with suspected CDI typically corresponds to one of the following three clinical syndromes (9,13–15):

1. Pocket site infection. Clinical evidence of CDI includes erythema, warmth, fluctuance, wound dehiscence, erosion, or tenderness at the generator site. These patients may also present with purulent discharge from the device pocket. This is the most common presentation, accounting for approximately 75% of patients on initial presentation (Fig. 12-1).

2. Bacteremia. These patients present with fever and other systemic signs of infection and have positive blood cultures. They may or may not have signs of pocket site infection. Approximately 20% of patients will fall into this category.

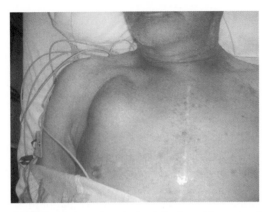

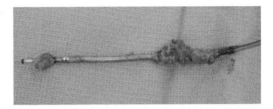

FIGURE 12-2. Extracted CIED lead with multiple attached vegetations. (Courtesy of Roger G. Carrillo, MD.)

FIGURE 12-1. Pocket device infection. (Courtesy of Roger G. Carrillo, MD.)

3. Unexplained fever. Patients in this category have an implanted cardiac device and present with fever and no clear source after initial workup. This is the least common presentation, accounting for 5% of patients with suspected CDI.

Some of these patients will have their infection recategorized after undergoing appropriate diagnostic workup including blood cultures, transesophageal echocardiography, complete device removal, and pocket and lead cultures. It is after this workup that device-associated endocarditis may be diagnosed. *Device-associated endocarditis* is defined as the presence of lead or valvular vegetation on surface or transesophageal echocardiography, associated with systemic signs of infection and positive blood cultures or if the Duke criteria for infective endocarditis are met (Fig. 12-2) (14).

Table 12-2 describes how the initial presentation relates to the final diagnosis. Overall, approximately 30% of subjects who present with local or systemic signs of cardiac device infection will in fact have underlying device-associated endocarditis. This estimate includes 19% of patients with seemingly uncomplicated pocket infections, 57% of patients with bacteremia, and 75% of patients with unexplained fever (15). To underscore the concept that local symptoms within the pocket are frequently associated with a deeper infection, Klug and colleagues described a series of 105 patients admitted for local complications of the pacemaker pocket, including inflammation or exteriorization of the device generator. Upon removal of the device, they found positive cultures in almost 80% of the intravascular portion and 92% of the extravascular portion of the extracted leads (16).

Most CDIs are caused by gram-positive organisms. Between 60% and 90% of cases are

TABLE 12-2 **Correlation Between Initial Presentation and Final Diagnosis of Device-Associated Infections**[a]

	Final Diagnosis			
	Pocket Infection	Bacteremia	Culture-Negative, Unexplained Fever	Device-Associated Endocarditis
	50.7	15.3	4.2	29.9
Initial presentation	Pocket infection ($n = 106$) 73.6 67.9	8.5	4.7	18.9
	Bacteremia ($n = 30$) 20.8 0	43.3	0	56.7
	Unexplained fever ($n = 8$) 5.6 12.5	0	12.5	75

[a]Values are presented as percentage.
(Adapted from Griffin AD, Carrillo RG, Chan JC. Correlation between presenting signs and final diagnosis in a retrospective review of 288 cardiac device related infections. Poster presented at: the 47th Annual Meeting of the Infectious Disease Society of America; 2009; Philadelphia, PA.)

caused by staphylococci (17,18). Three out of four of these staphylococci are resistant to methicillin (17). The most common organism isolated is *S. epidermidis*, followed by other coagulase-negative staphylococci. *S. aureus* is responsible for approximately 15% of infections. Other microorganisms, causing a minority of CDIs include a variety of gram-negative aerobic bacilli and species of *Candida, Aspergillus, Propionibacterium,* and *Corynebacterium.* Approximately 10% to 15% of patients have negative cultures (17,18), and approximately 25% of infected leads grow more than one microorganism (18).

Diagnostic Tests

Microbiology Tests

Blood cultures are positive in only 12.5% to 50% of patients with CDIs, making this an insensitive method to make this diagnosis (18,19). On the other hand, more than two positive blood cultures are a reliable criterion for the diagnosis of device lead-related infection, with 80% to 90% of patients with positive blood cultures culturing the same organism from the explanted leads (18,19). When a single blood culture is positive, there is a concordance of approximately 50% with the lead culture result (18).

Lead cultures, especially if multiple segments are sent to the laboratory, clearly increase the diagnostic sensitivity of local and systemic infections associated with cardiac devices. Lead cultures also have the best concordance with blood cultures when these are positive (19).

Pocket tissue cultures have a better yield than pocket swab cultures for the microbiologic diagnosis of pocket infections (19,20). A study by Chua et al. (20) found a sensitivity of 69% and 31% for pocket tissue and swab cultures, respectively. Pocket cultures should not be taken routinely in patients without signs or symptoms of infection, as up to a third of patients undergoing generator replacement or lead revision have an asymptomatic bacterial colonization of generator pockets (21). Almost all of these colonizing bacteria are normal components of skin flora, such as coagulase-negative staphylococci and *Propionibacterium* species (21). After revision of the device, however, 7.5% of these asymptomatically colonized patients develop a device infection with the same species of microorganism, compared with 2.4% of patients with a negative culture (21).

The American Heart Association recommends that all patients have at least two sets of blood cultures drawn at the initial evaluation before prompt initiation of antimicrobial therapy for CIED infection and that generator-pocket tissue Gram stain and culture and lead-tip culture be obtained when the CIED is explanted (22).

Echocardiography

A transesophageal echocardiogram (TEE) is indicated in the evaluation of all patients with suspected or confirmed device-associated infection, prior to the extraction of the device and/or intraoperatively (Fig. 12-3) (22). TEE has a reported sensitivity in the detection of lead vegetations of >90% (23). TEE results, however, should be interpreted in the context of clinical and microbiological data, as 5% of patients with CIED undergoing TEE will have incidental masses on the pacing leads that do not represent infection (23). Transthoracic echocardiograms (TTEs), on the other hand, have poor sensitivity in the detection of lead-associated vegetations. In a recent study, Zamora and colleagues (24) compared the accuracy of TTE with that of TEE. Using TEE as a "gold standard"—all vegetations detected by TEE were confirmed visually after lead extraction—they found that TTE detected only 28.6% of lead vegetations (24). This is consistent with other studies that reported that TTE detects between 22% and 30% of vegetations (25).

Echocardiograpy is useful for several reasons. Before removing device leads, the operator needs to know about the presence and/or size of vegetations on the leads. Leads with vegetations larger than 1 cm in longest dimension have been

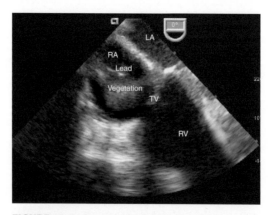

FIGURE 12-3. Transesophageal echocardiogram showing a large vegetation attached to an endocardial lead. (Courtesy of Roger G. Carrillo, MD.)

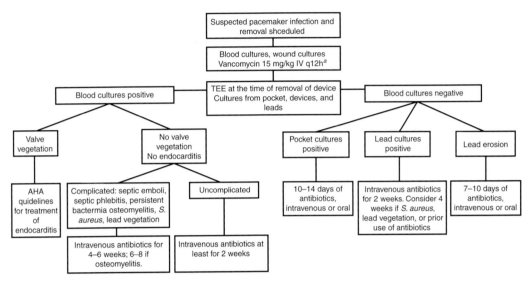

FIGURE 12-4. University of Miami algorithm of cardiac device infection management. Length of therapy is counted from the day of explanation. [a]Consider adding empirical antibiotics active against gram negative bacteria in patients with sepsis or if febrile despite antibiotics against gram positive organisms. TEE, transesophageal echocardiogram; AHA, American Heart Association. (Courtesy of Maria L. Alcaide, MD.)

safely and successfully extracted via the transvenous route. However, vegetations larger than 2 cm may embolize into a main pulmonary artery should they become dislodged from the lead, and those should be extracted via an open procedure with extracorporeal circulation unless the patient has high perioperative risk (26).

Echocardiography will also evaluate the presence of valvular vegetations, valvular anatomy, and valvular function. Patients with severe valvular destruction may need valvular reconstruction and/or replacement, and for them, an open lead extraction may be indicated (26). In addition, the presence of valvular endocarditis will change the timing of device reimplantation after removal. While patients with no vegetations and no further evidence of systemic infection may have their device reimplanted relatively early (3 days), it is advisable to delay reimplantation of a new system for at least 14 days, and possibly longer, if a valvular vegetation is present (27).

Management

Cure of cardiac device-associated infection is best achieved by complete removal of the device, including the generator, all the leads, adapters, caps, sutures, and as much of the infected tissue as possible, in combination with pathogen-directed antibiotic therapy (22,27–29). Several algorithms have been proposed for the management of cardiac associated infections (22,29). Figure 12-4 shows an algorithm used at the University of Miami.

Conservative Treatment Versus Complete Device Removal

There are no published randomized controlled trials comparing retention and extraction strategies with cure device-associated infections. Some case reports and small series have reported successful treatment of pacemaker infections using a conservative approach with systemic and local antibiotics and generator pocket debridement without hardware removal (30–32). However, most published studies have shown unacceptably high rates of failure with conservative treatment. Lewis et al. described 75 patients (including 10 with epicardial systems) presenting with pocket abscess or erosion, including 17 patients with positive blood cultures. Out of 32 patients treated conservatively (antibiotics, limited debridement, and irrigation or aspiration of the infected site), only 1 patient was cured. In the other 43 patients, primary removal of all hardware led to successful resolution of infection in all. Also, the 31 patients who failed conservative treatment were cured after removal of the pacing system (33). A study from the Cleveland Clinic showed relapse of infection in 1 of 117 patients in whom the device had been removed and in 3 of 6 patients who did not have complete hardware removal (14). Another study from Spain showed that conservative treatment of patients with device-associated endocarditis failed in all 7 patients in whom it was attempted, whereas 20 out of 24 were cured with surgical explantation of the device. In this study, however, devices and leads were removed by manual traction or open thoracotomy, and 3 of 24 patients died during the perioperative period (34). So, complete device extraction is usually recommended in the management of infected cardiac devices, unless the patient's overall prognosis is so poor as to favor chronic suppression with antibiotics instead of extraction (27,35). The Heart Rhythm Society's recommendations for transvenous lead extraction in the setting of a suspected or confirmed infection—endorsed by the American Heart Association—are described in Table 12-3 (27).

Antibiotic Therapy

Antimicrobial therapy is adjunctive in patients with CIED infection, and complete device removal should be done without delay. Unless the patient is clinically unstable, and provided that extraction can be done promptly, it is preferable to avoid empiric antibiotic therapy until the patient has been taken for device extraction and cultures have been taken, maximizing the yield of microbiological testing. After cultures of blood, pocket, and leads have been sent, it is reasonable to administer empirical antibiotics directed against gram-positive bacteria, including methicillin-resistant strains (28). For most patients, vancomycin at 15 mg/kg every 12 hours is an appropriate initial regimen (28). The dose needs to be adjusted for any renal insufficiency and further titrated to

---

TABLE 12-3 **Indications for Transvenous Lead Extraction for Suspected or Confirmed Infection[a]**

Class I

1. Complete device and lead removal is recommended in all patients with definite cardiovascular implantable electronic device (CEID) system infection, as evidenced by valvular endocarditis, lead endocarditis, or sepsis.
2. Complete device and lead removal is recommended in all patients with CEID pocket infection as evidenced by pocket abscess, device erosion, skin adherence, or chronic draining sinus without clinically evident involvement of the transvenous portion of the lead system.
3. Complete device and lead removal is recommended in all patients with valvular endocarditis without definite involvement of the lead(s) and/or device.
4. Complete device and lead removal is recommended in patients with occult gram-positive bacteremia (not contaminant).

Class IIa

1. Complete device and lead removal is reasonable in patients with persistent occult gram-negative bacteremia.

Class III

1. CIED removal is not indicated for a superficial or incisional infection without involvement of the device and/or leads.
2. CEID removal is not indicated to treat chronic bacteremia due to a source other than the CEID, when long-term suppressive antibiotics are required.

[a]Classification of recommendations and level of evidence are expressed in the American College of Cardiology/American Heart Association format:

Class I: Conditions for which there is evidence and/or general agreement that a given procedure or treatment is useful and effective.

Class II: Conditions for which there is conflicting evidence and/or a divergence of opinion about the usefulness/efficacy of a procedure or treatment.

IIa: Weight of evidence/opinion is in favor of usefulness/efficacy.

IIb: Usefulness/efficacy is less well established by evidence/opinion.

Class III: Conditions for which there is evidence and/or general agreement that the procedure/treatment is not useful or effective and in some cases may be harmful.

(Reprinted from Wilkoff BL, Love CJ, Byrd CL, et al. Transvenous lead extraction: heart rhythm society expert consensus on facilities, training, indications, and patient management: This document was endorsed by the American Heart Association (AHA). *Heart Rhythm.* 2009;6:1085–1104, with permission from Elsevier.)

achieve a trough level of 15 to 20 μg/mL (36). As soon as the cultures results are received, the antibiotic regimen should be tailored to the isolated pathogen(s). Specifically, if the cultures grow oxacillin-susceptible staphylococci, vancomycin should be discontinued and the patient treated with oxacillin, nafcillin, or cefazolin (22).

There are no studies to guide a recommendation for the duration of antibiotic therapy for patients with infected cardiac devices. In general terms, however, these patients should be treated in a similar fashion to patients with other forms of soft tissue or bacteremic infections. Provided that the device is fully removed, antibiotic regimens after device removal of 10 to 14 days for uncomplicated pocket infections and 28 days for patients with deep infections (positive lead or vegetation cultures or bacteremia) are associated with a risk of relapse of less than 2% and seem to be adequate (37).

Device Reimplantation

Every patient who undergoes removal of an infected CIED must be thoroughly evaluated for the continuous need of the device. In most series, 13% to 52% of patients whose devices are removed due to infection do not need to have the device replaced (28). The timing of reimplantation is very important, given that there are few sites where replacement CIEDs may be placed. Device reimplantation should be at a new site and when the patient is no longer bacteremic (28). Patients with no vegetations and no further evidence of systemic infection may have their device reimplanted relatively early (3 days). It is advisable to delay reimplantation of a new system for at least 14 days, and possibly longer, if a valvular vegetation is present (27).

Prevention

Implementation of a comprehensive infection control program is very effective at preventing CDIs (38). All the preventive interventions described in the "Infection Control in the Cardiovascular Interventional Suite" section, apply to the implantation of CIEDs. In addition, certain precautions should be taken to prevent infectious complications of these devices.

1. Perioperative antimicrobial prophylaxis. The administration of systemic antibiotics significantly reduces the risk of infectious complications after cardiac device implantations. In a meta-analysis of 2023 patients in seven trials, Da Costa and colleagues (39) found a significant protective effect of perioperative antibiotic prophylaxis (OR, 0.256; 95 CI, 0.10–0.656). There is no need, however, for a prolonged course of preventive antibiotics. In fact, a single dose of cefazolin has been found to be safe and effective as prophylaxis, with an infection rate of less than 1% in a cohort of 852 patients followed for more than 2 years (40). In another study, 48 hours of antibiotics were as effective as 7 days in preventing device-associated infections (41). The chosen antibiotic should be active against common skin organisms. A cephalosporin with moderately long serum half-life, such as cefazolin, is an appropriate choice. Alternatively, vancomycin or clindamycin may be used in individuals who are allergic to β-lactam antibiotics. Prophylactic antibiotics must be infused 30 to 60 minutes prior to the incision for maximum efficacy. Vancomycin should be started 60 to 120 minutes before the incision (2).

2. Prevention of hematoma formation. Hematoma within the pocket has been identified as a risk factor for CIED infection. Therefore, the operator should pay meticulous attention to hemostasis. Some providers pack the pockets with antibiotic-soaked sponges to provide compression while the leads are being placed, and consideration should be taken to the use of thrombin, especially in patients receiving anticoagulants. It is also recommended that low-molecular-weight heparin be avoided in the immediate postoperative period. Last, a pressure dressing applied for 12 to 24 hours after skin closure may further decrease the risk of hematoma formation (22).

3. Pocket irrigation. Irrigation of the pocket has been used in an attempt to

decrease CDIs. Different practices have used saline, disinfectants, or antibiotic solutions. There are no data, however, that this practice has any significant impact on the incidence of CDI. Lakkireddy and colleagues (42) published their experience on a large cohort of patients who underwent CIED implantation, about half of whom had saline irrigations and the other half had povidone iodine irrigations. They found no difference in the incidence of infection between both groups (0.6% and 0.7% in the saline and povidone-iodine groups, respectively) (42).

4. Antibiotic prophylaxis is not routinely recommended after device placement for patients who undergo dental, respiratory, gastrointestinal, or genitourinary procedures. Antibiotics should be administered, however, to patients with CIEDs who will undergo drainage of infection at other sites or replacement of an infected device (28).

■ INFECTIONS OF CORONARY AND NONCORONARY VASCULAR STENTS

Bacteremia occurs after 0.11% to 0.64% of percutaneous coronary interventions (43,44). Nevertheless, infections of intracoronary stents are exceedingly rare. In 2005, Kaufman and colleagues (45) reviewed all cases of stent infections reported in the literature to that date and found only 10 reported cases. When stent infections occur, though, they are frequently associated with serious complications, including stent occlusions with myocardial infarction, coronary abscess (46), coronary perforation (47), mycotic aneurism (48,49), rupture into an adjacent heart chamber, purulent pericarditis (50), and multiple organ septic emboli (45). It is unclear whether these infections occur at the time of the stent placement or via hematogenous seeding of the stent at a later time.

Patients with coronary stent infection typically present within 4 weeks after the procedure. Fever is the only consistent clinical manifestations, and chest pain is reported by about half of the patients. These patients all have positive blood cultures (45). The infection may be verified with echocardiography, computed tomography, and magnetic resonance imaging, but there are not enough data to assess the relative accuracy of each of these modalities; and therefore, no recommendation can be given. *S. aureus* is the most common causative microorganism. Coagulase-negative *Staphylococcus* and *Pseudomonas aeruginosa* have also been described to cause coronary stent infections (45).

Coronary stent infections must be treated with intravenous antibiotics. On the basis of the predominance of gram-positive bacteria, vancomycin is an adequate initial empirical antibiotic. Selection of the definitive antibiotic is based on the organism isolated from blood cultures. Surgical debridement and/or stent removal may be required as well (45). Mortality of patients with coronary stent infections is high, in the order of 40% to 50% even with optimal medical care (45).

Infection of noncoronary vascular stents occur infrequently, with an estimated incidence of less than 1 in 10,000 cases. However, when they occur, noncoronary stent infections may be associated with severe complications, which include pseudoaneurysms, mycotic aneurysms, abscess, arterial necrosis, and septic emboli (28,51,52).

Vascular stent infections tend to occur early (<2 weeks) after placement, although late infections account for approximately 25% of cases (51–53). *S. aureus* is responsible for most cases. Optimal treatment requires antibiotics and surgical removal of the infected stent (54). In cases where surgical intervention is not feasible, long-term suppressive antibiotic therapy is used (28).

Given the rarity of stent-associated infections, antibiotic prophylaxis is not routinely recommended for stent placement, coronary and noncoronary. Likewise, it is not recommended that patients with stents receive antimicrobial prophylaxis when undergoing other invasive procedures, including those likely to generate bacteremia (27,55).

■ INFECTIONS FOLLOWING THE USE OF VCDs

VCDs are used frequently after cardiac catheterization and other percutaneous procedures.

They are preferred over manual compression because they decrease the time to hemostasis and ambulation and are more comfortable for the patients (28). The frequency of local access site infection after coronary angiography is extremely low, in the order of 0% to 0.05% (56). The widespread use of VCD appears to have raised the risk of access site complications after percutaneous procedures, although the frequency of such infections continues to be rare (57,58). Most of the literature describing soft tissue and arterial infections associated with the use of VCD is composed by case reports and small case series describing single-center experiences (59–62). In most large series, the infection rate ranges from 0% to 3% (56). Risk factors for VCD-associated infections include groin hematomas and presence of a foreign body at the site, such as sheaths or intra-aortic balloon pumps.

Most infections associated with VCDs are caused by *S. aureus*. An ultrasound is useful to determine the presence of abscess, hematoma, and pseudoaneurysms. Compared with groin infections following catheterization with manual compression—that are frequently uncomplicated and treated with antibiotics alone—VCD-associated infections tend to manifest later, be more severe, and require surgical intervention. Surgery should be considered when there is persistent bacteremia, symptomatic relapse after appropriate antibiotics, abscess formation, or hemorrhage ± pseudoaneurysm formation (63). This may include open drainage, surgical device removal, and arterial reconstruction. Antibiotic therapy is directed initially against *S. aureus* and should continue for at least 4 weeks when the arterial wall is involved. Vancomycin is an appropriate empirical choice. Once the culture results are reported, the antibiotics must be tailored as needed.

Some authors have advocated the administration of antibiotic prophylaxis prior to the procedure when a VCD is used (58,60). The current consensus is that antibiotic prophylaxis should be decided on a case-by-case basis when VCD is expected to be used. A single dose of an antistaphylococcal antibiotic, such as cefazolin, may be used in high-risk patients, such as diabetic or immunocompromised individuals, repeated procedures, prolonged use of sheath, or access through a vascular graft (28,56).

■ INFECTION CONTROL IN THE CARDIOVASCULAR INTERVENTIONAL SUITE

Prevention of infections associated with cardiovascular procedures requires strict adherence to good infection control practices and procedures. The Society for Cardiovascular Angiography and Interventions published infection control guidelines for the cardiac catheterization laboratory in 2006 (1). These comprehensive guidelines are based in Centers for Disease Control and Prevention recommendations and other published literature and the reader is referred to them for a comprehensive discussion of the various interventions. The most salient points are described below:

1. Avoid hair removal unless it directly interferes with the procedure. If hair removal is done, utilize clippers or depilatory creams and avoid shaving. Hair removal should be done on the day of the procedure, and not before, to prevent dermal abrasions and bacterial overgrowth.

2. The skin at the puncture or incision site must be thoroughly cleaned. A product containing 2% chlorhexidine is preferred, although alcohol- and iodophor-based products are also acceptable.

3. Full barrier precautions shall be used when performing a cardiovascular procedure. These include a cap, a mask, a long-sleeved and cuffed sterile gown, and sterile gloves.

4. Drapes must be sterile, nonporous, and water-resistant. Drapes must cover the entire body and any equipment attached to the table that may come in contact with long catheters or wires.

5. Antibiotic prophylaxis is not generally indicated for cardiac catheterization and other procedures performed in the catheterization laboratory. An exception is the implantation of CIEDs (Table 12-4).

6. Remote infections should be treated, when possible, prior to cardiac procedures. When it is not possible to wait, patient should be receiving treatment appropriate to that infection.

TABLE 12-4   **Recommendations for Administration of Periprocedural Prophylactic Antibiotics for Cardiovascular Procedures**

Procedure	Antibiotic Recommended	Dose/Frequency/Comments
Coronary angiography without VCD	No	
Coronary angiography with VCD	Consider on a case-by-case basis for immunosuppressed patients, diabetic patients, repeated procedures, prolonged use of sheath, or access through a vascular graft.	Cefazolin 1 gm IV 30–60 min prior to the procedure. One dose. Vancomycin 15 mg/kg IV may be substituted for patients intolerant of β-lactams or known to be colonized or infected with MRSA.
Coronary and noncoronary vascular stent placement	No	
Placement of devices for atrial septal closure, patent ductus arteriosus, and ventricular septal defect occlusion	No	Some experts recommend perioperative prophylaxis, although there are no data to support this practice and infections associated to these devices are exceedingly rare (28).
Percutaneous mitral or aortic valvuloplasty	No	
CIED placement	Yes	Cefazolin 1 gm IV 30–60 min prior to the procedure. One dose. Vancomycin 15 mg/kg IV may be substituted for patients intolerant of β-actams or known to be colonized or infected with MRSA.

VCD, vascular closure device; CIED, cardiovascular implantable electronic device; MRSA, methicillin-resistant *Staphylococcus aureus*.
(Adapted from Baddour L, Bettmann M, Bolger A, et al. AHA scientific statement: nonvalvular cardiovascular device–related infections. *Circulation.* 2003;108:2015–2031.)

References

1. Chambers C, Eisenhauer M, McNicol L, et al. Infection control guidelines for the cardiac catheterization laboratory. *Catheter Cardiovasc Interv.* 2006;67:78–86.

2. Voigt A, Shalaby A, Saba S. Rising rates of cardiac rhythm management device infections in the United States: 1996 through 2003. *J Am Coll Cardiol.* 2006;48(3):590–591.

3. Voigt A, Shalaby A, Saba S. Continued rise in rates of cardiovascular implantable electronic device infections in the United States: temporal trends and causative insights. [published online ahead of print September 30, 2009]. *Pacing Clin Electrophysiol.* 2010;33(4):414–419.

4. Cabell C, Heidenreich P, Chu V, et al. Increasing rates of cardiac device infections among Medicare beneficiaries: 1990–1999. *Am Heart J.* 2004;147:582–586.

5. Uslan DZ, Sohail MR, St. Stauver JL, et al. Permanent pacemaker and implantable cardioverter defibrillator infection: a population-based study. *Arch Intern Med.* 2007;167:669–675.

6. Klug D, Balde M, Pavin D, et al. Risk factors related to infections of implanted pacemakers and cardioverter-defibrillators: results of a large prospective study. *Circulation.* 2007;116: 1349–1355.

7. Duval X, Selton-Suty C, Alla F, et al. Endocarditis in patients with a permanent pacemaker: a 1-year

epidemiological survey on infective endocarditis due to valvular and/or pacemaker infection. *Clin Infect Dis.* 2004;39:68–74.

8. Karchmer AW, Longworth DL. Infections of intracardiac devices. *Cardiol Clin.* 2003;21:253–271.

9. Chamis AL, Peterson GE, Cabell CH, et al. *Staphylococcus aureus* bacteremia in patients with permanent pacemakers or implantable cardioverter-defibrillators. *Circulation.* 2001;104:1029–1033.

10. Uslan DZ, Sohail MR, Friedman PA, et al. Frequency of permanent pacemaker or implantable cardioverter-defibrillator infection in patients with gram-negative bacteremia. *Clin Infect Dis.* 2006;43:731–736.

11. Sohail M, Uslan D, Khan A, et al. Risk factor analysis of permanent pacemaker infection. *Clin Infect Dis.* 2007;45:166–173.

12. Marschall J, Hopkins-Broyles D, Jones M, Fraser V, Warren D. Case-control study of surgical site infections associated with pacemakers and implantable cardioverter-defibrillators. *Infect Control Hosp Epidemiol.* 2007;28(11):1299–1304.

13. Chua JD, Wilkoff BL, Lee I, Juratli N, Longworth DL, Gordon SM. Diagnosis and management of infections involving implantable electrophysiologic cardiac devices. *Ann Intern Med.* 2000;133(8):604–608.

14. Sohail MR, Uslan DZ, Khan AH, et al. Infective endocarditis complicating permanent pacemaker and implantable cardioverter-defibrillator infection. *Mayo Clin Proc.* 2008;83(1):46–53.

15. Griffin AD, Carrillo RG, Chan JC. Correlation between presenting signs and final diagnosis in a retrospective review of 288 cardiac device related infections. Poster presentd at: the 47th Annual Meeting of the Infectious Disease Society of America; October 29 to November 1, 2009; Philadelphia, PA.

16. Klug D, Wallet F, Lacroix D, et al. Local symptoms at the site of pacemaker implantation indicate latent systemic infection. *Heart.* 2004;90:882–886.

17. Anselmino M, Vinci M, Comoglio C, et al. Bacteriology of infected extracted pacemaker and ICD leads. *J Cardiovasc Med.* 2009;10:693–698.

18. Klug D, Wallet F, Kacet S, Courcol RJ. Detailed bacteriologic tests to identify the origin of transvenous pacing system infections indicate a high prevalence of multiple organisms. *Am Heart J.* 2005;149:322–328.

19. Golzio PG, Vinci M, Anselmino M, et al. Accuracy of swabs, tissue specimens, and lead samples in diagnosis of cardiac rhythm management device infections. *Pacing Clin Electrophysiol.* 2009; 32(suppl 1):S76–S80.

20. Chua JD, Abdul-Karim A, Mawhorter S, et al. The role of swab and tissue culture in the diagnosis of implantable cardiac device infection. *Pacing Clin Electrophysiol.* 2005;28:1276–1281.

21. Kleeman T, Becker T, Strauss M, et al. Prevalence of bacterial colonization of generator pockets in implantable cardioverter defibrillator patients without signs of infection undergoing generator replacement or lead revision [published online ahead of print October 27, 2009]. *Europace.* 2010;12(1):58–63.

22. Baddour L, Epstein A, Erickson C, et al. Update on cardiovascular implantable electronic device infections and their management: a scientific statement from the American Heart Association. *Circulation.* 2010;121:458–477.

23. Lo R, D'Anca M, Cohen T, Kerwin T. Incidence and prognosis of pacemaker lead-associated masses: a study of 1,569 transesophageal echocardiograms. *J Invasive Cardiol.* 2006;18(12):599–601.

24. Zamora CR, Griffin AD, Nascimento F, Chan JC, Carrillo R. Comparison of transthoracic and transesophageal echocardiography in detection of vegetations. Poster presented at: the 47th Annual Meeting of the Infectious Disease Society of America; October 29 to November 1, 2009; Philadelphia, PA.

25. Dumont E, Camus C, Victor F, et al. Suspected pacemaker or defibrillator transvenous lead infection: prospective assessment of a TEE-guided therapeutic strategy. *Eur Heart J.* 2003; 24:1779–1787.

26. Ruttmann E, Hangler HB, Kilo J, et al. Transvenous pacemaker lead removal is safe and effective even in large vegetations: an analysis of 53 cases of pacemaker lead endocarditis. *Pacing Clin Electrophysiol.* 2006;29:231–236.

27. Wilkoff BL, Love CJ, Byrd CL, et al. Transvenous lead extraction: Heart Rhythm Society expert consensus on facilities, training, indications, and patient management. *Heart Rhythm.* 2009;6(7):1085–1104.

28. Baddour L, Bettmann M, Bolger A, et al. AHA scientific statement: nonvalvular cardiovascular device–related infections. *Circulation.* 2003;108:2015–2031.

29. Sohail MR, Uslan DZ, Khan AH, et al. Management and outcome of permanent pacemaker and implantable cardioverter-defibrillator infections. *J Am Coll Cardiol.* 2007;49:1851–1859.

30. Hurst LN, Evans HB, Windle B, Klein GJ. The salvage of infected cardiac pacemaker pockets using a closed irrigation system. *Pacing Clin Electrophysiol.* 1986;9:789–792.

31. Lee JH, Geha AS, Rattehalli NM, et al. Salvage of infected ICDs: management without removal. *Pacing Clin Electrophysiol.* 1996;19:437–442.

32. Turkisher V, Priel I, Dan M. Successful management of an infected implantable cardioverter defibrillator with oral antibiotics and without removal of the device. *Pacing Clin Electrophysiol.* 1997;20:2268–2270.

33. Lewis A, Hayes D, Holmes D, Vlietstra R, Pluth J, Osborn M. Update on infections involving permanent pacemakers: characterization and management. *J Thorac Cardiovasc Surg.* 1985;89:785–763.

34. Del Rio A, Anguera I, Miro JM, et al. Surgical treatment of pacemaker and defibrillator lead endocarditis the impact of electrode lead extraction on outcome. *Chest.* 2003;124:1451–1459.

35. Bracke FA, Meijer A, van Gelder LM. Pacemaker lead complications: when is extraction appropriate and what can we learn from published data? *Heart.* 2001;85:254–259.

36. Rybak M, Lomaestro B, Rotschafer JC, et al. Therapeutic monitoring of vancomycin in adult patients: a consensus review of the American Society of Health-System Pharmacists, the Infectious Diseases Society of America, and the Society of Infectious Diseases Pharmacists. *Am J Health Syst Pharm.* 2009;66:82–98.

37. Griffin AD, Carrillo RG, Chan JC. Outcomes of infected cardiac devices removed by laser lead extraction. Poster presented at: the 47th Annual Meeting of the Infectious Disease Society of America; October 29 to November 1, 2009; Philadelphia, PA.

38. Borer A, Gilad J, Hyam E, et al. Prevention of infections associated with permanent cardiac antiarrhythmic devices by implementation of a comprehensive infection control program. *Infect Control Hosp Epidemiol.* 2004;25:492–497.

39. Da Costa A, Kirkorian G, Cucherat M, et al. Antibiotic prophylaxis for permanent pacemaker implantation : a meta-analysis. *Circulation.* 1998; 97:1796–1801.

40. Bertaglia E, Zerbo F, Zardo S, Barzan D, Zoppo F, Pascotto P. Antibiotic prophylaxis with a single dose of cefazolin during pacemaker implantation: incidence of long-term infective complications. *Pacing Clin Electrophysiol.* 2006;29: 29–33.

41. Dwivedi SK, Saran RK, Khera P, et al. Short-term (48 hours) versus long-term (7 days) antibiotic prophylaxis for permanent pacemaker implantation. *Indian Heart J.* 2001;53(6):740–742.

42. Lakkireddy D, Valasareddi S, Ryshon K, et al. The impact of povidone-iodine pocket irrigation use on pacemaker and defibrillator infections. *Pacing Clin Electrophysiol.* 2005;28:789–794.

43. Samore MH, Wessolossky MA, Lewis SM, Shubrooks SJ, Karchmer AW. Bacteremia after percutaneous transluminal coronary angiography. *Am J Cardiol.* 1997;79:873–877.

44. Muñoz P, Blanco JR, Rodriguez-Creixems M, Garcia E, Delcan JL, Bouza E. Bloodstream infections after invasive nonsurgical cardiologic procedures. *Arch Intern Med.* 2001;161:2110–2115.

45. Kaufmann BA, Kaiser C, Pfisterer ME, Bonetti PO. Coronary stent infection: a rare but severe complication of percutaneous coronary intervention. *Swiss Med Wkly* 2005;135(33/34):483–487.

46. Liu JC, Cziperle DJ, Kleinman B, Loeb H. Coronary abscess: a complication of stenting. *Catheter Cardiovasc Interv.* 2003;58(1):72.

47. Carg RK, Sear JE, Hockstad ES. Spontaneous coronary artery perforation secondary to a sirolimus-eluting stent infection. *J Invasive Cardiol.* 2007;19(10):E303–E306.

48. Marcu CB, Balf DV, Donahue TJ. Post-infectious pseudoaneurysm after coronary angioplasty using drug eluting stents. *Heart Lung Circ.* 2005; 14(2):85–86.

49. Le MQ, Narins CR. Mycotic pseudoaneurysm of the left circumflex coronary artery: a fatal complication following drug-eluting stent implantation. *Catheter Cardiovasc Interv.* 2007;69(4): 508–512.

50. Shoenkerman AB, Lundstrom RJ. Coronary stent infections: a case series. *Catheter Cardiovasc Interv.* 2009;73:74–76.

51. Ghosh J, Murray D, Khwaja N, Murphy MO, Halka A, Walker MG. Late infection of an endovascular stent graft with septic embolization, colonic perforation, and aortoduodenal fistula. *Ann Vasc Surg.* 2006;20:263–266.

52. Kondo Y, Muto A, Ando M, Nishibe T. Late infected pseudoaneurysm formation after uneventful iliac artery stent placement. *Ann Vasc Surg.* 2007;21:222–224.

53. Sternbergh WC, Money SR. Iliac artery stent infection treated with superficial femoral vein. *J Vasc Surg.* 2005;41:348.

54. Fiorani P, Speziale F, Calisti A, et al. Endovascular graft infection: preliminary results of an international enquiry. *J Endovasc Ther.* 2003;10:919–927.

55. American Society for Gastrointestinal Endoscopy. Antibiotic prophylaxis for GI endoscopy. *Gastrointest Endosc.* 2008;67(6):791–798.

56. Lewis-Carey MB, Kee ST. Complications of arterial closure devices. *Tech Vasc Interv Radiol.* 2003;6(2):103–106.

57. Boulos Toursarkissian MA. Changing patterns of access site complications with the use of percutaneous closure devices. *Vasc Surg.* 2001;35:203–206.

58. Wilson JS, Johnson BL, Parker JL, Back MR, Bandyk DF. Management of vascular complications following femoral artery catheterization with and without percutaneous arterial closure devices. *Ann Vasc Surg.* 2002;16:597–600.

59. Smith TP, Cruz CP, Moursi MM, Eidt JF. Infectious complications resulting from use of hemostatic puncture closure devices. *Am J Surg.* 2001; 182:658–662.

60. Pipkin W, Brophy C, Nesbit R, Mondy JS. Early experience with infectious complications of percutaneous femoral artery closure devices. *J Vasc Surg.* 2000;32:205–208.

61. Johanning JM, Franklin DP, Elmore JR, Han DC. Femoral artery infections associated with percutaneous arterial closure devices. *J Vasc Surg.* 2001;34:983–985.

62. Geary K, Landers JT, Fiore W, Riggs P. Management of infected femoral closure devices. *Cardiovasc Surg.* 2002;10(2):161–163.

63. Kalapatapu VR, Ali AT, Masroor F, Moursi MM, Eidt JF. Techniques for managing complications of arterial closure devices. *Vasc Surg.* 2006;40:399–408.

13

Complications of Contrast Media: Contrast-Induced Nephropathy, Allergic Reactions, and Other Idiosyncratic Reactions

MAURO MOSCUCCI AND ROXANA MEHRAN

Adverse reactions to radiocontrast can be divided into the two broad categories of contrast-induced nephropathy (CIN), leading to acute deterioration of renal function, and hypersensitivity reactions.

Acute deterioration of renal function can occur in a small but significant proportion of patients undergoing coronary angiography, percutaneous coronary intervention (PCI), and other invasive diagnostic and therapeutic vascular procedures. Several studies have shown that renal function deterioration is associated with significant morbidity and increased risk of in-hospital and long-term mortality. Thus, identification of patients at increased risk of acute deterioration of renal function and institution of the appropriate interventions aimed toward its prevention are important components of the overall approach to patients requiring diagnostic or therapeutic cardiovascular procedures.

■ DEFINITIONS OF NEPHROPATHY

Different terminology and definitions of nephropathy have been used in the literature. Most studies have used the terminology "contrast-induced nephropathy" to indicate deterioration in renal function following diagnostic or therapeutic cardiovascular procedures including

the use of contrast media. Other studies have used the terminology "acute deterioration of renal function," (1) which is perhaps more appropriate given that not only contrast media nephrotoxicity but also cholesterol embolism can lead to such deterioration. In addition, three separate definitions of nephropathy have been used in the literature. The first definition is any increase in serum creatinine level of 0.5 mg/dL over the baseline (or preprocedure) value (2–4). The second and currently recommended definition is any increase in serum creatinine level 25% above the baseline (1,5–7). The third and more consistent definition is an acute deterioration of renal function requiring temporary or permanent dialysis support (2,8).

■ EPIDEMIOLOGY OF CONTRAST-INDUCED NEPHROPATHY

Incidence

Differences in definitions and postprocedure surveillance might explain why the reported incidence of nephropathy after cardiac catheterization, PCI, or other vascular procedures varies among studies. In a single-center analysis of 8,357 PCIs, Mehran et al. (6) reported an incidence of CIN of 13.1%, with nephropathy being defined as a 25% increase of serum creatinine over baseline. In a more recent analysis of 29,409 patients undergoing PCI, Khanal et al. (3) reported an incidence of CIN of 5.4%. In that analysis, CIN was defined as an increase in peak postprocedure serum creatinine level of 0.5 mg/dL or more over baseline.

While the overall occurrence of nephropathy following diagnostic and therapeutic cardiac catheterization is relatively common, the occurrence of nephropathy requiring dialysis is less common. McCullough et al. (5) reported an incidence of nephropathy requiring dialysis of 0.21% and 0.77% in two consecutive data sets (1,826 patients and 1,869 patients, respectively). In another series of 7,741 patients referred for PCI, the incidence of nephropathy requiring dialysis was 0.66% (8). Similar event rates have also been recently reported in other registry analyses (2).

Risk Factors

The identification of patients at increased risk of deterioration of renal function plays an important role in the management strategies aimed toward its prevention. Several studies have identified risk factors for the development of nephropathy. These risk factors include patient comorbidities and the volume of contrast media administered during the procedure (Table 13-1).

The relationship between baseline renal dysfunction and the development of nephropathy has been well established in numerous studies. In an analysis of a large multicenter registry of contemporary PCI, baseline renal insufficiency defined as a preprocedure creatinine level of more than 2 mg/dL was identified as a strong independent predictor of postprocedure nephropathy requiring dialysis (2). A similar result was found in another large analysis, targeting as end point the development of any nephropathy, defined as an increase in serum creatinine level 25% above baseline and/or 0.5 mg/dL over baseline. In that analysis, a baseline creatinine more than 1.5 mg/dL was identified as a risk factor for further deterioration of renal function (6). Other studies have evaluated baseline creatinine clearance, glomerular filtration rate (GFR), or baseline creatinine as a continuous variable (5). Although creatinine clearance and GFR are more accurate measurements of

TABLE 13-1	Risk Factors for the Development of Contrast-Induced Nephropathy, Independently from the Amount of Contrast Administered

Renal insufficiency (any degree of renal insufficiency)

Peripheral vascular disease

Diabetes mellitus

History of hypertension

Cardiogenic shock

Congestive heart failure

Dehydration

Hyponatremia

Diuretic usage

Hypoalbuminemia

Blood transfusion requirement

History of bypass surgery

Intra-aortic balloon pump use

renal function when compared with serum creatinine level alone, regardless of how baseline renal function was evaluated in each analysis, all studies have consistently confirmed the relationship between baseline renal dysfunction and an increased risk for the development of CIN. Other risk factors include underlying peripheral vascular disease (2), history of hypertension (8), diabetes mellitus (6), cardiogenic shock (2), congestive heart failure (2,6), dehydration, hyponatremia, diuretic usage, hypoalbuminemia, blood transfusion requirement, history of bypass surgery (8), and intra-aortic balloon pump use (6). It remains to be determined whether the relationship between intra-aortic balloon pump use and deterioration of renal function following invasive procedures is secondary to an association between intra-aortic balloon pump use and an increased risk of cholesterol embolism or whether intra-aortic balloon pump use is just a marker of disease severity and/or reduced renal blood flow.

Beyond patient's risk factors, the total amount of contrast media administered during the procedure has been found to be an important predictor of CIN (2,5,6). While some studies have evaluated the role of any contrast amount as a predictor of CIN and nephropathy requiring dialysis, other studies have highlighted the importance of a contrast dose threshold. In a study of patients with serum creatinine level more than 2 mg/dL, the incidence of CIN was only 2% if the amount of contrast received was less than 125 mL (the mean contrast dose) and increased to 19% if the amount received was more than 125 mL (9). Cigarroa et al. (10) evaluated the role of exceeding a weight- and creatinine-adjusted contrast dose in a group of patients with renal dysfunction, defined as a baseline creatinine more than 1.8 mg/dL. In their study, the contrast dose threshold was calculated using the formula (5 cc of contrast × body weight in kg/serum creatinine in mg/dL). Renal dysfunction postprocedure occurred in 2% of patients when the contrast dose did not exceed the threshold but increased to 38% of patients when the contrast dose threshold was exceeded. Two large registry analyses of contemporary PCIs recently confirmed the critical role that exceeding this weight- and creatinine-adjusted contrast dose has in the occurrence of postprocedure renal dysfunction (2,11). In the first analysis, a dramatic increase in the development of nephropathy requiring dialysis was observed once the weight- and baseline serum creatinine-adjusted contrast dose was exceeded (2). In the second analysis, a reduction in the frequency of CIN and of nephropathy requiring dialysis was observed in association with a reduction in total amount of contrast per case and with a reduction in the percentage of patients exceeding the weight- and creatinine-adjusted contrast dose (11). In the study by Merhan et al., a further increase in the risk of CIN was observed for each 100 cc of contrast administered (6). Intuitively a "threshold" effect depending on baseline creatinine level and body weight rather than a simple linear dose–effect relationship independent of baseline creatinine level and body weight seems understandable. A 300 mL contrast dose given to a young man with a serum creatinine level of 1.0 mg/dL and weighing 90 kg is likely not biologically equivalent to the same dose given to an elderly woman with a creatinine level of 1.5 mg/dL and weighing 55 kg.

In an attempt to provide an aid toward a rapid, bedside identification of patients at increased risk for contrast nephropathy, several risk prediction tools for CIN have been recently developed (2,6,11,12) (Figs. 13-1–13-3). These risk prediction tools have been used both for the identification of patients at increased risk and for the institution of quality improvement interventions aimed toward the reduction of contrast nephropathy and nephropathy requiring dialysis (11).

Prognostic Implications

Unfortunately, while mild renal dysfunction following PCIs is more common and is often reversible, development of severe nephropathy requiring in-hospital dialysis carries significant mortality risk, with reported in-hospital mortality rates as high as 39% (Fig. 13-4) (2,5), and 1-year mortality rates as high as 54.5% (8). In addition, other studies have shown that even in the absence of dialysis requirement, patients who develop acute deterioration of renal function following PCI have worse long-term survival (Fig. 13-5) (1,13).

■ MECHANISMS OF ACUTE DETERIORATION OF RENAL FUNCTION

There are two currently recognized mechanisms leading to acute deterioration of renal function in patients undergoing invasive therapeutic and cardiovascular procedures. The first mechanism is renal embolization of atherosclerotic plaque during catheter exchange, and the second mechanism is a direct nephrotoxic effect of contrast media, leading to a CIN. Although the focus of this chapter is on CIN and on other adverse reactions secondary to radiocontrast administration, we will outline in brief key issues surrounding cholesterol embolism, given its relevance on morbidity and mortality.

Cholesterol Embolism

Cholesterol embolism can occur spontaneously in patients with severe atherosclerosis but is more commonly induced by cardiovascular procedures. It is caused by disruption of atheromatous plaque in the aorta during advancement of catheters or during catheter exchanges and leads to distal embolization of cholesterol crystals. It is important to emphasize that the disruption of atheromatous plaque during catheter exchange and collection of debris inside the catheter is a common occurrence. In a systematic analysis of guiding catheter aspirates, Keeley and colleagues showed that atheromatous particles could be

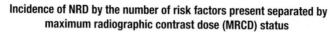

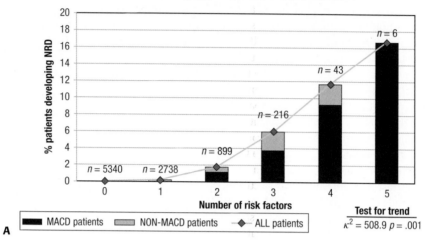

Incidence of NRD by the number of risk factors present separated by maximum radiographic contrast dose (MRCD) status

y-axis: % patients developing NRD

x-axis: Number of risk factors

$n = 5340$ $n = 2738$ $n = 899$ $n = 216$ $n = 43$ $n = 6$

MACD patients   NON-MACD patients   ALL patients

Test for trend
$\kappa^2 = 508.9$ $p = .001$

A

**High risk patient characteristics
for contrast nephropathy**

Diabetes
Creatinine ≥2 mg/dL
Peripheral vascular disease
Cardiogenic shock
Congestive heart failure

Proposed guidelines for high-risk patients

A. Aggressive hydration **before** contrast administration. Measuring the LVEDP or PCWP before
contrast administration might help in further determining volume status. It is not uncommon to
find low PCWP/LVEDP in patients who have been admitted for preprocedure "IV hydration."

B. Determine "maximum allowed contrast dose" according to the following formula:

5 cc × kg body weight/creatinine

C. Avoid exceeding this amount. Use of biplane coronary angiography and avoidance of
unnecessary images (i.e., left ventriculogram or other images) might help in minimizing total
amount of contast used.

D. Consider staged procedures. When planning a staged procedure, current recommendations
are to perform the second procedure several days after the first.

E. Use of smaller catheters might help in decreasing amount of contrast.

F. Use of low osmolar or nonionic contrast might decrease the risk in high-risk patients.

G. In view of a recent study showing a significant benefit from acetylcysteine, and given its
safety, consider acetylcysteine 600 mg bid on the day before and on the day of contrast

B   administration (*New Engl J Med.* 2000;343:180–184).

FIGURE 13-1. Bedside risk prediction tool for the prediction (**A**) and prevention (**B**) of nephropathy requiring dialysis (NRD). The risk factors for NRD include (1) diabetes mellitus, (2) creatinine > 2 mg/dL, (3) peripheral vascular disease, (4) cardiogenic shock, and (5) history of congestive heart failure. Within each risk factor number group, the relative proportion of patients exceeding a weight- and creatinine-adjusted maximum radiographic contrast dose (MRCD) is represented by the darker bar. (From Moscucci M, Rogers EK, Montoye C, et al. Association of a continuous quality improvement initiative with practice and outcome variations of contemporary percutaneous coronary interventions. *Circulation.* 2006;113:814–822. ©2001 University of Michigan Board of Regents. All Rights Reserved.)

retrieved from more than 50% of guiding catheter aspirates, suggesting a high frequency of the substrate needed for cholesterol embolism (14). The clinical manifestation of cholesterol embolism varies considerably, from a completely asymptomatic status to a syndrome including skin lesions, acute renal failure, and other clinical findings consistent with embolization in other end organs. The most common skin lesions include livedo reticularis (Fig. 13-6), followed by

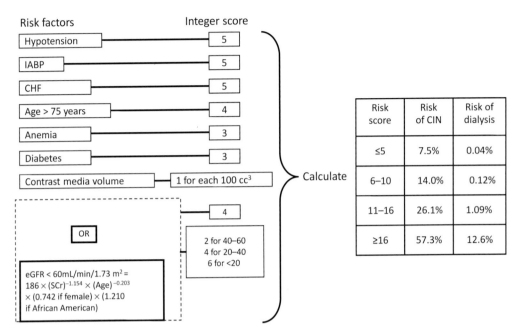

FIGURE 13-2. Risk score for prediction of contrast-induced nephropathy after percutaneous coronary intervention. CHF, congestive heart failure; IABP, intra-aortic balloon pump; CIN, contrast-induced nephropathy. (Reprinted from Mehran R, et al. A simple risk score for prediction of contrast-induced nephropathy after percutaneous coronary intervention: development and initial validation. *J Am Coll Cardiol.* 2004;44:1393–1399, with permission from Elsevier.)

cyanosis, gangrene, ulceration, skin nodules, and purpura. Other findings secondary to embolization in other organs include gastrointestinal bleeding, pancreatitis, ischemic bowel syndrome, weight loss, and retinal embolization. From a diagnostic perspective, the development of progressive renal failure with gradual increase in serum creatinine and blood urea nitrogen levels, in association with skin lesions and eosinophilia,

is pathognomonic of cholesterol embolism. Renal failure due to CIN usually presents with a rapid rise in serum creatinine level (within 1 or 2 days) that peaks within 4 to 5 days and that is often at least partially reversible. Renal failure secondary to cholesterol embolism tends to present with a delayed and progressive rise in serum creatinine level, which is often irreversible. The incidence of cholesterol embolism has been estimated to be as

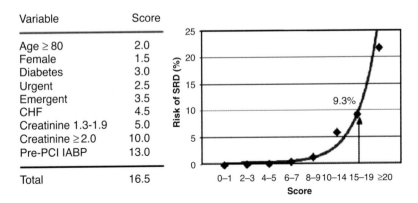

FIGURE 13-3. Northern New England risk score and nomogram for serious renal dysfunction (SRD). CHF, coronary heart failure; IABP, intra-aortic balloon pump; PCI, percutaneous coronary intervention. (Reprinted from Brown JR, et al. Serious renal dysfunction after percutaneous coronary interventions can be predicted. *Am Heart J.* 2008;155:260–266, with permission from Elsevier).

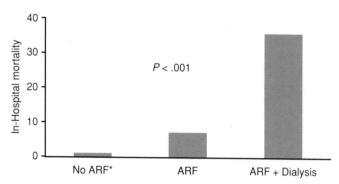

FIGURE 13-4. In-hospital mortality in patients developing acute renal failure (ARF) and ARF requiring dialysis. (Based on data from McCullough PA, et al. Acute renal failure after coronary intervention: incidence, risk factors, and relationship to mortality. *Am J Med.* 1997;103:368–375.)

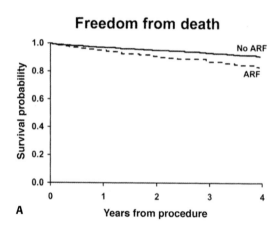

FIGURE 13-5. Kaplan–Meier survival analysis, estimated probability of freedom from death (**A**) and freedom from death and Myocardial Infarction (MI) (**B**) among patients surviving to hospital dismissal, stratified by presence or absence of acute renal failure (ARF) occurring in hospital, defined as increase in serum creatinine ≥ 0.5 mg/dL from baseline. MI, myocardial infarction. (From Rihal CS, et al. Incidence and prognostic importance of acute renal failure after percutaneous coronary intervention. *Circulation.* 2002;105:2259–2264).

low as 0.15% to 1.4% in clinical studies (15,16) and as high as 30% in pathological series (17). Given that cutaneous findings are not present in every case, it is likely that clinical series underestimate the true incidence of cholesterol embolism. In a study evaluating the incidence of cholesterol embolism following left heart catheterization, Fukumoto and colleagues (16) evaluated 1,786 consecutive patients undergoing cardiac catheterization. They defined *definite* cholesterol embolism as the development of peripheral cutaneous signs with or without renal insufficiency, while *probable* cholesterol embolism was defined as the development of renal insufficiency without cutaneous signs. In that study, definite cholesterol embolism occurred in 12/1,786 patients (0.67%), whereas probable cholesterol embolism occurred in 25/1,786 (1.4%). The eosinophil count increased significantly from 220 to 330 cells/μL in patients with renal dysfunction, while 9 patients without renal dysfunction did not show an increase. The observed in-hospital mortality rate

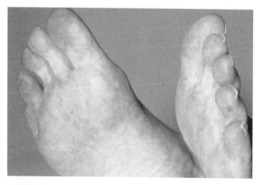

FIGURE 13-6. Livedo reticularis. (From Smeltzer SC, Bare BG. *Textbook of Medical-Surgical Nursing.* 9th ed. Philadelphia, PA: Lippincott Williams & Wilkins; 2000). (See color insert.)

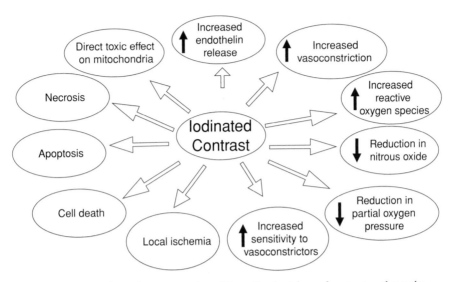

FIGURE 13-7. Schematic representation of the pathophysiology of contrast nephropathy.

in patients with renal dysfunction was 25%. At this time, supportive measures are the only therapy available for cholesterol embolism, and beyond meticulous over-the-wire catheter advancement and catheter flushing after exchanges, there is no protocol for prevention.

Contrast-Induced Nephropathy

Contrast-induced nephropathy is defined as a deterioration of renal function secondary to administration of contrast media and should be differentiated from cholesterol embolism. The majority of studies on CIN have been performed on patients undergoing invasive procedures. Because of the possibility of underlying cholesterol embolism, it is not currently possible to determine the contribution of cholesterol embolism to the deterioration of renal function observed following contrast administration in the absence of cutaneous skin findings. The pathophysiology of CIN has not yet been completely elucidated (18). Overall, administration of radiographic contrast media is associated with a reduction in renal perfusion and with a possible direct toxic effect on tubular cells. It has been suggested that the synthesis of "reactive oxygen species" plays an important role in the development of CIN (19,20). By acting as scavengers for nitric oxide (NO), "reactive oxygen species" including superoxide, hydrogen peroxide, and hydroxyl radicals lead to a reduction of partial oxygen pressure and an in increase in vascular

reactivity to various vasoconstrictors, including angiotensin II, thromboxane, endothelin, adenosine, and norepinephrine (21). In addition, contrast media can have a direct toxic effect on tubular cells mediated by a direct effect on mitochondrial activity (22) (Fig. 13-7). This effect seems to be more pronounced with ionic and dimeric iso-osmolar compounds when compared with monomeric low-osmolar compounds (22). It has been suggested that the differences in nephrotoxicity observed between dimeric iso-osmolar and monomeric low-osmolar compounds might be due to differences in viscosity of the contrast agent (23). Also, a recent systematic review has suggested the existence of differences in the incidence of CIN with different low-osmolar contrast agents having similar osmolarity (24). Thus, it has been suggested that factors other than the osmolarity of the contrast agent might play an important role in the development of CIN (18,24). The complex pathophysiology surrounding the development of CIN has led to the assessment of several pharmacological and nonpharmacological interventions aimed toward its prevention.

■ CLINICAL COURSE AND PREVENTION OF CIN

As discussed earlier, CIN has a broad spectrum clinical presentation ranging from a transient increase in serum creatinine level with rapid return to baseline, to acute renal failure with oliguria requiring transient or permanent dialysis support.

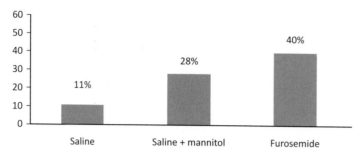

FIGURE 13-8. Incidence of renal failure stratified by treatment allocation in patients receiving 0.9% normal saline or 0.9% normal saline plus mannitol and in patients receiving furosemide. $P = .02$ for saline vs. furosemide group; $P = $ NS for mannitol vs. furosemide group. (Based on data from Solomon R, et al. Effects of saline, mannitol, and furosemide to prevent acute decreases in renal function induced by radiocontrast agents. *N Engl J Med.* 1994;331:1416–1420.)

Prevention

All patients receiving intravenous (IV) or intra-arterial contrast media should undergo assessment of baseline renal function and clinical assessment for the identification of additional risk factors for the development of CIN. It is also recommended that in high-risk patients, a follow-up serum creatinine be obtained between 24 and 72 hours from contrast exposure (25,26).

Hydration and Sodium Bicarbonate Infusion

Preprocedure hydration continues to be the mainstay in the prevention of CIN. Its key role has been supported both by observation data and by the results of recent randomized clinical trials, which have shown that hydration through the administration of IV fluids is superior to oral administration of fluids alone (27) and is also superior to volume

supplementation with the addition of mannitol or furosemide (Fig. 13-8) (28). In addition, one landmark clinical trial has shown that hydration with normal isotonic 0.9% saline is superior to hydration with half-isotonic (0.45%) saline (29) (Fig. 13-9). The difference in efficacy between the two regimens might be due to a more effective expansion of intravascular volume and to inhibition of renin release with 0.9% isotonic saline when compared with 0.45% half-isotonic saline.

More recently, bicarbonate infusion has emerged as an alternative regimen for preprocedure hydration (30) (Fig. 13-10). The hypothesis behind the use of bicarbonate is that alkalinization of renal tubular fluid with bicarbonate may reduce the formation of free radicals and thus reduce tubular injury (Fig. 13-11). In a prospective, single-center trial, 119 patients with stable serum creatinine levels of at least 1.1 mg/dL were randomized to receive a 154 mEq/L

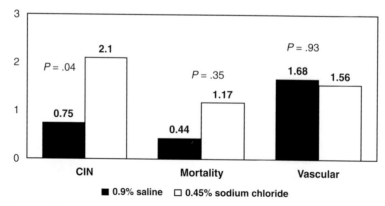

FIGURE 13-9. Optimal hydration protocols: 0.9% normal saline compared with 0.45% normal saline. CIN, contrast-induced nephropathy. (Based on data from Mueller C, et al. Prevention of contrast media-associated nephropathy: randomized comparison of 2 hydration regimens in 1620 patients undergoing coronary angioplasty. *Arch Intern Med.* 2002;162:329–336.)

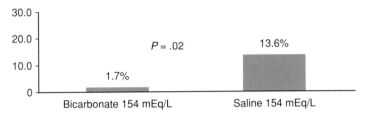

FIGURE 13-10. Frequency of contrast nephropathy in patients receiving sodium bicarbonate and in patients receiving normal saline in the initial study supporting a beneficial effect of sodium bicarbonate in the prevention of contrast nephropathy. Contrast-induced nephropathy defined as 25% increase of serum creatinine level over baseline. (Based on data from Merten GJ, et al. Prevention of contrast-induced nephropathy with sodium bicarbonate: a randomized controlled trial. *JAMA.* 2004;291:2328–2334.)

infusion of either sodium chloride ($n = 59$) or sodium bicarbonate as a bolus of 3 mL/kg ($n = 60$) 1 hour before iopamidol contrast (370 mg iodine/mL), followed by an infusion of 1 mL/kg per hour for 6 hours after the procedure (30). The main outcome measure was CIN, defined as an increase of 25% or more in serum creatinine level within 2 days after contrast administration. Baseline serum creatinine level was 1.71 ± 0.42 mg/dL in patients receiving sodium chloride and 1.89 ± 0.69 mg/dL in patients receiving sodium bicarbonate; $P = .09$. In this study, CIN occurred in eight patients (13.6%) who received sodium chloride and in only 1 patient (1.7%) who received sodium bicarbonate (mean difference, 11.9%; 95% confidence interval, 2.6%21.2%; $P = .02$).

A similar effect was observed in a more recent single-center trial including 111 consecutive patients with acute coronary syndromes undergoing emergency PCI (31). In that study, 56 patients (group A) received an infusion of sodium bicarbonate plus *N*-acetylcysteine (NAC) started just before contrast injection and continued for 12 hours after PCI, and 55 patients (group B) received IV isotonic saline for 12 hours after PCI. In the sodium bicarbonate group, NAC was administered IV at a dose of 2,400 mg over

Alkalinization of renal tubular fluid
↓
Reduction in the formation of free radicals
↓
Reduction of tubular injury
↓
Reduction in the incidence of CIN

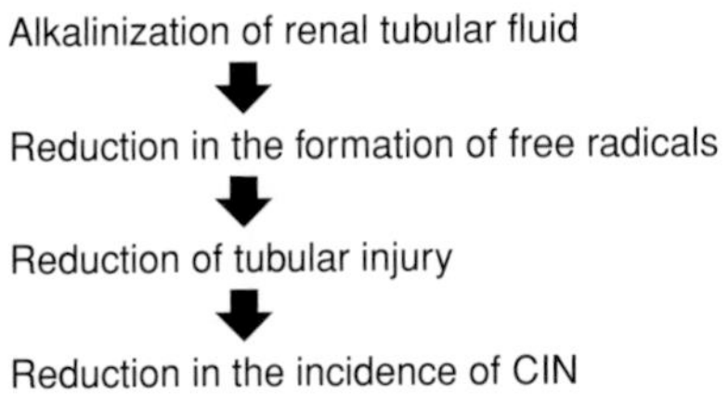

FIGURE 13-11. Rational surrounding the use of bicarbonate in the prevention of contrast-induced nephropathy (CIN).

1 hour in the same solution. In both groups, two doses of oral NAC were administered the next day. CIN was defined as an increase in creatinine concentration of 0.5 mg/dL from baseline. In that study, CIN was observed after emergency PCI in 1 patient in the group receiving bicarbonate (1.8%) and in 12 patients in group receiving isotonic saline (21.8%; $P = .001$), whereas acute anuric renal failure was observed in 1 patient in the group receiving bicarbonate (1.8%) and in 7 patients in the group receiving isotonic saline (12.7%) ($P = .032$). Unfortunately, the results of this study are difficult to interpret given that the control group received hydration only after the procedure and therefore was treated with a suboptimal protocol. The additional effect of IV NAC also remains to be determined. On the other hand, it could be argued that in an emergency situation, prolonged preprocedure hydration with isotonic saline would not be feasible; and therefore, in the setting of emergency, PCI bicarbonate represents a valid treatment for the prevention of CIN.

Briguori et al. randomized 326 consecutive patients with chronic renal failure (preprocedure creatinine ≥ 2.0 mg/dL and/or estimated GFR < 40 mL × min(–1) × 1.73 min(–2) to three different treatment regimens: (1) prophylactic administration of 0.9% saline infusion plus NAC ($n = 111$), (2) sodium bicarbonate infusion plus NAC ($n = 108$), and (3) 0.9% saline plus ascorbic acid plus NAC ($n = 107$) (32) (Figs. 13-12 and 13-13). In all cases, iodixanol was the contrast agent used. The primary end point was an increase of ≥ 25% in the serum creatinine level 48 hours after the procedure. CIN occurred in 11 of 111 patients (9.9%) in the saline plus NAC group, in 2 of 108 (1.9%) in the bicarbonate plus NAC group ($P = .019$), and in 11 of 107 (10.3%) in the saline plus

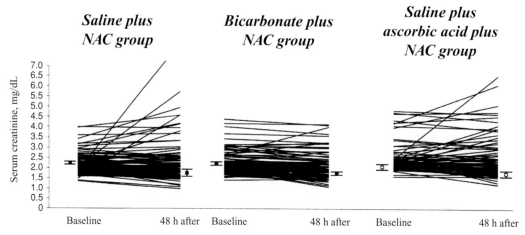

FIGURE 13-12. Serum creatinine concentrations before and after contrast administration in the three groups receiving saline plus N-acetylcysteine (NAC), bicarbonate plus NAC, and saline plus NAC plus ascorbic acid (error bars indicate median). All patients received NAC orally at a dose of 1,200 mg twice daily on the day before and the day of administration of the contrast agent (total of 2 days). Isotonic saline (0.90%) was given intravenously at a rate of 1 mL/kg body weight per hour (0.5 mL/kg for patients with left ventricular ejection fraction <40%) for 12 hours before and 12 hours after administration of the contrast agent. The initial intravenous bolus of bicarbonate was 3 mL/kg/h for 1 hour immediately before contrast injection followed by 1 mL/kg/h during contrast exposure and for 6 hours after the procedure. Patients randomized to ascorbic acid received 3 g ascorbic acid intravenously 2 hours before followed by 2 g the night and the morning after the procedure. h, hour. (From Briguori C, et al. Renal Insufficiency Following Contrast Media Administration Trial [REMEDIAL]: a randomized comparison of 3 preventive strategies. *Circulation.* 2007;115:1211–1217).

ascorbic acid plus NAC group (P = 1.00 vs. saline plus NAC group; see Fig. 13-12). Also, this study was consistent with a superiority of sodium bicarbonate plus NAC over the combination of NS with NAC alone or with the addition of ascorbic acid in preventing CIN in patients at medium to high risk (Fig. 13-13). Importantly, the results of this study suggest that the addition of ascorbic acid to NAC in patient receiving isotonic saline does not provide further benefit in the prevention of CIN. The effect of bicarbonate has been further assessed in a meta-analysis of seven trials including 1,307 patients (33). Preprocedural hydration with sodium bicarbonate was associated with a significant decrease in the rate of CIN (5.96% in the bicarbonate arm vs. 17.23% in the isotonic saline arm, summary response rate (RR) 0.37; 95% CI, 0.18–0.714; P = .005). No difference in the rates of postprocedure hemodialysis or death was observed. Formal testing revealed moderate heterogeneity and a strong likelihood of publication bias. As for any meta-analysis, these results should be interpreted within the important context of publication bias, which is bias derived by lack of publication of negative results.

However, two more recent large randomized clinical trials have questioned the value of bicar-

bonate. In the first study (34), Maioli et al. randomized 502 patients with estimated creatinine clearance less than 60 mL/min to receive an infusion of 0.9% NS (1 mL/kg/h) for 12 hours before and after the procedure or to receive sodium bicarbonate (154 mEq/L in dextrose and water) 3 mL/kg for 1 hour before contrast injection, followed by an infusion of 1 mL/kg/h for 6 hours after the procedure. All patients received oral NAC 600 mg twice a day. CIN was defined as an absolute increase of serum creatinine level higher than 0.5 mg/dL measured within 5 days. In that study, CIN developed in 10% of patients treated with sodium bicarbonate and 11.5% of patients treated with saline (P = .60). The conclusion from this study is that hydration with sodium bicarbonate plus NAC before contrast medium exposure is not more effective than prolonged hydration with isotonic saline plus NAC for prophylaxis of CIN, but it might provide an advantage due to its shorter duration. However, in the second study (35), Brar et al. randomized 353 patients undergoing coronary angiography with a baseline GFR higher than 60 mL/min per 1.73 m^2 to receive either 0.9% NS (n = 178) or sodium bicarbonate (n = 175). Both infusions were administered at 3 mL/kg for

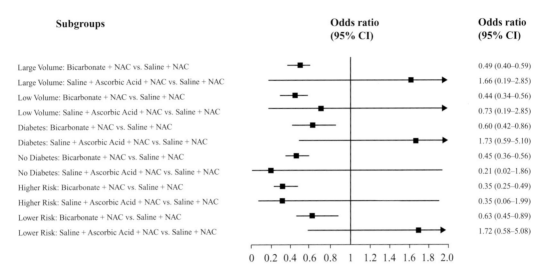

Subgroups	Odds ratio (95% CI)	Odds ratio (95% CI)
Large Volume: Bicarbonate + NAC vs. Saline + NAC		0.49 (0.40–0.59)
Large Volume: Saline + Ascorbic Acid + NAC vs. Saline + NAC		1.66 (0.19–2.85)
Low Volume: Bicarbonate + NAC vs. Saline + NAC		0.44 (0.34–0.56)
Low Volume: Saline + Ascorbic Acid + NAC vs. Saline + NAC		0.73 (0.19–2.85)
Diabetes: Bicarbonate + NAC vs. Saline + NAC		0.60 (0.42–0.86)
Diabetes: Saline + Ascorbic Acid + NAC vs. Saline + NAC		1.73 (0.59–5.10)
No Diabetes: Bicarbonate + NAC vs. Saline + NAC		0.45 (0.36–0.56)
No Diabetes: Saline + Ascorbic Acid + NAC vs. Saline + NAC		0.21 (0.02–1.86)
Higher Risk: Bicarbonate + NAC vs. Saline + NAC		0.35 (0.25–0.49)
Higher Risk: Saline + Ascorbic Acid + NAC vs. Saline + NAC		0.35 (0.06–1.99)
Lower Risk: Bicarbonate + NAC vs. Saline + NAC		0.63 (0.45–0.89)
Lower Risk: Saline + Ascorbic Acid + NAC vs. Saline + NAC		1.72 (0.58–5.08)

FIGURE 13-13. Effect of the three preventive approaches in selected subsets according to volume of contrast media, risk score, and presence of diabetes mellitus. Large volume indicates contrast ratio >1 or exceeding the weight and creatinine contrast dose calculated as 5 cc of contrast × kg body weight/serum creatinine (mg/dL); higher risk, risk score >11. All patients received *N*-acetylcysteine (NAC) orally at a dose of 1,200 mg twice daily on the day before and the day of administration of the contrast agent (total of 2 days). Isotonic saline (0.90%) was given intravenously at a rate of 1 mL/kg body weight per hour (0.5 mL/kg for patients with left ventricular ejection fraction <40%) for 12 hours before and 12 hours after administration of the contrast agent. The initial intravenous bolus of bicarbonate was 3 mL/kg/h for 1 hour immediately before contrast injection followed by 1 mL/kg/h during contrast exposure and for 6 hours after the procedure. Patients randomized to ascorbic acid received 3 g ascorbic acid intravenously 2 hours before followed by 2 g the night and the morning after the procedure. The symbols indicate the unadjusted odds ratios; horizontal lines, 95% confidence intervals. (From Briguori C, et al. Renal Insufficiency Following Contrast Media Administration Trial [REMEDIAL]: a randomized comparison of 3 preventive strategies. *Circulation.* 2007;115:1211–1217.)

1 hour before coronary angiography, and at 1.5 ml/kg/h during the procedure and for 4 hours after the completion of the procedure. CIN was defined as a 25% or more decrease in GFR within 4 days from contrast exposure. In this study, CIN occurred in 13.3% of the sodium bicarbonate group and 14.6% of the NS group (*P* = .82). There was also no difference in the rates of death, dialysis, myocardial infarction, and cerebrovascular events at 30 days or 6 months between the two groups. Thus, on the basis of these two last large randomized clinical trials, hydration with bicarbonate might not provide an additional advantage when compared with optimal and equivalent hydration with 0.9% NS. However, according to the most recent meta-analysis, even after adding these latest clinical trials, there might still be an additional benefit with bicarbonate when compared with NS in the prevention of contrast nephropathy (36) (Fig. 13-14). In addition, there is a suggestion of a higher benefit in patients receiving low-osmolar contrast when compared with

those receiving iso-osmolar contrast (Fig. 13-15) and in patients undergoing emergency procedures (Fig. 13-16). No study so far has shown a deleterious effect of bicarbonate on the development of CIN when compared with NS, and the negative studies still show a nonsignificant trend toward a lower incidence of CIN in patients treated with bicarbonate. Therefore, bicarbonate seems to be a valid and perhaps superior alternative to NS as a periprocedure hydration solution.

The optimal duration and timing of fluid administration remains to be determined. Currently, results from small clinical trials suggest that a regimen of 1 mL/kg/h starting 12 hours before the procedure and continued for 12 hours after the procedure is superior to administration of oral fluid before beginning the procedure plus a fluid bolus during contrast administration (37,38). However, another study has suggested that an outpatient protocol including 1,000 cc of oral fluid administration over 10 hours prior to the procedure, followed

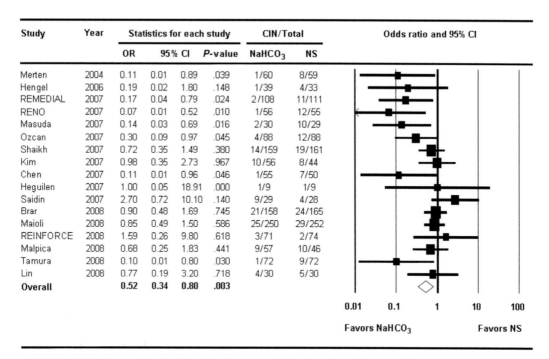

Study	Year	OR	95% CI		P-value	NaHCO₃	NS
Merten	2004	0.11	0.01	0.89	.039	1/60	8/59
Hengel	2006	0.19	0.02	1.80	.148	1/39	4/33
REMEDIAL	2007	0.17	0.04	0.79	.024	2/108	11/111
RENO	2007	0.07	0.01	0.52	.010	1/56	12/55
Masuda	2007	0.14	0.03	0.69	.016	2/30	10/29
Ozcan	2007	0.30	0.09	0.97	.045	4/88	12/88
Shaikh	2007	0.72	0.35	1.49	.380	14/159	19/161
Kim	2007	0.98	0.35	2.73	.967	10/56	8/44
Chen	2007	0.11	0.01	0.96	.046	1/55	7/50
Heguilen	2007	1.00	0.05	18.91	.000	1/9	1/9
Saidin	2007	2.70	0.72	10.10	.140	9/29	4/28
Brar	2008	0.90	0.48	1.69	.745	21/158	24/165
Maioli	2008	0.85	0.49	1.50	.586	25/250	29/252
REINFORCE	2008	1.59	0.26	9.80	.618	3/71	2/74
Malpica	2008	0.68	0.25	1.83	.441	9/57	10/46
Tamura	2008	0.10	0.01	0.80	.030	1/72	9/72
Lin	2008	0.77	0.19	3.20	.718	4/30	5/30
Overall		0.52	0.34	0.80	.003		

FIGURE 13-14. Forest plot of odds ratios of contrast-induced nephropathy. Sizes of data markers are proportional to the weight of each study in the meta-analysis. Studies are stratified by year of presentation and/or publication. Horizontal bars, 95% confidence interval (CI). CIN, contrast-induced nephropathy; NaHCO₃, sodium bicarbonate; NS, normal saline; OR, odds ratio. (From Meier P, et al. Sodium bicarbonate-based hydration prevents contrast-induced nephropathy: a meta-analysis. *BMC Med.* 2009;7:23.)

by 0.45% half-isotonic IV saline 300 mL/h administered 30 to 60 minutes prior to the procedure and continued for a total of 6 hours after the procedure, might be as effective as 24 hours of IV 0.45% half-isotonic saline at a rate of 75 mL/h (39) However, given that 0.45% half-isotonic saline is inferior to 0.9% saline (see Fig. 13-9), the value of this protocol on the basis of the most recent data is questionable. All the studies that have evaluated bicarbonate have used a rapid preprocedure infusion protocol over 1 hour, followed by infusion during the procedure and for 4 to 6 hour thereafter at a lower rate. Overall, on the basis of the results of the most recent clinical trials evaluating bicarbonate, it appears that a rapid hydration protocol is a valid alternative to preprocedure hydration with NS over a 12-hour period. Table 13-2 summarizes different hydration protocols that have been proposed and that have been shown to be effective for the prevention of CIN. Concentrations in mEq/L of stock solutions and preparation of the bicarbonate solution as used in randomized clinical trials are listed in Tables 13-3 and 13-4.

N-Acetylcysteine

NAC is a potent antioxidant that also has vasodilatatory effects. In animal studies, acetylcysteine has been shown to inhibit cell death induced by ischemia reperfusion injury in the kidney (40), to increase the expression of nitric oxide synthase, and to reduce the effect of oxygen free radicals by scavenging them. Given these beneficial effects and its high safety profile, the use of NAC initially appeared to be an attractive intervention for the prevention of CIN. In the first study to evaluate the use of NAC in the prevention of CIN (4), Tepel et al. randomized 83 patients with chronic renal insufficiency (mean [±SD] serum creatinine concentration, 2.4 ± 1.3 mg/dL) who were undergoing computed tomography (CT) with a nonionic low-osmolarity contrast agent. One patient group received acetylcysteine (600 mg orally twice daily) and 0.45% saline IV before and after administration of the contrast agent, whereas the second patient group received placebo and saline. The primary end point was CIN, which was defined as an increase in serum creatinine level of at least

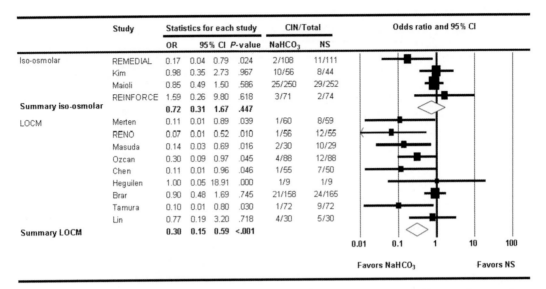

	Study	Statistics for each study			CIN/Total		Odds ratio and 95% CI
		OR	95% CI	P-value	NaHCO₃	NS	
Iso-osmolar	REMEDIAL	0.17	0.04 0.79	.024	2/108	11/111	
	Kim	0.98	0.35 2.73	.967	10/56	8/44	
	Maioli	0.85	0.49 1.50	.586	25/250	29/252	
	REINFORCE	1.59	0.26 9.80	.618	3/71	2/74	
Summary iso-osmolar		**0.72**	**0.31 1.67**	**.447**			
LOCM	Merten	0.11	0.01 0.89	.039	1/60	8/59	
	RENO	0.07	0.01 0.52	.010	1/56	12/55	
	Masuda	0.14	0.03 0.69	.016	2/30	10/29	
	Ozcan	0.30	0.09 0.97	.045	4/88	12/88	
	Chen	0.11	0.01 0.96	.046	1/55	7/50	
	Heguilen	1.00	0.05 18.91	.000	1/9	1/9	
	Brar	0.90	0.48 1.69	.745	21/158	24/165	
	Tamura	0.10	0.01 0.80	.030	1/72	9/72	
	Lin	0.77	0.19 3.20	.718	4/30	5/30	
Summary LOCM		**0.30**	**0.15 0.59**	**<.001**			

0.01   0.1   1   10   100

Favors NaHCO₃   Favors NS

FIGURE 13-15. Forest plot of stratified analysis by studies using iso-osmolar (iodixanol) versus low-osmolar contrast media. Sizes of data markers are proportional to the weight of each study in the meta-analysis. Horizontal bars, 95% confidence interval (CI). CIN, contrast-induced nephropathy; LOCM, low osmolar contrast media; NaHCO₃, sodium bicarbonate; NS, normal saline; OR, odds ratio. (From Meier P, et al. Sodium bicarbonate-based hydration prevents contrast-induced nephropathy: a meta-analysis. *BMC Med.* 2009;7:23.)

0.5 mg/dL over the baseline. The primary end point was reached in 1 of the 41 patients in the acetylcysteine group (2%) and 9 of the 42 patients in the control group (21%; $P = .01$; RR, 0.1; 95% CI, 0.02–0.9). Since this study was published, there have been numerous other clinical trials that have evaluated the use of acetylcysteine for the prevention of contrast-related nephropathy and that have reported mixed results. The results of these trials have been summarized in several meta-analyses that have suggested that acetylcysteine might be beneficial in reducing the incidence of CIN, although with inconsistencies across currently available trials. More recently, a randomized clinical trial has shown that an IV dose of NAC (1,200 mg) prior to PCI followed by 1,200 mg orally twice daily for 48 hours after PCI is superior to placebo, and it might be superior to a lower IV dose of NAC (600 mg) prior to PCI followed by 600 mg orally twice daily for 48 hours after PCI (41). Thus, despite some of the inconsistencies, given the overall safety and low cost of acetylcysteine, its routine use in high-risk patients seems justified.

Aminophylline

Aminophylline is a phosphodiesterase inhibitor and a competitive adenosine antagonist. In animal studies, aminophylline has been found to increase renal blood flow, particularly in the medulla, and to increase GFR. In view of its effects on renal hemodynamics, aminophylline has been proposed as a potential agent in the prevention of CIN; however, its effect in preventing or reducing a rise in serum creatinine level following contrast administration appears to be marginal (42). In addition, a recent randomized clinical trial was unable to show any effect of aminophylline in reducing the incidence of CIN (43). Thus, the use of aminophylline for the prevention of CIN is currently not recommended.

Dopamine Receptor Agonists

Currently, there are five different identified types of dopamine receptors (44–46). The dopamine-1–like receptor group includes the D_1 and D_5 subtypes (45,46). Activation of dopamine-1 subtype receptor leads to an increase in intracellular cyclic adenosine monophosphate (AMP), whereas activation of dopamine-2 subtype receptor leads to a decrease in intracellular cyclic AMP. D_1 receptors are particularly prominent in the renal vasculature, renal tubules, mesenteric vasculature, and peripheral vessels. Activation of D_1 receptors results in vasodilatation of the renal, mesenteric, and peripheral circulation, and it leads to a decrease in blood pressure and

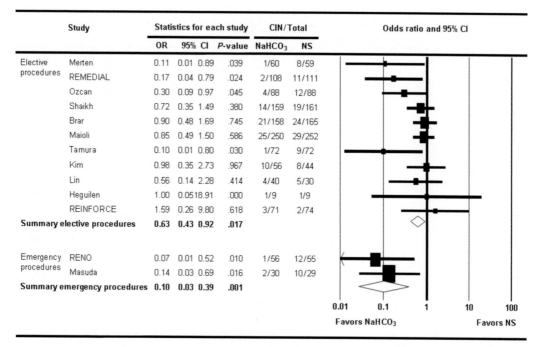

FIGURE 13-16. Forest plot of odds ratios of contrast-induced nephropathy. This is stratified by studies with elective procedures versus those including only emergency procedures. Sizes of data markers are proportional to the weight of each study in the meta-analysis. Horizontal bars, 95% confidence interval (CI). CIN, contrast-induced nephropathy; NaHCO₃, sodium bicarbonate; NS, normal saline; OR, odds ratio. (From Meier P, et al. Sodium bicarbonate-based hydration prevents contrast-induced nephropathy: a meta-analysis. *BMC Med.* 2009;7:23.)

an increase in renal blood flow. In addition, stimulation of the D_1 receptors in the tubules causes an increase in sodium excretion.

Fenoldopam is a specific agonist for the D_1 receptor that has potent vasodilatatory effects and was developed for the management of hypertensive urgencies and emergencies (47). In animal studies, fenoldopam has been shown to

decrease significantly renal vascular resistance and to increase renal blood flow. Because of these characteristics, it has been suggested that fenoldopam might have renal protective effects against noxious stimuli that lead to renal vasoconstriction and to a reduction in renal blood flow. Initial animal and human data suggested that fenoldopam might have a renoprotective

TABLE 13-2 Hydration Protocols for the Prevention of Contrast-Induced Nephropathy

0.9% normal saline (NS) 1 mL/kg/h starting 12 hours before the procedure and continued for 12 hours after the procedure

Outpatient protocol: 1000 cc of oral fluid over 10 hours prior to the procedure, followed by 0.45% saline at 300 cc/h 30 to 60 minutes prior to the procedure and continued for a total of 6 hours after the procedure. Note: this protocol includes the use of 0.45% half-isotonic saline, which is inferior to 0.9% NS.

Sodium bicarbonate: 3 mL/kg bolus infusion of 154 mEq/L of sodium bicarbonate 1 hour before contrast administration, followed by an infusion of 1 mL/kg/h during the procedure and for 6 hours thereafter.

Sodium bicarbonate: 3 mL/kg bolus infusion of 154 mEq/L of sodium bicarbonate 1 hour before contrast administration, followed by an infusion of 1.5 mL/kg/h during the procedure and for 4 hours thereafter is an alternative to 0.9% NS, but it does not appear to provide any significant advantage.

0.9% NS: 3 mL/kg bolus infusion of 0.9 NS 1 hour before contrast administration, followed by an infusion of 1.5 mL/kg during the procedure and for 4 hours thereafter.

TABLE 13-3 Preprepared Vials of Sodium Bicarbonate and Concentrations in mg/mL and mEq/mL

List No.	Dosage Form	Concentration (%)	NaHCO$_3$ (mg/mL)	Na$^+$ (mEq/mL)	HCO$_3^-$ (mEq/mL)	mEq/ Container Size (mL)	mOsm/mL
3495	Plastic Ansyr II Syringe	8.4	84	1	1	50/50	2
3486	Plastic Ansyr II Syringe	7.5	75	0.9	0.9	44.6/50	1.79

(Reproduced from http://dailymed.nlm.nih.gov/dailymed/drugInfo.cfm?id=2854#nlm34069-5. Rev: January, 2006.)

effect in the prevention of CIN (48,49). The efficacy of fenoldopam in this setting was recently assessed in the CONTRAST trial, a prospective, placebo-controlled, double-blind, multicenter trial in which 315 patients with creatinine clearance less than 60 mL/min were randomized to receive fenoldopam mesylate (0.05 μg/kg/min titrated to 0.10 μg/kg/min) ($n = 157$) or placebo ($n = 158$) (50). In this study, the main outcome measure was CIN, which was defined as an increase of 25% or more in serum creatinine level within 96 hours postprocedure. The results of the study were rather disappointing given that the primary end point of CIN occurred in 33.6% of patients assigned to receive fenoldopam versus 30.1% assigned to receive placebo (RR, 1.11; 95% CI, 0.79–1.57; $P = .61$). In addition, there were also no significant differences in 30-day mortality (2.0% vs. 3.8%, $P = .50$), dialysis (2.6% vs. 1.9%, $P = .72$) or rehospitalization (17.6% vs. 19.9%, $P = .66$). Two more recent studies comparing fenoldopam with NAC were also unable to show any benefit of fenoldopam when compared with NAC (51). Based on these data,

fenoldopam administration is not currently recommended for the prevention of CIN.

Contrast Media

Available contrast media can be classified in three major groups: high osmolar (1,500–2,000 mOsm/kg), low osmolar (600–1,000 mOsm/kg), and iso-osmolar (280–290 mOsm/kg; see Table 13-2). In a meta-analysis of clinical trials comparing high-osmolar contrast media with low-osmolar contrast media, Barrett et al. found that while there were no differences in the incidence of CIN in patients with normal renal function, in patients with renal insufficiency, the incidence of CIN was significantly higher with high-osmolar contrast media than with low-osmolar contrast media (52). In view of these findings and the fact that high-osmolar contrast media have additional adverse hemodynamic effects, high-osmolar contrast media are rarely used today. Whether the use of iso-osmolar contrast media results in further reduction in the incidence of CIN remains controversial. In a

TABLE 13-4 Characteristics of Intravenous (IV) Solutions Commonly Used for IV Hydration in the Prevention of Contrast-Induced Nephropathy

IV Solution	Concentration	Stock Solution (mEq/L)	Preparation
0.45% Normal saline	4.5 g NaCl/L	77	Stock solution
0.9 Normal saline	9 g NaCl/L	154	Stock solution
Sodium bicarbonate	84 mg/mL 75 mg/mL	1,000 900	IV solution prepared by adding 154 mL of 1,000 mEq/L sodium bicarbonate to 846 mL of 5% dextrose in H$_2$O

recent clinical trial, high-risk patients undergoing angiography were randomized to receive the iso-osmolar nonionic contrast medium iodixanol or the low-osmolar nonionic, monomeric contrast medium iohexol. In that study, the incidence of CIN was significantly lower in the group of patients who received iodixanol when compared with the group of patients who received iohexol (53). However, a recent systematic review of controlled randomized clinical trials has suggested that factors other than osmolarity might play an important role in the development of CIN. In that analysis, Solomon (24) evaluated clinical trials either comparing low-osmolar and iso-osmolar contrast media or evaluating the efficacy of various interventions aimed toward the prevention of CIN. In that analysis, the incidence of CIN was similar with the iso-osmolar nonionic contrast medium iodixanol and the low-osmolar nonionic media iopamidol but was significantly higher with the low-osmolar nonionic contrast medium iohexol (24).

Sang-Ho Jo and colleagues (54) compared iodixanol with ioxaglate in a prospective, randomized trial including 300 patients with creatinine clearance ≤ 60 mL/min and undergoing coronary angiography with or without PCI. The

primary end point was the incidence of CIN, defined in this trial as an increase in serum creatinine level by more than ≥25% or ≥0.5 mg/dL. In that study, the incidence of CIN was significantly lower with iodixanol (7.9%) than with ioxaglate (17.0%; $P = .021$). The reduction in the incidence of CIN was observed also in patients with severe renal impairment, in patients with diabetes, and in patients receiving ≥ 140 mL of contrast media. Importantly, multivariate analysis identified use of ioxaglate, baseline serum creatinine level (mg/dL), and left ventricular ejection fraction as independent risk factors for CIN. In contrast, in the CARE trial, no difference was observed between iodixanol and iopamidol (55). Similarly, no difference was observed between iodixanol and iomeprol in another recent clinical trial (Figs. 13-17 and 13-18) (56).

One more recent meta-analysis has further assessed the relative value of iso-osmolar contrast media when compared with low-osmolar contrast media and the additional interrelationship with the viscosity (57). In that study, there was a reduction in CIN when iodixanol was compared with ioxaglate (RR, 0.58; 95% CI, 0.37–0.92; $P = .022$) and iohexol (RR, 0.19; 95% CI, 0.07–0.56; $P = .002$), but no difference when

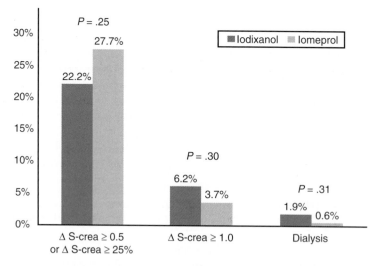

FIGURE 13-17. Randomized trial of iodixanol versus iomeprol in the prevention of contrast nephropathy). Contrast-induced nephropathy (CIN) associated with the use of iodixanol (*black bars*) or iomeprol (*gray bars*). The incidence of CIN is defined as an increase of S-creatinine level of more than 0.5 mg/dL or more than 25% of the value before contrast exposure is shown on the left. The bars in the center display the incidence of severe CIN, defined as an increase in S-creatinine level by 1 mg/dL or more. The bars on the right reveal the rate of dialysis that was required subsequent to percutaneous coronary intervention. (From Wessely R, et al. Choice of contrast medium in patients with impaired renal function undergoing percutaneous coronary intervention. *Circ Cardiovasc Interv.* 2009;2:430–437.)

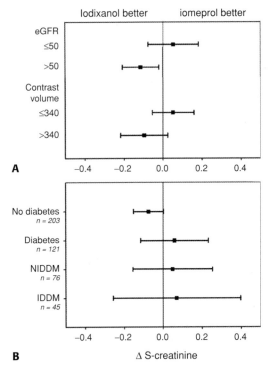

FIGURE 13-18. Randomized trial of iodixanol versus iomeprol in the prevention of contrast nephropathy). **A:** Subgroup analysis of the study population regarding nephrotoxicity associated with the grade of impairment of renal function and amount of contrast exposure. **B:** Comparison of outcome according to the presence of diabetes. eGFR (mL/min/1.73 m^2), amount of contrast volume delivered during coronary angiography, and percutaneous coronary intervention (mL). NIDDM, non–insulin-dependent diabetes mellitus; IDDM, insulin-dependent diabetes mellitus. (From Wessely R, et al. Choice of contrast medium in patients with impaired renal function undergoing percutaneous coronary intervention. *Circ Cardiovasc Interv.* 2009;2:430–437.)

compared with iopamidol (RR, 1.20; 95% CI, 0.66–2.18; $P = .55$), iopromide (RR, 0.93; 95% CI, 0.47–1.85; $P = .84$), or ioversol (RR, 0.92; 95% CI, 0.60–1.39; $P = .68$).

In summary, while there seems to be adequate evidence supporting the use of low-osmolar or iso-osmolar contrast agents in high-risk patients, controversy remains whether there are significant differences between iso-osmolar and low-osmolar contrast media and whether there are differences among currently available low-osmolar contrast media. Table 13-5 provides a summary of physical characteristics of contrast media available for intravascular administration.

Hemodialysis and Hemofiltration

Iodinated contrast media are hydrosoluble, are excreted primary by glomerular filtration, and can be removed by hemodialysis (58,59). These pharmacokinetic properties have led to the development of clinical trials and registry analysis aimed at assessing the effect of hemodialysis in the prevention of CIN (60–67). Unfortunately, none of the randomized clinical trials performed so far has been able to show a beneficial effect of hemodialysis in the prevention of CIN. It has been suggested that the lack of benefit of hemodialysis might be due to the fact that the nephrotoxic effects of contrast administration are of rapid onset and would begin before the institution of hemodialysis (68). In addition, hemodialysis does not reduce peak concentrations of contrast media. Finally, it has also been suggested that hemodialysis itself might be nephrotoxic in this setting (60,64,68).

More recently, ultrafiltration has been proposed as an additional intervention that could reduce the incidence of CIN in high-risk patients. Marenzi et al. (7) randomized 114 patients with chronic renal failure who were undergoing coronary interventions to either hemofiltration (58 patients, mean serum creatinine concentration of 3.0 ± 1.0 mg/dL) or iso-tonic-saline hydration at a rate of 1 mL/kg of body weight per hour (56 patients, mean serum creatinine concentration of 3.1 ± 1.0 mg/dL) (7). Hemofiltration (fluid replacement rate, 1000 mL/h without weight loss) and saline hydration were initiated 4 to 8 hours before the coronary intervention and were continued for 18 to 24 hours after the procedure. Both groups received a rather high contrast dose (247 ± 125 mL in the hemofiltration group and 258 ± 132 mL in the control group). In that study, an increase in serum creatinine concentration of more than 25% from the baseline value occurred in 5% of patients in the hemofiltration group and in 50% of patients in the saline group ($P <$ .001). In addition, temporary renal replacement therapy with hemodialysis or hemofiltration was required in 25% of the control patients and in 3% of the patients in the hemofiltration group. In-hospital mortality was 2% in the hemofiltration group and 14% in the control group ($P =$ .02), and the cumulative 1-year mortality was 10% and 30%, respectively (0.01). Although

TABLE 13-5 Characteristics of Contrast Media Available for Intravascular Use

Product	Chemical Structure	Anion	Cation	Salt Concentration (%)	Iodine Concentration (%)	Iodine+ (mgI/mL)	Viscosity+ C (cps)25°	Viscosity+ C (cps)37°	Osmolality (mOsm/kg H₂O)
Omnipaque® 140 (GE Healthcare)	Iohexol	Nonionic	Nonionic	None	14	140	2.3[a]	1.5	322
Conray™ 30 (Covidien)	Ionic	Iothalamate	Meglumine	30	14.1	141	2	1.5	600
Ultravist® 150 (Bayer Healthcare)	Iopromide	Nonionic	Nonionic	<0.1	15	150	2.3[a]	1.5	328
Optiray™ 160 (Covidien)	Ioversol 34%	Nonionic	Nonionic	None	16	160	2.7	1.9	355
Isovue® -200 (Bracco)	Iopamidol 40.8%	Nonionic	Nonionic	None	20	200	3.3[a]	2	413
Conray™ 43 (Covidien)	Ionic	Iothalamate	Meglumine	43	20.2	202	3	2	1,000
Omnipaque® 240 (GE Healthcare)	Iohexol 51.8%	Nonionic	Nonionic	None	24	240	5.8[a]	3.4	520
Optiray™ 240 (Covidien)	Ioversol 51%	Nonionic	Nonionic	None	24	240	4.6	3	502
Ultravist® 240 (Bayer Healthcare)	Iopromide	Nonionic	Nonionic	<0.1	24	240	4.9[a]	2.8	483
Isovue® -250 (Bracco)	Iopamidol 51%	Nonionic	Nonionic	None	25	250	5.1[a]	3	524

Visipaque® 270 (GE Healthcare)	Iodixanol	Nonionic	Nonionic	None	27	12.7[a]	270	6.3	290
Conray™ (Covidien)	Ionic	Iothalamate	Meglumine	60	28.2	6	282	4	1,400
Isovue® -300 (Bracco)	Iopamidol 61.2%	Nonionic	Nonionic	None	30	8.8[a]	300	4.7	616
Omnipaque® -300 (GE Healthcare)	Iohexol 64.7%	Nonionic	Nonionic	None	30	11.8[a]	300	6.3	672
Optiray™ 300 (Covidien)	Ioversol 64%	Nonionic	Nonionic	None	30	8.2	300	5.5	651
Oxilan® 300 (Guerbet)	Ioxilan 62.3%	Nonionic	Nonionic	None	30	9.4[a]	300	5.1	585
Ultravist® 300 (Bayer Healthcare)	Iopromide	Nonionic	Nonionic	<0.1	30	9.2[a]	300	4.9	607
Hexabrix™ (Covidien)	Ionic	Ioxaglate	Meglumine Sodium	39.3 19.6	32	15.7[a]	320	7.5	~600
Optiray™ 320 (Covidien)	Ioversol 68%	Nonionic	Nonionic	None	32	9.9	320	5.8	702
Visipaque® -320 (GE Healthcare)	Iodixanol	Nonionic	Nonionic	None	32	26.6	320	11.8	290
Optiray™ 350 (Covidien)	Ioversol 74%	Nonionic	Nonionic	None	35	14.3	350	9	792

(continued)

TABLE 13-5 Characteristics of Contrast Media Available for Intravascular Use (*Continued*)

Product	Chemical Structure	Anion	Cation	Salt Concentration (%)	Iodine Concentration (%)	Iodine+ (mgI/mL)	Viscosity+ C (cps)25°	Viscosity+ C (cps)37°	Osmolality (mOsm/ kg H₂O)
Omnipaque® -350 (GE Healthcare)	Iohexol 75.5%	Nonionic	Nonionic	None	35	350	20.4[a]	10.4	844
Oxilan® 350 (Guerbet)	Ioxilan 72.7%	Nonionic	Nonionic	None	35	350	16.3[a]	8.1	695
Isovue® -370 (Bracco)	Iopamidol 75.5%	Nonionic	Nonionic	None	37	370	20.9[a]	9.4	796
MD-76™ R (Covidien)	Ionic	Diatrizoate	Meglumine Sodium	66 10	37	370	16.4	10.5	1,551
Ultravist® 370 (Bayer Healthcare)	Iopromide	Nonionic	Nonionic	<0.1	37	370	22.0	10	774
Cholografin® (Bracco)	Ionic	Iodipamide	Meglumine	52	25.7	257	6.6	5.6	664

(Adapted from Manual of Contrast Media, Committee on Drugs and Contrast Media, American College of Radiology, Version 7 2010. [a]Measured at 20°C.)

these preliminary results are promising, they are in disagreement with the results of other studies that have shown no benefit of hemodialysis in the prevention of CIN. In addition, hemofiltration has only a modest effect on the clearance of radio-contrast material, and in that study, it was stopped during the procedure and restarted after contrast injection. Thus, until confirmed by other randomized clinical trials, hemofiltration cannot be recommended as a frontline therapy in the prevention of CIN.

Statins

Preprocedure statins use has been shown to reduce the risk of non–Q-wave myocardial infarction associated with PCIs (69–71). In addition, several studies have shown an association between preprocedure statin use and a reduction in the incidence of CIN (3,72,73). Plaque stabilization and a pleiotropic effect (beyond lipid lowering) are among the proposed mechanisms surrounding the beneficial effect of statins in this setting. In general, the available evidence supports the use of periprocedure statins in patients undergoing PCI and in patient undergoing other peripheral vascular interventions.

Investigational Devices and Interventions

There are several investigational devices that are currently undergoing evaluation. These devices include among others the "Be*nephi*t system" for "targeted renal therapy" (FlowMedica, Inc, Freemont, CA), which involves bilateral renal artery cannulation for direct infusion of various agents including fenoldopam mesylate, sodium bicarbonate, alprostadil, or B-type natriuretic peptide (74), and a coronary sinus contrast removal system (75). The future clinical and widespread application of these devices remains to be determined.

Modification of Procedure Strategy

The importance of the relationship between the total amount of contrast administered and the development of CIN has been confirmed by numerous studies. Therefore, steps should be undertaken to affect a reduction in the total amount of contrast administered within a procedure. These steps include avoidance of unnecessary views, limiting the quantity of contrast to only the amount needed for adequate opacification and visualization of the vessels imaged, and consideration of performing staged procedures. It is important to note that with the introduction of CT coronary angiography, patients might be referred for coronary angiography and for PCI immediately after having been evaluated with CT coronary angiography. This approach might expose the patient to an increased risk related to the additional administration of contrast media. It might be advisable in stable patients to postpone the second procedure until baseline renal function has been evaluated and until appropriate hydration has been administered. In patients with severe baseline renal insufficiency, a strategy of diagnostic angiography followed by percutaneous intervention at a later stage (if clinically indicated) would be more advantageous than diagnostic angiography followed by ad hoc PCI within the same setting, although no studies so far have systematically addressed such strategy. In addition, while left ventriculography is included in the standard cardiac catheterization protocol, it appears that in patients with renal insufficiency, a noninvasive assessment of left ventricular function followed by coronary angiography can provide the same information but without the additional risk associated with the larger amount of contrast needed for left ventriculography. In addition, a recent registry analysis has shown that the use of smaller catheters is associated with a lower amount of contrast/case and, not surprisingly, with a lower incidence of contrast nephropathy (76). Several studies have also suggested using special angiographic techniques to reduce the amount of contrast used during the procedure, including rotational and biplane angiography. Furthermore, given the importance of avoiding exceeding contrast thresholds, and in particular, weight- and creatinine-adjusted contrast dose thresholds, estimating these contrast dose thresholds in high-risk patients referred for invasive procedure is advisable. Figure 13-1 shows a bedside tool that can be used to rapidly identify patients at increased risk of CIN and which includes recommendations for the prevention of CIN, and Table 13-6 provides a summary of a practical approach toward the prevention of CIN.

In conclusion, the development of CIN is associated with an increased risk of morbidity and

> **TABLE 13-6**   **A Practical Approach to the Prevention of Contrast-Induced Nephropathy**

Patients at Risk and Procedure Strategy—Minimize Contrast Amount

All patients receiving intravenous or intra-arterial contrast media should undergo assessment of baseline renal function and clinical assessment for the identification of additional risk factors for the development of CIN.

Several studies have shown increasing risk of CIN with increasing contrast doses, and the additional importance of a contrast dose threshold, including either <125 mL or a weight- and creatinine-adjusted contrast dose calculated using the formula (5 cc of contrast/serum creatinine in mg/dL) × body weight in kg.

Minimize the total amount of contrast media by avoiding unnecessary views or unnecessary tests, e.g., left ventriculography when ejection fraction is already available from noninvasive tests, and by using biplane angiography if available.

Use of smaller catheter might be associated with a lower amount of contrast per case

Hydration Protocols

Isotonic 0.9% normal saline (NS) is superior to 0.45% half

0.9% NS 1 mL/kg/h starting 12 hours before the procedure and continued for 12 hours after the procedure.

An "outpatient" protocol that has been proposed includes 1,000 cc oral fluid over 10 hours prior to the procedure, followed by IV 0.45% saline 300 cc/h 30 to 60 minutes prior to the procedure and continued for a total of 6 hours after the procedure. However, this protocol includes the use of 0.45% half-isotonic saline, which is inferior to 0.9% NS.

A 3 mL/kg bolus infusion of 154 mEq/L of sodium bicarbonate 1 hour before contrast administration, followed by an infusion of 1.5 mL/kg/h during the procedure and for 4 hours thereafter is an alternative to 0.9% NS, but on the basis of most recent data, it does not appear to provide any advantage.

A 3 mL/kg bolus infusion of 154 mEq/L of NaCl (0.9% NS) 1 hour before contrast administration, followed by an infusion of 1.5 mL/kg/h during the procedure and for 4 hours thereafter

Role of Contrast Media and of Pharmacological Interventions

Among the characteristics of contrast media, a higher viscosity and higher osmolarity appear to be associated with an increased risk of CIN. Thus, low-osmolar contrast media should be used.

It remains to be determined whether the use of iso-osmolar (280–290 mOsm/kg) contrast media is associated with additional benefits.

Of the many pharmacological interventions tested in the prevention of CIN, N-acetylcysteine at a dose of 600 mg bid 24 hours prior to the procedure, followed by 600 mg bid 24 hours after the procedure, seems to be promising.

An additional protocol that has been shown to be effective includes the administration of N-acetylcysteine at a dose of 1,200-mg IV bolus prior to contrast administration and 1200 mg orally bid for the 48 hours after contrast administration. This protocol might be superior to a 600-mg intravenous bolus before contrast administration and 600 mg orally twice daily for the 48 hours after contrast administration.

For emergency procedures, a protocol including bicarbonate infusion plus N-acetylcysteine (2,400 mg IV over 1 hour) in the same infusion started immediately before the procedure has been shown to be more effective than postprocedure hydration with isotonic saline.

Preprocedure statins use has also been found to be associated with a lower incidence of CIN and other complications of PCI.

mortality. Identification of patients at increased risk, modification of procedure strategies to minimize the total amount of contrast administered to the patient, preprocedure hydration with 0.9% NS or with bicarbonate infusion, the use of low-osmolar contrast media, and possibly the use of NAC are currently the most important interventions that have shown to reduce the incidence of CIN.

■ HYPERSENSITIVITY REACTIONS TO RADIOCONTRAST

Hypersensitivity reactions can be classified into two broad categories—anaphylactic and anaphylactoid reactions. Anaphylactic reactions are IgE-mediated and are the results of the development of immune complex. Anaphylactoid reactions are non–IgE-mediated, and they can occur

TABLE 13-7	Classification of Hypersensitivity Reactions	
	Classification #1 (78)	Classification #2 (79)
Mild	Single episode of emesis, nausea, sneezing, or vertigo	Cough, erythema, hives, nasal congestion, pruritus, scratchy throat, sneezing
Moderate	Hives, erythema, emesis more than once, or fever or chills (or both)	Bradycardia, bronchospasm, chest pain, dyspnea, facial edema, hypertension, transient hypotension, mild hypoxemia, tachycardia, diffuse urticaria
Severe	Shock, bronchospasm, laryngospasm or laryngeal edema, loss of consciousness, convulsions, fall or rise in blood pressure, cardiac arrhythmia, angina, angioedema, or pulmonary edema	Cardiopulmonary arrest, refractory hypotension, moderate or severe hypoxemia, laryngeal edema

unpredictably, as they do not require previous exposure to the antigen. Thus, anaphylactoid reactions can also occur at the time of first exposure. Available evidence suggests that the majority of contrast reactions are anaphylactoid, rather than IgE-mediated (77). Regardless of the pathophysiology surrounding the development of the reactions, the downstream mechanism and clinical presentation are similar, and they are characterized by degranulation of mast cells and basofils, complement activation, modulation of enzymes and proteolytic cascades in plasma, and release of histamine, leading to a variety of systemic reactions. These reactions range from mild urticaria and pruritus to life-threatening reactions including laringospasm, bronchospasm, nausea, vomiting, and cardiovascular collapse, and they can be classified on the basis of the severity into three categories—mild, moderate, and severe (Table 13-7).

Immediate and Delayed Reactions

Acute reactions include reactions that occur within 1 hour of the contrast administration, whereas delayed reactions include those reactions that occur beyond 1 hour and up to 7 days (80). In an analysis of 107 patients with immediate reactions and known time from contrast administration to symptom onset, 67% of patients had a reaction within 1 to 5 minutes from contrast injection and 17.7%, 12%, and 2.8% had a reaction within 10 to 15 minutes, 20 to 30 minutes, and 45 to 60 minutes, respectively. Thus, consistent with other studies, the majority of immediate reactions occur within

15 minutes from contrast administration. The spectrum of acute reactions ranges from itching and hives, to angioedema, bronchospasm, hypotension, and shock.

In general, the majority of delayed reactions are cutaneous. Usually, these reactions are self-limited and resolve within 7 days. It is currently difficult to estimate the true frequency of delayed reactions, given that a "placebo" or "procedure" effect cannot be excluded in some of the reported series. For example, in one study, the incidence of delayed reactions in patients undergoing CT was 12.4%. However, in the same study, 10.3% of patients who underwent CT evaluation without contrast media also reported delayed reactions (81).

Itching, urticaria, skin rash, headache, and nausea are common symptoms and signs associated with delayed reactions. A generalized maculopapular exanthema developing 7 days after cardiac catheterization, oropharyngeal edema 4 to 6 hours following sialography, and hypotension with hyperthermia following a CT scan have also been described (82).

Risk Factors for Reactions

Risk factors for hypersensitivity reactions include a history of adverse reaction, history of allergy and/or asthma, younger age, and concomitant treatment with β-blockers. In addition, concomitant treatment with interleukin 2 has been shown to increase the risk of both delayed and immediate reactions. The issue of concomitant treatment with β-blockers deserves further comments. The development of bronchospasm has been associated with history of asthma and prior treatment with β-blockers (81). In addition, β-blockade has been shown in animal studies to lead to hypersensitivity to histamine (83), and in case of anaphylaxis, it can blunt the response to epinephrine. Thus, it is strongly recommended to withhold β-blocker prior to contrast administration in patients with history of contrast reactions.

Clinical Presentation

As stated earlier, the spectrum of hypersensitivity reactions to radiocontrast is quite broad, and ranges from pruritus and congestion of mucous membranes (eyes, nose, and mouth) to cardiovascular collapse and shock. Laryngeal edema leading to upper airways obstruction, bronchospasm, and gastrointestinal symptoms including nauseas and vomiting are additional symptoms in the clinical presentation. A classification of hypersensitivity reaction based on severity, with corresponding symptoms, is listed in Table 13-7.

Prevention

The critical steps to prevent adverse reactions to contrast media and their consequences include a thorough medical history, the identification of patients at increased risk, and readiness in managing severe adverse reactions as they occur.

Although it is not uncommon to administer IV hydrocortisone to patients immediately before the procedure, prior studies have shown that single doses of steroid might be ineffective in reducing risk. In a prospective clinical trial, Ring et al. (78) randomized 800 patients undergoing IV urography to pretreatment with IV

prednisolone (250 mg 5 minutes prior to the infusion of contrast), the H1-antagonist clemastine, a combination of clemastine and the H2-antagonist cimetidine or to 0.9% saline. When compared with saline, there was a significant reduction in the frequency of adverse reactions in the combination clemastine/cimetidine (6% vs. 12%), whereas there was no significant reduction in the clemastine or prednisolone groups (78). In a landmark study by Lasser et al., 6,763 patients receiving IV contrast media were randomized to two doses of oral corticosteroids (methylprednisolone, 32 mg) approximately 12 hours and 2 hours before challenge with contrast, one dose of oral prednisolone approximately 2 hours before challenge, or placebo (79). The two-dose corticosteroid regimen significantly reduced the incidence of reactions of all types ($P < .05$), except for a group of reactions dominated by hives ($P = .055$), while the one dose regimen was ineffective (Fig. 13-19). Although that study triggered a controversy about the method used for statistical analysis, the current consensus is that an appropriate oral regimen should include a minimum of two oral doses of steroids. The effect of steroids use in patient receiving nonionic contrast (ioversol) was further assessed in another randomized study. In this study, the overall incidence of adverse reactions to contrast administration was 1.7% in a two-dose regimen of methylprednisolone (32 mg 6–12 hours before and 2 hours before contrast administration) when compared with 4.8% in the placebo group ($P = .05$) (84). Overall, the evidence from randomized clinical trials suggests that a two-dose regimen is more effective than a single-dose regimen in preventing adverse reactions (Fig. 13-20).

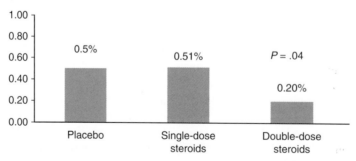

FIGURE 13-19. Effect of a single dose and a double dose of steroids on the development of severe hypersensitivity reactions to contrast media. (Based on data from Lasser EC, et al. Pretreatment with corticosteroids to alleviate reactions to intravenous contrast material. *N Engl J Med.* 1987;317:845–849.)

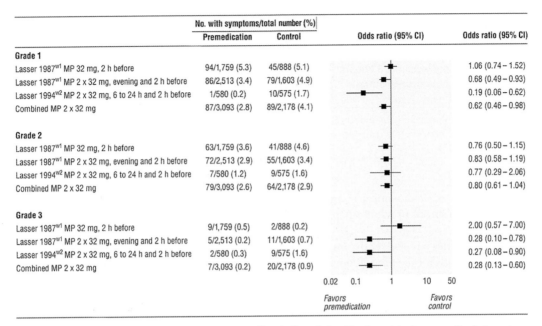

	No. with symptoms/total number (%)		Odds ratio (95% CI)	Odds ratio (95% CI)
	Premedication	Control		
Grade 1				
Lasser 1987[w1] MP 32 mg, 2 h before	94/1,759 (5.3)	45/888 (5.1)		1.06 (0.74 – 1.52)
Lasser 1987[w1] MP 2 x 32 mg, evening and 2 h before	86/2,513 (3.4)	79/1,603 (4.9)		0.68 (0.49 – 0.93)
Lasser 1994[w2] MP 2 x 32 mg, 6 to 24 h and 2 h before	1/580 (0.2)	10/575 (1.7)		0.19 (0.06 – 0.62)
Combined MP 2 x 32 mg	87/3,093 (2.8)	89/2,178 (4.1)		0.62 (0.46 – 0.98)
Grade 2				
Lasser 1987[w1] MP 32 mg, 2 h before	63/1,759 (3.6)	41/888 (4.6)		0.76 (0.50 – 1.15)
Lasser 1987[w1] MP 2 x 32 mg, evening and 2 h before	72/2,513 (2.9)	55/1,603 (3.4)		0.83 (0.58 – 1.19)
Lasser 1994[w2] MP 2 x 32 mg, 6 to 24 h and 2 h before	7/580 (1.2)	9/575 (1.6)		0.77 (0.29 – 2.06)
Combined MP 2 x 32 mg	79/3,093 (2.6)	64/2,178 (2.9)		0.80 (0.61 – 1.04)
Grade 3				
Lasser 1987[w1] MP 32 mg, 2 h before	9/1,759 (0.5)	2/888 (0.2)		2.00 (0.57 – 7.00)
Lasser 1987[w1] MP 2 x 32 mg, evening and 2 h before	5/2,513 (0.2)	11/1,603 (0.7)		0.28 (0.10 – 0.78)
Lasser 1994[w2] MP 2 x 32 mg, 6 to 24 h and 2 h before	2/580 (0.3)	9/575 (1.6)		0.27 (0.08 – 0.90)
Combined MP 2 x 32 mg	7/3,093 (0.2)	20/2,178 (0.9)		0.28 (0.13 – 0.60)

0.02   0.1   1   10   50

Favors premedication   Favors control

FIGURE 13-20. Arbitrary symptom combinations ("grades") as defined in the original reports. Grade 1 = single episode of emesis, nausea, sneezing, or vertigo; grade 2 = hives, erythema, emesis more than once, or fever or chills (or both); grade 3 = shock, bronchospasm, laryngospasm or laryngeal edema, loss of consciousness, convulsions, fall or rise in blood pressure, cardiac arrhythmia, angina, angioedema, or pulmonary edema. Grade 3 was considered to be potentially life-threatening. CI, confidence interval; h, hour; MP, methylprednisolone (oral). (From Tramer MR, et al. Pharmacological prevention of serious anaphylactic reactions due to iodinated contrast media: systematic review. *BMJ.* 2006;333:675.)

Additional studies have compared low-osmolar and high-osmolar contrast media. Greenberger et al. evaluated the incidence of immediate generalized reactions to repeated contrast administration in pretreated high-risk patients who received the low-osmolar radiocontrast media iopamidol or iohexol during 200 procedures (181 intravascular). All patients had experienced a previous adverse reaction to a conventional radiocontrast media. Pretreatment consisted of prednisone, 50 mg, 13, 7, and 1 hour before the procedure and diphenhydramine, 50 mg, 1 hour before the procedure in 140 intravascular infusions. Ephedrine, 25 mg, 1 hour before the infusion was added to prednisone–diphenhydramine in 41 cases. Only 1 (0.7%) urticarial reaction occurred in 141 procedures with prednisone–diphenhydramine, and no repeated reactions occurred with the three-drug regimen. They compared these rates with the reaction rates in an historical control group of patients pretreated with prednisone–diphenhydramine or prednisone–diphenhydramine–ephedrine and undergoing procedures

using conventional, high-osmolar contrast media during 800 intravascular procedures. In the historical control group, the incidence of adverse reactions was 9.1%, when compared with an incidence of 0.5% in patients pretreated with prednisone–diphenhydramine or prednisone–diphenhydramine–ephedrine and lower osmolality contrast media ($P < .001$) (85). The regimen including 3 oral 50 mg doses of prednisone plus 50 mg of diphenhydramine is currently one of the recommended regimens (Table 13-7).

For emergency procedure in high-risk patient, Greeenberg et al. have reported a small case series of 9 high-risk patients (history of anaphylactoid reactions) requiring emergency administration of radiocontrast. The patients were pretreated with 200 mg IV dose of hydrocortisone immediately and at every 4 hours until the procedure was completed and 50 mg IV diphenhydramine 1 hour before the procedure. No reactions occurred in these patients. The authors suggest that this pretreatment regimen may be valuable for patients requiring emergency

TABLE 13-8 Premedication Regimens for the Prevention of Adverse Reactions to Contrast Media

1. Prednisone 50 mg by mouth 13 hours, 7 hours, and 1 hour before contrast administration	Diphenhydramine (Benadryl) 50 mg intravenously, intramuscularly, or by mouth 1 hour before contrast injection	± H_2 blockers
2. Methylprednisolone 32 mg by mouth 12 hours and 2 hours before contrast administration	± Diphenhydramine (Benadryl) 50 mg intravenously, intramuscularly, or by mouth 1 hour before contrast injection	± H_2 blockers

administration of radiocontrast media and who have experienced previous anaphylactoid reactions (86).

Antihistamines are currently included in standard protocols for the prevention of adverse reactions to contrast. Available evidence supports the benefit of antihistamines in reducing the incidence of adverse reactions, and particularly of cutaneous symptoms (87) (Fig. 13-21). One randomized clinical trial has suggested the added benefit of combining H1 and H2 blockers (78). In addition, it is recommended to withhold β-blockers prior to the procedure in patients with a history of adverse reactions. Preprocedure protocols that are currently used are summarized in Table 13-8.

Breakthrough Reactions

Breakthrough reactions are reactions that occur despite premedication in patients with a history

			No. with symptoms/total number (%)		Odds ratio (95% CI)	Odds ratio (95% CI)
			Premedication	Control		
Haemodynamic symptoms						
Chevrot 1988[w4]	Betamethasone	Hypotension	0/109 (0.0)	1/112 (0.9)		0.14 (0.00–7.01)
Lasser 1994[w2]	Methylprednisolone	Hypotension	0/580 (0.0)	2/575 (0.3)		0.13 (0.01–2.14)
		Steroid combined	0/689 (0.0)	3/687 (0.4)		0.14 (0.01–1.30)
Respiratory symptoms						
Bertrand 1992[w3]	Hydroxyzine	Bronchospasm	0/200 (0.0)	1/200 (0.5)		0.14 (0.00–6.82)
Ring 1985[w6]	Clemastine	Angio-edema	4/191 (2.1)	8/194 (4.1)		0.51 (0.16–1.61)
		Anti-H_1 combined	4/391 (1.0)	9/394 (2.3)		0.46 (0.15–1.39)
Lasser 1994[w2]	Methylprednisolone	Laryngeal edema	0/580 (0.0)	3/575 (0.5)		0.13 (0.01–1.29)
Ring 1985[w6]	Prednisolone	Angio-edema	3/198 (1.5)	8/194 (4.1)		0.39 (0.12–1.28)
		Steroid combined	3/778 (0.4)	11/769 (1.4)		0.31 (0.11–0.88)
Cutaneous symptoms						
Bertrand 1992[w3]	Hydroxyzine	Urticaria	0/200 (0.0)	17/200 (8.5)		0.12 (0.05–0.33)
Smith 1995[w8]	Dimenhydrinate	Pruritus	7/150 (4.7)	9/149 (6.0)		0.76 (0.28–2.09)
Small 1982[w7]	Chlorpheniramine	Hives, pruritus	1/78 (1.3)	15/142 (10.6)		0.25 (0.09–0.73)
Wicke 1975[w9]	Clemastine	Urticaria	0/92 (0.0)	2/116 (1.7)		0.17 (0.01–2.71)
Ring 1985[w6]	Clemastine	Flush	6/191 (3.1)	6/194 (3.1)		1.02 (0.32–3.20)
		Anti-H_1 combined	14/711 (2.0)	49/801 (6.1)		0.36 (0.22–0.60)[a]
Ring 1985[w6]	Prednisolone	Flush	2/198 (1.0)	6/194 (3.1)		0.35 (0.09–1.43)
Lasser 1994[w2]	Methylprednisolone	Hives	3/580 (0.5)	9/575 (1.6)		0.36 (0.12–1.13)
		Steroid combined	5/778 (0.6)	15/769 (2.0)		0.36 (0.15–0.87)

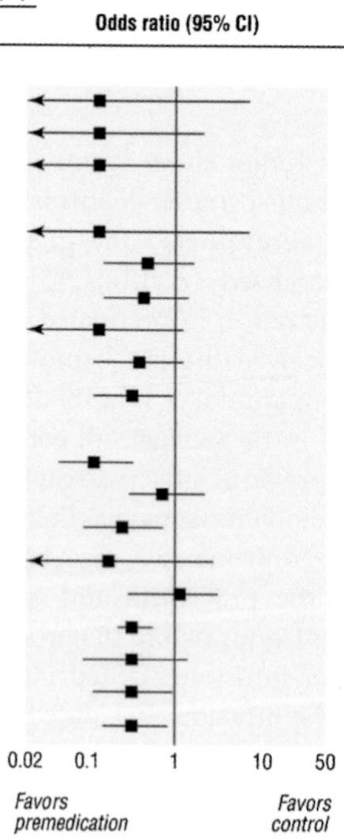

0.02 0.1 1 10 50

Favors premedication · · · *Favors control*

FIGURE 13-21. Systematic review of clinical trials evaluating various pharmacological interventions in the prevention of hypersensitivity reactions to contrast media. Distinct hemodynamic, respiratory, and cutaneous symptoms. Hypotension, bronchospasm, angioedema, and laryngeal edema were considered to be potentially life-threatening. Anti-H, antihistamine; CI, confidence interval. [a]P for heterogeneity = .03, I2 = 62%. (From Tramer MR, et al. Pharmacological prevention of serious anaphylactic reactions due to iodinated contrast media: systematic review. *BMJ.* 2006;333:675.)

of an adverse reaction. Davemport et al. evaluated 175 patients with a history of contrast media reactions and who had 195 breakthrough reactions (88). The severity of the index reaction could be identified in 128 cases, and it was mild in 81% of cases, moderate in 15% of cases, and severe in 5% of cases (see Table 13-7, Classification 2, for the definition of severity). In this group of patients for whom the severity of the index reaction was known, the breakthrough reaction was mild in 85% of cases, moderate in 14%, and severe in 2%. Patients who had a mild index reaction had a very low risk of a severe breakthrough reaction (0%). In the group of patients who had a moderate index reaction, 37% had a moderate breakthrough reaction and 5.3% had a severe reaction, whereas in the group of patients with a severe index reaction, the incidence of moderate and severe breakthrough reactions was 33.3% each. History of severe allergies, allergies to any four or more allergens, any drug allergy, and chronic use of corticosteroid were associated with a significantly higher risk of a moderate or severe breakthrough reaction. Importantly, of the 175 patients with a breakthrough reaction, 58 patients underwent 197 CT evaluations involving the IV administration of low-osmolar contrast medium. All patients were premedicated according to a protocol including three doses of prednisone (50 mg 13 hours, 7 hours, and 1 hour prior to the study) and 50 mg of diphenhydramine 1 hour prior to the study. No breakthrough reactions were observed in 88% of these repeat procedures, suggesting that a history of breakthrough reaction is not an absolute contraindication to subsequent low-osmolar contrast administration.

Management

Management of hypersensitivity reaction depends on the severity of the reaction. Mild reactions, including all skin reactions, do not require any therapy, although most operators tend to manage those reactions with histamine receptor blockers (diphenhydramine).

Moderate reactions require treatment but do not require hospital admission. Severe reactions require treatment and hospital admission. The recommended treatment for severe reactions includes diphenhydramine, corticosteroids, and epinephrine (89). Guidelines for treatment according to the type of reaction are provided in Table 13-9.

■ USE OF RADIOCONTRAST IN PATIENTS RECEIVING METFORMIN

There have been several case reports of severe lactic acidosis in patients who received contrast agents while on metformin, a biguinide oral antihyperglycemic agent (90). Lactic acidosis is a rare adverse effect of metformin, with an overall reported incidence of approximately 3 cases/100,000 patient-years and a fatality rate of approximately 50%. The mechanism of lactic acidosis is complex. It appears that metformin increases production of lactic acid by the intestinal wall while decreasing its liver uptake. The interaction metformin-contrast media is not a drug–drug interaction, but it is rather due to the change in excretion of metformin in those few patients who will develop CIN following contrast administration (91). Metformin, which is renally excreted, will accumulate in these patients. The higher metformin blood level will then lead to increased production of lactic acid and reduced liver uptake (92,93). Any other condition associated with an increased production or reduced metabolism of lactic acid, such as sepsis, severe heart failure, liver failure, or alcohol abuse, will further enhance this effect. The current recommendation is to hold metformin at the time of the procedure and 48 hours thereafter. Metformin should be resumed only after renal function has been reevaluated and found to be normal. There is no need to withhold metformin in advance before contrast administration, because even if the patient develops renal failure, serum levels of metformin will remain stable as long as the patient does not receive additional doses. Products currently available in the United States and that include metformin are listed in Table 13-10.

■ CORTICAL BLINDNESS

Cortical blindness is a very rare complication of contrast administration, and it is characterized by bilateral amblyopia or amaurosis, by a normal fundoscopic examination, by a normal pupillary light reflex, and by normal extraocular movements. It has been described both with high-osmolar and low-osmolar contrast

TABLE 13-9 Recommended Management of Adverse Reactions

Urticaria and Skin Itching	(1) No treatment (2) Diphenhydramine 25–50 mg IV ***Unresponsive:*** (3) Epinephrine 0.3 cc of 1:1,000 solution sub-Q q 15 min up to 1 cc (4) Cimetidine 300 mg or ranitidine 50 mg in 20 cc NS IV over 15 minute
Bronchospasm	(a) 02, by mask (b) Oximetry ***Mild:*** Albuterol inhaler-2 puffs ***Moderate:*** Epinephrine 0.3 cc of 1:1,000 solution sub-Q q 15 minutes up to 1 cc ***Severe:*** (1) Epinephrine IV as a bolus(es) of 10 mcg/min and then an infusion of 1 to 4 mcg/min; observe for desired effect with blood pressure and electrocardiogram monitoring (2) Diphenyhydramine 50 mg IV (3) Hydrocortisone 200–400 mg IV (4) Optional: H_2 blocker as outlined ***Preparation of Epinephrine IV:*** Bolus dose: 0.1 cc of 1:1,000 solution or 1 cc of 1:10,000 diluted to 10 cc (10 mcg/cc) Infusion dose: 1 cc of 1:1,000 or 10 cc of 1:10,000) in 250 cc NS (4 mcg/cc)
Facial Edema and Laryngeal Edema	Call anesthesia Assess airway (a) O_2 by mask (b) Intubation (c) Tracheostomy tray ***Mild:*** Epinephrine 0.3 cc of 1:1,000 solution sub-Q q 15 minutes up to 1 cc ***Moderate/Severe:*** (1) Epinephrine IV as outlined (2) Diphenhydramine 50 mg IV (3) Oximetry/Arterial Blood Gases (4) Optional: H_2 blocker as outlined

Hypotension/Shock	Call anesthesia
	Assess airway
	    (a) O_2 by mask
	    (b) Oximetry/ABG
	    (c) Intubation
	    (d) Tracheostomy tray
	(1) Simultaneous administration:
	    (a) Epinephrine IV—bolus(es) 10 mcg/min IV until desired blood pressure response obtained, then infuse 1–4 mcg/min to maintain desired BP. Preparation of solution as outlined earlier.
	    (b) Large volumes of 0.9% NS (1–3 liters in first hour).
	(2) Diphenhydramine 50–100 mg IV.
	(3) Hydrocortisone 400 mg IV.
	(4) CVP/Swan-Ganz 6
	Unresponsive:
	(5) H_2 blocker as outlined
	(6) Dopamine 2–15 mcg/kg/min IV
	(7) ACLS support

ACLS, advanced cardiac life support. (Adapted from Goss JE, Chambers CE, Heupler FA Jr. Systemic anaphylactoid reactions to iodinated contrast media during cardiac catheterization procedures: guidelines for prevention, diagnosis, and treatment. Laboratory Performance Standards Committee of the Society for Cardiac Angiography and Interventions. *Cathet Cardiovasc Diagn.* 1995;34:99–104, with permission.)

TABLE 13-10 Available Prescription Medications Including Metformin as a Single Agent or in Combination with Another Agent

Brand Name	Composition
ActosPlus Met	Pioglitizone and metformin
Avandamet	Rosiglitazone maleate and metformin hydrochloride
Fortamet	Metformin
Glipizide + Metformin	Glipizide and metformin
Glucophage	Metformin
Glucovance	Glyburide and metformin
Glumetza	Metformin
Janumet	Sitagliptin phosphate and metformin
Metaglip	Glipizide and metformin
Prandi-Met	Repaglinide and metformin
Riomet	Metformin

media (94,95). Selective injection of contrast in the vertebral artery and cerebral angiography are the most common causes of cortical blindness (95–98), although it has also been described following injection of contrast in the subclavian artery during angiography of the left internal mammary artery (99) and following coronary angiography (100,101). The proposed mechanism includes an alteration of the blood–brain barrier, resulting in increased permeability and a direct neurotoxic effect (94,102–104). CT imaging in patients who developed cortical blindness following angiography has shown extravasation of contrast, which is felt to be due to disruption of the blood–brain barrier. Associated symptoms might include headache, mental status changes, memory loss, seizures, and hallucinations. The onset of cortical blindness is between minutes and 12 hours from angiography, and its course is usually relatively benign, with most cases (if not all) recovering gradually within few days. There is no specific treatment other than ruling out other causes of visual loss and establishing the appropriate diagnosis.

■ CONCLUSION

The past two decades have been characterized by a major progress in the understanding of risk factors associated with adverse reactions to contrast media, by the development of contrast media with a higher safety profile, and by further advancements in the prevention and management of adverse reactions. However, administration of contrast is still associated with some risks, and it is only through a meticulous history, optimization of angiographic technique and optimization of periprocedural management that those risks can be reduced.

References

1. Gruberg L, et al. The prognostic implications of further renal function deterioration within 48 h of interventional coronary procedures in patients with pre-existent chronic renal insufficiency. *J Am Coll Cardiol.* 2000;36(5):1542–1548.
2. Freeman RV, et al. Nephropathy requiring dialysis after percutaneous coronary intervention and the critical role of an adjusted contrast dose. *Am J Cardiol.* 2002;90(10):1068–10673.
3. Khanal S, et al. Statin therapy reduces contrast-induced nephropathy: an analysis of contemporary percutaneous interventions. *Am J Med.* 2005;118(8):843–849.
4. Tepel M, et al. Prevention of radiographic-contrast-agent-induced reductions in renal function by acetylcysteine. *N Engl J Med.* 2000;343(3):180–184.
5. McCullough PA, et al. Acute renal failure after coronary intervention: incidence, risk factors, and relationship to mortality. *Am J Med.* 1997;103(5):368–375.
6. Mehran R, et al. A simple risk score for prediction of contrast-induced nephropathy after percutaneous coronary intervention: development and initial validation. *J Am Coll Cardiol.* 2004;44(7):1393–1399.
7. Marenzi G, et al. The prevention of radiocontrast-agent-induced nephropathy by hemofiltration. *N Engl J Med.* 2003;349(14):1333–1340.
8. Gruberg L, et al. Acute renal failure requiring dialysis after percutaneous coronary interventions. *Catheter Cardiovasc Interv.* 2001;52(4):409–416.
9. Taliercio CP, et al. Risks for renal dysfunction with cardiac angiography. *Ann Intern Med.* 1986;104(4):501–504.

10. Cigarroa RG, et al. Dosing of contrast material to prevent contrast nephropathy in patients with renal disease. *Am J Med.* 1989;86(6, pt 1): 649–652.

11. Moscucci M, et al. Association of a continuous quality improvement initiative with practice and outcome variations of contemporary percutaneous coronary interventions. *Circulation.* 2006;113(6):814–822.

12. Brown JR, et al. Serious renal dysfunction after percutaneous coronary interventions can be predicted. *Am Heart J.* 2008;155(2):260–266.

13. Rihal CS, et al. Incidence and prognostic importance of acute renal failure after percutaneous coronary intervention. *Circulation.* 2002;105(19): 2259–2264.

14. Keeley EC, Grines CL. Scraping of aortic debris by coronary guiding catheters: a prospective evaluation of 1,000 cases. *J Am Coll Cardiol.* 1998;32(7):1861–1865.

15. Drost H, et al. Cholesterol embolism as a complication of left heart catheterisation: report of seven cases. *Br Heart J.* 1984;52(3):339–342.

16. Fukumoto Y, et al. The incidence and risk factors of cholesterol embolization syndrome, a complication of cardiac catheterization: a prospective study. *J Am Coll Cardiol.* 2003;42(2): 211–216.

17. Ramirez G, et al. Cholesterol embolization: a complication of angiography. *Arch Intern Med.* 1978;138(9):1430–1432.

18. Persson PB, Tepel M. Contrast medium-induced nephropathy: the pathophysiology. *Kidney Int Suppl.* 2006;(100):S8–S10.

19. Bakris GL, Gaber AO, Jones JD. Oxygen free radical involvement in urinary Tamm-Horsfall protein excretion after intrarenal injection of contrast medium. *Radiology.* 1990;175(1):57–60.

20. Bakris GL, et al. Radiocontrast medium-induced declines in renal function: a role for oxygen free radicals. *Am J Physiol.* 1990;258(1Pt 2):F115–F120.

21. Schnackenberg CG. Physiological and pathophysiological roles of oxygen radicals in the renal microvasculature. *Am J Physiol Regul Integr Comp Physiol.* 2002;282(2):R335–342.

22. Hardiek K, et al. Proximal tubule cell response to radiographic contrast media. *Am J Physiol Renal Physiol.* 2001;280(1):F61–F70.

23. Persson PB, Hansell P, Liss P. Pathophysiology of contrast medium-induced nephropathy. *Kidney Int.* 2005;68(1):14–22.

24. Solomon R. The role of osmolality in the incidence of contrast-induced nephropathy: a systematic review of angiographic contrast media in high risk patients. *Kidney Int.* 2005;68(5): 2256–2263.

25. Solomon R, Barrett B. Follow-up of patients with contrast-induced nephropathy. *Kidney Int Suppl.* 2006;(100):S46–S50.

26. Solomon R, Deray G. How to prevent contrast-induced nephropathy and manage risk patients: practical recommendations. *Kidney Int Suppl.* 2006;(100):S51–S53.

27. Trivedi HS, et al. A randomized prospective trial to assess the role of saline hydration on the development of contrast nephrotoxicity. *Nephron Clin Pract.* 2003;93(1):C29–C34.

28. Solomon R, et al. Effects of saline, mannitol, and furosemide to prevent acute decreases in renal function induced by radiocontrast agents. *N Engl J Med.* 1994;331(21):1416–1420.

29. Mueller C, et al. Prevention of contrast media-associated nephropathy: randomized comparison of 2 hydration regimens in 1620 patients undergoing coronary angioplasty. *Arch Intern Med.* 2002;162(3):329–336.

30. Merten GJ, et al. Prevention of contrast-induced nephropathy with sodium bicarbonate: a randomized controlled trial. *JAMA.* 2004;291(19): 2328–2334.

31. Recio-Mayoral A, et al. The reno-protective effect of hydration with sodium bicarbonate plus N-acetylcysteine in patients undergoing emergency percutaneous coronary intervention: the RENO Study. *J Am Coll Cardiol.* 2007;49(12): 1283–1288.

32. Briguori C, et al. Renal Insufficiency Following Contrast Media Administration Trial (REMEDIAL): a randomized comparison of 3 preventive strategies. *Circulation.* 2007;115(10):1211–1217.

33. Hogan SE, L'Allier P, Chetcuti S, et al. Current role of sodium bicarbonate-based pre-procedural hydration for the prevention of contrast-induced acute kidney injury: a meta-analysis. *Am Heart J.* 2008;156(3):414–421.

34. Maioli M, et al. Sodium bicarbonate versus saline for the prevention of contrast-induced nephropathy in patients with renal dysfunction undergoing coronary angiography or intervention. *J Am Coll Cardiol.* 2008;52(8):599–604.

35. Brar SS, et al. Sodium bicarbonate vs sodium chloride for the prevention of contrast

medium-induced nephropathy in patients undergoing coronary angiography: a randomized trial. *JAMA.* 2008;300(9):1038–1046.

36. Meier P, et al. Sodium bicarbonate-based hydration prevents contrast-induced nephropathy: a meta-analysis. *BMC Med.* 2009;7:23.

37. Bader BD, et al. What is the best hydration regimen to prevent contrast media-induced nephrotoxicity? *Clin Nephrol.* 2004;62(1):1–7.

38. Krasuski RA, et al. Optimal timing of hydration to erase contrast-associated nephropathy: the OTHER CAN study. *J Invasive Cardiol.* 2003;15(12):699–702.

39. Taylor AJ, et al. PREPARED: Preparation for Angiography in Renal Dysfunction: a randomized trial of inpatient vs outpatient hydration protocols for cardiac catheterization in mild-to-moderate renal dysfunction. *Chest.* 1998;114(6):1570–1574.

40. DiMari J, et al. N-acetyl cysteine ameliorates ischemic renal failure. *Am J Physiol.* 1997;272(3 Pt 2):F292–F298.

41. Marenzi G, et al. N-acetylcysteine and contrast-induced nephropathy in primary angioplasty. *N Engl J Med.* 2006;354(26):2773–2782.

42. Bagshaw SM, Ghali WA. Theophylline for prevention of contrast-induced nephropathy: a systematic review and meta-analysis. *Arch Intern Med.* 2005;165(10):1087–1093.

43. Dussol B, et al. A randomized trial of saline hydration to prevent contrast nephropathy in chronic renal failure patients. *Nephrol Dial Transplant.* 2006;21(8):2120–2126.

44. Jackson DM, Westlind-Danielsson A. Dopamine receptors: molecular biology, biochemistry and behavioural aspects. *Pharmacol Ther.* 1994;64(2):291–370.

45. Sidhu A. Coupling of D1 and D5 dopamine receptors to multiple G proteins: implications for understanding the diversity in receptor-G protein coupling. *Mol Neurobiol.* 1998;16(2):125–134.

46. Emilien G, et al. Dopamine receptors-physiological understanding to therapeutic intervention potential. *Pharmacol Ther.* 1999;84(2):133–156.

47. Asif A, Epstein DL, Epstein M. Dopamine-1 receptor agonist: renal effects and its potential role in the management of radiocontrast-induced nephropathy. *J Clin Pharmacol.* 2004;44(12):1342–1351.

48. Bakris GL, Lass NA, Glock D. Renal hemodynamics in radiocontrast medium-induced renal dysfunction: a role for dopamine-1 receptors. *Kidney Int.* 1999;56(1):206–210.

49. Tumlin JA, et al. Fenoldopam mesylate blocks reductions in renal plasma flow after radiocontrast dye infusion: a pilot trial in the prevention of contrast nephropathy. *Am Heart J.* 2002;143(5):894–903.

50. Stone GW, et al. Fenoldopam mesylate for the prevention of contrast-induced nephropathy: a randomized controlled trial. *JAMA.* 2003;290(17):2284–2291.

51. Ng TM, et al. Comparison of N-acetylcysteine and fenoldopam for preventing contrast-induced nephropathy (CAFCIN). *Int J Cardiol.* 2006;109(3):322–328.

52. Barrett BJ, Carlisle EJ. Meta-analysis of the relative nephrotoxicity of high- and low-osmolality iodinated contrast media. *Radiology.* 1993;188(1):171–178.

53. Aspelin P, et al. Nephrotoxic effects in high-risk patients undergoing angiography. *N Engl J Med.* 2003;348(6):491–499.

54. Jo SH, et al. Iodixanol vs ioxaglate for preventing contrast nephropathy: who is winner? *Kidney Int.* 2007;71(8):828, author reply 828–829.

55. Solomon RJ, et al. Cardiac Angiography in Renally Impaired Patients (CARE) study: a randomized double-blind trial of contrast-induced nephropathy in patients with chronic kidney disease. *Circulation.* 2007;115(25):3189–3196.

56. Wessely R, et al. Choice of contrast medium in patients with impaired renal function undergoing percutaneous coronary intervention. *Circ Cardiovasc Interv.* 2009;2(5):430–437.

57. Reed M, et al. The relative renal safety of iodixanol compared with low-osmolar contrast media: a meta-analysis of randomized controlled trials. *JACC Cardiovasc Interv.* 2009;2(7):645–654.

58. Furukawa T, et al. Permeability of contrast media through hemodialysis membrane. *Acta Radiol.* 1997;38(5):918–921.

59. Furukawa T, et al. Elimination of low-osmolality contrast media by hemodialysis. *Acta Radiol.* 1996;37(6):966–971.

60. Berger ED, et al. [Contrast media-induced kidney failure cannot be prevented by hemodialysis]. *Dtsch Med Wochenschr.* 2001;126(7):162–166.

61. Huber W, et al. [Contrast medium-induced renal failure can not be prevented by hemodialysis]. *Dtsch Med Wochenschr.* 2002;127(1/2): 45–47.

62. Kawashima S, et al. Prophylactic hemodialysis does not prevent contrast-induced nephropathy after cardiac catheterization in patients with chronic renal insufficiency. *Circ J.* 2006;70(5): 553–558.

63. Moon SS, et al. Hemodialysis for elimination of the nonionic contrast medium iohexol after angiography in patients with impaired renal function. *Nephron.* 1995;70(4):430–437.

64. Reinecke H, et al. A randomized controlled trial comparing hydration therapy to additional hemodialysis or N-acetylcysteine for the prevention of contrast medium-induced nephropathy: the Dialysis-versus-Diuresis (DVD) Trial. *Clin Res Cardiol.* 2007;96(3):130–139.

65. Sterner G, et al. Does post-angiographic hemodialysis reduce the risk of contrast-medium nephropathy? *Scand J Urol Nephrol.* 2000;34(5):323–326.

66. Takebayashi S, Hidai H, Chiba T. No need for immediate dialysis after administration of low-osmolarity contrast medium in patients undergoing hemodialysis. *Am J Kidney Dis.* 2000; 36(1):226.

67. Woo GC, et al. Effect of hemodialysis on contrast sensitivity in renal failure. *Am J Optom Physiol Opt.* 1986;63(5):356–361.

68. Deray G. Dialysis and iodinated contrast media. *Kidney Int Suppl.* 2006;(100):S25–S29.

69. Briguori C, et al. Statin administration before percutaneous coronary intervention: impact on periprocedural myocardial infarction. *Eur Heart J.* 2004;25(20):1822–1828.

70. Auguadro C, et al. Protective role of chronic statin therapy in reducing myocardial damage during percutaneous coronary intervention. *J Cardiovasc Med (Hagerstown).* 2006;7(6):416–421.

71. Merla R, et al. Meta-analysis of published reports on the effect of statin treatment before percutaneous coronary intervention on periprocedural myonecrosis. *Am J Cardiol.* 2007;100(5): 770–776.

72. Patti G, et al. Usefulness of statin pretreatment to prevent contrast-induced nephropathy and to improve long-term outcome in patients undergoing percutaneous coronary intervention. *Am J Cardiol.* 2008;101(3):279–285.

73. Attallah N, et al. The potential role of statins in contrast nephropathy. *Clin Nephrol.* 2004;62(4): 273–278.

74. Weisz G, et al. Safety and performance of targeted renal therapy: the Be-RITe! Registry. *J Endovasc Ther.* 2009;16(1):1–12.

75. Michishita I, Fujii Z. A novel contrast removal system from the coronary sinus using an adsorbing column during coronary angiography in a porcine model. *J Am Coll Cardiol.* 2006;47(9):1866–1870.

76. Grossman PM, et al. Percutaneous coronary intervention complications and guide catheter size: bigger is not better. *JACC Cardiovasc Interv.* 2009;2(7):636–644.

77. Greenberger PA, Patterson R. Adverse reactions to radiocontrast media. *Prog Cardiovasc Dis.* 1988;31(3):239–248.

78. Ring J, Rothenberger KH, Clauss W. Prevention of anaphylactoid reactions after radiographic contrast media infusion by combined histamine H1- and H2-receptor antagonists: results of a prospective controlled trial. *Int Arch Allergy Appl Immunol.* 1985;78(1):9–14.

79. Lasser EC, et al. Pretreatment with corticosteroids to alleviate reactions to intravenous contrast material. *N Engl J Med.* 1987;317(14): 845–849.

80. Yasuda R, Munechika H. Delayed adverse reactions to nonionic monomeric contrast-enhanced media. *Invest Radiol.* 1998;33(1):1–5.

81. Lang DM, et al. Elevated risk of anaphylactoid reaction from radiographic contrast media is associated with both beta-blocker exposure and cardiovascular disorders. *Arch Intern Med.* 1993; 153(17):2033–2040.

82. Idee JM, et al. Allergy-like reactions to iodinated contrast agents. A critical analysis. *Fundam Clin Pharmacol.* 2005;19(3):263–281.

83. Matsumura Y, Tan EM, Vaughan JH. Hypersensitivity to histamine and systemic anaphylaxis in mice with pharmacologic beta adrenergic blockade: protection by nucleotides. *J Allergy Clin Immunol.* 1976;58(3):387–394.

84. Lasser EC, et al. Pretreatment with corticosteroids to prevent adverse reactions to nonionic contrast media. *AJR Am J Roentgenol.* 1994; 162(3):523–526.

85. Greenberger PA, Patterson R. The prevention of immediate generalized reactions to radiocontrast media in high-risk patients. *J Allergy Clin Immunol.* 1991;87(4):867–872.

86. Greenberger PA, et al. Emergency administration of radiocontrast media in high-risk patients. *J Allergy Clin Immunol.* 1986;77(4):630–634.

87. Tramer MR, et al. Pharmacological prevention of serious anaphylactic reactions due to iodinated contrast media: systematic review. *BMJ.* 2006;333(7570):675.

88. Davenport MS, et al. Repeat contrast medium reactions in premedicated patients: frequency and severity. *Radiology.* 2009;253(2):372–379.

89. Goss JE, Chambers CE, Heupler FA Jr. Systemic anaphylactoid reactions to iodinated contrast media during cardiac catheterization procedures: guidelines for prevention, diagnosis, and treatment. Laboratory Performance Standards Committee of the Society for Cardiac Angiography and Interventions. *Cathet Cardiovasc Diagn.* 1995;34(2):99–104.

90. Safadi R, et al. Metformin-induced lactic acidosis associated with acute renal failure. *Am J Nephrol.* 1996;16(6):520–522.

91. McCartney MM, et al. Metformin and contrast media—a dangerous combination? *Clin Radiol.* 1999;54(1):29–33.

92. Nawaz S, et al. Clinical risk associated with contrast angiography in metformin treated patients: a clinical review. *Clin Radiol.* 1998;53(5):342–344.

93. Rasuli P, Hammond DI. Metformin and contrast media: where is the conflict? *Can Assoc Radiol J.* 1998;49(3):161–166.

94. Saigal G, et al. MR findings of cortical blindness following cerebral angiography: is this entity related to posterior reversible leukoencephalopathy? *AJNR Am J Neuroradiol.* 2004;25(2):252–256.

95. Studdard WE, Davis DO, Young SW. Cortical blindness after cerebral angiography. Case report. *J Neurosurg.* 1981;54(2):240–244.

96. Prendes JL. Transient cortical blindness following vertebral angiography. *Headache.* 1978;18(4):222–224.

97. Shyn PB, Bell KA. Transient cortical blindness following cerebral angiography. *J La State Med Soc.* 1989;141(11):35–37.

98. Till V, et al. Transient cortical blindness following vertebral angiography in a young adult with cerebellar haemangioblastoma. *Pediatr Radiol.* 2009;39(11):1223–1226.

99. Henzlova MJ, et al. Cortical blindness after left internal mammary artery to left anterior descending coronary artery graft angiography. Cathet Cardiovasc Diagn. 1988;15(1):37–39.

100. Tatli E, Buyuklu M, Altun A. An unusual but dramatic complication of coronary angiography: transient cortical blindness. *Int J Cardiol.* 2007;121(1):e4–e6.

101. Kinn RM, Breisblatt WM. Cortical blindness after coronary angiography: a rare but reversible complication. *Cathet Cardiovasc Diagn.* 1991;22(3):177–179.

102. Junck L, Marshall WH. Neurotoxicity of radiological contrast agents. *Ann Neurol.* 1983;13(5):469–484.

103. Lantos G. Cortical blindness due to osmotic disruption of the blood-brain barrier by angiographic contrast material: CT and MRI studies. *Neurology.* 1989;39(4):567–571.

104. Parry R, Rees JR, Wilde P. Transient cortical blindness after coronary angiography. *Br Heart J.* 1993;70(6):563–564.

14

Local Arterial and Venous Vascular Access Site Complications

STANLEY J. CHETCUTI, MAURICIO G. COHEN, AND MAURO MOSCUCCI

T he ever-evolving landscape of interventional cardiology has seen dramatic improvement in procedural outcomes and widening of the procedural spectrum tackled by operators in the field. While the refining of access techniques and downsizing of interventional equipment have lead to an overall decrease in access site complications, widening of the horizons in the field of cardiac interventional procedures relating to structural heart disease and the use of percutaneous cardiac assist devices has led to a trend in the opposite direction in terms of equipment size and the occurrence of vascular issues. However, available data suggest that a thorough understanding of factors related to an increased risk of vascular access complications and optimization of procedure and postprocedure strategy can play an important role in reducing the incidence of vascular complications in patients undergoing cardiovascular procedures. In general, a broad classification of vascular complications includes arterial access complications and venous access complications.

■ ARTERIAL ACCESS COMPLICATIONS

Arterial access vascular complications may be divided into three main subgroups: (1) vessel thrombosis, (2) distal embolization, and (3) hemorrhagic complications at the vascular access site.

Arterial Thrombosis

Although more commonly seen in the pediatric population, this complication may occur also in adults. Predisposing factors to this complication include small common femoral arteries (females, severe peripheral arterial disease (PAD), small body habitus), large arterial sheaths, prolonged dwell time especially with larger sheaths, prolonged compression postsheath removal, and "unroofing" of plaque during sheath site insertion.

The clinical presentation tends to be acute and examination reveals a painful white extremity with varying levels of decreased sensorium and motor function. The treatment is one that removes the obstruction and restores blood flow to the effected limb. For many years, the treatment of choice was surgical extraction of the thrombotic material by using a Fogarty catheter (1). Thrombus removal may also be attempted using various percutaneous aspiration devices (2,3). Time is the essence, and delay of more than 6 hours may lead to extensive muscle necrosis and reperfusion injury when the blood flow is restored. Delayed reperfusion is associated with reperfusion injury that may necessitate fasciotomy, varying degrees of amputation, and also predispose to renal failure (4).

Atheroembolism

Microembolization of atherosclerotic debris and small cholesterol crystals may result from catheter manipulation in any arterial bed, but patients with extensive atherosclerosis are at the highest risk of developing this complication. The embolic material may result in occlusion of small arteries (100–300 μm in diameter). The incidence of this complication is reported to be around 0.08% (5); however, it is felt that this

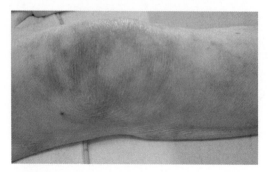

FIGURE 14-1. Livedo reticularis.

complication is underdiagnosed (6). The clinical presentation depends on the origin of the debris and on the vascular bed in which it lodges. When related to access site embolization, the extremities are involved in isolation, with the cutaneous manifestations of livedo reticularis, acrocyanosis, and gangrene comprising the clinical spectrum (7) (Fig. 14-1). The triad of leg and foot pain, livedo reticularis, and intact peripheral pulses is pathognomonic for cholesterol/athero embolization (6). Ancillary laboratory tests that may point toward this diagnosis include eosinophilia, eosinophiluria (when the kidneys are involved), elevated sedimentation rate, and decreased complement levels (8,9). The differential diagnosis includes various types of vasculitis and cutaneous manifestations of bacterial endocarditis. Treatment of this condition consists of supportive care for its complications such as hypertension, gangrene, renal failure, and mesenteric ischemia. Analgesia control is a critical part of the management especially in the early stages when the pain syndrome may be very intense. Unfortunately, there is no cure for this disease, with thrombolytic therapy and anticoagulation having no effect and even considered contraindicated. When the manifestations are diffuse and involve the gastrointestinal tract, the central nervous system, and the kidneys together with peripheral cutaneous manifestations, the prognosis is poor with reported mortality rates as high as 72% to 80% (7,10).

Hemorrhagic Complications at the Vascular Access Site

Bleeding after percutaneous coronary interventional procedures, especially if in the retroperi-

toneal space, remains a significant source of morbidity and mortality (11,12). Although the bleeding seen post percutaneous coronary intervention (PCI) may be due to a varying etiology, access site complications remain a significant factor in postprocedural bleeding (13–15) and may occur in 1% to 12% of cases (16–18). As the interventional community continues to expand the boundaries of coronary interventions (19), increased awareness of the importance of periprocedural bleeding from access site complications has led to renewed focus in limiting this complication. Strategies employed to this end have included using fluoroscopy to guide femoral artery access (20), ultrasound guided access of the femoral artery and vein (21,22), downsizing sheath sizes (23,24), use of vascular closure devices (VCDs) (25) or dedicated sheath pulling teams, and minimizing heparin use for the intervention. Suggested pharmacological interventions to reverse or blunt the effect of antiplatelet and antithrombotic agents are discussed in Chapter 6. Poorly controlled bleeding at the vascular access site can demonstrate in one of the following clinical scenarios.

Free Hemorrhage

Uncontrolled bleeding from the arterial puncture site is the most common complication encountered after femoral cardiac catheterization (26). Free bleeding around a still intact sheath may be caused by a laceration of the femoral artery. This complication may be more common with heavily calcified and scarred arteries. The free bleeding may respond to replacing the sheath with the next larger French-sized sheath. Failure to control the bleeding may necessitate firm compression over the sheath insertion site, while obtaining a type and cross-match for transfusion if clinically indicated. Once anticoagulation has been reversed, the sheath should be removed and prolonged compression should be applied to compensate for the larger sheath and any possible tear in the vessel. Direct surgical repair may be necessary if the bleeding fails to be controlled.

Femoral Hematoma

A femoral hematoma is a collection of blood within the soft tissues of the upper thigh. Groin hematomas are the next most common compli-

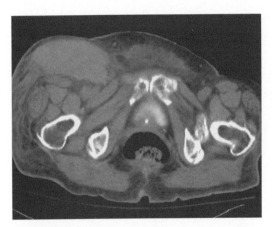

FIGURE 14-2. Computed tomography scan in a patient following the development of a femoral hematoma. There is no evidence of extension to the retroperitoneal space.

cation of femoral arterial puncture. Groin hematomas smaller than 6 cm in diameter occur with an incidence of 5% to 23%. Hematomas larger than 6 cm occur in 6% to 12% of cases (27). The clinical presentation is heralded by a tender mass of varying size at the femoral puncture site. Hematomas may compress the femoral vein, predisposing to femoral vein thrombosis. Local nerve compression (femoral nerve or the lateral cutaneous nerve of the thigh) may result in neuropathies that may be symptomatic for months. The diagnosis is confirmed by a Doppler ultrasound revealing the absence of flow from the artery into the hematoma, thus differentiating the hematoma from a pseudoaneurysm (28). A computed tomography (CT) scan is also useful to measure the extent of the hematoma and to exclude a retroperitoneal bleed (Fig. 14-2). Treatment consists of controlling the bleeding source with repeated compression, analgesia, and blood transfusion if clinically indicated.

Pseudoaneurysm

A femoral pseudoaneurysm develops if a hematoma remains in continuity with the femoral artery lumen by a neck or sinus tract at the needle puncture site. It is contained within the overlying fibromuscular tissue. Blood tends to flow into it during systole and out during diastole. Pseudoaneurysms can be differentiated from a hematoma by the presence of a pulsatile sensation in the mass, and they are often associ-

ated with an audible bruit. They become symptomatic when they compress an adjacent nerve (29). Thrombus layers may develop within the pseudoaneurysm, potentially causing distal embolic phenomenon compromising the distal circulation and even septic endarteritis if the thrombus becomes infected (30). In addition, there is a substantial risk of rupture of the pseudoaneurysm leading to massive bleeding. The diagnosis of a pseudoaneurysm is confirmed with Duplex ultrasound (28). Small pseudoaneurysms, less than 2 cm in diameter, may close spontaneously (31,32); however, as most continue to enlarge and possibly rupture, repair is usually recommended. Nonsurgical closure can be successfully achieved with ultrasound-guided compression of the narrow neck for 30 to 60 minutes in more than 90% of cases attempted (31,32). Contraindications for ultrasound-guided compression include skin ischemia, severe discomfort during compression, large hematomas with compartment syndrome, and injury above the inguinal ligament (33). The false aneurysm cavity may also be injected with thrombin or similar procoagulant material and occluded flow through the neck (34) (Figs. 14-3 and 14-4). It is important that this technique that is vastly replacing simple ultrasound compression of the pseudoaneurysm neck be performed by experienced operators to avoid embolism of the thrombotic material down the femoral artery. This may lead to an acute thrombosis of the vessel that may be treated with rheolytic thrombectomy and systemic or local thrombolytic therapy (35).

Retroperitoneal Hemorrhage

A retroperitoneal hemorrhage is a rare but potentially catastrophic complication of coronary interventional procedures (36). The incidence of this complication is 0.15% to 0.5% and tends to occur more frequently in the presence of more aggressive anticoagulation regimens (5,37). The reported mortality rate can be as high as 10% (12). The most likely mechanism is puncture of the femoral artery above the inguinal ligament and above the inferior epigastric artery, allowing the resultant bleeding to extend into the retroperitoneal space (Fig. 14-5). However, it has also been shown that adoption of a common femoral artery puncture site does not necessarily

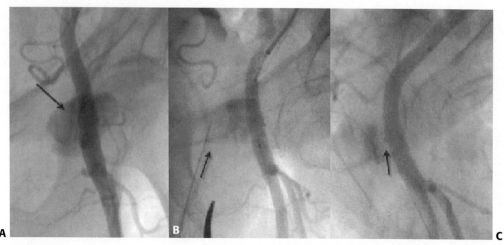

FIGURE 14-3. Femoral pseudoaneurysm. (**A**) To evaluate a pulsatile mass in the left groin following a catheterization, crossover angiography was performed from the right groin showing a large pseudoaneurysm over the common femoral artery. (**B**) An angioplasty balloon was positioned under the prior puncture site as a needle (*arrow*) was advanced to puncture the pseudoaneurysm cavity confirmed by contrast injection. (**C**) After occlusion of the common femoral by inflation of the angioplasty balloon, thrombin was injected through the needle into the pseudoaneurysm cavity, causing it to clot, as shown by the absence of further contrast flow into it on the postprocedure angiogram (*arrow*). (Case courtesy of Dr. Andrew Eisenhauer, Brigham and Women's Hospital. From Baim DS. *Grossman's Cardiac Catheterization, Angiography, and Intervention.* 7th ed. Philadelphia, PA: Lippincott Williams & Wilkins, 2006.)

prevent the development of a retroperitoneal hematoma. In addition, inadvertent trauma or perforation of the inferior epigastric artery can also lead to the formation of a retroperitoneal hematoma (Fig. 14-6). The bleeding may not always be clinically evident in the early stages, and a high index of suspicion is warranted in patients who develop hypotension, falling hematocrit, severe flank pain, abdominal pain, back pain, and even lower extremity pain from

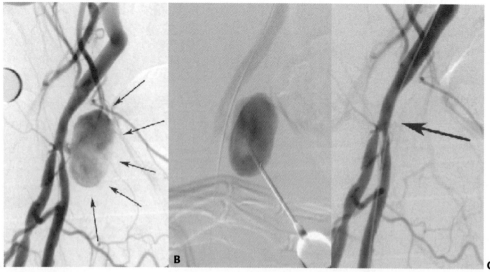

FIGURE 14-4. (**A**) Angiographic appearance of a pseudoaneurysm sac (outlined by *arrows*). The hole in the artery is between the sac and the common femoral artery. (**B**) Using roadmapping and fluoroscopy, a needle is inserted percutaneously into the pseudoaneurysm sac. Once pulsatile flow is obtained, contrast is injected to confirm location, followed by very slow injection of thrombin a tenth of a cc at a time. (**C**) Final angiography demonstrates closure of the hole in the common femoral artery and obliteration of the pseudoaneurysm (*arrow*). (From Baim DS. *Grossman's Cardiac Catheterization, Angiography, and Intervention.* 7th ed. Philadelphia, PA: Lippincott Williams & Wilkins, 2006.)

TABLE 14-1	Common Symptoms and Signs Associated with a Retroperitoneal Hematoma

- Back pain
- Flank pain
- Diaphoresis
- Abdominal pain
- Unexplained hypotension
- Declining hemoglobin levels
- Femoral neuropathy
- "Vasovagal" reactions (hypotension with bradycardia)
- Flank ecchymosis

femoral nerve compression (38) (Table 14-1). The diagnosis may be confirmed by CT scanning or abdominal ultrasound. A noncontrast CT may show shifting of organs from their regular position by the collection of blood at the site (Fig. 14-7). The treatment is initially conservative with close hemodynamic monitoring, reversal of anticoagulation, bed rest, and volume expansion if clinically indicated. Catheter-based therapies are becoming the favored approach when patients fail conservative management. A contralateral approach is usually favored for localization and tamponade of the retroperitoneal bleeding site, with an appropriately sized angioplasty balloon followed by placement of a covered stent to cover the perforation (39) (Figs. 14-5 and 14-6). Coil embolization is another effective treatment modality in case of laceration or perforation of small side branches (Figs. 14-8 and 14-9). Figure 14-10 illustrates a suggested algorithm for the management of patients with suspected retroperitoneal hematoma.

Femoral Neuropathy

Femoral neuropathy is a rare complication of femoral artery access with a reported incidence of 0.21% (40). Femoral neuropathy can result from direct trauma during femoral artery access, from compression by a hematoma or a pseudoaneurysm (40), or from prolonged local compression during removal of the arterial sheaths (41). The femoral nerve originates from the lumbar plexus and enters the pelvic region through the fibers of the psoas major. As it continues to descend, it has a course between the iliacus muscle and the lateral aspect of the psoas; after exiting beneath the inguinal ligament, the femoral nerves give rise to the anterior cutaneous branches. Femoral neuropathy can present with two different clinical syndromes (40). The first syndrome is a lumbar plexopathy involving the femoral, obturator, or lateral femoral cutaneous nerves and is associated with a large retroperitoneal hematoma. The clinical presentation is usually with paresthesias and

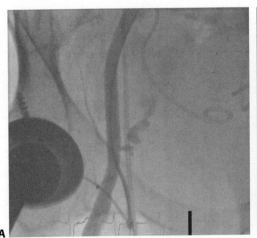
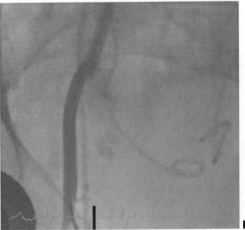

FIGURE 14-5. Angiography of the right femoral artery. (**A**) The arterial sheath has been inserted above the inguinal ligament, and there is extravasation of contrast in the retroperitoneal space. (**B**) Repeat angiography after deployment of a covered stent. There is no further extravasation of contrast in the retroperitoneal space.

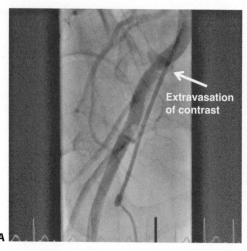 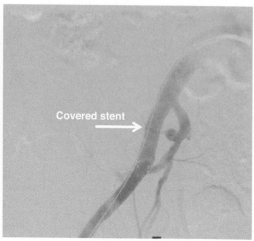

FIGURE 14-6. (**A**) Angiography of the right femoral artery showing extravasation of contrast from the inferior epigastric artery. (**B**) Repeat angiography following deployment of a covered stent.

with the inability to bear weight upon ambulation following sheath removal. Although there often is recovery, a mild persistent sensory neuropathy and a persistent motor deficit have been reported (40). The second syndrome is characterized by paresthesias involving the medial and intermediate cutaneous branches of the femoral nerve, in association with a groin hematoma or a false aneurysm. Decompression through evacuation of large hematoma or repair of a pseudoaneurysm is usually indicated in these cases.

Arteriovenous Fistula

An arteriovenous (AV) fistula results when bleeding from an arterial puncture site communicates with an adjacent venous puncture

site (Fig. 14-11) (42). Any of the two puncture sites may be inadvertent and not obvious at the time of the procedure. The incidence of this complication after cardiac catheterization is approximately 1% with reported risk factors

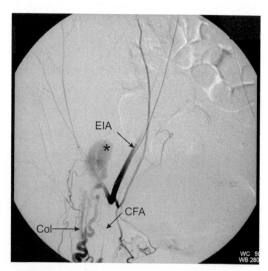

FIGURE 14-8. Retroperitoneal bleeding demonstrated by selective catheterization of the right internal and external iliac branches with contrast extravasation (*) around a prominent collateral (Col) running from the right distal external iliac artery (EIA) to the femoral bifurcation. CFA, chronic subtotal occlusion of the common femoral artery. (From Morris GM, O'Grady EA, Wynn GJ, Davis GK. Retroperitoneal hematoma after diagnostic coronary angiography caused by collateralization of a chronic common femoral artery occlusion secondary to childhood femoral cannulation. *Circ Cardiovasc Interv.* 2009;2:580–581.)

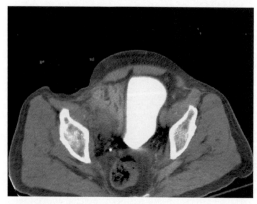

FIGURE 14-7. Pelvic computed tomography scan showing a large retroperitoneal hematoma.

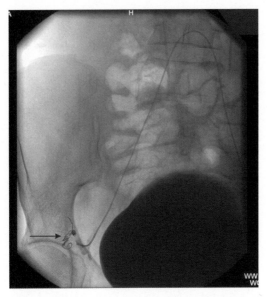

FIGURE 14-9. Treatment of bleeding point by coil embolization (*arrow*). (From Morris GM, O'Grady EA, Wynn GJ, Davis GK. Retroperitoneal hematoma after diagnostic coronary angiography caused by collateralization of a chronic common femoral artery occlusion secondary to childhood femoral cannulation. *Circ Cardiovasc Interv.* 2009;2:580–581.)

including arterial hypertension, female gender (possible because of smaller arteries), multiple punctures, left groin access, aggressive anticoagulation regimens, and impaired hemostasis (43,44). In addition, a low puncture site can be associated with an increased incidence of AV fistula. AV fistula can be clinically recognized by a continuous bruit over the femoral puncture site, which may be evident only after many days following the procedure. As the volume of blood shunted is usually low (160–510 mL/min—significantly less than the flow associated with dialysis fistulae), the more ominous complications of distal arterial insufficiency, heart failure exacerbation, and painful lower extremity are rarely seen (42,43). The diagnosis is confirmed by Doppler ultrasound (42). Although the fistulae may enlarge with time, one-third of them close spontaneously within 1 year. Three therapeutic options are available for persistent AV fistulae

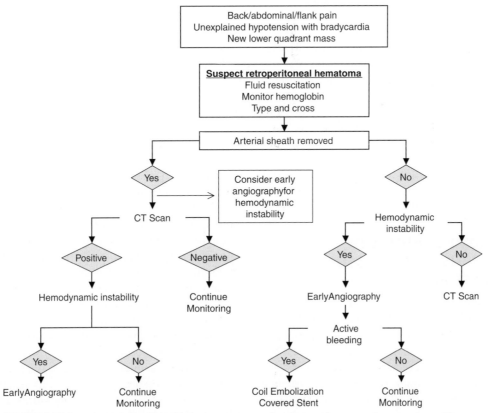

FIGURE 14-10. Suggested algorithm for the management of patients with suspected retroperitoneal hematoma. CT, computed tomography.

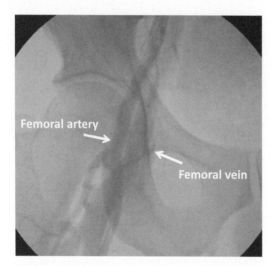

FIGURE 14-11. Femoral arteriovenous fistula. During angiography of the femoral artery, there is simultaneous visualization of the femoral vein.

that have not closed spontaneously: (1) ultrasound-guided compression, (2) endovascular implantation of covered stents, and (3) surgical repair. Ultrasound-guided compression should be applied first. It is a relatively benign and noninvasive procedure although its success rate is less than when it is applied for the treatment of pseudoaneurysms (33,45). Covered stents may be implanted, although the repetitive movements encountered at the common femoral results in outcomes that are less favorable than stenting in other areas (46). Surgical intervention should be reserved for patients who have not closed spontaneously at 1 year or for the less likely scenario when the AV fistula precipitates a further complication (47).

■ COMPLICATIONS OF TRANSRADIAL VASCULAR ACCESS

Femoral access complications accounts for approximately 60% to 70% of cases of bleeding complications following PCI (48). Switching access site to a smaller and easily compressible vessel, such as the radial artery, can potentially maximize safety, improve patient comfort, and eliminate access-related bleeding. As a matter of fact, all published comparisons between transfemoral and transradial catheterization demon-

strate in aggregate that transradial access is associated with a substantial 73% reduction in major bleeding and a 30% trend toward a reduction in the incidence of death, myocardial infarction, or stroke (49). On the other hand, transradial catheterization is associated with a slightly higher radiation exposure to the operator and requires specific skills usually acquired after a learning curve of 50 to 80 cases (50,51). For these reasons, transradial catheterization has not gained widespread acceptance in the United States (52).

Despite improved overall patient safety, transradial vascular access is not without specific complications. These include vascular spasm, hematoma, vascular perforations, postprocedural radial occlusion, and abscess development at the puncture site.

Radial Artery Spasm

This is by far the most common complication of transradial access and a frequent reason for crossover to transfemoral access. It is manifested with excruciating forearm pain and unusually difficult manipulation of the catheters and the sheath. Independent predictors of radial artery spasm include the presence of radial artery anomalies, multiple catheter exchanges, pain during radial cannulation, catheter diameter, and radial artery caliber (53). In extreme cases, eversion radial endarterectomy has been reported after forceful removal of the radial sheath (54). Spasm should be routinely prevented using a hydrophilic-coated sheath with the injection of a single vasodilator or a cocktail of vasodilators through the sidearm of the sheath immediately after obtaining access in every case. Most commonly used vasodilators in order of frequency include verapamil, nicardipine, nitroglycerin, lidocaine, and papaverine (55). In addition, it is important to maintain good sedation to avoid the release of catecholamines associated with the emotional stress and fear that patients usually experience before the procedure. When spasm occurs, measures such as the administration of additional doses of intra-arterial vasodilators, sedation, and use of smaller size catheters (5F or 4F), are usually recommended. If after these measures the patient still complains of substantial pain and the catheters are difficult to manipulate, a

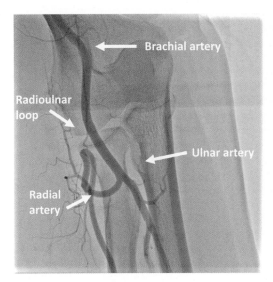

FIGURE 14-12. Angiography of the radial artery showing the presence of a radioulnar loop.

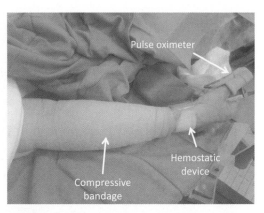

FIGURE 14-14. Prevention of compartment syndrome with compression bandage.

limited upper extremity angiography is recommended to rule out vascular anomalies such as radioulnar loops (Fig. 14-12).

Forearm Hematoma—Vascular Perforations

Most commonly, this complication is caused by accidental advancement of the wire into small radial side branches causing perforation. As full anticoagulation is usually administered during transradial procedures, a small branch perforation can result in significant hematoma formation. In other circumstances, forceful advancement of the wire against resistance can cause main radial artery perfo-

ration, especially in the presence of radioulnar loops (Fig. 14-13).

Forearm bleeding and hematoma formation should be suspected in the presence of significant postprocedural pain and swelling. Awareness and early detection in the catheterization laboratory or the holding area is important to prevent compartment syndrome. Circumferential compression to the forearm should be applied as soon as the diagnosis is suspected. This is usually accomplished by wrapping the forearm with an elastic bandage or a blood pressure cuff inflated up to 15 mm Hg below the systolic blood pressure, until the coagulation parameters return to normal values, usually after 1 or 2 hours. A pulse oximeter should be placed in the ipsilateral thumb to monitor for hand ischemia (Fig. 14-14). In cases of large perforations, vascular ultrasound is recommended to rule out the

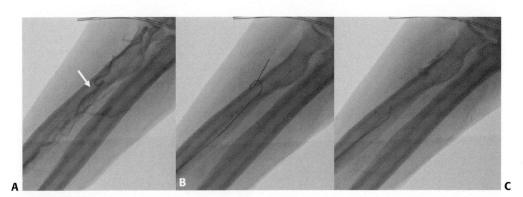

FIGURE 14-13. Radial artery perforation. (**A**) An extremely tortuous radial artery with diffuse spasm (*arrow*). (**B**) Advancement of a 0.018-in. wire was attempted but the wire perforated the radial artery. (**C**) Frank extravasation of contrast in the forearm.

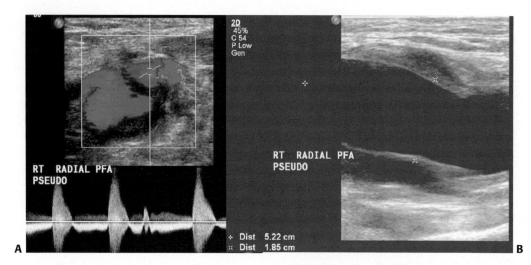

FIGURE 14-15. Radial artery pseudoaneurysm (Pseudo). RT, right. (See color insert.)

presence of a pseudoaneurysm in the forearm, as shown in Figure 14-15. In extreme cases, compartment syndrome can develop with a need for surgical fasciotomy of the forearm (56).

Vascular perforations or avulsions can also occur with forceful advancement of more rigid guiding catheters through tortuous or anomalous vessels. In rare occasions, a radial artery with a high takeoff from the brachial artery in the upper arm can be avulsed by the passage of a guiding catheter, as depicted in Figure 14-16.

Radial Artery Occlusion

This complication occurs in approximately 5% to 10% of transradial procedures and is manifested as asymptomatic loss of radial pulse. Lack of anticoagulation use during the procedure and prolonged occlusive compression for hemostasis increase the risk of radial artery occlusion. Hand ischemia after transradial cardiac catheterization has not been described in the literature and is unlikely to occur after radial artery occlusion due to the extensive collateral circulation through the ulnar artery. A few cases of hand ischemia have been reported after radial cannulation for blood pressure monitoring in critically ill patients treated with vasopressors (57,58). The actual concern about radial artery occlusion is that it limits the possibility for future transradial access and for using the radial artery as an arterial conduit for coronary artery bypass graft surgery.

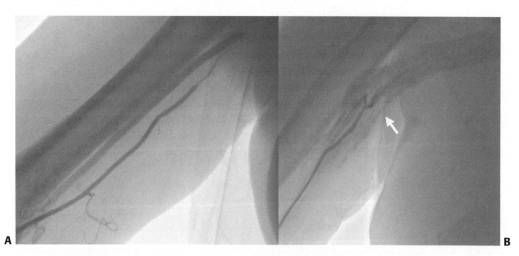

FIGURE 14-16. (**A**) High origin of the radial artery. (**B**)Perforation of a radial artery with high origin in the brachial artery.

This complication can be prevented by using full anticoagulation during the procedure, usually with 60 to 70 IU/kg of unfractionated heparin and a lower duration and intensity of compression during hemostasis. A technique for "patent" hemostasis has been described to minimize radial occlusion. Before sheath removal, a compression device with an inflatable balloon that applies selective pressure on the radial artery (TR Band, Terumo Medical, Somerset, NJ) is placed around the wrist. While the sheath is being removed, the device balloon is fully inflated with 15 to 18 cc of air to completely occlude the radial artery. A pulse oximeter is placed in the thumb, and the device is slowly deflated while applying manual pressure on the ulnar artery. Patent hemostasis is achieved when oximetry in the fingertips becomes positive and a waveform is visualized with plethysmography. Two hours later, 5 cc of air can be released every 15 minutes, until the device is completely deflated and removed. With this technique, late occlusion rates are approximately 2% (59).

Local Inflammatory Reaction

This complication occurs in less than 2% of the cases, it usually appears 2 to 3 weeks after the procedure, and its incidence has been related to the use of a particular brand of hydrophilic-coated sheaths (AQ Hydrophilic coated sheaths, Cook Medical Inc., Bloomington, Indiana). The hydrophilic coating strips off the sheath used during the procedure and it can remain in the subcutaneous tissue, leading to a granulomatous inflammatory reaction, sometimes with abscess formation (Fig. 14-17). No bacteria could be isolated from these reactions in the cases reported in the literature (60). Conservative management ruling out the presence of infection, local wound care with drainage in case of abscess formation, and reassurance are recommended for the management of this complication.

■ PREDICTORS OF VASCULAR COMPLICATIONS

In the early era of coronary stenting and aggressive antithrombotic treatment including heparin, dextran, aspirin and warfarin, the overall incidence of vascular complications was as high as 10% to 15% (44,61); with the introduction of dual antiplatelet therapy, weight-adjusted heparin dosing, new antithrombotic agents, and smaller catheters, there has been a progressive decline in the incidence of vascular complications (18). In general, clinical risk factors for vascular access site complications appear to be consistent across single center or multicenter registry analysis and include excessive anticoagulation, female gender, more aggressive antithrombotic therapy, renal failure, peripheral vascular disease, advanced age, small body surface area, indication for the procedure (emergency vs. elective), duration of arterial sheaths, history of hypertension and catheter size (Table 14-2) (16,18,23,44,61–64). In addition, several studies have shown a significantly lower incidence of vascular complications and transfusion in patients undergoing cardiac catheterization and PCI through the radial artery approach when compared with patients undergoing the same procedures through the femoral artery approach (49).

■ PREVENTION OF VASCULAR ACCESS SITE COMPLICATIONS

The identification of risk factors for complications has led to modification of procedure strategies aimed toward reducing the rate of vascular complications. As of today, weight-adjusted heparin dosing, early arterial sheath removal, avoidance of excessive anticoagulation, and use of smaller arterial sheath have become part of the standard of care. In addition, wider adoption of the radial artery approach and the choice of antithrombotic therapy have the potential to further reduce the rate of vascular complications. The value of weight-adjusted unfractionated heparin (UFH) dosing cannot be

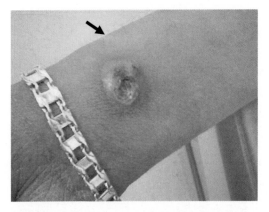

FIGURE 14-17. Radial access site inflammation. (See color insert.)

TABLE 14-2 Overview of Risk Factors and Frequency of Access Site Complications Across Single-Center and Multicenter Registry Analysis (1992–2003)

Reference	Popma et al. (61)	Moscucci et al. (44)	Blankenship et al. (64)	Mandak et al. (63)	Piper et al. (18)	Tavris et al. (62)	Applegate et al. (16)
Data source	Single center registry	Single center registry	Multicenter clinical trial (EPIC)	Multicenter clinical trial	Multicenter registry (NNE) (IMPACT II)	Multicenter registry	Single center registry
Publication date/N	1992 N = 1,413 New device angioplasty	1994 N = 688 Directional atherectomy and stenting	1997 N = 2,058	1998 N = 4,010 PCI	2003 (1997–1999) N = 18,137 PCI	2004 (2001) N = 156,853 PCI + diagnostic	2006 (1998–2003) N = 21,841 PCI + diagnostic
Complication rate	5.9%	11.7%	5.2% (major)	8.5%	2.98%	1.56%	1.8% PCI 1.1% diagnostic
Variables							
Demographic							
Age	…	X	X	X	X	X	X
Female Sex	…	X	X	X	X	X	X
BMI or BSA or weight	…	…	X	…	X		
Comorbidities							
Diabetes	…	…	…	…	…	X	X (protective)
PVD*	…	…	…	…	X	X	X
COPD	…	…	…	…	X		
Renal function	X	X	…	…	X	X	X
Cardiac history and function							
NYHA Class	…	…	…	…	…	X	
Hypertension	…	X	…	…	…	X	X

(continued)

	1	2	3	4	5	6
Priority (elective, urgent, emergent, salvage)			…	…	X	…	X
Indication							
STEMI, no-STEMI	…	X	…	X	X	X
Shock and/or VF arrest	…	…	…	…	X	X
Treatment							
Thrombolysis	X	…	X	…	…	…
Gp IIb/IIIa blockers	…	…	X	X	X	…
Heparin dose	…	…	…	X	…	…
Procedure							
Coronary stenting	X	…	X	…	X	…
TEC atherectomy	X	…	…	…	…	…
Repeat procedure	X	…	…	…	…	…
Multivessel PCI	…	X	…	X	…	…
Catheter size	…	X	…	…	…	…
Venous sheath	…	…	X	X	X	…
Coronary dissection/lesion complexity	…	…	…	…	X	…
Sheath duration	X	X	X	X	…	…
ACT-guided sheath removal	X	…	…	…	…	…
Use of VCD	…	…	…	…	…	X (protective)
Unsuccessful VCD	…	…	…	…	…	X
Laboratory results							
Nadir platelet count	X	…	X	…	…	…
Baseline platelet count	…	…	X	…	…	…
Excessive anticoagulation	X	…	X	…	…	…

BMI, body mass index; BSA, body surface area; PVD, peripheral vascular disease; COPD, chronic obstructive pulmonary disease; NYHA, New York Heart Association; STEMI, ST-segment elevation myocardial infarction; VF, ventricular fibrillation; TEC, transluminal extraction coronary; PCI, percutaneous coronary intervention; VCD, vascular closure device; ACT, activated clotting time.

overemphasized. The current recommendations include an initial dose of 60 IU/kg with a target activated clotting time (ACT) of 250 seconds in patients not receiving a Gp IIb/IIIa inhibitor and a target ACT of 200 seconds in patients receiving a Gp IIb/IIIa inhibitor. Continuous treatment with UFH is not indicated following completion of PCI, given that the continuous treatment does not reduce ischemic complications and is associated with a higher risk of bleeding (65). In addition, ACT-guided early removal of arterial sheaths can result in a lower rate of complications when compared with prolonged sheaths dwelling and non–ACT-guided removal (44,61). The identification of the appropriate femoral artery puncture site deserves further comments. As the common femoral artery exit beneath the inguinal ligament, it has a course in front of the femoral head, and it then bifurcates into the superficial and profunda femoral arteries at the level of the lower border of the femoral head. It has been proposed that the ideal puncture site should be between the center and the upper margin of the femoral head (66,67) (Fig. 14-18). This site will be below the inguinal ligament and before the bifurcation of the femoral artery into the superficial and profunda branches. A puncture site above the femoral head could lead to a retroperitoneal hematoma following sheath removal, whereas a puncture site too low could lead to bleeding due to inability to compress the artery against a hard plane and to an increased risk of pseudoaneurysm formation and of AV fistula. Given that the inguinal skin crease can be misleading and that it might be difficult in some cases to identify anatomical landmarks and the inguinal ligament, several operators have advocated the routine use of fluoroscopic guidance for the identification of the femoral head. A recent registry analysis has suggested that routine use of this practice (fluoroscopic guidance) can result in a lower incidence of vascular access complications (68). In addition, a recent randomized clinical trial comparing fluoroscopic guidance with ultrasound guidance has shown that ultrasound guidance can have a role in further reducing complications rates and particularly in avoiding inadvertent puncture of the femoral vein during vascular access (Femoral Arterial Access with Ultrasound Trial [FAUST], data presented at the 2009 Transcatheter Cardiovascular Therapeutic Meeting).

■ VASCULAR CLOSURE DEVICES

VCDs have emerged as an alternative to the traditional manual mechanical compression after coronary interventional procedures. They offer the potential of earlier ambulation postprocedure and decreased human resources that would otherwise be needed for manual compression (69,70). Complications associated with these devices may vary slightly from the complications associated with mechanical compression and include an increased risk of local infection with possible endarteritis, embolization of closure device, vessel closures (directly or by embolization), possible increased bleeding related to sheath removal while the patient is still fully anticoagulated, and femoral artery thrombosis. Although early data suggested that these devices were associated with increased bleeding and vascular complications (71), a more recent meta-analysis has shown that in the setting of coronary interventional procedures, the outcomes with two of the commonly use VCD (Angioseal and Perclose) were similar to the outcomes of mechanical compression (72). In addition, in the ACUITY trial, the use of VCD was found to be associated with a lower incidence of vascular complications when compared with manual compression (73). In the same trial, the lowest incidence of vascular complications (0.7%) was found in the group of patients treated with bivalirudin and managed with a VCD (Fig. 14-19). Patient selection and technique used are key elements in reducing complications associated with VCDs. *Device failure*, defined as failure to deploy the device or failure to achieve hemostasis, is a specific issue of VCD that might be related to a learning curve and to the type of device used. In a recent single-center analysis, device failure occurred in 2.7% of patients (2.3% of diagnostic cases and 3.0% of PCI) (74). Independent predictors of device failure included advance age, the use of Perclose, the use of VCD in patients undergoing PCI, and diabetes mellitus (Table 14-3). Unfortunately, failure of deployment of VCD is also associated with a higher incidence of major and minor access site complications (74) (Fig. 14-20). Prior to device deployment, femoral angiography should be performed in all patients to ensure that the arterial access entry point is in the common femoral artery, rather than in the

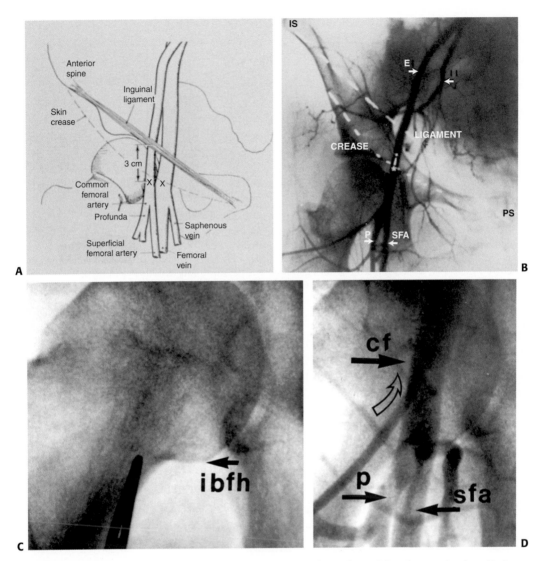

FIGURE 14-18. Regional anatomy relevant to percutaneous femoral arterial and venous catheterization. (**A**) Schematic diagram showing the right femoral artery and vein coursing underneath the inguinal ligament, which runs from the anterior superior iliac spine to the pubic tubercle. The arterial skin nick (indicated by X) should be placed approximately 3 cm below the ligament and directly over the femoral arterial pulsation, and the venous skin nick should be placed at the same level but approximately one fingerbreadth more medial. Although this level corresponds roughly to the skin crease in most patients, anatomic localization relative to the inguinal ligament provides a more constant landmark (see text for details). (**B**) Corresponding radiographic anatomy as seen during abdominal aortography. (**C**) Fluoroscopic localization of skin nick (marked by clamp tip) to the inferior border of the femoral head (ibfh). (**D**) Catheter (*open arrow*) inserted via this skin nick has entered the common femoral artery (cf), safely above its bifurcation into the superficial femoral (sfa) and profunda branches (67). (From Baim DS. *Grossman's Cardiac Catheterization, Angiography, and Intervention.* 7th ed. Philadelphia, PA: Lippincott Williams & Wilkins, 2006.)

superficial femoral artery or in the iliac artery. Femoral angiography can also disclose the presence of significant peripheral vascular disease, which is a contraindication to the use of VCDs. In addition, the use of VCDs includes leaving a foreign body (Angiosel, Vasoseal, Starclose) or a suture (Perclose) at the arteriotomy entry site. This will increase the risk of local infections, which will be difficult to manage. Thus, the use of thorough sterile techniques (use of hats and mask, repeat sterile prep of the entry site) is mandatory.

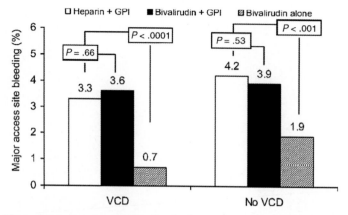

FIGURE 14-19. Thirty-day major access site bleeding in the ACUITY trial by randomized antithrombin treatment in patients with and without VCD use. VCD, vascular closure device; GPI, glycoprotein inhibitors. (From Sanborn TA, Ebrahimi R, Manoukian SV, et al. Impact of femoral vascular closure devices and antithrombotic therapy on access site bleeding in acute coronary syndromes: The Acute Catheterization and Urgent Intervention Triage Strategy (ACUITY) trial. *Circ Cardiovasc Interv.* 2010;3:57–62.)

■ VASCULAR COMPLICATIONS OF CENTRAL VENOUS ACCESS

Central venous catheters are still an excellent means of measuring hemodynamic parameters that are not easily obtained by noninvasive means. They are generally used in the intensive care setting but are also useful in the short term for hemodynamic monitoring during complex interventional procedures. In addition, all electrophysiology procedures require central venous access and, often, the placement of more than one catheter in more than one vein or in the same vein. The internal jugular vein, subclavian vein, and the femoral vein are the three main sites that are used for central venous access. Unfortunately each site is associated with a spectrum of mechanical complications,

TABLE 14-3   Univariate and Multivariate Predictors of Vascular Closure Device Failure

Parameter	Odds Ratio	95% CI	P
Univariate predictors			
Age	1.02	1.01–1.03	<.0001
Age > 70 y	1.79	1.41–2.29	<.0001
Men	1.27	0.98–1.63	.066
Diabetes mellitus	1.41	1.09–1.82	.010
Dyslipidemia	1.25	0.97–1.61	.083
Peripheral arterial disease	1.54	1.05–2.27	.028
Percutaneous coronary intervention	1.33	1.03–1.72	.029
Myocardial infarction	1.30	0.96–1.76	.094
Perclose device	6.67	5.21–8.54	<.0001
Procedure duration	1.002	1.000–1.004	.017
Multivariable predictors			
Age	1.02	1.01–1.03	.001
Perclose device	6.56	5.04–8.54	<.0001
Percutaneous coronary intervention	1.34	1.01–1.79	.045
Myocardial infarction	1.38	0.99–1.92	.060
Diabetes mellitus	1.28	0.97–1.71	.085

(From Bangalore S, Arora N, Resnic FS. Vascular closure device failure: frequency and implications: a propensity-matched analysis. *Circ Cardiovasc Interv.* 2009;2:549–556).

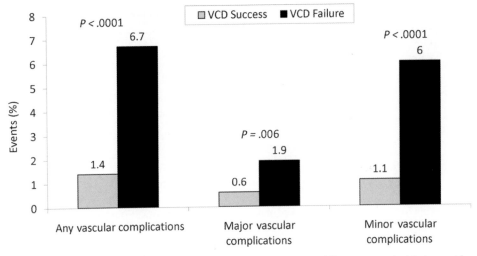

FIGURE 14-20. Incidence of vascular complications in patients with VCD failure compared with those with successful deployment of VCD. The incidence of any, major, or minor vascular complication was substantially higher in the group with VCD failure compared with the group with successful deployment of VCD. VCD, vascular closure device. (From Bangalore S, Arora N, Resnic FS. Vascular closure device failure: frequency and implications: a propensity-matched analysis. *Circ Cardiovasc Interv.* 2009;2:549–556).

some of which are site specific. Arterial injury (or inadvertent arterial cannulation), hematoma formation, and pneumothorax are the most common mechanical complications of central venous access and are reported to occur in 5% to 19% of patients undergoing these procedures (75–77). The subclavian site is more likely to be associated with the complications of pneumothorax and hemothorax and should be avoided in patients with compromised pulmonary function, whereas arterial puncture is more commonly associated with femoral and internal jugular vein access. Ultrasound guidance has been shown to be very useful in internal jugular vein access, reducing the procedure time and the complication rates (78,79). It allows for direct visualization of the vein, whereby the operator can plot its course, plot the depth from the skin, exclude the presence of thrombus, and visualize the vein's relationship to adjacent carotid artery.

Inadvertent Arterial Puncture during Central Venous Access

The dreaded complication of sheath insertion in the subclavian artery (a noncompressible vessel) used to be invariably a surgical issue. However, newer VCDs now offer a percutaneous approach that has negated the need of surgical intervention. Successful vascular closure with the Angioseal device, with Perclose, and with Starclose has been reported, thus suggesting that with the technology currently available, this complication can be managed with nonsurgical techniques (80–82). The general recommendation is to avoid access of noncompressible vessels in patients who are fully anticoagulated. In addition, should a patient develop a neck hematoma following inadvertent puncture of the carotid artery, it is strongly recommended not to attempt vascular access on the other site of the neck, given that a bilateral neck hematoma could lead to a compromised airway.

Femoral Vein Thrombosis

Femoral vein thrombosis and its dreaded association of pulmonary embolism are rare complications of cardiac catheterization. When studied systematically, however, these complications may be more frequent than anticipated, and lung scan abnormalities have been reported in as many as 10% of patients after diagnostic cardiac catheterization (83).

Risk factors for these complications include prolonged bed rest postprocedure, multiple lines placed in the same vein (more common during electrophysiology procedures), injury at the time of sheath removal, and compression by a neighboring hematoma that alters the flow in the vein.

TABLE 14-4	System Approach toward Reducing Vascular Access Complications
Domain	Variable
Vascular access	• Fluoroscopy guidance • Ultrasound guidance • Radial artery access, particularly in high-risk patients • Avoid additional venous sheaths if not needed
Sheaths size	• In general, complication rates are lower with 6F sheaths when compared with 7F or larger sheaths
Antithrombotic therapy	• Weight-adjusted heparin dosing • ACT monitoring during the procedure • Avoidance of excessive anticoagulation • Use of alternative antithrombotic therapy (bivalirudin)
Arterial sheaths management	• Early arterial sheaths removal • Management of hypertension • ACT-guided sheaths removal • Dedicated staff members for the management of patients with vascular sheaths

ACT, activated clotting time.

Treatment of this complication is standard for venous thromboembolic disease although it may complicate an already complex anticoagulation regimen and increase the risk of nonaccess site bleeding. Newer techniques for decreasing clot burden via percutaneous techniques are well described, but they do not seem to alter the need for additional antithrombotic therapy (84).

■ CONCLUSION

There has been tremendous progress toward a better understanding of risk factors of vascular complications and of procedure variables the modification of which can result in a decreased risk of complications. A system approach, as summarized in Table 14-4, including access site selection, optimization of antithrombotic therapy, and optimization of arterial sheaths management (and removal) can have an important role in reducing the rate of access site complications. Once complications have occurred, the appropriate and timely application of newly developed minimally invasive techniques can minimize the adverse clinical outcomes associated with complications.

References

1. Fogarty TJ, et al. Experience with balloon catheter technic for arterial embolectomy. *Am J Surg.* 1971;122(2):231–237.

2. Rilinger N, et al. Mechanical thrombectomy of embolic occlusion in both the profunda femoris and superficial femoral arteries in critical limb ischaemia. *Br J Radiol.* 1997;70:80–84.

3. Silva JA, et al. Rheolytic thrombectomy in the treatment of acute limb-threatening ischemia: immediate results and six-month follow-up of the multicenter AngioJet registry. Possis Peripheral AngioJet Study AngioJet Investigators. *Cathet Cardiovasc Diagn.* 1998;45(4):386–393.

4. Yassin MM, et al. Lower limb ischemia-reperfusion injury triggers a systemic inflammatory response and multiple organ dysfunction. *World J Surg.* 2002;26(1):115–121.

5. Johnson LW, et al. Peripheral vascular complications of coronary angioplasty by the femoral and brachial techniques. *Cathet Cardiovasc Diagn.* 1994;31(3):165–172.

6. Om A, Ellahham S, DiSciascio G. Cholesterol embolism: an underdiagnosed clinical entity. *Am Heart J.* 1992;124(5):1321–1326.

7. Falanga V, Fine MJ, Kapoor WN. The cutaneous manifestations of cholesterol crystal embolization. *Arch Dermatol.* 1986;122(10):1194–1198.

8. Cosio FG, Zager RA, Sharma HM. Atheroembolic renal disease causes hypocomplementaemia. *Lancet* 1985;2(8447):118–121.

9. Kasinath BS, Lewis EJ. Eosinophilia as a clue to the diagnosis of atheroembolic renal disease. *Arch Intern Med.* 1987;147(8):1384–1385.

10. Fine MJ, Kapoor W, Falanga V. Cholesterol crystal embolization: a review of 221 cases in the English literature. *Angiology.* 1987;38(10):769–784.

11. Rao SV, et al. A comparison of the clinical impact of bleeding measured by two different classifications among patients with acute coronary syndromes. *J Am Coll Cardiol.* 2006;47(4):809–816.

12. Ellis SG, et al. Correlates and outcomes of retroperitoneal hemorrhage complicating percutaneous coronary intervention. *Catheter Cardiovasc Interv.* 2006;67(4):541–545.

13. Lincoff AM, et al. Long-term efficacy of bivalirudin and provisional glycoprotein IIb/IIIa blockade vs heparin and planned glycoprotein IIb/IIIa blockade during percutaneous coronary revascularization: REPLACE-2 randomized trial. *JAMA.* 2004;292(6):696–703.

14. Moscucci M, et al. Predictors of major bleeding in acute coronary syndromes: the Global Registry of Acute Coronary Events (GRACE). *Eur Heart J.* 2003;24(20):1815–1823.

15. Stone GW, et al. Bivalirudin for patients with acute coronary syndromes. *N Engl J Med.* 2006; 355(21):2203–2216.

16. Applegate RJ, et al. Propensity score analysis of vascular complications after diagnostic cardiac catheterization and percutaneous coronary intervention 1998–2003. *Catheter Cardiovasc Interv.* 2006;67(4):556–562.

17. Berry C, et al. Comparison of femoral bleeding complications after coronary angiography versus percutaneous coronary intervention. *Am J Cardiol.* 2004;94(3):361–363.

18. Piper WD, et al. Predicting vascular complications in percutaneous coronary interventions. *Am Heart J.* 2003;145(6):1022–1029.

19. Lee TH, Hillis LD, Nabel EG. CABG vs. stenting—clinical implications of the SYNTAX trial. *N Engl J Med.* 2009;360(8):e10.

20. Turi ZG. Optimizing vascular access: routine femoral angiography keeps the vascular complication away. *Catheter Cardiovasc Interv.* 2005; 65(2):203–204.

21. Marcus AJ, Lotzof K, Howard A. Access to the superficial femoral artery in the presence of a "hostile groin": a prospective study. *Cardiovasc Intervent Radiol.* 2007;30(3):351–354.

22. Yeow KM, et al. Sonographically guided antegrade common femoral artery access. *J Ultrasound Med.* 2002;21(12):1413–1416.

23. Grossman PM, et al. Percutaneous coronary intervention complications and guide catheter size: bigger is not better. *JACC Cardiovasc Interv.* 2009;2(7):636–644.

24. Metz D, et al. Comparison of 6F with 7F and 8F guiding catheters for elective coronary angioplasty: results of a prospective, multicenter, randomized trial. *Am Heart J.* 1997;134(1):131–137.

25. Koreny M, et al. Arterial puncture closing devices compared with standard manual compression after cardiac catheterization: systematic review and meta-analysis. *JAMA.* 2004;291(3):350–357.

26. Skillman JJ, Kim D, Baim DS. Vascular complications of percutaneous femoral cardiac interventions. Incidence and operative repair. *Arch Surg.* 1988;123(10):1207–1212.

27. Nasser TK, et al. Peripheral vascular complications following coronary interventional procedures. *Clin Cardiol.* 1995;18(11):609–614.

28. Sheikh KH, et al. Utility of Doppler color flow imaging for identification of femoral arterial complications of cardiac catheterization. *Am Heart J.* 1989;117(3):623–628.

29. Rapoport S, et al. Pseudoaneurysm: a complication of faulty technique in femoral arterial puncture. *Radiology.* 1985;154(2):529–530.

30. Frazee BW, Flaherty JP. Septic endarteritis of the femoral artery following angioplasty. *Rev Infect Dis.* 1991;13(4):620–623.

31. Agarwal R, et al. Clinically guided closure of femoral arterial pseudoaneurysms complicating cardiac catheterization and coronary angioplasty. *Cathet Cardiovasc Diagn.* 1993;30(2):96–100.

32. Kresowik TF, et al. A prospective study of the incidence and natural history of femoral vascular complications after percutaneous transluminal coronary angioplasty. *J Vasc Surg.* 1991;13(2): 328–333, discussion 333–335.

33. Fellmeth BD, et al. Postangiographic femoral artery injuries: nonsurgical repair with US-guided compression. *Radiology.* 1991;178(3):671–675.

34. Sackett WR, et al. Ultrasound-guided thrombin injection of iatrogenic femoral pseudoaneurysms: a prospective analysis. *Am Surg.* 2000;66(10): 937–940, discussion 940–942.

35. Sadiq S, Ibrahim W. Thromboembolism complicating thrombin injection of femoral artery pseudoaneurysm: management with intraarterial thrombolysis. *J Vasc Interv Radiol.* 2001;12(5): 633–636.

36. Witz M, Cohen Y, Lehmann JM. Retroperitoneal haematoma—a serious vascular complication of cardiac catheterisation. *Eur J Vasc Endovasc Surg.* 1999;18(4):364–365.

37. Kent KC, et al. Retroperitoneal hematoma after cardiac catheterization: prevalence, risk factors, and optimal management. *J Vasc Surg.* 1994; 20(6):905–910, discussion 910–913.

38. Farouque HM, et al. Risk factors for the development of retroperitoneal hematoma after percutaneous coronary intervention in the era of glycoprotein IIb/IIIa inhibitors and vascular closure devices. *J Am Coll Cardiol.* 2005;45(3):363–368.

39. Mak GY, et al. Percutaneous treatment of post catheterization massive retroperitoneal hemorrhage. *Cathet Cardiovasc Diagn.* 1993;29(1):40–43.

40. Kent KC, et al. Neuropathy after cardiac catheterization: incidence, clinical patterns, and long-term outcome. *J Vasc Surg.* 1994;19(6):1008–1013, discussion 1013–1014.

41. Kuruvilla A, Kuruttukulam G, Francis B. Femoral neuropathy following cardiac catheterization for balloon mitral valvotomy. *Int J Cardiol.* 1999; 71(2):197–198.

42. Lamar R, Berg R. Rama K. Femoral arteriovenous fistula as a complication of percutaneous transluminal coronary angioplasty: a report of five cases. *Am Surg.* 1990;56(11):702–706.

43. Kelm M, et al. Incidence and clinical outcome of iatrogenic femoral arteriovenous fistulas: implications for risk stratification and treatment. *J Am Coll Cardiol.* 2002;40(2):291–297.

44. Moscucci M, et al. Peripheral vascular complications of directional coronary atherectomy and stenting: predictors, management, and outcome. *Am J Cardiol.* 1994;74(5):448–453.

45. Schaub F, et al. New aspects in ultrasound-guided compression repair of postcatheterization femoral artery injuries. *Circulation.* 1994;90(4):1861–1865.

46. Waigand J, et al. Percutaneous treatment of pseudoaneurysms and arteriovenous fistulas after invasive vascular procedures. *Catheter Cardiovasc Interv.* 1999;47(2):157–164.

47. Toursarkissian B, et al. Spontaneous closure of selected iatrogenic pseudoaneurysms and arteriovenous fistulae. *J Vasc Surg.* 1997;25(5):803–808, discussion 808–809.

48. Kinnaird TD, et al. Incidence, predictors, and prognostic implications of bleeding and blood transfusion following percutaneous coronary interventions. *Am J Cardiol.* 2003;92(8):930–935.

49. Jolly SS, et al. Radial versus femoral access for coronary angiography or intervention and the impact on major bleeding and ischemic events: a systematic review and meta-analysis of randomized trials. *Am Heart J.* 2009;157(1):132–140.

50. Spaulding C, et al. Left radial approach for coronary angiography: results of a prospective study. *Cathet Cardiovasc Diagn.* 1996;39(4):365–370.

51. Brasselet C, et al. Comparison of operator radiation exposure with optimized radiation protection devices during coronary angiograms and ad hoc percutaneous coronary interventions by radial and femoral routes. *Eur Heart J.* 2008;29(1):63–70.

52. Rao SV, et al. Trends in the prevalence and outcomes of radial and femoral approaches to percutaneous coronary intervention: a report from the National Cardiovascular Data Registry. *JACC Cardiovasc Interv.* 2008;1(4):379–386.

53. Ruiz-Salmeron RJ, et al. Assessment of the efficacy of phentolamine to prevent radial artery spasm during cardiac catheterization procedures: a randomized study comparing phentolamine vs. verapamil. *Catheter Cardiovasc Interv.* 2005;66(2):192–198.

54. Dieter RS, Akef A, Wolff M. Eversion endarterectomy complicating radial artery access for left heart catheterization. *Catheter Cardiovasc Interv.* 2003;58(4):478–480.

55. Kiemeneij F. Prevention and management of radial artery spasm. *J Invasive Cardiol.* 2006; 18(4):159–160.

56. Tizon-Marcos H, Barbeau GR. Incidence of compartment syndrome of the arm in a large series of transradial approach for coronary procedures. *J Interv Cardiol.* 2008;21(5):380–384.

57. Lee KL, Miller JG, Laitung G. Hand ischaemia following radial artery cannulation. *J Hand Surg Br.* 1995;20(4):493–495.

58. Wallach SG. Cannulation injury of the radial artery: diagnosis and treatment algorithm. *Am J Crit Care.* 2004;13(4):315–319.

59. Pancholy S, et al. Prevention of radial artery occlusion-patent hemostasis evaluation trial (PROPHET study): a randomized comparison of traditional versus patency documented hemostasis after transradial catheterization. *Catheter Cardiovasc Interv.* 2008;72(3):335–340.

60. Kozak M, et al. Sterile inflammation associated with transradial catheterization and hydrophilic sheaths. *Catheter Cardiovasc Interv.* 2003;59(2):207–213.

61. Popma JJ, et al. Vascular complications after balloon and new device angioplasty. *Circulation.* 1993;88(4, pt 1):1569–1578.

62. Tavris DR, et al. Risk of local adverse events following cardiac catheterization by hemostasis device use and gender. *J Invasive Cardiol.* 2004;16(9):459–464.

63. Mandak JS, et al. Modifiable risk factors for vascular access site complications in the IMPACT II Trial of angioplasty with versus without eptifibatide. Integrilin to Minimize Platelet Aggregation and Coronary Thrombosis. *J Am Coll Cardiol.* 1998;31(7):1518–1524.

64. Blankenship JC, et al. Vascular access site complications after percutaneous coronary intervention with abciximab in the Evaluation of c7E3 for the Prevention of Ischemic Complications (EPIC) trial. *Am J Cardiol.* 1998;81(1):36–40.

65. Friedman HZ, et al. Randomized prospective evaluation of prolonged versus abbreviated intravenous heparin therapy after coronary angioplasty. *J Am Coll Cardiol.* 1994;24(5):1214–1219.

66. Schnyder G, et al. Common femoral artery anatomy is influenced by demographics and comorbidity: implications for cardiac and peripheral invasive studies. *Catheter Cardiovasc Interv.* 2001;53(3):289–295.

67. Kim D, Orron DE, Skillman JJ, et al. Role of superficial femoral artery puncture in the development of pseudoaneurysm and arteriovenous fistula complicating percutaneous transfemoral cardiac catheterization. *Cathet Cardiovasc Diagn.* 1992;25:91

68. Fitts J, et al. Fluoroscopy-guided femoral artery puncture reduces the risk of PCI-related vascular complications. *J Interv Cardiol.* 2008;21(3):273–278.

69. Ward SR, et al. Efficacy and safety of a hemostatic puncture closure device with early ambulation after coronary angiography: Angio-Seal Investigators. *Am J Cardiol.* 1998;81(5):569–572.

70. Gerckens U, et al. Management of arterial puncture site after catheterization procedures: evaluating a suture-mediated closure device. *Am J Cardiol.* 1999;83(12):1658–1663.

71. Cura FA, et al. Safety of femoral closure devices after percutaneous coronary interventions in the era of glycoprotein IIb/IIIa platelet blockade. *Am J Cardiol.* 2000;86(7):780–782, A9.

72. Nikolsky E, et al. Vascular complications associated with arteriotomy closure devices in patients undergoing percutaneous coronary procedures: a meta-analysis. *J Am Coll Cardiol.* 2004;44(6):1200–1209.

73. Sanborn TA, et al. Impact of femoral vascular closure devices and antithrombotic therapy on access site bleeding in acute coronary syndromes: The Acute Catheterization and Urgent Intervention Triage Strategy (ACUITY) trial. *Circ Cardiovasc Interv.* 2010;3(1):57–62.

74. Bangalore S, Arora N, Resnic FS. Vascular closure device failure: frequency and implications: a propensity-matched analysis. *Circ Cardiovasc Interv.* 2009;2(6):549–556.

75. McGee DC, Gould MK. Preventing complications of central venous catheterization. *N Engl J Med.* 2003;348(12):1123–1133.

76. Sznajder JI, et al. Central vein catheterization: failure and complication rates by three percutaneous approaches. *Arch Intern Med.* 1986;146(2):259–261.

77. Merrer J, et al. Complications of femoral and subclavian venous catheterization in critically ill patients: a randomized controlled trial. *JAMA.* 2001;286(6):700–707.

78. Teichgraber UK, et al. A sonographically guided technique for central venous access. *AJR Am J Roentgenol.* 1997;169(3):731–733.

79. Randolph AG, et al. Ultrasound guidance for placement of central venous catheters: a meta-analysis of the literature. *Crit Care Med.* 1996;24(12):2053–2058.

80. Fraizer MC, et al. Use of a percutaneous vascular suture device for closure of an inadvertent subclavian artery puncture. *Catheter Cardiovasc Interv.* 2003;59(3):369–371.

81. Tran V, et al. Use of the StarClose device for closure of inadvertent subclavian artery punctures. *Ann Vasc Surg.* 2009;23(5):688.e11–688.e13.

82. Dowling K, et al. Use of a collagen plug device to seal a subclavian artery puncture secondary to intraarterial dialysis catheter placement. *J Vasc Interv Radiol.* 1999;10(1):33–35.

83. Gowda S, et al. Incidence of new focal pulmonary emboli after routine cardiac catheterization comparing the brachial to the femoral approach. *Cathet Cardiovasc Diagn.* 1984;10(2):157–161.

84. Kasirajan K, Gray B, Ouriel K. Percutaneous AngioJet thrombectomy in the management of extensive deep venous thrombosis. *J Vasc Interv Radiol.* 2001;12(2):179–185.

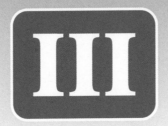
Specific Complications of Coronary Interventions

15

Coronary Dissection, Side Branch Occlusion, and Abrupt Closure

MAURICIO G. COHEN AND JOSEPH S. ROSSI

T he introduction of drug-eluting stents (DESs) has led to markedly improved patency rates for complex percutaneous coronary interventions (PCIs). Consequently, more operators are choosing to perform PCI on complex lesions, thereby increasing the overall risk profile of the PCI patient population. Although restenosis is often a primary consideration when contemplating an interventional strategy, it is also a treatable and usually stable complication of PCI. Abrupt vessel closure, coronary artery dissection, and side branch occlusions are more likely to cause myocardial necrosis, which is directly correlated with long-term survival (1). However, the risk of these complications is not usually foremost in the mind of the operator. In this chapter, we will focus on these important complications of coronary intervention, with an emphasis on prevention strategies and therapeutic options.

■ IDENTIFICATION OF HIGH-RISK PATIENTS

After balloon angioplasty became a commonly performed procedure in the early 1990s, retrospective reviews of procedural complications suggested that the angiographic characteristics of coronary lesions were powerful predictors of adverse outcomes, most importantly periprocedural myocardial infarction (MI) and emergency coronary artery bypass grafting (CABG). The most consistent, powerful indicators of abrupt closure and acute MI were stenosis severity and lesion morphology (2,3). Specific lesion characteristics were found to be associated with abrupt closure, which occurred in 3% to 5% of procedures in the balloon angioplasty era (2,4,5). Early American College of Cardiology/ American Heart Association guidelines reflected these concerns and recommended increased caution in patients with high-degree stenoses, heavily calcified, diffuse, or tortuous lesions. Early risk stratification was described using the "A–B–C" classification. Type A lesions were focal without complex characteristics, Type B lesions were of moderate complexity, and Type C classification was reserved for total occlusions or lesions that were diffuse in nature or heavily calcified or angulated. This initial classification system allowed operators to accurately describe coronary lesions and appropriately discuss the procedural risks with the patient prior to intervention. However, as operators became more proficient and complication rates dropped significantly, particularly in the stent era, it is now recognized that risk stratification is also changing. Specifically, there has been a marked decrease in postprocedural dissection and abrupt closure due to stent implantation. As a result, main vessel patency rates have continued to improve. In the modern era, there is now an increased focus on the treatment of complex lesions, including diffuse lesions, heavily calcified lesions, lesions with side branch involvement, and bifurcation lesions.

The most recent ACC/AHA guidelines for coronary revascularization no longer reference the A–B–C classification that was based on previous studies of balloon angioplasty. Instead, the current guidelines focus on "high-risk" angiographic features that are described in

TABLE 15-1 Angiographic Risk Assessment

Low Risk	Moderate Risk	High Risk
Discrete (length <10 mm)	Tubular (length 10–20 mm)	Diffuse (length >20 mm)
Concentric	Eccentric	Excessive tortuosity of proximal segment
Readily accessible	Moderate tortuosity of proximal segment	Extremely angulated segments >90 degree
Nonangulated segment (<45 degree)	Moderately angulated segment (>45 degree, <90 degree)	Total occlusions >3 months old and/or bridging collaterals
Smooth contour	Irregular contour	Inability to protect major side branches
Little or no calcification	Moderate or heavy calcification	Degenerated vein grafts with friable lesions
Less than totally occlusive	Total occlusions <3 months old	
Not ostial in location	Ostial in location	
No major side branch involvement	Bifurcation lesions requiring double guidewires	
Absence of thrombus	Some thrombus present	

Table 15-1 (6). There has been a precipitous drop in the rate of emergency CABG following PCI, and this is likely due to increased operator experience in the high-volume stent era and improved recognition of high-risk angiographic features (7). In general, mortality after PCI is highly correlated to baseline comorbidities rather than angiographic factors. Increasing age and baseline renal insufficiency are particularly important predictors of death following PCI (8). Nonetheless, angiographic predictors of adverse outcomes are well defined and remain an important component of complete risk stratification. Inability to protect a major side branch can lead to MI, and highly angulated and complex lesions are more likely to result in dissection and closure. The highest risk of MI continues to be intervention on degenerated saphenous vein grafts, and the treatment of this particular disease is discussed in detail elsewhere.

■ CLINICAL FACTORS ASSOCIATED WITH COMPLICATIONS OF PCI

It is now well recognized that clinical factors are strongly associated with the risk of adverse events following PCI. The exact mechanism by which some factors increase risk is not exactly understood, but it is likely that some features, such as increased age and renal insufficiency, increase the risk of postprocedural bleeding, which has been associated with increased risk of death (see Chapter 14 for discussion of bleeding complications of PCI). Clinical presentation with unstable features, such as congestive heart failure and acute MI, significantly increase the risk of 30-day mortality following PCI, perhaps by identifying patient subsets with large amounts of injured myocardium who are at increased risk of death from heart failure or sudden cardiac death. Elevated levels of cardiac biomarkers, such as C-reactive protein and interleukin 6, are also associated with poor prognosis (9,10).

Although it is unclear how these clinical predictors are related to mechanical complications of PCI, this association may be partially explained by thrombosis. In particular, increasing age and renal insufficiency may increase the risk of thrombotic events after PCI, which may manifest as side branch occlusion or main vessel closure. These vulnerable populations may also be predisposed to intimal injury if they present with more advanced disease and high-risk features such as calcification, tortuosity, and diffuse stenosis. Clinical predictors may therefore translate into morphologic complexity, increasing the risk of coronary dissection, side branch occlusion, and acute closure.

SIDE BRANCH OCCLUSION

There is much controversy surrounding the management of side branches at the time of PCI. Although there is no evidence that side branch intervention improves clinical outcomes, every operator has clinical experience suggesting that side branch occlusions can be clinically important and problematic, and significant cardiac enzyme level elevation following PCI has been associated with poor prognosis. Complications can range from minor chest pain and/or mild cardiac enzyme level elevation to transmural MI and cardiogenic shock. It is imperative that all side branches be evaluated carefully and appropriate precautions be taken to prevent acute closure. In the case of significant side branch occlusion, there are several techniques that can be considered for salvage. However, prevention of side branch occlusion should be foremost in the mind of the operator.

Risk Factors for Side Branch Occlusion

Common sense dictates that larger side branches should be protected, whereas small side branches are likely clinically insignificant and can be safely occluded without consequence. The natural history of side branch occlusion following stent placement is controversial. However, previous studies have suggested that a large portion remain patent on follow-up angiography at 6 months after PCI (11–14). Factors associated with the increased risk of side branch occlusion include severe ostial stenosis and large volume of plaque at the treated site. In an early study comparing different bare metal stents, Cho and colleagues found that only the degree of stenosis within a side branch was predictive of side branch patency after 6 months (15). Percutaneous transluminal coronary angioplasty (PTCA) and stent placement likely result in a "snowplow" effect that causes plaque shifting into a diseased segment (Fig. 15-1) and that is more common after high-pressure postdilation (16). Overlapping stents in the main vessel have been found to be associated with increased occlusion rates of side branches. In the TAXUS-V trial, paclitaxel-eluting stent use was associated with an increased incidence of non–Q-wave MI at 30 days (8.3% vs. 3.3%; $P = .047$), in comparison with bare metal stents. Blinded core laboratory angiographic analysis in patients who received more than one stent demonstrated more frequent occurrence of side branch flow compromise and complete occlusion. It was speculated that side branch compromise was caused by the thicker polymer-coated stent struts (17). As a general principle, the operator should avoid overlapping either bare metal or DESs at the origin of side branches because of higher chance of side branch occlusion and difficulty for reaccessing the vessel in case of need of rescue.

A study examined the fractional flow reserve (FFR) across 97 "stent-jailed" side branches of more than 2.0 mm diameter. None of the side branches with stenoses less than 75% severity had a FFR less than 0.75. Only a third of side branches with stenosis 75% or more had a FFR less than 0.75. This study highlights the lack of correlation between "jailed" side branch stenosis

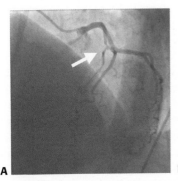 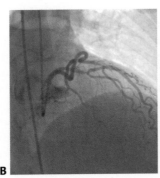 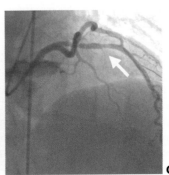

FIGURE 15-1. Severe, eccentric septal side branch stenosis and occlusion after stent placement. (**A**) Eccentric septal stenosis. (**B**) Orthogonal view prior to percutaneous transluminal coronary angioplasty. (**C**) Occlusion after stent placement.

severity and physiologic relevance and therefore suggests that FFR assessment should be considered before treatment of a "jailed" side branch (18). With side branches of less than 2.0 mm diameter, particularly those that perfuse a small territory of myocardium, conservative management is generally recommended to preserve an optimal main branch result.

Prevention of Side Branch Occlusion

The BBC-ONE trial evaluated two separate strategies for side branch stenoses. Patients were randomized to a strategy of provisional versus planned side branch intervention. Patients who received only main branch stenting followed by provisional side branch intervention based on FFR had decreased risk of MI and target vessel revascularization at 9 months (19). Other randomized clinical trials have evaluated strategies of provisional versus planned side branch intervention, and the results have generally favored the strategy of single stent placement with provisional side branch intervention. A recent retrospective analysis suggested that when controlling for patient factors, there is no difference in clinical outcomes between the two strategies (20).

Recent clinical trial data have resulted in a general consensus that complex interventions are associated with increased risk of early mortality, restenosis, and late stent thrombosis. A recent meta-analysis of randomized trials evaluating simple versus complex strategies of revascularization with DESs found that simple strategies were associated with similar restenosis and lower early mortality compared with planned complex intervention (21). However, a uniform strategy of main vessel intervention only should not be recommended for all patients, as this has been associated with increased risk of large periprocedural MI (22). Instead, it is the responsibility of the operator to develop a strategy for each individual patient, with the understanding that provisional side branch stenting is feasible in most cases. For complex bifurcation lesions where the side branch requires intervention, an experienced interventionalist should have several strategies in mind to obtain an acceptable result.

Rotational atherectomy is an attractive adjunct to balloon dilation for lesions with large, diseased side branches. Rotational atherectomy is thought to cause "plaque modification" that debulks the ostial side branch, thereby increasing the patency rate following main vessel stenting (23). Most experience with this technique is anecdotal, and it requires operator proficiency with rotational atherectomy and appropriate patient selection. The largest study of a debulking strategy for bifurcation lesions was performed in the era of balloon angioplasty and demonstrated improved acute results and improved long-term patency (24). It is unknown whether these results would be replicated in the era of DESs. Most centers now perform rotational atherectomy only in selected cases where there is high likelihood that a stent would not be expanded optimally in a highly calcified vessel. In general, increased burr:artery ratios (>0.8) should be avoided, as this is thought to increase the risk of vessel perforation (see Chapter 16). Rotational atherectomy should not be performed after predilation unless intravascular ultrasound (IVUS) suggests absence of dissection.

Kissing balloon inflations are recommended for the treatment of hemodynamically significant side branch lesions following main vessel PCI. This technique can now be performed with low-profile balloons through a 6F or 7F system and requires accurate estimation of the main vessel diameter and effective balloon size in the proximal vessel. This can be determined by calculating the square root of the sum of the squares of the individual balloon diameters (25). For quick reference, Figure 15-2 displays the estimated diameter reached in the parent vessel by kissing inflation of the most used balloon combinations in the main and side branches. Underestimation of the effective parent-vessel balloon diameter can lead to dissection or perforation, and care should be taken to perform a safe but effective terminal kissing inflation. The use of kissing inflation is controversial, particularly for small side branches that supply relatively small areas of myocardium. Kissing inflations are generally recommended for all large side branches and true bifurcations lesions, particularly when two stents are deployed. In cases where a single stent is used, the primary objective should be to maintain main vessel patency, and kissing balloon inflation can be avoided if the main vessel result is satisfactory and there is TIMI 3 flow in the side branch. Dedicated bifurcation stent designs are cur-

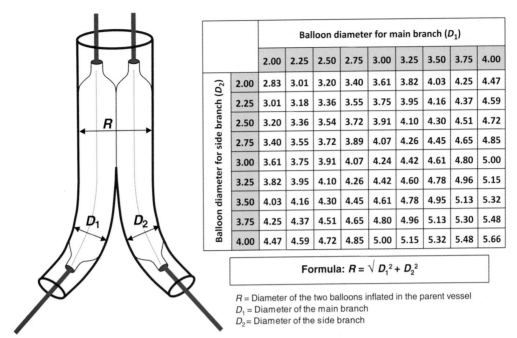

		Balloon diameter for main branch (D_1)								
		2.00	2.25	2.50	2.75	3.00	3.25	3.50	3.75	4.00
Balloon diameter for side branch (D_2)	2.00	2.83	3.01	3.20	3.40	3.61	3.82	4.03	4.25	4.47
	2.25	3.01	3.18	3.36	3.55	3.75	3.95	4.16	4.37	4.59
	2.50	3.20	3.36	3.54	3.72	3.91	4.10	4.30	4.51	4.72
	2.75	3.40	3.55	3.72	3.89	4.07	4.26	4.45	4.65	4.85
	3.00	3.61	3.75	3.91	4.07	4.24	4.42	4.61	4.80	5.00
	3.25	3.82	3.95	4.10	4.26	4.42	4.60	4.78	4.96	5.15
	3.50	4.03	4.16	4.30	4.45	4.61	4.78	4.95	5.13	5.32
	3.75	4.25	4.37	4.51	4.65	4.80	4.96	5.13	5.30	5.48
	4.00	4.47	4.59	4.72	4.85	5.00	5.15	5.32	5.48	5.66

Formula: $R = \sqrt{D_1{}^2 + D_2{}^2}$

R = Diameter of the two balloons inflated in the parent vessel
D_1 = Diameter of the main branch
D_2 = Diameter of the side branch

FIGURE 15-2. Quick reference for effective diameter estimation of the parent vessel prior to kissing balloon inflation. (Adapted from Morino Y, Yamamoto H, Mitsudo K, et al. Functional formula to determine adequate balloon diameter of simultaneous kissing balloon technique for treatment of bifurcated coronary lesions: clinical validation by volumetric intravascular ultrasound analysis. *Circ J.* 2008;72:886–892.)

rently available for clinical use outside of the United States, and multiple new stent designs are undergoing clinical investigation. Preliminary data are encouraging (26).

Side Branch Occlusion: Rescue

Wire trapping has been advocated by some operators as a method to maintain side branch patency during stent inflation in the main vessel. The trapped coronary wire may prevent complete occlusion of the side branch and provide a marker for the placement of a separate coronary wire through the stent struts for balloon inflation in the case of a significant side branch stenosis following PCI. This technique is widely practiced, particularly outside of the United States. The risk of permanent wire entrapment is very small, and almost all 0.014 wires can be easily removed from the native vessel after stent placement. In general, high-pressure initial inflations should be avoided to decrease the risk of wire entrapment in calcified plaque, and coated wires should not be used. For cases where the side branch is a large vessel that requires protection, the trapping of a guidewire during main-vessel stenting allows the operator the option of per-

forming a "rescue reverse crush" if unable to advance a wire through the struts of the main vessel (27). This technique involves advancing a small balloon (1.5–2.0 mm) along the side branch wire that has been trapped by the main vessel stent. Inflation of the low-profile balloon allows for a channel through which a larger diameter balloon can be advanced to crush the main vessel stent and allow for placement of a stent into the side branch. The crushed main vessel stent is then opened with a kissing balloon.

There is an increased risk of side branch occlusion following stent implantation compared with balloon angioplasty, due to the snowplow effect of the stent struts, causing the plaque shift into the ostium of the side branch (16). This is more likely to occur when the ostium of the side branch has angiographic evidence of severe stenosis. In the event of inadvertent side branch occlusion, recovery through the deployed stent can often be accomplished with a standard 0.014-in guidewire. If this is not successful, a hydrophilic wire can be used with or without balloon support. A small-diameter balloon may be needed to cross the stent struts overlying the occluded side branch. In cases where multiple

TABLE 15-2	**Clinical Features Associated with Side Branch Occlusion and Suggested Prophylactic Techniques**
Clinical Feature	Useful Techniques
Ostial side branch stenosis	Side branch balloon angioplasty before main vessel stenting, consider rescue for larger branches
Large plaque volume in main vessel	Consider rotational atherectomy
In stent-restenosis of main branch	Consider rotational atherectomy
Main branch dissection after initial balloon inflation	Hydrophilic wire to rescue side branch followed by balloon angioplasty and stenting of main branch
Large side branch occlusion after PCI	Consider wire trapping and rescue-reverse crush

PCI, percutaneous coronary intervention.

wires have been attempted without success, reinflation of the main vessel stent may open further the struts and change the geometry of the occlusion, thereby allowing recovery. This should be attempted only as a "last resort," as this technique can also result in further plaque shift into the side branch and make recovery less likely. Table 15-2 displays a summary of recommendations for side branch rescue in different clinical scenarios.

Side Branch Occlusion: Conclusions

In general, planned side branch intervention should be considered for large arteries (>2.0 mm) where the ostium of the side branch arises from the stenotic segment of the main branch or when the ostium of the side branch itself is severely diseased. For smaller side branches, the clinical consequences of closure may be negligible, and intervention may need to be avoided to preserve the angiographic result of the main vessel intervention. Many side branches open spontaneously after initial closure as evidenced by retrospective analysis of serial angiograms (28). Intervention is generally recommended only when the amount of myocardium at risk is deemed to be of clinical importance.

■ CORONARY DISSECTION

In the modern stent era, there has been a decrease in coronary perforation and emergency CABG as operator techniques and equipment have improved (7). However, as interventional cardiologists continue to treat high-risk patients, coronary dissection will continue to occur, both before and after stent placement. Although the incidence of coronary artery dissection requir-

ing emergency surgery in the stent era is less than 0.2% (29), it remains imperative that this complication be recognized during the initial procedure, as early treatment improves vessel patency and patient outcomes. Coronary dissection resulting from balloon angioplasty was described with comprehensive morphology criteria in the balloon angioplasty era, and these criteria were used to determine risk of closure and to determine appropriate therapies (30). After the development of intracoronary stents, postballoon angioplasty dissection is usually treated effectively, and it is not present at the end of most interventions. However, the classic Type A–F classification remains useful to describe the severity of luminal injury (Table 15-3).

In the modern era, there are generally three causes of iatrogenic coronary dissection, localized guide catheter–induced dissection, spiral dissection, and stent edge dissection. Proper treatment requires angiographic and IVUS imaging coupled with appropriate intervention to avoid progression and maintain vessel patency.

Guide Catheter Dissection

Guide catheter dissection is seen in less than 1% of PCIs. A number of factors have been reported to increase the risk of guide catheter dissection, and a recent review by Boyle and colleagues is summarized in Table 15-4 (31). Generally, guide catheter dissection is often associated with deep-seating of large catheters into smaller, diseased arteries. Proximal dissection can cause acute closure and is the most common indication for emergency surgery during PCI. If localized dissections are noticed

TABLE 15-3	National Heart, Lung and Blood Institute Morphologic Classification of Coronary Dissections
Classification	Description
Type A	Minor radiolucent areas in the lumen without impairment of flow or persistent dye staining after contrast runoff
Type B	Luminal flap that is radiolucent and that runs parallel to the vessel wall with contrast injection but without impairment of flow or persistent dye staining after contrast runoff
Type C	Contrast appears outside of the vessel lumen as an "extraluminal cap." The staining appears even after contrast clears the lumen
Type D	Spiral radiolucent luminal filling defects. Often persistent staining after contrast clears from the vessel.
Type E	New and persistent filling defects in the vessel lumen.
Type F	Lesions that progress to impaired flow or total occlusion.

(Adapted from Huber MS, Mooney JF, Madison J, Mooney MR. Use of a morphologic classification to predict clinical outcome after dissection from coronary angioplasty. *Am J Cardiol.* 1991;68:467–471.)

early, conservative management has been reported to be successful in some instances (32). However, stenting of the affected segment can prevent migration of the intimal flap and prevent closure and should be the preferred method of treatment when it can be accomplished safely. Left main coronary artery (LMCA) dissection can result in cardiovascular collapse; however, there have been case reports of successful LMCA stenting during cardiac arrest with reperfusion and survival with good outcome. Similarly, CABG has been performed with excellent results (33). When left main dissection is recognized, immediate deployment of coronary guidewires into the major bifurcation vessels of the LMCA should be attempted. If the true lumen cannot be wired, a different catheter curve is generally recommended. After protecting the left circumflex and left anterior descending artery, an angiogram should be performed to assess for propagation. If flow is not compromised, the ramus intermedius should be also protected if it is a large vessel (>2.5 mm). For localized LMCA dissection, a single stent should be placed with the intention of covering the entire abnormal segment. If the dissection flap has propagated into a major branch artery, a stent should be placed directly into that artery while protecting the other major arteries with guidewires. After stenting all affected territories, repeat angiography

should be performed in multiple views to assess for progression prior to guidewire removal.

Spiral Dissection

Spiral dissection is fortunately a rare occurrence in contemporary PCI. The etiology of spiral dissection is controversial, and it is possible that this rare entity is more common among patients with connective tissue disease. Spontaneous coronary dissection is a rare event but is likely responsible for a small percentage of sudden cardiac deaths and acute coronary syndromes. Iatrogenic coronary dissection is much more common. In some

TABLE 15-4	Factors Associated with Guide Catheter Dissection	
Definite	Possible
Left main coronary stenosis	Catheter manipulation
Amplatz guide catheters	Vigorous contrast injections
Acute myocardial infarction	Deep intubation Variant anatomy of coronary ostia Vigorous, deep inspiration

(Adapted from Boyle AJ, Chan M, Dib J, Resar J. Catheter-induced coronary artery dissection: risk factors, prevention and management. *J Invasive Cardiol.* 2006;18:500–503.)

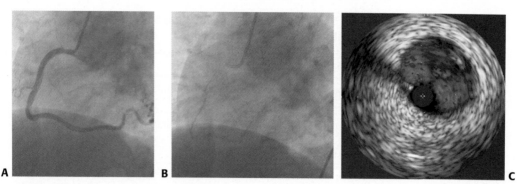

FIGURE 15-3. Angiographic appearance of a Type D spiral dissection, during and after contrast injection. Intravascular ultrasound (IVUS) images show the true and false lumen. (**A**) A thin spiral dissection line can be visualized throughout the length of the vessel. (**B**) False lumen staining becomes apparent after injection of contrast. (**C**) IVUS demonstration of true and false lumen. It can be noticed that the IVUS catheter is located in the false lumen. (See color insert.)

cases, spiral dissection may result from forceful injection of contrast into an unrecognized tissue plane following catheter induced injury. This phenomenon is fortunately rare and, when noted, should be treated with immediate advancement of a coronary wire into the true lumen to protect the distal vessel. Rapid stenting can prevent distal propagation and side branch occlusion and is necessary to preserve distal flow. Figures 15-3 and 15-4 show cases in which aggressive cannulation of the right coronary artery caused large spiral dissections with inability to regain access into

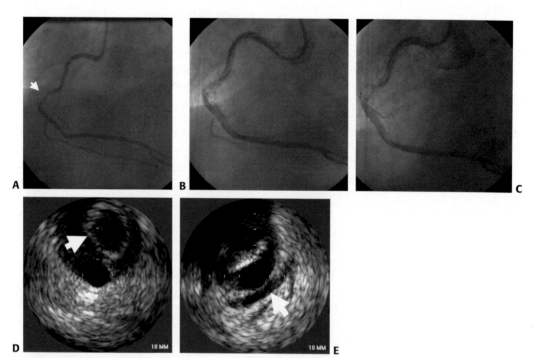

FIGURE 15-4. Spiral dissection caused by aggressive manipulation of a guiding catheter. (**A**) Diagnostic right coronary contrast injection demonstrates a severe stenosis in the mid-vessel (*arrow*). (**B**) Aggressive manipulation of an Amplatz guiding-catheter caused a spiral dissection that extended throughout the length of the vessel. (**C**) The true lumen could not be wired despite exchanging the guiding catheter for a Judkins right shape. (**D**) The round shape in the IVUS indicates that the wire and catheter were in the false lumen. (**E**) The true lumen (*arrow*) is compressed by the false lumen.

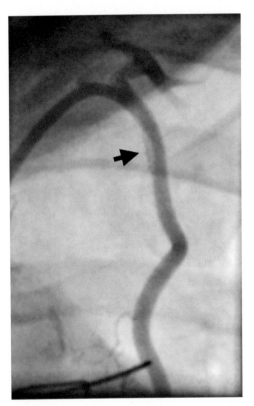

FIGURE 15-5. Proximal dissection of a left internal mammary artery caused by aggressive manipulation of a 0.035-in guidewire.

the true lumen. Careless manipulation of the 0.035-in. guidewire can also result in dissection of either proximal coronary vessels or left internal mammary grafts, as depicted in Figure 15-5.

IVUS imaging has an important role in the management of spiral dissection, as it can confirm whether the guidewire has entered true lumen or the false lumen during advancement through the dissection planes (see Fig. 15-4).

Stenting of the entire dissected segment has been performed with good angiographic result; however, this approach is likely to result in side branch occlusion. Figure 15-6 illustrates a case of guiding-catheter–induced occlusive dissection of the left circumflex coronary artery that was successfully managed with stent placement. It is generally accepted that stenting can result in scaffolding of the involved segment and support vessel patency while preventing progression. For cases where stent delivery is not possible, advancement of a balloon perfusion catheter into the distal dissection can maintain coronary perfusion until surgical intervention is performed. Unfortunately because of their relatively rare use in the current era, many laboratories do not currently stock perfusion balloons, and prolonged, conventional balloon inflation may be the only available option to prevent distal propagation

There have been case reports of proximal propagation of a dissection into the ascending aorta. This is a rare complication with an incidence of 0.02% of cardiac catheterization procedures but can result in catastrophic outcomes. The management of this complication depends on the extension of the dissection. Isolated involvement of the ipsilateral

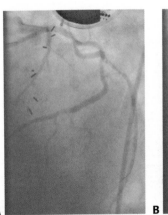
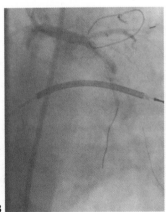
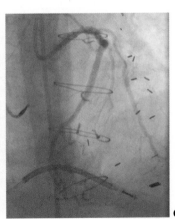

FIGURE 15-6. Guide catheter-induced coronary dissection and treatment with stent placement. (**A**) Cranial left anterior oblique image showing the aggressive selective cannulation of the left circumflex coronal artery with an extra backup catheter. (**B**) Occlusive dissection and contrast staining in the left circumflex in right anterior oblique. Note that the wire position was preserved throughout the case. (**C**) Final result with complete restoration of flow after stent placement.

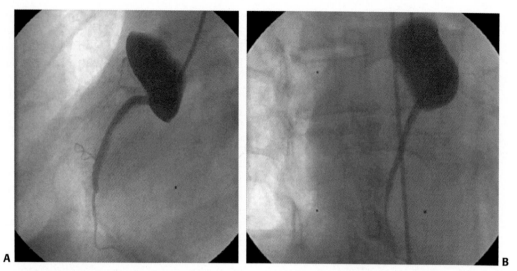

FIGURE 15-7. Guiding-catheter dissection of the right coronary ostium extending into sinus of Valsalva and the aortic root. Orthogonal views obtained with a biplane angiographic equipment show a large dissection of the right sinus of Valsalva. The patient presented clinical instability with hypotension and severe chest pain and was immediately referred for surgical repair of the aortic root.

cusp or extension into the aortic root of less than 4 cm can be conservatively managed with stenting of the coronary ostium and close observation. Dissections extending more than 4 cm into the aortic root require surgical intervention. Conditions predisposing to iatrogenic aortic dissection include hypertension, Marfan syndrome, congenitally unicuspid and bicuspid aortic valves, and cystic medial necrosis (34). Figures 15-7 and 15-8 display two cases of coronary dissection extending into the right and left sinuses of Valsalva, respectively.

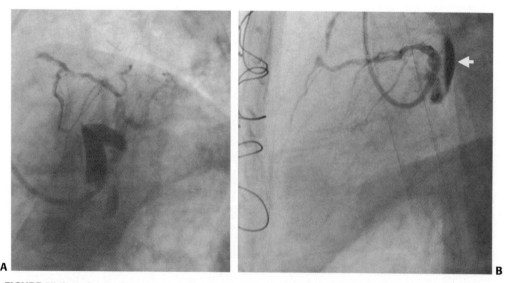

FIGURE 15-8. Left main dissection extending into the left coronary and noncoronary aortic cusps. (**A**) Left main dissection extending into the aortic cusps caused by aggressive manipulation of the guiding catheter to place a stent in a diffusely diseased left anterior descending artery. (**B**) Final angiographic images after a stent was placed in the left main coronary artery, sealing the dissection. The patient remained stable throughout the procedure. The *arrow* indicates residual contrast staining in the ipsilateral coronary cusp in a straight lateral view.

Edge Dissection Following Stent Placement

Post-PCI stent edge dissection is a common finding on IVUS, with a reported incidence of approximately 10% based on cases series from the early stent era (5%–23% based on abstract references in the ACC/AHA guidelines) (35,36). A recent large series by Liu et al. described the incidence of stent edge dissection among 977 native arteries treated with DES implantation. They found the overall incidence of edge dissection to be 8.4% and evenly distributed between the proximal and distal stent edge (37). The exact mechanism of stent edge dissection is unknown, but it has been hypothesized that a false lumen is created after intimal disruption from stent struts deployed at relatively high pressure (36). The natural history of stent edge dissection is somewhat controversial. Data from the early stent era suggest that many cases of localized dissections heal without consequence and are not associated with increased risk of adverse events (36). These data conflicts somewhat with published case series suggesting that coronary dissection can be seen in many cases of acute stent thrombosis. In a seminal series of 53 cases of early stent thrombosis from the Predic-

tors and Outcomes of Stent Thrombosis (POST) registry, Uren and colleagues found that 94% of cases had at least one abnormality on IVUS, and dissection was seen in 26%, as displayed in Figure 15-9 (35).

When a localized proximal dissection is seen and there is no flow limitation, the risk of acute closure is probably small. However, serial angiography more than 30 days after initial stent implantation has suggested that these areas of localized vessel trauma can be associated with restenosis in DESs (38). Distal edge dissections, which can propagate and result in acute vessel closure, are also associated with increased risk of restenosis. It is now common to perform IVUS on all suspected cases of edge dissection and to treat most dissections with an additional stent if technically feasible. Figure 15-10 illustrates the IVUS confirmation of a proximal edge dissection after stent placement. The risk of restenosis associated with segmental stenting of localized dissections should be weighed against the long-term risk of stent thrombosis when multiple stents are used, particularly first-generation DESs. Small, limited dissections can probably be managed conservatively with good results in selected cases. Table 15-5 summarizes suggested

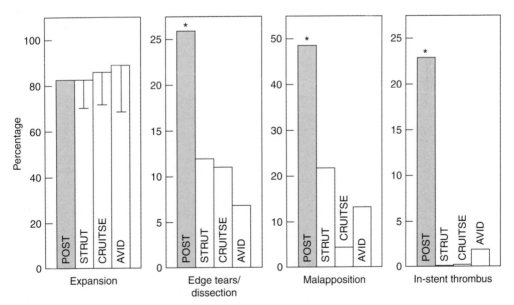

FIGURE 15-9. Etiology of acute stent thrombosis. AVID, Angiography Versus Intravascular ultrasound Directed stent placement; POST, Predictors and Outcomes of Stent Thrombosis; CRUISE, Can Routine Ultrasound Influence Stent Expansion?; STRUT, Stent Treatment Region assessed by Ultrasound Tomography; *p < 0.05 vs STRUT, CRUISE, and AVID. (From Uren NG, Schwarzacher SP, Metz JA, et al. Predictors and outcomes of stent thrombosis: an intravascular ultrasound registry. *Eur Heart J.* 2002;23(2):124–132, by permission of Oxford University Press.)

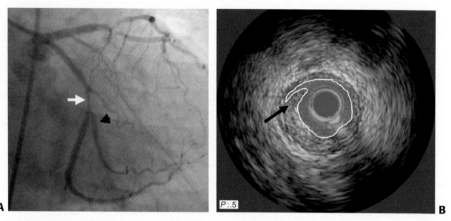

FIGURE 15-10. Stent edge dissection with intravascular ultrasound imaging. (**A**) A narrowed segment (*white arrow*) in the main left circumflex became apparent after placement of a stent in a moderate-sized second obtuse marginal branch (*black arrow*). (**B**) Intravascular ultrasound demonstrated the presence of a proximal edge stent dissection (*arrow*) that was treated with placement of an additional stent. (See color insert.)

interventions for the management of different types of dissections.

ABRUPT CLOSURE

Acute vessel closure from mechanical complication following PCI should be differentiated from the "no-reflow" phenomenon, which is usually associated with distal embolization or microvascular occlusion (39). This topic is discussed in detail in Chapter 17. Like no-reflow, mechanical acute vessel closure at the site of PCI results in acute ischemia that can lead to myocardial injury, cardiogenic shock, and death. Fortunately, the incidence of closure in the modern era is very low due to improved antiplatelet and anticoagulation therapies and the use of intracoronary stents. The primary responsibility of the interventional cardiologist is to differentiate between medical and mechanical factors leading to acute vessel closure. All patients should be expected to be free of angina following coronary intervention, and early chest pain postprocedure should suggest acute vessel closure until proven otherwise. Chest pain following coronary intervention has been shown to

TABLE 15-5 **Coronary Dissection Type and Suggested Interventions**

Dissection Type	Interventions
Guide catheter dissection	Protect main branches
	Avoid repeat contrast injections until distal stent is placed
	Cover injured segment with stent
	Assess for propagation
	Consider switching to a different guiding catheter curve if unable to wire true lumen
Spiral dissection	Wire main branches
	Stent distal edge first to minimize propagation
	Cover entire involved segment
Stent edge dissection	IVUS to assess stent deployment
	Consider stenting if tissue flap is apparent on IVUS or for any flow limitation
	Conservative management for small, localized dissections when additional stent is contraindicated

IVUS, intravenous ultrasound.

TABLE 15-6 **Causes of Abrupt Closure and Treatments Available**

Cause	Treatment
No-reflow	1. Confirm effective anticoagulation 2. Consider intracoronary adenosine 3. Consider 2b3a inhibitor
Dissection	1. Repeat PTCA 2. IVUS to confirm presence and extent of dissection
Acute Thrombosis	1. Confirm effective anticoagulation 2. Administer 2b3a inhibitor 3. Repeat PTCA 4. IVUS to confirm stent apposition and rule out dissection

PTCA, percutaneous transluminal coronary angioplasty; IVUS, intravenous ultrasound.

be the strongest predictor of large creatine kinase-myocardial band level elevation (40).

The incidence of acute closure following PCI prior to the widespread use of intracoronary stents was approximately 5% (41). This was usually due to PTCA-induced dissection. Routine IVUS imaging of coronary lesions following PCI has previously suggested a very high rate of undiagnosed dissection, and this finding has been associated with a fivefold increase in abrupt closure (2). For patients in whom stent placement is not possible for technical reasons, careful technique can minimize the risk of dissection and closure. Slow balloon inflation and stepwise increases in balloon diameter may help to avoid unnecessary trauma. Most importantly, observation of the treated vessel for at least 10 minutes after final balloon inflation is warranted to rule out flow-limiting dissection. If dissection is present and surgery is required to restore flow, a balloon perfusion catheter can be advanced into the distal vessel to provide limited coronary perfusion and minimize ischemia prior to CABG. Prolonged balloon inflations with perfusion catheters have also been shown to reverse abrupt closure (42).

Similar to dissection, the presence of post-procedure thrombus is highly correlated with acute vessel closure. The role of acute thrombus formation in acute closure is also supported by the decreased incidence of ischemic complications in patients receiving intravenous glycoprotein 2b3a inhibitors during PCI. In addition, patients who receive subtherapeutic anticoagulation, as evidenced by low Activated Clotting Time (ACT) values during the procedure, have also been shown to have an increased

risk of acute closure. In general, for patients receiving 2b3a inhibitors, a target ACT of greater than 200 seconds is recommended. For patients who receive heparin only, a target ACT of 250 is likely to prevent acute thrombus formation within the treated artery and on or within the interventional equipment (43).

Control of anticoagulation is of paramount importance to avoid thrombotic occlusion of the stented artery. Anticoagulation is most important at the time of PCI, when interventional equipment including guide catheters, guidewires, stents, and balloons provide a nidus for clot formation. Heparin dosing is unreliable, particularly in chronically ill patients and those with low or high body weight. ACT should be measured at intervals of 30 minutes to avoid over- and underdosing. For patients who receive weight-based bivalirudin infusion, ACT should be measured with 10 minutes of the infusion and initial bolus to confirm appropriate drug delivery. Newer agents under development have the potential to provide more reliable anticoagulation during PCI, which should help to decrease the incidence of both thrombotic and hemorrhagic complications (44). Table 15-6 outlines different management strategies for different suspected causes of abrupt closure.

■ CONCLUSIONS

Contemporary PCI is associated with a relatively low risk of dissection, closure, and side branch occlusion. Randomized trials have not provided good evidence for blanket recommendations, and the avoidance of these feared complications of PCI is best accomplished by operator experience and appropriate preventive techniques. For cases of coronary dissection, the long-term patency of modern stents suggests that diseased segments should be treated with a stent to prevent progression and avoid abrupt closure. Side branch occlusion can be avoided in most cases with proper risk stratification and pretreatment, but when it occurs, treatment should be based on the amount of myocardium in jeopardy and the relative size of the side branch and main branch vessel. Abrupt closure is rare in the modern era. When it occurs, it is important to differentiate mechanical from embolic causes. No-reflow due to distal embolization is best treated with medical therapies, whereas dissection resulting in abrupt closure is most effectively treated with stent deployment. Case reports have provided a large amount of anecdotal experience regarding novel treatment strategies, and continued education in the evolving field of PCI will allow further improvement in patient outcomes.

References

1. Milani RV, Fitzgerald R, Milani JN, Lavie CJ. The impact of micro troponin leak on long-term outcomes following elective percutaneous coronary intervention. *Catheter Cardiovasc Interv.* 2009;74: 819–822.

2. Ellis SG, Roubin GS, King SB III, et al. Angiographic and clinical predictors of acute closure after native vessel coronary angioplasty. *Circulation.* 1988;77:372–379.

3. Ellis SG, Vandormael MG, Cowley MJ, et al. Coronary morphologic and clinical determinants of procedural outcome with angioplasty for multivessel coronary disease: implications for patient selection: Multivessel Angioplasty Prognosis Study Group. *Circulation.* 1990;82:1193–1202.

4. Gaul G, Hollman J, Simpfendorfer C, Franco I. Acute occlusion in multiple lesion coronary angioplasty: frequency and management. *J Am Coll Cardiol.* 1989;13:283–288.

5. Hartzler GO, Rutherford BD, McConahay DR, et al. "High-risk" percutaneous transluminal coronary angioplasty. *Am J Cardiol.* 1988;61:33G–37G.

6. King SB III, Smith SC Jr, Hirshfeld JW Jr, et al. 2007 Focused Update of the ACC/AHA/SCAI 2005 Guideline Update for Percutaneous Coronary Intervention: a report of the American College of Cardiology/American Heart Association Task Force on Practice Guidelines: 2007 Writing Group to Review New Evidence and Update the ACC/AHA/SCAI 2005 Guideline Update for Percutaneous Coronary Intervention, Writing on Behalf of the 2005 Writing Committee. *Circulation.* 2008;117:261–295.

7. Yang EH, Gumina RJ, Lennon RJ, et al. Emergency coronary artery bypass surgery for percutaneous coronary interventions: changes in the incidence, clinical characteristics, and indications from 1979 to 2003. *J Am Coll Cardiol.* 2005;46: 2004–2009.

8. Qureshi MA, Safian RD, Grines CL, et al. Simplified scoring system for predicting mortality after percutaneous coronary intervention. *J Am Coll Cardiol.* 2003;42:1890–1895.

9. Mueller C, Buettner HJ, Hodgson JM, et al. Inflammation and long-term mortality after non-ST elevation acute coronary syndrome treated with a very early invasive strategy in 1042 consecutive patients. *Circulation.* 2002;105:1412–1415.

10. Buffon A, Liuzzo G, Biasucci LM, et al. Preprocedural serum levels of C-reactive protein predict early complications and late restenosis after coronary angioplasty. *J Am Coll Cardiol.* 1999;34: 1512–1521.

11. Mazur W, Grinstead WC, Hakim AH, et al. Fate of side branches after intracoronary implantation of the Gianturco-Roubin flex-stent for acute or threatened closure after percutaneous transluminal coronary angioplasty. *Am J Cardiol.* 1994;74: 1207–1210.

12. Tanabe K, Serruys PW, Degertekin M, et al. Fate of side branches after coronary arterial sirolimus-eluting stent implantation. *Am J Cardiol.* 2002;90: 937–941.

13. Fischman DL, Savage MP, Leon MB, et al. Fate of lesion-related side branches after coronary artery stenting. *J Am Coll Cardiol.* 1993;22:1641–1646.

14. Alfonso F, Hernandez C, Perez-Vizcayno MJ, et al. Fate of stent-related side branches after coronary intervention in patients with in-stent restenosis. *J Am Coll Cardiol.* 2000;36:1549–1556.

15. Cho GY, Lee CW, Hong MK, et al. Effects of stent design on side branch occlusion after coronary stent placement. *Catheter Cardiovasc Interv.* 2001; 52:18–23.

16. Aliabadi D, Tilli FV, Bowers TR, et al. Incidence and angiographic predictors of side branch occlusion following high-pressure intracoronary stenting. *Am J Cardiol.* 1997;80:994–997.

17. Stone GW, Ellis SG, Cannon L, et al. Comparison of a polymer-based paclitaxel-eluting stent with a bare metal stent in patients with complex coronary artery disease: a randomized controlled trial. *JAMA*. 2005;294:1215–1223.

18. Koo BK, Kang HJ, Youn TJ, et al. Physiologic assessment of jailed side branch lesions using fractional flow reserve. *J Am Coll Cardiol*. 2005; 46:633–637.

19. Hildick-Smith D, de Belder AJ, Cooter N, et al. Randomized trial of simple versus complex drug-eluting stenting for bifurcation lesions: the British Bifurcation Coronary Study: old, new, and evolving strategies. *Circulation*. 2010; 121(10):1235–1243.

20. Zhang F, Dong L, Ge J. Simple versus complex stenting strategy for coronary artery bifurcation lesions in the drug-eluting stent era: a meta-analysis of randomised trials. *Heart* 2009;95: 1676–1681.

21. Gilchrist IC. Seal it to heal it: potential option for distal wire perforation. *Catheter Cardiovasc Interv*. 2009;73:795–796.

22. Chaudhry EC, Dauerman KP, Sarnoski CL, et al. Percutaneous coronary intervention for major bifurcation lesions using the simple approach: risk of myocardial infarction. *J Thromb Thrombolysis*. 2007;24:7–13.

23. Tran T, Brown M, Lasala J. An evidence-based approach to the use of rotational and directional coronary atherectomy in the era of drug-eluting stents: when does it make sense? *Catheter Cardiovasc Interv*. 2008;72:650–662.

24. Dauerman HL, Higgins PJ, Sparano AM, et al. Mechanical debulking versus balloon angioplasty for the treatment of true bifurcation lesions. *J Am Coll Cardiol*. 1998;32:1845–1852.

25. Morino Y, Yamamoto H, Mitsudo K, et al. Functional formula to determine adequate balloon diameter of simultaneous kissing balloon technique for treatment of bifurcated coronary lesions: clinical validation by volumetric intravascular ultrasound analysis. *Circ J*. 2008;72: 886–892.

26. Legrand V, Thomas M, Zelisko M, et al. Percutaneous coronary intervention of bifurcation lesions: state-of-the-art: insights from the second meeting of the European Bifurcation Club. *EuroIntervention*. 2007;3:44–49.

27. Furuichi S, Airoldi F, Colombo A. Rescue inverse crush: a way of get out of trouble. *Catheter Cardiovasc Interv*. 2007;70:708–712.

28. Poerner TC, Kralev S, Voelker W, et al. Natural history of small and medium-sized side branches after coronary stent implantation. *Am Heart J*. 2002;143:627–635.

29. Roy P, de Labriolle A, Hanna N, et al. Requirement for emergent coronary artery bypass surgery following percutaneous coronary intervention in the stent era. *Am J Cardiol*. 2009;103:950–953.

30. Huber MS, Mooney JF, Madison J, Mooney MR. Use of a morphologic classification to predict clinical outcome after dissection from coronary angioplasty. *Am J Cardiol*. 1991;68:467–471.

31. Boyle AJ, Chan M, Dib J, Resar J. Catheter-induced coronary artery dissection: risk factors, prevention and management. *J Invasive Cardiol*. 2006;18:500–503.

32. Nikolsky E, Boulos M, Amikam S. Spontaneous healing of long, catheter-induced right coronary artery dissection. *Int J Cardiovasc Intervent*. 2003; 5:211.

33. Awadalla H, Sabet S, El Sebaie A, et al. Catheter-induced left main dissection incidence, predisposition and therapeutic strategies experience from two sides of the hemisphere. *J Invasive Cardiol*. 2005;17:233–236.

34. Dunning DW, Kahn JK, Hawkins ET, O'Neill WW. Iatrogenic coronary artery dissections extending into and involving the aortic root. *Catheter Cardiovasc Interv*. 2000;51:387–393.

35. Uren NG, Schwarzacher SP, Metz JA, et al. Predictors and outcomes of stent thrombosis: an intravascular ultrasound registry. *Eur Heart J*. 2002;23: 124–132.

36. Sheris SJ, Canos MR, Weissman NJ. Natural history of intravascular ultrasound-detected edge dissections from coronary stent deployment. *Am Heart J*. 2000;139:59–63.

37. Liu X, Tsujita K, Maehara A, et al. Intravascular ultrasound assessment of the incidence and predictors of edge dissections after drug-eluting stent implantation. *JACC Cardiovasc Interv*. 2009; 2:997–1004.

38. Lemos PA, Saia F, Ligthart JM, et al. Coronary restenosis after sirolimus-eluting stent implantation: morphological description and mechanistic analysis from a consecutive series of cases. *Circulation*. 2003;108:257–260.

39. Klein LW, Kern MJ, Berger P, et al. Society of cardiac angiography and interventions: suggested management of the no-reflow phenomenon in the cardiac catheterization laboratory. *Catheter Cardiovasc Interv*. 2003;60:194–201.

40. Cai Q, Skelding KA, Armstrong AT Jr, et al. Predictors of periprocedural creatine kinase-myocardial band elevation complicating elective percutaneous coronary intervention. *Am J Cardiol.* 2007;99:616–620.

41. Black AJ, Namay DL, Niederman AL, et al. Tear or dissection after coronary angioplasty: morphologic correlates of an ischemic complication. *Circulation.* 1989;79:1035–1042.

42. de Muinck ED, den Heijer P, van Dijk RB, et al. Autoperfusion balloon versus stent for acute or threatened closure during percutaneous transluminal coronary angioplasty. *Am J Cardiol.* 1994;74:1002–1005.

43. Smith SC Jr, Feldman TE, Hirshfeld JW Jr, et al. ACC/AHA/SCAI 2005 guideline update for percutaneous coronary intervention: a report of the American College of Cardiology/American Heart Association Task Force on Practice Guidelines (ACC/AHA/SCAI Writing Committee to Update 2001 Guidelines for Percutaneous Coronary Intervention). *Circulation.* 2006;113:e166–e286.

44. Hirsh J, O'Donnell M, Eikelboom JW. Beyond unfractionated heparin and warfarin: current and future advances. *Circulation.* 2007;116:552–560.

16

Coronary Perforation, Aneurysm Formation, Covered Stents, and Coil Embolization

JOSEPH S. ROSSI AND MAURICIO G. COHEN

isruption of the coronary artery intima is inherent to all percutaneous coronary interventions (PCIs). The vast majority of intimal tears are limited and covered by stent placement without consequence. In more severe cases of coronary injury, disruption of the media and adventitia can cause perforation of the artery and presents with acute findings including contrast extravasation and cardiac tamponade. More limited disruptions may be recognized as localized dissections or contained perforations. Long-term consequences of these disruptions are well described and include aneurysm formation and delayed healing that may increase the risk of stent restenosis and/or thrombosis.

The evolving techniques of contemporary PCI have been unable to completely eliminate coronary injury and consequent mechanical complications. In addition, the introduction of stiff hydrophilic guidewires and the development of new anterograde and retrograde techniques allow the treatment of complex coronary artery stenosis and chronic total occlusions that were previously thought to be untreatable (1,2). Thus, the risk profile of the population undergoing PCI in the modern era is markedly increased, and coronary perforation will continue to be encountered. This chapter outlines the clinical features and acute management of coronary perforation, and its late manifestations including aneurysm formation.

■ CORONARY PERFORATION
Incidence and Risk Factors

Fortunately, coronary perforation remains relatively uncommon in the modern era of PCI, with most recent series suggesting an incidence of less than 1.0% (3–11). Nonetheless, catastrophic perforation continues to occur and is currently responsible for approximately 20% of cases referred for emergency coronary artery bypass surgery (12). Interventional cardiologists should therefore be familiar with strategies and equipment used to treat this potentially catastrophic complication with three primary goals: avoid emergency surgery, maintain systemic perfusion, and minimize myocardial necrosis.

Coronary artery perforation during PCI can present along a spectrum of severity, ranging from inconsequential side branch perforation induced by coronary guidewires to large and catastrophic proximal vessel perforation following atherectomy or overly aggressive balloon or stent inflation. Coronary perforation was initially described during the early experience with balloon angioplasty in the 1980s. A review of angioplasty procedures by Ellis in 1994 described an overall incidence of approximately 0.5%, with a significantly increased risk during atheroablative procedures such as directional atherectomy, rotational atherectomy, and excimer laser procedures (4). In another large series including more than 6,000 patients, the likelihood of developing a large and clinically significant perforation was almost seven times greater following use of an atheroablative device (1.49% of 489 procedures vs. 0.05% of 5,725 nonatheroablative procedures; $P < .001$) (13). Other risk factors reported include older age, female gender, device to artery ratio greater than 1.2, high complexity lesion, chronic total occlusion, routine use of intravascular ultrasound (IVUS) to maximize stented luminal area, and use of hydrophilic wires (3,5–8,10,13,14). Table 16-1 lists the incidence and risk factors for perforation in published case series.

There are no convincing data suggesting that glycoprotein IIb/IIIa inhibitors increase the frequency or the risk of perforation (15). A recent review of more than 12,000 patients found that the incidence of coronary perforation was 0.26% among patients receiving a glycoprotein IIb/IIIa inhibitor compared with 0.3% among patients who did not receive these agents (9). However, the use of glycoprotein IIb/IIIa inhibitors can potentiate bleeding. Therefore, in selected patients, small perforations may become angiographically apparent and cause pericardial effusions resulting in serious hemodynamic compromise and adverse clinical outcomes (7,13). In a series of 36 perforations at the Kings College Hospital in London, Gunning et al. (7) showed that abciximab was used in 9 of the 10 cases that developed significant pericardial effusion. In the Mayo Clinic database, 33 of 95 patients were on glycoprotein IIb/IIIa inhibitors at the time of coronary perforation. These patients were more likely to require placement of a covered stent or undergo emergency cardiac surgery (33.3% vs. 3.2%) (6). It must be noted that in the presence of glycoprotein IIb/IIIa inhibitors, small guidewire perforations thought to be resolved by the end of the procedure may manifest a few hours later as pericardial tamponade.

Bivalirudin, a direct thrombin inhibitor, has gained popularity among interventional cardiologists over the past few years because of its association with reduced bleeding risk (16,17). Even though this agent has a short half-life of approximately 20 minutes, the interventionalist should be cautious in choosing this agent for intervening on lesions at high risk of perforation because of the inability to monitor the intensity of anticoagulation and the lack of a specific reversal agent. However, a recent report from a high-volume institution showed excellent outcomes after wire perforations in patients treated with bivalirudin in comparison with heparin. Of the 50 patients who experienced a wire perforation, 30 were treated with heparin and 20 with bivalirudin. Three patients died and 12 patients required pericardiocentesis, covered stents, or coil embolization in the heparin group and none in the bivalirudin group, who responded very well to discontinuation of bivalirudin and prolonged balloon inflations (11). Of note, the report did not include outcome details on 32 nonwire perforations that occurred during the study period. Nonwire perforations have a more dramatic presentation and are usually caused by vessel rupture by either atheroablative device or an oversized stent.

In summary, it is now accepted that while medical therapies may have an effect on the presentation and/or progression of coronary perforation, they likely do not represent a causal factor.

Classification

A classification based on morphology and severity has previously been proposed by Ellis (Table 16-2) (4). The frequency distribution by type of perforation is illustrated in Figure 16-1. Type I coronary perforations are defined as crater formation or linear collection without extravasation of contrast within a treated segment, and may be impossible to distinguish from localized dissection (Fig. 16-2). These complications are likely underreported because of lack of clinical significance. In a review published by Dippel examining more than 6,000 cases, no type I perforations were noted (13). It has therefore been suggested that type I perforations are of descriptive but not prognostic significance. The most common etiology of this relatively minor complication is likely wire advancement through the media and adventitia creating a shelf without contrast extravasation; another possible etiology is balloon inflation within a calcified artery resulting in extramural hematoma. Stent placement often results in scaffolding of the artery and prevents extension.

Type II perforations are defined by pericardial or myocardial blush without active contrast extravasation. This is most commonly seen following distal wire advancement into the pericardial space. The amount of contrast extravasation

TABLE 16-1 Incidence and Predictors of Coronary Perforation in Different Series

	Aljuni et al.(3)	Ellis et al.(4)	Dippel et al.(13)	Gunning et al.(7)	Fasseass et al.(6)	Stankovic et al.(8)	Witzke et al.(9)	Javaid et al.(10)
Study period	1988–1992	1990–1991	1995–1999	1995–2001	1990–2001	1993–2001	1995–2003	1996–2005
Incidence	0.4% (35/8,932)	0.5% (62/12,900)	0.58% (36/6,214)	0.8% 52/6,245	0.58% 95/16,298	1.47% (84/5,728)	0.3% (39/12,658)	0.19% (72/38,559)
Risk factors								
Older age		X						
Female gender		X						
Prior CABG					X			
High-risk lesion (ACC/AHA B2 or C)	X			X	X	X		X
Chronic total occlusion	X			X				
Balloon:artery > 1.2:1	X	X				X		X
Atheroablative techniques	X	X	X		X	X		X
Hydrophilic wires							X	X
IVUS guidance for stent sizing								X

CABG, coronary artery bypass graft; ACC, American College of Cardiology; AHA, American Heart Association; IVUS, intravascular ultrasound.

TABLE 16-2 **Ellis Classification of Coronary Artery Perforation**

Type	Morphology	Clinical Sequelae
I	Extraluminal crater without extravasation	Almost always benign, treated effectively with stent placement
II	Pericardial or myocardial blush without contrast jet extravasation and without a > 1-mm exit hole	Can result in late presentation of tamponade, requires close observation
III	Extravasation through a frank perforation with a ≥ 1-mm exit hole	High risk of tamponade, requires reversal of anticoagulation and immediate treatment
III—cavity spilling	Perforation into an anatomic chamber, such as coronary sinus, atria, or ventricles	Can often have a benign course, may result in fistulae formation, large perforation requires repair to avoid coronary steal

(From Ellis SG, Ajluni S, Arnold AZ, et al. Increased coronary perforation in the new device era: incidence, classification, management, and outcome. *Circulation*. 1994;90:2725–2730.)

is often barely noticeable, and pericardial effusion therefore tends to be inconsequential when 0.014-in. guidewires are used. Type II perforations can be managed conservatively in most cases. When the direction of perforation is into the myocardium, a small staining artifact may be recognized that remains stable (intramyocardial hematoma). When the direction of perforation is into the pericardium, there can be localized collection of contrast within the pericardial sac. Management of type II perforations where the

exit hole is smaller than 1 mm is dependent on the underlying clinical scenario.

Type III perforations are defined by active contrast extravasation through an exit hole greater than 1 mm in diameter and are the most likely to result in pericardial tamponade and hemodynamic compromise. Figures 16-3 to 16-5 illustrate several cases of type III perforations in native coronary arteries and saphenous vein grafts. Type III perforations can result from high pressure balloon inflation causing a tear through

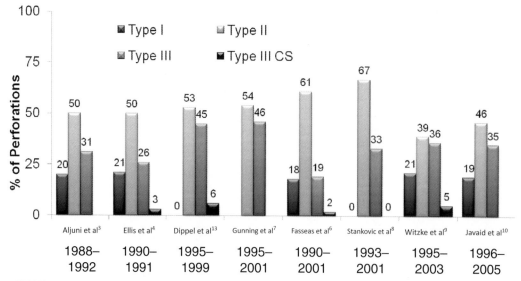

FIGURE 16-1. Type of perforation reported in different series. Different series demonstrated a low prevalence (20%) of type I perforations, most likely related to underreporting. Approximately half of the perforations were type II and a third were type III. Despite the different time periods, the distribution of the type of perforation did not show significant secular variation. CS, cavity spilling.

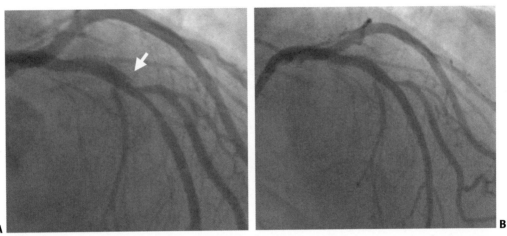

FIGURE 16-2. Type 1 coronary perforation. (**A**) The *arrow* indicates an extraluminal crater after balloon angioplasty of a 90% lesion in the left anterior descending coronary artery. (**B**) The perforation is completely sealed poststent placement

the full thickness of the arterial wall, although stiff guidewire perforation can also result in type III perforation morphology, particularly when stiff or hydrophilic guidewire is advanced through an area of tortuosity or severe calcification, where the underlying support matrix of the artery may be weakened. Active extravasation into the pericardial space through a large perforation requires immediate action, as shown in a treatment algorithm that appropriately describes current clinical practice (13) (Fig. 16-6). Severe coronary perforations have consistently been associated with adverse outcomes.

A unique classification that is rarely seen is commonly referred to as "type III cavity

spilling." On rare occasion, coronary artery perforation may be directionally oriented into a cavity other than the pericardial space or myocardium, causing contrast extravasation to be seen in the coronary sinus or possibly a ventricular or atrial chamber. If these perforations are small in caliber, they may be of little clinical significance. However, if the amount of cavity spilling is large enough, it may result in coronary steal phenomenon and resulting myocardial ischemia. Large cavity spilling perforations should be treated immediately with catheter-based or surgical therapies.

In particular, coronary perforation resulting in cardiac tamponade has a very high risk of

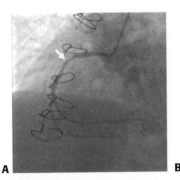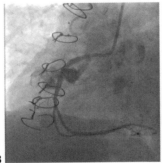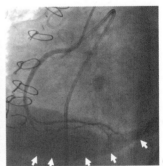

FIGURE 16-3. Type III perforation in a native right coronary artery causing tamponade. (**A**) Right coronary perforation in an 82-year-old woman with a 75% lesion in the right coronary artery. A 3.5 × 15 mm bare metal stent, which had a stent-to-artery ratio greater than 1.2 was directly deployed at the lesion causing a large type III perforation with contrast extravasation in the pericardial space (**B**). A JOMED covered stent was successfully inserted sealing the perforation (**C**). (*Arrows* indicate the presence of a substantial amount of contrast in the pericardial space.)

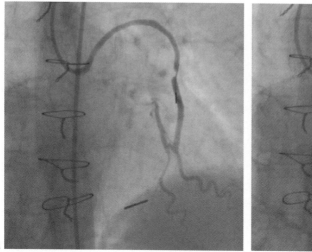
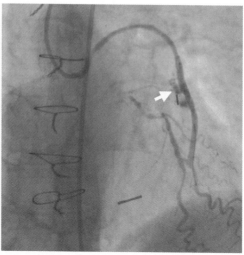

A   B

FIGURE 16-4. Mediastinal hemorrhage after direct stenting of a saphenous vein graft with a bare metal stent. (**A**) Severe 95% stenosis in a saphenous vein graft to an obtuse marginal. (**B**) After direct deployment of a bare metal stent, a type III perforation causing mediastinal hemorrhage became apparent (*arrow*). The patient suffered profound hypotension and had to be intubated and started on inotropic support. Multiple attempts to deliver a JOMED covered stent were unsuccessful due to lack of guiding catheter support. The stent came off balloon as it was being retrieved in the guiding catheter and finally embolized to the profunda femoral artery. In the end, the perforation was sealed with prolonged low-pressure balloon inflation.

mortality and need for emergency cardiac surgery (4,13). When performed, cardiac surgery is also associated with poor outcomes as these patients often had prolonged cardiogenic shock and are at high risk for bleeding due to the administration of antiplatelet agents such as thienopyridines and glycoprotein IIb/IIIa inhibitors. Emergency cardiac surgery has been associated with markedly increased risk of death, myocardial infarction, cerebral ischemia, and acute renal failure (18). The proper response to coronary perforation is dependent on the specific details of the underlying clinical scenario, but there are general procedural guidelines that should enable

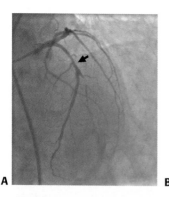
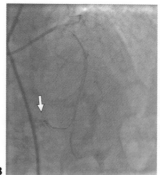
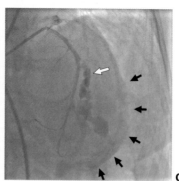

A   B   C

FIGURE 16-5. Type III cavity spilling and type III perforations with tamponade in the same patient. Angiographic images of a 76-year-old woman admitted through the emergency department with chest pain and left bundle branch block. There was a 95% lesion in the proximal-mid left anterior descending that was initially stented. (**A**) A second stent was deemed necessary as there was a significant residual stenosis proximal to the stented segment. (**B**) A stent is being positioned in the proximal left anterior descending artery (LAD). Notice the position of the wire in the a septal perforator and contrast spilling in the right ventricle. (**C**) After deployment of the stent a large perforation was noticed at the origin of a diagonal branch (*large arrow*). The *small arrows* indicate the rapid accumulation of contrast in the pericardial space causing tamponade. The patient collapsed rapidly and was taken emergently to the operating room. The patient did not survive.

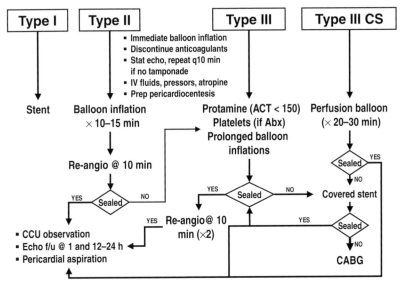

FIGURE 16-6. Algorithm for management of coronary perforations. (Modified from Dippel EJ, Kereiakes DJ, Tramuta DA, et al. Coronary perforation during percutaneous coronary intervention in the era of abciximab platelet glycoprotein IIb/IIIa blockade: an algorithm for percutaneous management. *Catheter Cardiovasc Interv.* 2001;52:279–286.)

all interventional cardiologists to effectively manage coronary perforation when it is recognized in a timely fashion.

■ MANAGEMENT STRATEGY FOR CORONARY PERFORATION

Guidewire advancement is a common cause of coronary perforation (usually type 1 or type 2). Fortunately, the use of 0.014-in. coronary guidewires usually ensures that the majority of small perforations do not become hemodynamically significant (4). The factors that increase the risk of side branch or distal vessel perforation are the use of hydrophilic wires and overaggressive distal advancement in cases where additional wire support is needed to deliver equipment. Unrecognized wire perforations can result in hemodynamic compromise, particularly in the presence of glycoprotein IIb/IIIa inhibitors or when anticoagulation is continued after the procedure. Small areas of myocardial staining should be watched carefully, and observation within the cardiac catheterization suite for a minimum of 20 minutes after all small perforations is generally recommended, even when there is no evidence of early expansion into the pericardial space. Echocardiography should be used to verify the absence of pericardial effusion

when perforation is noted. In all cases where myocardial staining from a small perforation is seen, the patient should be observed in the coronary care unit for a minimum of 24 hours, with prompt echocardiography available for bedside diagnosis and pericardiocentesis if tamponade is suspected or develops. Anticoagulation and glycoprotein IIb/IIIa inhibitors should be discontinued immediately and reversal considered for any evidence of clinical progression.

Large perforations causing frank bleeding into the pericardial space can result in rapid cardiovascular collapse. These episodes are often the result of increased balloon:artery ratios (>1.2:1) causing longitudinal avulsion of the arterial wall. Oversizing of stents is more common among women and the elderly, and caution is particularly important in heavily calcified lesions. Large perforation can sometimes be treated with a covered stent (19). Alternatively, if the perforation is in a distal vessel or in an epicardial vessel with a relatively small amount of myocardium at risk, prolonged balloon occlusion can be attempted to achieve hemostasis. Rapid reversal of anticoagulation should be achieved when possible, and transfusion of platelets can be considered. Because covered stents are not approved for use in the coronary circulation by the U.S. Food and Drug Administration

TABLE 16-3	Avoiding Coronary Perforation with High-Risk Devices
Device Type	Methods Important to Avoid Perforation
Rotational atherectomy	Low burr:artery ratio (<0.8); avoid angulated segments
Stiff wires	Careful distal advancement; check wire position in multiple views to maintain distal tip in true lumen
Hydrophilic wires	Careful distal advancement to avoid side branches; maintain tip mobility to avoid subintimal advance
Angioplasty balloon	Low balloon:artery ratio; avoid high-pressure predilation
Stent	Plan for postdilation in heavily calcified arteries (avoid high-pressure initial inflation and oversizing)

(FDA), compassionate use documentation after implantation is required in the United States. Current accepted clinical practice is well described in an algorithm published by Dippel et al. (13), as illustrated in Figure 16-6.

In general, small coronary perforations (type 1) that do not progress can be managed conservatively, and antiplatelet agents can be continued if staining is not seen following stent placement. In the most severe cases, such as large type 2 and all type 3 perforations, culprit artery occlusion is necessary while other measures are considered. Specific treatment steps should be determined on case-by-case basis. Table 16-3 provides recommendations to avoid coronary perforations according to the type of device used in PCI. The following sections describe a summary of separate actions that have been proven successful in the treatment of coronary perforation.

Perforation Sealing: Stents and Balloon Inflation

In the era of balloon-only angioplasty, acute closure and dissections were both common complications. Perfusion balloons were designed to allow for distal coronary perfusion while also providing balloon pressure to treat dissected segments of coronary artery (20). This was also a widely used technique for the treatment of coronary artery perforation. A perfusion balloon was inflated at low pressure to allow for sealing of a perforated segment while preserving distal coronary flow. Unfortunately, because these devices are used so infrequently in the modern era, very few catheterization laboratories currently stock this equipment. Vessel occlusion is

generally now performed with standard angioplasty balloons within distal arteries to treat wire perforations, and covered stents are preferred for the treatment of perforations within larger arteries. For distal artery perforations from inadvertent guidewire advancement, a small-caliber balloon should be advanced into the distal artery and inflated at low pressure to occlude flow. Efforts should be made to ensure that the smallest amount of territory is in jeopardy during these inflations. Particular attention should be given to large side branches and short balloons are often preferred in these circumstances. In most cases of type I perforations, a bare metal stent will usually seal the coronary perforation. In larger perforations (type II or III) that do not respond to prolonged balloon occlusion, other strategies such as a covered stent or coil embolization should be considered. These strategies are further discussed in the last section of the chapter.

Reversal of Anticoagulation and Antiplatelet Agents

Heparin should be used for anticoagulation in all cases where perforation is thought to be more likely to occur, including degenerated vein grafts, chronic total occlusions, and lesions requiring atheroablative techniques. In cases of severe perforation, protamine sulfate provides rapid reversal of heparin anticoagulation and should be dosed at a standard of 1 mg per 100 units of heparin given. Patients with a history of insulin exposure (protamine insulin and Neutral Protamine Hagedorn (NPH) in particular), fish protein allergy, or vasectomy are more likely to experience adverse reactions to protamine, but these reactions are fortunately rare. Diphenhydramine should be given to all patients receiving protamine to minimize the effects of histamine release associated with infusion. Protamine–heparin complexes are cleared by the reticuloendothelial system and are not dependent on liver or renal function. Protamine is not titratable and can induce direct mast cell degranulation, complement activation, and antibody formation leading to potentially catastrophic adverse reactions, such as myocardial depression, cardiac arrest, bronchospasm, pulmonary hypertension, pulmonary edema, and shock (21). Systematic reversal with protamine post-PCI has been tested but not widely adopted because of its toxicity profile. Therefore, protamine use in the catheterization laboratory is restricted to the management of severe life-threatening bleeds associated with vascular perforations (22,23).

For patients receiving glycoprotein IIb/IIIa inhibitors, the infusion should be stopped immediately when type II or type III perforation is noted. In patients receiving abciximab, platelet transfusion can overcome the antiplatelet effect of this irreversible antibody to the glycoprotein IIb/IIIa receptor. Random donor platelets should be transfused when there is ongoing bleeding that does not resolve after endovascular treatment with balloon inflations or covered stent placement. Eptifibatide and tirofiban are reversible inhibitors of the glycoprotein IIb/IIIa receptor, and their action cannot be overcome by platelet transfusion. In this situation, the infusion should be discontinued while alternative actions are taken to treat the perforation (13).

Cardiac Surgery

Type III perforations are associated with an increased risk of death and emergency coronary artery bypass graft (10). These complications are often associated with immediate hemodynamic compromise and require emergency pericardiocentesis. The cardiac surgery team should be notified immediately of all type III perforations in order to prepare an operating room immediately while percutaneous therapy is attempted. Because of the high risk associated with type III perforations, anticoagulation should be immediately reversed. Platelet transfusion should be considered for patients receiving abciximab infusion on the way to the operating room, and

aggressive fluid resuscitation should be encouraged to maintain right ventricular filling. For patients proceeding to the operating room, prophylactic pericardial drain placement may prevent the development of clinical tamponade while the operating suite is being prepared. The interventional cardiologist should remain a critical member of the team in the operating room to assist in the management of antithrombotic therapies, to maintain communication with the surgeon regarding the nature and location of the perforation, and to hold discussions with the patient's family (24).

Pericardiocentesis

Pericardiocentesis should be performed prophylactically for large pericardial effusions before tamponade develops. Early drainage should be encouraged to avoid the formation of organized clot. There have been recent case reports of pericardial tamponade with unsuccessful drainage due to clot formation in the pericardial space among patients receiving anticoagulation with bivalirudin (25). Although clot formation is likely to complicate pericardial drainage, it may also result in sealing of the perforation and might indicate a favorable characteristic of direct thrombin inhibitors in this setting. Bivalirudin has also been associated with a lower risk of severe complications after wire perforation compared with heparin, possibly due to its short half-life (11).

The subxyphoid approach is likely the most accessible while the patient is on the catheterization table. In some cases, where localized pericardial blood accumulation is thought to cause hemodynamic compromise, pericardiocentesis with echocardiographic guidance should be considered, particularly for lateral or apical perforations.

It is important to emphasize that a large percentage of coronary perforations resulting in tamponade may not be diagnosed during the interventional procedure. The incidence of delayed tamponade varies across different studies. In a case series from England, 5 of the 24 patients (21%) who developed tamponade presented clinical manifestations more than 2 hours after the procedure. Hydrophilic wires and glycoprotein IIb/IIIa inhibitors were used in three and four of these cases, respectively (7). In a case

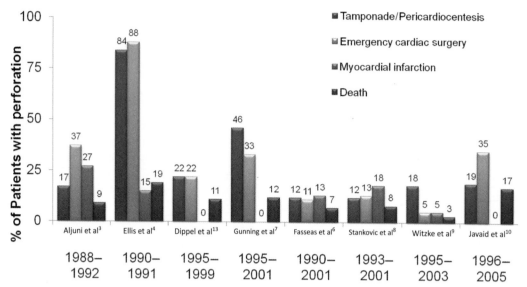

FIGURE 16-7. Outcomes after perforation in different series. Reported case series demonstrated a disparate rates of tamponade/pericardiocentesis (12%–84%), emergency surgery (5%–88%), myocardial infarction (5%–27%), and death (3%–17%). In general, lower rate of complications were noted in the more contemporary series.

series from William Beaumont Hospital, cardiac tamponade presented late in 14 of 31 (45%) patients at a mean time of 4.4 hours after the conclusion of PCI and was treated with volume expanders, reversal of anticoagulation with protamine, and pericardiocentesis. The overall cardiac mortality in patients with tamponade was high (42%). However, early tamponade occurring in the catheterization laboratory was associated with higher mortality in comparison with delayed tamponade (59% vs. 21%, $P = .036$) (26). The diagnosis of tamponade once the patient has left the catheterization laboratory is a challenge and should be considered in all patients with new-onset hypotension, engorged jugular veins, and/or chest pain following PCI. A goal-directed, abbreviated bedside echocardiography should be promptly performed to avoid delays in the diagnosis. Classic echocardiographic findings include the presence of a pericardial effusion, right atrial compression during late diastole, right ventricular collapse in early diastole, and dilated inferior vena cava without inspiratory collapse.

Rescue echo-guided pericardiocentesis can be successfully performed in an unstable patient in most cases. The largest collection of pericardial fluid in proximity to the chest wall can be easily identified with the transducer. As described in Chapter 23, a polytef-sheathed needle (16 to 18 gauge) is then advanced with the same angulation of the transducer. Subsequently, the steel core of the needle is withdrawn and a small volume of agitated saline can be injected through the sheath to confirm the position in the pericardial space. In a series of 92 patients who developed acute tamponade in relation to catheter-based procedures, this approach was successful at relieving the hemodynamic compromise in 99% of the cases (27). Patients with delayed tamponade should be brought back to the catheterization laboratory, as the cause of pericardial effusion can be potentially treated percutaneously by a prolonged balloon inflations, stent deployment or occlusion with a covered stent, or coil embolization. Figure 16-7 summarizes outcomes after perforation in different series.

■ CORONARY ARTERY ANEURYSM

The incidence of coronary artery aneurysm in the era of high volume diagnostic angiography has been reported in the range of 1.5% to 5% (28). The accepted definition of aneurysm formation is a widening of the arterial lumen greater than 1.5 times the normal native vessel diameter.

Etiology

Although the formation of coronary artery aneurysm is generally associated with the presence of risk factors for atherosclerosis, cases of coronary aneurysm in young patients without risk factors have also been reported. In a review of the published data prior to high volume stenting in 1998, it was suggested that approximately 50% of coronary aneurysms were atherosclerotic in nature and the remaining cases were the result of a combination of inflammatory and/or connective tissue diseases such as Kawasaki disease, Marfan syndrome, Ehler–Danlos disease, and syphilis (28).

Iatrogenic Coronary Aneurysm

Coronary aneurysm and pseudoaneurysm following perforation have been reported, although they are a rare occurrence (29,30). The pathophysiology of iatrogenic coronary aneurysm is likely related to small caliber perforations followed by abnormal healing and inflammation. Trauma from balloon angioplasty can also be associated with aneurysm formation, with series from the balloon angioplasty era suggesting an incidence of up to 4.0% (31,32). While the incidence of coronary aneurysm formation following contemporary stent implantation appears to be small, and no large cases series have been published to suggest that this is a common phenomenon, a recent review has suggested that coronary artery aneurysm can be seen in 1.25% of patients receiving drug-eluting stents for de novo coronary artery disease (33). The exact mechanism of coronary aneurysm formation following stent implantation has not been elucidated, but there are several plausible explanations. Previous studies have suggested that the incidence of aneurysm formation may be similar after bare metal stent (BMS) implantation compared with drug eluting stent (DES) (34). Direct perforation of the vessel during high-pressure inflation has often been associated with "crater" formation, and aneurysm may simply represent the later stages of these initial arterial injuries. Drug-eluting stents may result in localized hypersensitivity reactions leading to inflammation and aneurysm formation (35). There has been suggestion of an increased incidence of coronary aneurysm associated with drug-eluting stents, and abnormal healing of the vessel wall has been proposed as a possible mechanism (36).

In the largest study to date, Alfonso et al. reported the incidence of coronary aneurysm formation among 1,197 consecutive patients undergoing late angiographic follow-up after DES placement at a single center (33). They found a total of 15 cases, correlating to an overall incidence of 1.25%. IVUS was used to evaluate the aneurysm in 13 of 15 patients. They found a high incidence of stent malapposition but found no cases suggestive of hypersensitivity reactions. All cases in which coronary aneurysm formation was associated with stent thrombosis or death occurred in cases where at least one antiplatelet agent had been discontinued. The authors also described six cases associated with stent implantation for myocardial infarction and four cases where coronary aneurysm was associated with stent overlap.

Management of Coronary Artery Aneurysms

Regardless of the cause, the treatment of coronary aneurysm has two specific goals: prevention of aneurysm expansion and maintenance of coronary artery patency.

The natural history of idiopathic coronary aneurysms is not well defined, and the treatment course is best determined on an individual basis. For patients with ischemic heart disease and associated coronary stenosis, the proper course of action is probably relief of ischemia and treatment of atherosclerotic risk factors. For patients with inflammatory conditions or connective tissue disorder and diagnosed large coronary aneurysm, treatment is recommended for large aneurysms (>3 mm in diameter) that are thought to be at higher risk of spontaneous rupture. Treatment options include the use of covered coronary stents and endovascular coiling using any of the currently available products. Endovascular coiling can be considered if rupture is thought to be likely based on rapid progression or compressive symptoms. The treatment of atherosclerotic coronary aneurysm is more controversial. A review of angiograms from the Coronary Artery Surgery Study (CASS) registry suggested that of more than 900 identified cases, there were no cases of spontaneous rupture. It has been demonstrated, however, that aneurysmal segments can lead to thrombosis and acute myocardial infarction (33,38).

In general, all aneurysms and pseudoaneurysms in the coronary circulation should be followed closely for progression, as large aneurysms may require surgical intervention, particularly when associated with symptoms of ischemia. In addition, there is evidence that coronary artery aneurysms can increase the risk of in-stent restenosis and late-stent thrombosis (33). Asymptomatic patients with small aneurysms can potentially be followed with a computed tomography or magnetic resonance coronary angiography.

Interventional management of coronary aneurysm should be reserved for patients with symptoms and those with large aneurysm who may be at increased risk of rupture. Platinum microcoil embolization has only rarely been reported in the literature but may be reasonable for large aneurysm in low-risk territories. However, this technique should be used only as a last resort, as unintended coil embolization into the native coronary can have disastrous consequences. A more appealing approach is the placement of a covered coronary stent, thereby excluding the aneurysmal segment and promoting spontaneous closure.

■ COVERED STENTS

The use of covered coronary stents, or "stent grafts" to treat perforation in the coronary circulation has become increasingly common as these devices have become widely available. Initial reports of the JOSTENT (Abbott Vascular, Redwood City, CA) covered stents began in 1998 after successful use in the treatment of iatrogenic coronary perforation following atherectomy (39). Shortly thereafter, a case report of JOSTENT use was published, demonstrating a successful treatment of a coronary artery aneurysm. The JOSTENT covered stent consists of an ultrathin polytetrafluoroethylene (PTFE) expandable layer sandwiched in between two coaxial 316L stainless steel, slotted-tube, balloon-expandable stents with a potential diameter of 2.5 to 5.0 mm. The device is rigid and requires a 7F guiding-catheter for delivery. Therefore, the use of 7F guiding catheters when technically feasible is recommended in cases at high risk of coronary perforation, such as degenerated saphenous vein grafts and highly calcified lesions or when the use of atheroablative devices or stiff hydrophilic wires is antici-

pated. If a life-threatening perforation occurs while using a smaller guiding catheter (6F or 5F), an angioplasty balloon should be immediately inflated at low pressure to occlude the perforation. Another operator should obtain access in the contralateral femoral artery and advance a 7F guiding catheter to selectively cannulate the coronary ostium after gently disengaging the smaller guiding catheter. A second guidewire should be advanced just proximal to the occluding balloon, which is then deflated and retracted, allowing passage of the new guidewire and covered stent for complete and definitive closure of the perforation (19).

Briguori et al. reported their experience in treating 12 coronary ruptures in which the JOSTENT covered stent was used. The device failed only in one case in which the coronary perforation was too distal in the coronary anatomy and could not be reached with the stent. The devices were deployed promptly in approximately 10 minutes at a mean pressure of 15 atmospheres causing a significant reduction in the development of cardiac tamponade and the need for cardiac surgery (40). An international voluntary registry reported encouraging results with the JOSTENT covered stent. A total of 52 devices were successfully deployed to treat 41 coronary perforations, resulting in a 93% complete perforation sealing, with none of the patients requiring surgery (19). Although the PTFE-covered stent has many theoretical advantages over uncovered stents, it has not proven to reduce the risk of restenosis in the coronary circulation under a variety of circumstances (41). The main advantage of the PTFE-covered stent-graft is the simple mechanical advantage of complete exclusion of the lumen in the stented segment.

Surprisingly, the technology of covered stents has progressed slowly over the past decade. The JOSTENT PTFE-covered stent is not currently approved for use in the coronary circulation in the United States, and compassionate use documentation is required at most institutions. Advancements are currently under way, and new technologies are making their way into the market. New pericardial covered stent are now available within a humanitarian device exemption in the United States. Fortunately, other investigational covered stents are currently under development that are designed to provide complete lumen exclusion in case of perforation

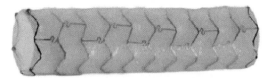

FIGURE 16-8. The Over and Under equine pericardium-covered stent graft sets a barrier between the blood vessel wall and its lumen. (Courtesy of ITGI Medical, Or Akiva, Israel.)

and may have the advantage of improved deliverability.

Jokhi et al. (42) recently reported the successful use of a pericardial covered stent to treat a localized type 3 coronary perforation. The Over and Under stent (ITGI Medical Ltd., Or Akiva, Israel) is a single layer of stainless steel stent covered by a treated layer of equine [GRC5]pericardium (Fig. 16-8). This device, and a second pericardial tissue-covered stent (Aneugraft) manufactured by ITGI Medical received a humanitarian device exemption (HDE) by the FDA in April of 2009. The same stent has also been described for use in the treatment of idiopathic coronary artery aneurysm exclusion (43) (Fig. 16-9). The eventual availability of devices such as the Over and Under stent will provide important options for coronary interventional procedures in the United States and will become increasingly important as operators choose to perform PCI on an increasing number of high-risk lesions.

The JOSTENT remains the most commonly used covered stent in the coronary circulation and is available in most laboratories. Recent HDE approval of the pericardial tissue-covered stents will likely result in a significant shift in clinical practice, as these devices can be delivered through a 6F system and offer improved flexibility.

■ VASCULAR COILS AND OTHER EMBOLIC MATERIALS

Despite appropriate acute management including reversal of anticoagulation, distal perforations may lead to progressive accumulation of pericardial blood, resulting in tamponade. The risk of distal perforation was higher in the era of balloon-only angioplasty, likely due to the use of stiffer, more lubricious guidewires (14). Because occlusion of side branches and distal vessels is least likely to cause transmural ischemia or significant myocardial infarction, perforations in these locations are most appropriately treated with prolonged balloon inflation and reversal and/or discontinuation of antiplatelet agents and anticoagulation. However, microcoil embolization has been performed with good success when these measures are unsuccessful, and it should be considered when the amount of myocardium at risk is small and not likely to result in hemodynamically significant ischemia and/or infarction (44). In general, arteries with a diameter of less than 1.5 mm are considered reasonable to treat with embolic devices, whereas larger arteries should be managed with the goal of preserving distal perfusion (45).

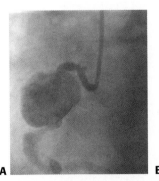
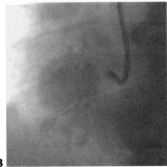
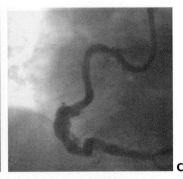

A   B   C

FIGURE 16-9. Large right coronary aneurysm treated with an Over and Under pericardium-covered stent (ITGI Medical, Or Akiva, Israel). (**A**) Large right coronary aneurysm with a diameter of 35 mm and a length of 40 mm and large right coronary aneurysm treated with an Over and Under pericardium-covered stent. (**B**) A 3.5 × 27 mm covered stent is positioned in the distal portion of the aneurysm. (**C**) Final result after placement of a proximal 3.5 × 23 mm covered stent and complete exclusion of the aneurysm. (Courtesy of Dr. E. Bramucci, Policlinico San Matteo, Pavia, Italy.)

The use of embolization coils in the coronary circulation is rare, and available devices are not currently approved for this indication. However, off-label use can be an important treatment for some patients, and the use of platinum coils to occlude distal coronary arteries following perforation after PCI has been reported (6,46,47). These devices have the advantage of allowing for precise occlusion of distal vessels. In general, all thrombotic vascular coils work in a similar way—by inducing thrombogenesis through platelet activation on a matrix consisting of prothrombotic agents. Stainless steel or platinum microcoils are currently manufactured by several companies and are generally compatible for delivery through most angiographic catheters and 3F microcatheters. Most devices are compatible with polyethylene and braided nylon catheters but should not be used with polyurethane catheters to avoid distal entrapment (47). Most devices are detachable and manufactured in a variety of coil lengths, diameters, and shapes. Many coils are supplied with a manufacturer-recommended microcatheter. The larger coils (0.035 mm thickness) are generally preferred for the peripheral circulation, and smaller diameter coils (0.018 mm thickness) are preferred for small vessel occlusion such as coronary or cerebral arteries.

The technical aspects of coil embolization vary somewhat among devices, and all practicing interventionalists should have a general familiarity with their use. Coil embolization should be attempted only when the amount of myocardium at risk is small and unlikely to result in significant myocardial dysfunction. In most cases, due to their relative stiffness, these devices require optimal guide catheter support when delivered into the coronary circulation through a microcatheter. The microcatheter is advanced over a previously placed coronary guidewire via the coronary guiding catheter into the distal vessel that requires thrombosis. Typically, a 0.014 guidewire can be used with any number of available microcatheter devices. The microcatheter should be delivered into the distal vessel to be embolized and then the guidewire withdrawn (or used for coil delivery depending on the device). Platinum microcoils are loaded in the microcatheter, and they can then be advanced through the microcatheter by pushing with a "coil-pushing wire," with careful attention paid to guiding catheter support and distal catheter position. It is generally acceptable to choose a microcoil from 120% to 150% of the diameter of the target vessel (48). Successful coil embolization has been reported after coronary artery injury during elective pericardiocentesis (49). Figure 16-10 displays an illustration of the Tornado Platinum Microcoil (Cook Medical).

Alternatives to metallic coil embolization include polyvinyl alcohol foam particles and direct thrombin injection. Gelfoam embolization has also been reported in the coronary circulation (50). Gelfoam use is appealing because of its availability, low cost, and flexibility in size

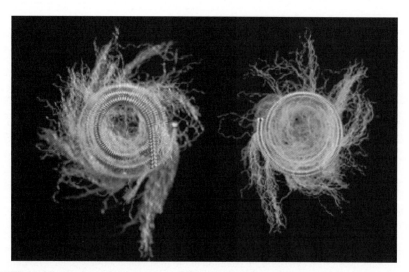

FIGURE 16-10. Tornado Platinum Microcoil. (Courtesy of Cook Medical, Bloomington, Indiana.)

and structure (51). Gelatin sponge particles have been developed for delivery through a microcatheter, and this technique has been frequently described for use in multiple circulatory beds. Similar to platinum microcoils, these materials are highly thromobogenic and should be delivered only into the distal circulation where the risk of proximal migration is small.

■ CONCLUSION

Coronary perforation is a rare but serious complication of PCI. As a rare complication, most of our knowledge derives from retrospective analyses of databases at high-volume single institutions. Type I perforation, because of its benign clinical course, is usually underreported (8,13). Distal wire perforations are generally not consequential if recognized early and treated appropriately. Larger perforations are typically the result of aggressive balloon or stent inflation in smaller, diseased arteries and/or degenerated vein grafts. Treatment is based on the specific features of each case with three common goals: maintain vital organ perfusion by preventing cardiac tamponade, maintain distal coronary circulation to avoid myocardial infarction, and avoid emergency cardiac surgery. All such events should be treated with reversal of anticoagulation and antiplatelet agents when feasible. Covered stents provide an important option for the treatment of large perforations that persist after conventional stent placement. Long-term, coronary aneurysm formation may result from inadequate healing of coronary perforations during PCI. The off-label use of platinum microcoils, gelfoam embolization, and other techniques of distal embolization have occasional application in the coronary circulation but should be considered only in situations where the distal coronary supplies a small territory and the risk of proximal migration of embolic material can be effectively minimized. Covered stents provide an important option in the treatment of iatrogenic coronary aneurysm and have been proven effective in excluding the aneurysmal segment while maintaining vessel patency.

References

1. Saito S. Different strategies of retrograde approach in coronary angioplasty for chronic total occlusion. *Catheter Cardiovasc Interv.* 2008;71:8–19.

2. Colombo A, Mikhail GW, Michev I, et al. Treating chronic total occlusions using subintimal tracking and reentry: the STAR technique. *Catheter Cardiovasc Interv.* 2005;64:407–411, discussion 412.

3. Ajluni SC, Glazier S, Blankenship L, et al. Perforations after percutaneous coronary interventions: clinical, angiographic, and therapeutic observations. *Cathet Cardiovasc Diagn.* 1994;32:206–212.

4. Ellis SG, Ajluni S, Arnold AZ, et al. Increased coronary perforation in the new device era: incidence, classification, management, and outcome. *Circulation.* 1994;90:2725–2730.

5. Gruberg L, Pinnow E, Flood R, et al. Incidence, management, and outcome of coronary artery perforation during percutaneous coronary intervention. *Am J Cardiol.* 2000;86:680–682, A8.

6. Fasseas P, Orford JL, Panetta CJ, et al. Incidence, correlates, management, and clinical outcome of coronary perforation: analysis of 16,298 procedures. *Am Heart J.* 2004;147:140–145.

7. Gunning MG, Williams IL, Jewitt DE, et al. Coronary artery perforation during percutaneous intervention: incidence and outcome. *Heart.* 2002;88:495–498.

8. Stankovic G, Orlic D, Corvaja N, et al. Incidence, predictors, in-hospital, and late outcomes of coronary artery perforations. *Am J Cardiol.* 2004;93:213–216.

9. Witzke CF, Martin-Herrero F, Clarke SC, et al. The changing pattern of coronary perforation during percutaneous coronary intervention in the new device era. *J Invasive Cardiol.* 2004;16:257–301.

10. Javaid A, Buch AN, Satler LF, et al. Management and outcomes of coronary artery perforation during percutaneous coronary intervention. *Am J Cardiol.* 2006;98:911–914.

11. Kini AS, Rafael OC, Sarkar K, et al. Changing outcomes and treatment strategies for wire induced coronary perforations in the era of bivalirudin use. *Catheter Cardiovasc Interv.* 2009;74:700–707.

12. Seshadri N, Whitlow PL, Acharya N, et al. Emergency coronary artery bypass surgery in the contemporary percutaneous coronary intervention era. *Circulation.* 2002;106:2346–2350.

13. Dippel EJ, Kereiakes DJ, Tramuta DA, et al. Coronary perforation during percutaneous coronary intervention in the era of abciximab platelet glycoprotein IIb/IIIa blockade: an algorithm for percutaneous management. *Catheter Cardiovasc Interv.* 2001;52:279–286.

14. Wong CM, Kwong Mak GY, Chung DT. Distal coronary artery perforation resulting from the use of hydrophilic coated guidewire in tortuous vessels. *Cathet Cardiovasc Diagn.* 1998;44:93–96.

15. Colombo A, Stankovic G. Coronary perforations: old screenplay, new actors! *J Invasive Cardiol.* 2004;16:302–303.

16. Lincoff AM, Bittl JA, Harrington RA, et al. Bivalirudin and provisional glycoprotein IIb/IIIa blockade compared with heparin and planned glycoprotein IIb/IIIa blockade during percutaneous coronary intervention: REPLACE-2 randomized trial. *JAMA.* 2003;289:853–863.

17. Stone GW, McLaurin BT, Cox DA, et al. Bivalirudin for patients with acute coronary syndromes. *N Engl J Med.* 2006;355:2203–2216.

18. Roy P, de Labriolle A, Hanna N, et al. Requirement for emergent coronary artery bypass surgery following percutaneous coronary intervention in the stent era. *Am J Cardiol.* 2009;103:950–953.

19. Lansky AJ, Yang YM, Khan Y, et al. Treatment of coronary artery perforations complicating percutaneous coronary intervention with a polytetrafluoroethylene-covered stent graft. *Am J Cardiol.* 2006;98:370–374.

20. Gorge G, Erbel R, Haude M, et al. Continuous coronary perfusion balloon catheters in coronary dissections after percutaneous transluminal coronary angioplasty: acute clinical results and 6-months follow-up. *Eur Heart J.* 1994;15:908–914.

21. Levy JH, Adkinson NF Jr. Anaphylaxis during cardiac surgery: implications for clinicians. *Anesth Analg.* 2008;106:392–403.

22. Cosgrave J, Qasim A, Latib A, et al. Protamine usage following implantation of drug-eluting stents: a word of caution. *Catheter Cardiovasc Interv.* 2008;71:913–914.

23. Antoniucci D. *ARNO: A Prospective Randomized Trial Comparison of Bivalirudin and Unfractionated Heparin Plus Protamine in Patients Undergoing Elective Percutaneous Coronary Intervention.* Washington, DC: Transcatheter Cardiovascular Therapeutics; 2008.

24. Bittl JA. Reducing the risk of emergency bypass surgery for failed percutaneous coronary interventions. *J Am Coll Cardiol.* 2005;46:2010–2012.

25. Al Shammeri OM, Crowell R, Stewart K, Fort S. Failed pericardiocentesis for acute cardiac tamponade: two cases associated with bivalirudin administration during PCI. *Catheter Cardiovasc Interv.* 2010;75(1):114–116.

26. Fejka M, Dixon SR, Safian RD, et al. Diagnosis, management, and clinical outcome of cardiac tamponade complicating percutaneous coronary intervention. *Am J Cardiol.* 2002;90:1183–1186.

27. Tsang TS, Freeman WK, Barnes ME, et al. Rescue echocardiographically guided pericardiocentesis for cardiac perforation complicating catheter-based procedures: the Mayo Clinic experience. *J Am Coll Cardiol.* 1998;32:1345–1350.

28. Syed M, Lesch M. Coronary artery aneurysm: a review. *Prog Cardiovasc Dis.* 1997;40:77–84.

29. Saito S, Arai H, Kim K, Aoki N. Pseudoaneurysm of coronary artery following rupture of coronary artery during coronary angioplasty. *Cathet Cardiovasc Diagn.* 1992;26:304–307.

30. Eshima K, Takemoto M, Inoue S, et al. Coronary aneurysm associated with coronary perforation after sirolimus-eluting stents implantation: close follow-up exceeding 2 years by coronary 3-dimensional computed tomography. *J Cardiol.* 2009;54:115–120.

31. Slota PA, Fischman DL, Savage MP, et al. Frequency and outcome of development of coronary artery aneurysm after intracoronary stent placement and angioplasty: STRESS Trial Investigators. *Am J Cardiol.* 1997;79:1104–1106.

32. Hill JA, Margolis JR, Feldman RL, et al. Coronary arterial aneurysm formation after balloon angioplasty. *Am J Cardiol.* 1983;52:261–264.

33. Alfonso F, Perez-Vizcayno MJ, Ruiz M, et al. Coronary aneurysms after drug-eluting stent implantation: clinical, angiographic, and intravascular ultrasound findings. *J Am Coll Cardiol.* 2009;53:2053–2060.

34. Aoki J, Kirtane A, Leon MB, Dangas G. Coronary artery aneurysms after drug-eluting stent implantation. *JACC Cardiovasc Interv.* 2008;1:14–21.

35. Joner M, Finn AV, Farb A, et al. Pathology of drug-eluting stents in humans: delayed healing and late thrombotic risk. *J Am Coll Cardiol.* 2006;48:193–202.

36. Bavry AA, Chiu JH, Jefferson BK, et al. Development of coronary aneurysm after drug-eluting stent implantation. *Ann Intern Med.* 2007;146:230–232.

37. Robertson T, Fisher L. Prognostic significance of coronary artery aneurysm and ectasia in the Coronary Artery Surgery Study (CASS) registry. *Prog Clin Biol Res.* 1987;250:325–339.

38. Daoud AS, Pankin D, Tulgan H, Florentin RA. Aneurysms of the coronary artery: report of ten cases and review of literature. *Am J Cardiol.* 1963;11:228–237.

39. Ramsdale DR, Mushahwar SS, Morris JL. Repair of coronary artery perforation after rotastenting by implantation of the JoStent covered stent. *Cathet Cardiovasc Diagn.* 1998;45:310–313.

40. Briguori C, Nishida T, Anzuini A, et al. Emergency polytetrafluoroethylene-covered stent implantation to treat coronary ruptures. *Circulation.* 2000; 102:3028–3031.

41. Schachinger V, Hamm CW, Munzel T, et al. A randomized trial of polytetrafluoroethylene-membrane-covered stents compared with conventional stents in aortocoronary saphenous vein grafts. *J Am Coll Cardiol.* 2003;42:1360–1369.

42. Jokhi PP, McKenzie DB, O'Kane P. Use of a novel pericardial covered stent to seal an iatrogenic coronary perforation. *J Invasive Cardiol.* 2009;21: E187–E190.

43. Hayat SA, Ghani S, More RS. Treatment of ruptured coronary aneurysm with a novel covered stent. *Catheter Cardiovasc Interv.* 2009;74:367–370.

44. Katsanos K, Patel S, Dourado R, Sabharwal T. Lifesaving embolization of coronary artery perforation. *Cardiovasc Intervent Radiol.* 2009;32: 1071–1074.

45. Klein LW. Coronary artery perforation during interventional procedures. *Catheter Cardiovasc Interv.* 2006;68:713–717.

46. Aslam MS, Messersmith RN, Gilbert J, Lakier JB. Successful management of coronary artery perforation with helical platinum microcoil embolization. *Catheter Cardiovasc Interv.* 2000;51:320–322.

47. Ponnuthurai FA, Ormerod OJ, Forfar C. Microcoil embolization of distal coronary artery perforation without reversal of anticoagulation: a simple, effective approach. *J Invasive Cardiol.* 2007;19:E222–E225.

48. Vance MS. Use of platinum microcoils to embolize vascular abnormalities in children with congenital heart disease. *Pediatr Cardiol.* 1998; 19:145–149.

49. Lee EW, Hung R, Kee ST, et al. Coronary artery perforation following pericardiocentesis managed by coil embolization. *Eur J Radiol Extra.* 2009;70:e57–e59.

50. Dixon SR, Webster MW, Ormiston JA, et al. Gelfoam embolization of a distal coronary artery guidewire perforation. *Catheter Cardiovasc Interv.* 2000;49:214–217.

51. Abada HT, Golzarian J. Gelatine sponge particles: handling characteristics for endovascular use. *Tech Vasc Interv Radiol.* 2007;10:257–260.

17

No-Reflow, Distal Embolization, and Embolic Protection

ELIAS V. HADDAD AND ROBERT N. PIANA

Coronary "no-reflow" is manifested by insufficient myocardial perfusion in the absence of flow-limiting epicardial vessel obstruction, dissection, spasm, or distal macroembolus (1,2). Interventionalists generally encounter two types of no-reflow in clinical practice: reperfusion-related no-reflow (RNR) and primary no-reflow (PNR) (3–5). The RNR phenomenon involves a baseline period of impaired myocardial perfusion due to epicardial coronary obstruction, as in the setting of acute ST-elevation myocardial infarction (STEMI) with complete coronary occlusion or under conditions of profound ischemia due to a subtotal occlusion with reduced but existent coronary flow. Even when the obstruction is relieved with either percutaneous coronary intervention (PCI) or pharmacologic intervention, distal myocardial tissue perfusion remains compromised. In PNR, PCI performed on a vessel with normal perfusion before the intervention acutely precipitates no-reflow.

■ PATHOPHYSIOLOGY

No-reflow was first described in cerebral ischemia and later demonstrated in animal models of coronary ischemia–reperfusion (1–2). Kloner (1) found that temporary occlusion of the canine coronary artery followed by release after 40 minutes yielded normal myocardial perfusion. However, after 90 minutes of coronary occlusion, the post-release perfusion was significantly impaired. Prolonged ischemia promotes cellular and interstitial edema, endothelial cell distortions, cellular contraction, and intravascular platelet–fibrin aggregates (Fig. 17-1). Together these cause microvascular compression, plugging, and constriction, inhibiting effective tissue perfusion even when epicardial flow is subsequently restored.

Despite the obvious benefits of epicardial coronary recanalization, the act of reperfusion also floods the downstream tissues with activated leukocytes and tissue factor, which further plug the microvasculature with microaggregates, generate oxygen free radicals, and escalate edema by increasing vascular permeability. The destruction of capillaries mediated by activated neutrophils and their proinflammatory products creates a vicious cycle of endothelial cell dysfunction and persistent vasoconstriction (1,6). Thus, reperfusion can amplify some of the adverse microvascular effects of prolonged ischemia.

In PNR, barotrauma from PCI is thought to precipitate distal microembolization of atheroma and thrombus and to induce the release of potent vasoconstrictors. Coronary aspirates after PCI complicated by no-reflow exhibit a greater burden of atheromatous plaque and more platelet-fibrin complex, macrophages, and cholesterol crystals than do aspirates from procedures with normal flow (7). It has been shown that obstruction of more than 50% of the microcirculatory bed is required to decrease myocardial blood flow irreversibly (8). These mechanisms are also important factors in RNR when the epicardial obstruction is dilated or lysed, leading to downstream embolization. The role of vasoconstriction is implicated by the known potential of multiple cellular elements involved to release vasoactive substances and the observed responsiveness of no-reflow to vasodilators.

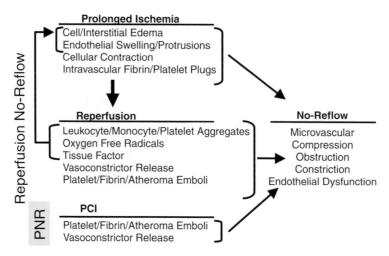

FIGURE 17-1. Mechanisms of no-reflow. PCI, percutaneous coronary intervention; PNR, primary no-reflow.

▪ RECOGNITION

Reperfusion no-reflow can be documented by using multiple imaging modalities. Scintigraphy, positron emission tomography, cardiac magnetic resonance imaging (MRI), and myocardial contrast echocardiography can all demonstrate zones of no-reflow and give direct evidence of impaired myocardial perfusion. Incomplete ST-segment resolution (defined as <70% resolution) after reperfusion for STEMI also correlates with tissue no-reflow.

The most immediate manifestation of no-reflow from the proceduralist's standpoint in the catheterization laboratory is angiographic evidence of delayed anterograde flow, often accompanied by ischemic electrocardiographic changes and angina (Fig. 17-2). To confirm no-reflow, mechanical obstruction should be excluded. Angiographic inspection can ensure no-flow–limiting residual lesion, dissection, or distal cutoff. Injection through the lumen of an-over-the-wire balloon positioned beyond the lesion can document absence of distal obstruction, and intravascular ultrasound of the vessel can be used to identify occult lesions not visualized angiographically.

The degree of angiographic no-reflow can be quantified using several methodologies. The Thrombolysis in Myocardial Infarction (TIMI) flow grade was designed to describe the rapidity of blood flow through an obstructed or severely stenosed artery in the setting of myocardial infarction (MI) (9) (Table 17-1). While TIMI flow grade is applied to coronary no-reflow as

well, by definition, no-reflow refers to impaired perfusion in the *absence* of obvious epicardial obstruction. The TIMI blush score may therefore be more applicable to no-reflow in that it grades the degree of tissue inflow and outflow, without reference to a site of upstream epicardial obstruction (10) (Table 17-2). The TIMI Frame Count can further quantify the speed of anterograde flow by counting the number of imaging frames required for contrast to reach a specified distal landmark. In this manner, perfusion can be incorporated into research analyses as a continuous variable. Finally, intracoronary (IC) Doppler measurements can detect a typical pattern during no-reflow of reduced or absent anterograde systolic flow, followed by a retrograde systolic flow and a rapid deceleration of diastolic flow (11).

▪ INCIDENCE

The incidence of no-reflow depends largely on the rigor of the surveillance, the detection method, and the completeness of reporting. Reperfusion no-reflow (TIMI flow ≤2) complicating primary PCI for MI was reported in 12% to 25% of cases in earlier single-center studies (12–13), but in only 4% to 7% of patients in the multicenter prospective PAMI and CADILLAC trials (14–15). Much higher rates of RNR have been noted with other modalities that can assess microvascular flow: 29% using the TIMI blush score (16), 34% using myocardial contrast echocardiography (17), and 39% with contrast-enhanced cardiac MRI (18).

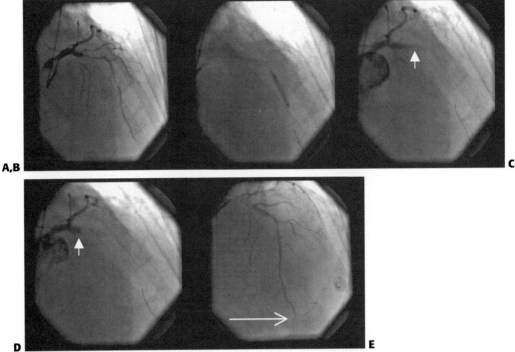

FIGURE 17-2. Angiographic appearance of no-reflow following percutaneous intervention to a critical stenosis (**A**) in the mid LAD. Following stent deployment (**B**), a column of contrast hangs up in the proximal vessel and does not progress beyond the stent (TIMI 0 flow). There was no evidence of distal vessel obstruction, using injection through the lumen of an over the wire balloon positioned in the distal vessel. Frames 28 (**C**) and 39 (**D**) from a single cine run indicate to-and-fro motion of contrast in the proximal vessel, characteristic of severe no-reflow. Note that the column of dye is further down the LAD in (C) than in (D). (**E**) Final result after multiple rounds of intracoronary calcium channel blockers and nitroprusside. There was still very slow anterograde flow with incomplete opacification of the apical vessel (*white arrow*).

PNR is likely significantly underreported in clinical practice unless it directly precipitates clinical complications. In a single-center, systematic retrospective review of more than 1,900 unselected PCI cases (including acute MI patients), Piana et al. (13) documented angiographic no-reflow in 2.0% in the overall cohort, with much higher rates of 11.5% in saphenous

TABLE 17-1 **TIMI Flow Classification**

TIMI Class	Definition
0	No anterograde flow beyond point of obstruction
1	Contrast passes the point of obstruction but fails to opacify the entire coronary bed
2	Contrast passes the point of obstruction and opacifies the distal coronary bed, but the rate of entry and clearance of contrast is slower than that seen in a comparable coronary bed not supplied by the occluded vessel
3	Brisk anterograde flow distal to the point of obstruction with rapid clearance of contrast comparable with that seen in an uninvolved coronary bed

(Adapted from Chesebro J, Knatterud G, Roberts R. Thrombolysis in Myocardial Infarction (TIMI) Trial, Phase I: a comparison between intravenous tissue plasminogen activator and intravenous streptokinase: clinical findings through hospital discharge. *Circulation*. 1987;76:142–154.)

| TABLE 17-2 | Myocardial Blush Grade Classification |

Myocardial Blush Grade	Definition
0	No myocardial blush or contrast density
1	Minimal myocardial blush or contrast density
2	Moderate myocardial blush or contrast density but less than that obtained with angiography of a contralateral or ipsilateral noninfarct-related artery
3	Normal myocardial blush or contrast density comparable with that obtained during angiography of a contralateral or ipsilateral noninfarct–related artery

(Adapted from vant Hof AW, Liem A, Suryapranata H, Hoorntje JC, de Boer MJ, Zijlstra F. Angiographic assessment of myocardial reperfusion in patients treated with primary angioplasty for acute myocardial infarction: myocardial blush grade. Zwolle Myocardial Infarction Study Group. *Circulation*. 1998;97: 2302–2306.)

vein graft (SVG) interventions and 4% in primary PCI for acute MI. The reported incidence is only 0.6%, using a more conservative definition of no-reflow as TIMI flow 1 or less (19). Importantly, the incidence of no-reflow has diminished substantially over the course of the last two decades. In an analysis of 21,000 patients, Mattichak et al. (20) reported no-reflow in only 1.7% in the pre-stent era, 2.8% with first generation stenting, and only 0.5% of contemporary stent cases (20). This trend parallels improved antithrombotic therapy, more refined interventional techniques, and lower profile, less traumatic devices for mechanical revascularization.

■ RISK FACTORS AND PREDICTORS

Clinical Features

Conditions that promote vascular inflammation, such as diabetes mellitus and hypercholesterolemia, have been suggested to predispose to no-reflow. Patients presenting with acute MI are at high risk, and this is exacerbated in patients with hyperglycemia (21). Similarly, renal dysfunction correlates with RNR (22,23). As a corollary, elevated levels of high sensitivity C-Reactive Protein (hsCRP) have also been associated with greater no-reflow (24).

Platelet hyperreactivity, an independent marker of risk for recurrent cardiovascular events following PCI, has now also been associated with an increased risk of no-reflow and impaired

myocardial reperfusion following PCI (25). However, since no consistent marker of in vivo platelet activation exists, routine platelet testing has not yet become standard of care to stratify risk of no-reflow and other adverse events during PCI. Interestingly, elevated plasma thromboxane A2 levels and higher mean platelet volumes have been shown to correlate with no-reflow, further supporting the contribution of platelet activity to the pathophysiology of no-reflow (25,26).

Angiographic and Procedural Factors

Thrombotic coronary occlusion in acute MI and acute coronary syndromes has consistently emerged as a potent risk for no-reflow. Angiographic features suggestive of high no-reflow risk include large thrombus burden with more than 5 mm of thrombus proximal to the obstruction, presence of mobile thrombus, persistent stasis of contrast distal to the obstruction, and a cutoff pattern of obstruction without a taper morphology (27) (Figs. 17-3–17-6). Other adverse prognostic features of the infarct-related artery include a reference luminal diameter of 4 mm or more and lesion length of more than 13.5 mm and an initial TIMI flow grade less than 3 (22,28).

Bypass grafts appear to be at particularly high risk. SVG lesions endured no-reflow at a rate of 4.0% in the study by Piana et al., compared with 1.5% in non-MI, non–vein graft patients (13) Device selection may also play a role. Rotational atherectomy (RA) was plagued with an incidence of no-reflow of 8% to 12% early on in its

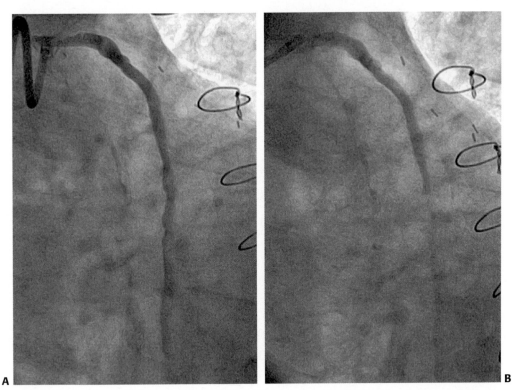

FIGURE 17-3. (**A**) Contrast progression at 33 frames into the injection before a stent is placed in the very distal portion of the graft (*not shown*). (**B**) Contrast progression at 33 frames into the injection after stent placement, showing marked impairment of flow. There is a suggestion in the right panel of a cutoff, but this is artifactual from the still frame.

adoption (19,29–31). Together, these data support the concept that distal embolization contributes significantly to the process of no-reflow. Finally, the timing of primary PCI factors prominently in the risk profile for RNR, with longer delays correlating with higher rates of RNR (27,28). In a single-center analysis, the incidence of RNR approached 20% when revascularization was delayed for 4 hours or more (27).

OUTCOMES

Left ventricular systolic dysfunction and infarct size are significantly increased in the setting of RNR (17,22,32). Moreover, angiographic evidence of no-reflow (such as reduced TIMI myocardial blush grade) is a potent independent predictor of reduced survival, with an odds ratio for cardiac death of 3.6 (33).

PREVENTION

The most efficacious approach to no-reflow is to prevent its occurrence in the first place. Case selec-

tion is critical. The interventionalist may be well advised to revascularize a territory through the native circulation when possible, rather than tackling a severely degenerated vein graft with multiple bulky filling defects, for example (Figs. 17-7 and 17-8). Minimizing the door-to-balloon time in acute MI should reduce the chances of RNR on the basis of current data. The interventionalist can also minimize barotrauma and distal embolization by limiting the number, diameter, and pressure of balloon inflations when stenting high-risk lesions. Techniques designed to prevent no-reflow during RA include avoiding lesions with IC thrombus, reducing burr to artery ratio to 0.6 or less, and lowering the rotational speed to approximately 140,000 rpm, as well as using the adjunctive pharmacologic measures described below.

Mechanical Prevention

Fortunately, when confronted with high-risk clinical scenarios, mechanical methods to prevent distal embolization are now available (see "Embolic Protection Devices" section later) (Tables 17-3

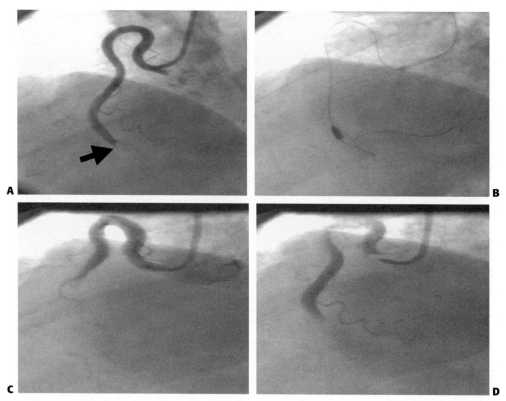

FIGURE 17-4. (**A**) Left anterior oblique view of thrombotic occlusion (*black arrow*) of the distal right coronary artery in a patient undergoing primary percutaneous intervention for acute ST-elevation myocardial infarction. Note the abrupt cutoff with a visible meniscus indicating thrombus. (**B**) Balloon inflation at the lesion. (**C**) Left anterior oblique view after balloon angioplasty showing TIMI 0 flow. (**D**) Even after prolonged angiographic run, there is no flow past the lesion (TIMI 0). Residual mechanical obstruction has not been excluded as the distal lesion was not stented, no intravascular ultrasound was performed, and no injection of the distal vessel beyond the lesion was performed through the lumen of an over the wire balloon positioned beyond the lesion. These maneuvers are important to confirm the diagnosis of no-reflow.

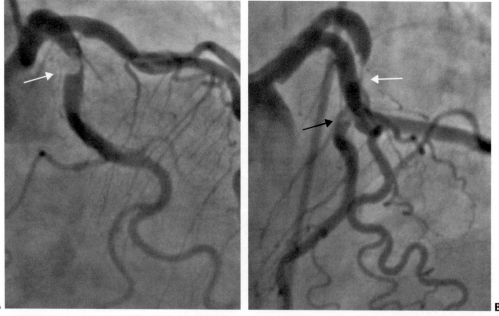

FIGURE 17-5. (**A**) Right anterior oblique caudal view of a large burden of thrombus (*white arrow*) in the proximal left circumflex artery. (**B**) Left anterior oblique cranial view showing a thrombotic lesion in the left anterior descending artery (*black arrow*).

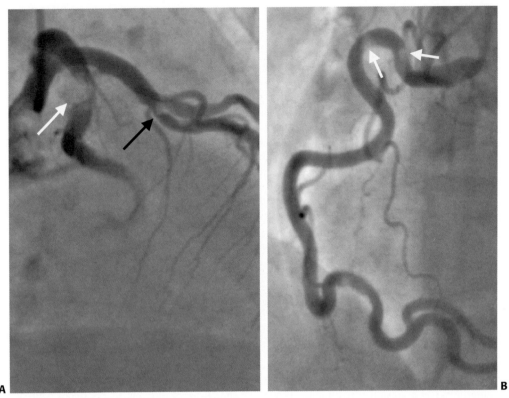

FIGURE 17-6. (**A**) Straight right anterior oblique view showing the thrombotic lesions in the left circumflex (*white arrow*) and left anterior descending arteries (*black arrow*). (**B**) Straight left anterior oblique view showing thrombotic lesion in the proximal right coronary artery (*white arrows*).

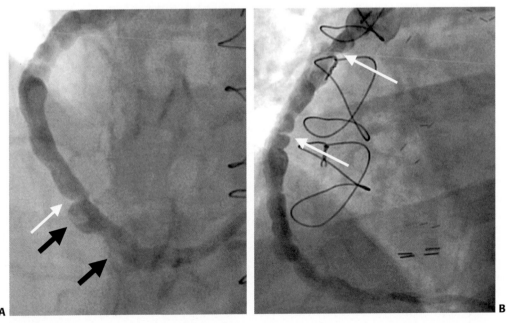

FIGURE 17-7. Degenerated vein graft with a multiple filling defects (*black arrows*), multiple moderate lesions (*white arrows*), diffuse haziness, and TIMI 2 flow.

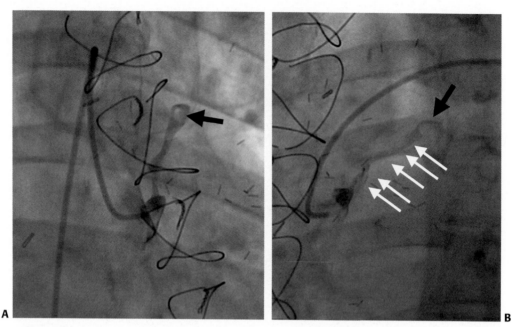

FIGURE 17-8. Degenerated (*white arrows*) vein graft with a large filling defect (*black arrow*) and TIMI 0 flow.

and 17-4). Embolic protection devices (EPDs) utilize conduit vessel occlusion (proximal or distal) with aspiration or distal filter capture of debris (34). Distal embolic protection is particularly useful in the setting of degenerated SVGs with a high embolic potential. In the SAFER (Saphenous vein graft Angioplasty Free of Emboli Randomized) trial, a strategy of distal embolic protection significantly reduced the incidence of no-reflow and MI, with an overall 42% relative risk reduction in major adverse cardiac events (35).

Interestingly, EPDs have not improved clinical outcomes in primary PCI for acute MI (36–38). Proposed explanations for this paradox include masking of any EPD-derived benefit by the much larger ischemic burden of the underlying infarction, distal embolization by the EPD insertion, embolization of distal material into side branches as it is aspirated back during certain EPD procedures, and inability of filters to capture debris smaller than the filtration pore size and vasoactive substances contributing to no-reflow. Rheolytic thrombectomy has also failed to improve outcomes in primary PCI (39). In the prospective, randomized "AngioJet® Rheolytic™ Thrombectomy In Patients Undergoing Primary Angioplasty for Acute Myocardial Infarction" (AiMI) trial, adjunctive AngioJet during primary PCI removed thrombus effectively but did not reduce infarct

size or improve TIMI flow grade, blush score, ST-segment resolution, or 30-day major adverse cardiac events. Proposed explanations have again included device-induced embolization, increased procedural time with thrombectomy, concurrent use of glycoprotein IIb/IIIa receptor inhibitors (GPI), and lower rates of baseline TIMI 3 flow in the thrombectomy group.

By contrast, adjunctive manual thrombectomy during primary PCI does improve TIMI 3 flow rates, myocardial blush grade, and resolution of ST-segment elevation compared with PCI alone (40–42). Moreover, the TAPAS (Thrombus Aspiration during Percutaneous coronary intervention in Acute myocardial infarction Study) correlated improvements in these indices of myocardial perfusion with reduced mortality 30 days following PCI (41–42). Perhaps, the lower profile of the manual aspiration catheters and the technique of continuous aspiration during initial advancement into the culprit lesion reduce device-induced embolization with this approach. The simplicity of these devices may also reduce door to balloon time compared with more complex rheolytic devices.

Pharmacologic Prevention

Pharmacologic strategies to prevent no reflow include use of vasodilators, inhibition of

TABLE 17-3 Embolic Protection Device Specifications

Device Type	FDA-Approved Devices	Manufacturer	Guide Compatibility	Guidewire Compatibility	Distal Landing Zone[a]	Advantages	Disadvantages
Distal filtration	SpiderFx	Ev3, Plymouth, Minnesota	6F	0.014 in.	20 mm	• Maintain anterograde flow • Allow angiography with device deployed • Rapid deployment and retrieval in most cases using techniques familiar to interventionalists	• Debris may embolize if smaller than filter pore size • Soluble factors not trapped • Filter crossing lesion may cause distal embolization • Possibly difficult to place in presence of tortuosity
	AngioGuard	Cordis, Miami, Florida	7F	Integrated wire	18 mm		
	FilterWire	Boston Scientific, Natick, Massachusetts	6F	0.014 in.	25 mm		
Distal occlusion	GuardWire	Medtronic, Santa Rosa, California	8F	0.014 in./0.018 in.	20 mm	• Lower profile than filter EPD • More easily delivered in tortuous anatomy	• Temporary flow obstruction may not be tolerated • Crossing lesion more challenging with device wire than with standard wire • Not applicable for very proximal lesions: risk debris embolization into the aorta • Crossing lesion may cause embolization • Risk of balloon induced dissection or injury • Limited lesion visualization with device deployed • Complex procedural steps less familiar to interventionalists • Potential for deflation failure
	TriActiv System	Kensey Nash, Exton, Pennsylvania	7F	0.014 in.	≥20 mm		
Proximal occlusion	Proxis System	Velocimed, Maple Grove, Minnesota	6F/7F	0.014 in.	12 mm (proximal)	• Device does not have to cross lesion • Protection of branch vessels • Protection in presence of tortuosity • Can be used for PCI on multiple separate lesions	• Temporary flow obstruction may not be tolerated • Risk of balloon-induced dissection or injury • Cannot be used for ostial/very proximal lesions

[a]Distal landing zone = disease-free segment distal to the lesion required to adequately deploy device.

TABLE 17-4 **Thrombectomy Devices**

Device	Guide Compatibility
Simple aspiration catheters	
Export (Medtronic)	6F/7F
Rescue (Boston Scientific)	7F
Diver CE (Invatec)	6F
Fetch (Medrad)	6F
Disruption plus aspiration systems	
X-Sizer (eV3, Inc.)	6F/8F
Angiojet (Possis/Medrad)	6F
Rinspiration (Kerberos)	6F

platelet activation with glycoprotein IIb/IIIa antagonists, and HMG-CoA reductase inhibitors (statins). The use of vasodilators and glycoprotein IIb/IIIa antagonists will be discussed in the section titled "Management and Bailout Techniques." Statins deserve brief mention as they have diverse actions beyond their lipid-lowering effect. They are known to be potent modulators of endothelial cell nitric oxide synthase (eNOS) and have been shown to upregulate NO synthesis (43). In addition, simvastatin specifically has been shown to activate mitrochondrial K_{ATP} channels, which play a role in protection from ischemia/reperfusion–induced injury (44).

Special interest has been given to the prevention of no-reflow during RA for the treatment of calcified plaque. It is in this setting the risk for no reflow is especially high, with an incidence of 6% to 12% (19,29–31). A number of pharmacologic cocktails have been postulated to mitigate against no-reflow during RA, including adenosine, nitroprusside, nitrates, calcium channel blockers (CCBs), GPIs, and potassium channel activators, as well as the use of Rotaglide lubricant. In a retrospective analysis, IC boluses of adenosine during RA were associated with a significant decrease in the incidence of no-reflow (30). However, data are limited, and at present, no uniform strategy has been put forward as superior for the prevention of no-reflow during RA.

Embolic Protection Devices

These devices can be divided into three types: (1) distal conduit occlusion, (2) proximal conduit occlusion, and (3) distal filtration. Table 17-3 summarizes the technical aspects of the devices currently available.

Distal Occlusion Devices

These devices interrupt anterograde flow by inflation of a balloon distal to the target lesion. Atherothrombotic debris and soluble substances liberated by PCI are therefore trapped in the epicardial vessel, avoiding distal embolization to the microvasculature. Following intervention, these components are aspirated from the vessel prior to balloon deflation and restoration of forward flow. The PercuSurge GuardWire (Medtronic, Minneapolis, MN) employs a balloon (2.5–5 mm or 3–6 mm) that is expanded with saline/contrast solution (Figs. 17-9 and 17-10). In contrast, the TriActiv System (Kensey Nash, Exton, PA) uses a gas (CO_2)-expandable balloon that allows for more rapid inflation and deflation. The advantage of distal occlusion is that debris of all sizes is captured and aspirated, and the risk of debris passing around the device is low. In theory, this approach also allows for the removal of soluble vasoactive or prothrombotic substances that would pass through alternative distal filtering devices.

The obvious disadvantage is the induction of ischemia during balloon occlusion of the conduit. The GuardWire requires a series of steps that can prolong the ischemic time if the interventionalist is not very familiar with this device. Patients dependent on perfusion through the graft undergoing intervention may therefore not tolerate this approach. Crossing the target lesion with the GuardWire is also generally more difficult than with standard coronary wires, and its crossing profile is 0.028 in. These factors lead to a risk of distal embolization during the unprotected period. Complete occlusion of anterograde flow during PCI of a very proximal or ostial lesion has the potential risk of embolization of debris back into the aorta and could increase the chances of stroke. Balloon inflation can traumatize the distal vessel, and balloon deflation failures can occur, mandating that the operator be very familiar with the technical steps required to troubleshoot swiftly in such a circumstance to relieve ischemia.

Distal occlusion devices have proven efficacious in the setting of SVG interventions. The SAFER trial assigned 801 patients to conventional stenting or graft intervention with the

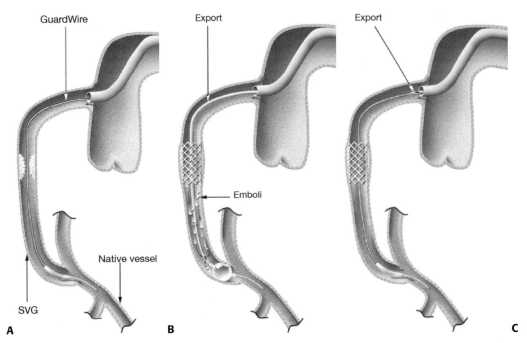

FIGURE 17-9. (**A**) GuardWire is advanced across the lesion and positioned approximately 2 cm distal to the lesion. (**B**) With balloon inflated, lesion is dilated and embolic debris is prevented from reaching the distal vessel due to the distal occlusion. Export catheter is used to aspirate the embolic debris and soluble factors. (**C**) Distal occlusion balloon is deflated and removed, restoring anterograde flow through the saphenous vein graft and into the native circulation. SVG, saphenous vein graft. (Adapted from Gorog DA, Foale RA, Malik I. Distal myocardial protection during percutaneous coronary intervention: When and Where? *J Am Coll Cardiol.* 2005;46:1434–1445.) (See color insert.)

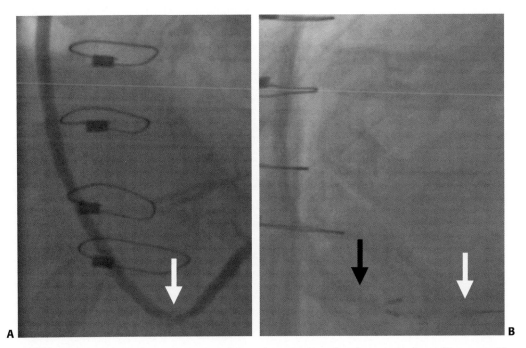

FIGURE 17-10. (**A**) Left anterior oblique view of the saphenous vein graft to the posterior descending artery with severe lesion in the distal graft (*white arrow*). (**B**) GuardWire is positioned and distal occlusion balloon inflated (*white arrow*) with stent positioned across the lesion (*black arrow*).

GuardWire distal occlusion device (35). Use of distal protection was shown to significantly decrease the incidence of no-reflow (3% vs. 9%) and MI (8.6% vs. 14.7%) and resulted in a 42% relative risk reduction in major adverse cardiac events (35). The benefit achieved with distal occlusion devices in vein graft intervention has not been duplicated with primary PCI in the setting of acute MI. The GuardWire was used in the EMERALD (Enhanced Myocardial Efficacy and Recovery by Aspiration of Liberated Debris) trial, which randomly assigned 501 patients with STEMI to primary PCI with or without embolic protection. There was no difference in the primary or secondary cardiovascular endpoints between those receiving distal protection versus conventional PCI (38).

Distal Filtration Devices

Filtration devices approach the problem of embolization using a nonocclusive basket with an elliptical mouth deployed distal to the target lesion (Fig. 17-11). This strategy benefits from the fact that the delivery and retrieval steps are familiar to most interventionalists. In the case of the SpiderFx, the lesion is crossed with any standard coronary wire rather than a less responsive, bulkier filter-wire or occlusion balloon-wire apparatus (Fig. 17-12). A distinct advantage of the filter approach is that flow through the conduit is preserved during the period of embolic protection. This allows good visualization of the target lesion and the distal vasculature during the procedure. Moreover, ischemia is minimized, rendering these devices more applicable to the critically ischemic patient.

Filter devices face several limitations. All distal filters must traverse the target lesion and thus incur some risk of device-induced distal embolization before protection is established. The completeness of debris capture is also variable. Good apposition of the basket against the vessel wall is critical for debris capture, and this is compromised with filter placement in tortuous segments (Figs. 17-13 and 17-14). The pore size of the filtration material also determines the completeness of capture. Available devices have a pore size ranging from 80 to 150 μm to allow passage of red blood cells and leucocytes through the filter. However, debris smaller than 80 μm and soluble factors will also pass through the filter and enter the microcirculation. Complete occlusion of the filter by embolic debris can occur, mimicking no-reflow. The operator must recognize this promptly and either use an aspiration catheter to clear the filter or retrieve the filter entirely to restore anterograde flow. In addition, instructions for use require a distal landing zone of approximately 18 to 30 mm from a graft anastomosis to accommodate the

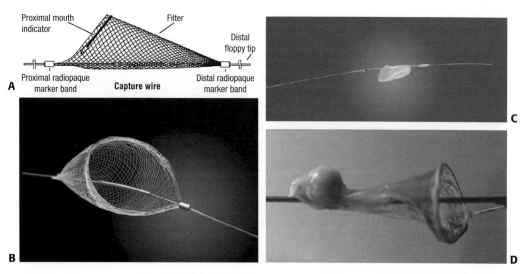

FIGURE 17-11. Several available Filter Devices. (**A**) Design of the SpiderFX device. (**B**) SpiderFX device. (**C**) Filter-Wire EZ device. (**D**) Captured embolic material in FilterWire EZ device. (**A** and **B:** Courtesy of ev3, Plymouth, Minnesota. **C** and **D:** Courtesy of Boston Scientific, Natick, Massachusetts.) (See color insert.)

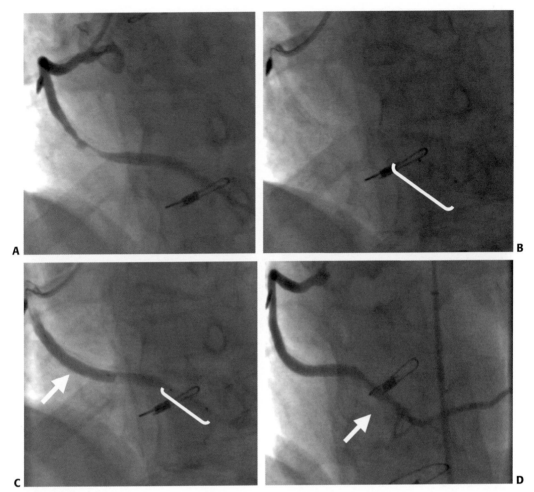

FIGURE 17-12. SpiderFx. (**A**) Left anterior oblique image of a saphenous vein graft to the posterior descending with a severe, ulcerated distal lesion. (**B**) Spider device in position (bracket) distal to the lesion. (**C**) Stent (*arrow*) being deployed across the lesion with Spider device in place (bracket). (**D**) Spider device removed. TIMI 3 flow. There may be some disruption (*arrow*) of the saphenous vein graft at the site of the Spider device positioning.

length of the device, thereby limiting the use of distal filtration in the setting of very distal lesions. However, in practice these devices are sometimes deployed in the native circulation beyond the distal graft anastomosis in the case of very distal lesions if the subtended coronary is of adequate diameter for proper device expansion. Filters also have the potential to traumatize the distal vessel, and advancement of filter retrieval sheaths through freshly deployed stents is sometimes difficult.

The data for benefit from distal filtration is similar to that seen with distal occlusion. The use of the FilterWire EX (Boston Scientific, Natick, Massachusetts) in the FIRE (FilterWire EX Randomized Evaluation) trial proved distal filtration noninferior to distal balloon occlusion for SVG intervention in terms of postprocedural myocardial perfusion and 30-day major adverse cardiac events (45). In the setting of STEMI, several trials have failed to show benefit from distal filtration during primary PCI in terms of infarct size, angiographic assessment of microcirculatory function, left ventricular function, and mortality.

Proximal Occlusion Devices

The Proxis (Velocimed, Maple Grove, Minnesota) device is useful when there is an inadequate distal landing zone. Similar to distal occlusion, this approach arrests anterograde flow while the intervention is performed, followed by

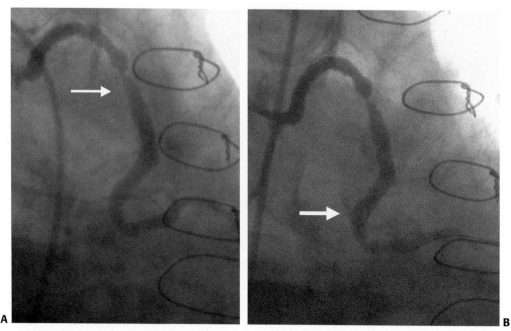

FIGURE 17-13. FilterWire EZ. (**A**) Critical lesion in saphenous vein graft to the left coronary system. (**B**) FilterWire EZ positioned beyond the lesion. Because of the tortuosity in the landing zone, the distal filter may not be optimally apposed. The arrow points to the proximal end of the FilterWire EZ seen as a thin circular black structure.

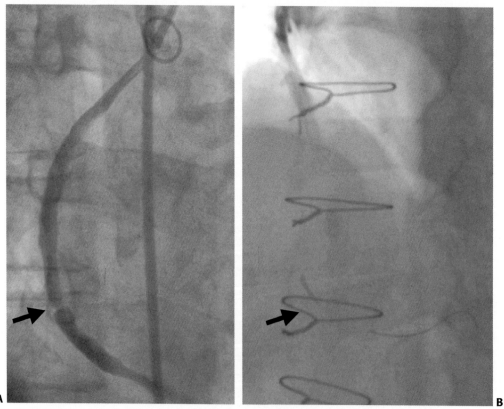

FIGURE 17-14. (**A**) Critical lesion (*black arrow*) in distal saphenous vein graft to the posterior descending artery. (**B**) FilterWire EZ within its delivery sheath before deployment (*black arrow*). (*continued*)

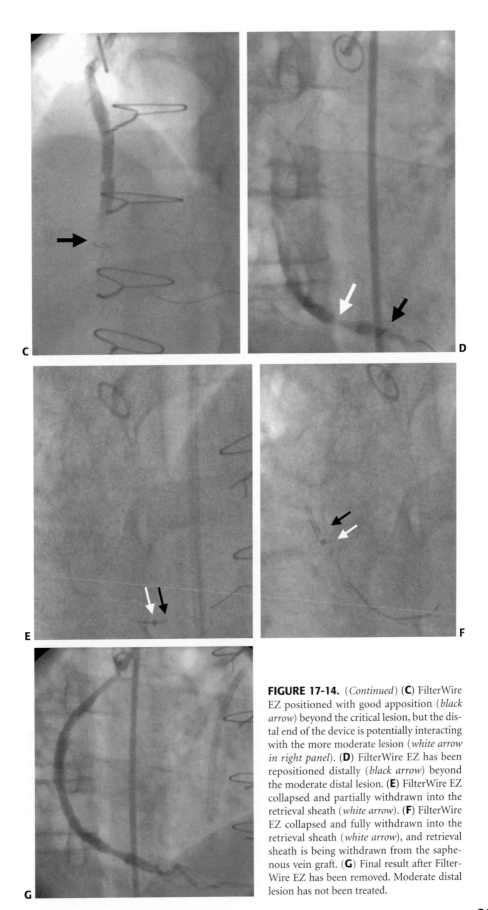

FIGURE 17-14. (*Continued*) (**C**) FilterWire EZ positioned with good apposition (*black arrow*) beyond the critical lesion, but the distal end of the device is potentially interacting with the more moderate lesion (*white arrow in right panel*). (**D**) FilterWire EZ has been repositioned distally (*black arrow*) beyond the moderate distal lesion. (**E**) FilterWire EZ collapsed and partially withdrawn into the retrieval sheath (*white arrow*). (**F**) FilterWire EZ collapsed and fully withdrawn into the retrieval sheath (*white arrow*), and retrieval sheath is being withdrawn from the saphenous vein graft. (**G**) Final result after FilterWire EZ has been removed. Moderate distal lesion has not been treated.

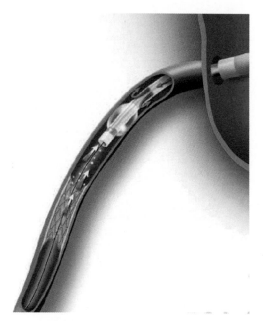

FIGURE 17-15. Schematic of Proxis system. (Courtesy of St. Jude Medical, St. Paul, Minnesota.) (See color insert.)

aspiration of the conduit to remove liberated debris, with subsequent deflation of the occlusion balloon and restoration of flow (Figs. 17-15 and 17-16). Since the lesion is not crossed with the device, the risk of distal embolization during an unprotected period is minimized. In addition, multiple downstream lesions can be addressed without the need for repeated catheter exchanges or repositioning of the device. Ischemia during the period of proximal occlusion is a limitation of Proxis, and trauma to the proximal landing zone by the device is also possible. A proximal landing zone of 12 mm is needed so that ostial and proximal lesions are not suitable for the Proxis system. Noninferiority of proximal occlusion to distal protection (mostly filtration) has been shown by the PROXIMAL (Proximal Protection During Saphenous Vein Graft Intervention) trial in which 594 patients undergoing SVG stenting were randomized to proximal or distal embolic protection (46) (Fig. 17-17).

The current American College of Cardiology (ACC)/American Heart Association/Society for Cardiac Angiography and Interventions and European Society of Cardiology guidelines provide a class I recommendation for EPD use in SVG intervention based on the results of the SAFER and FIRE trials. Despite this, only 22% of SVG PCIs are currently supported with EPD according to an ACC-National Cardiovascular Database Registry analysis (47). Clearly, there is

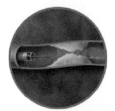

The Proxis sealing balloon is positioned proximal to the lesion, The interventional device is advanced to the distal end of the Proxis catheter.

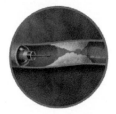

The Proxis sealing balloon is inflated, temporarily suspending antegrade blood flow and protecting all downstream vessels during lesion crossing.

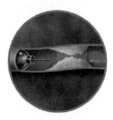

With the blood flow suspended, contrast medium can be injected into the vessel to provide better visualization and give you a visual "road map" for the intervention.

Treat

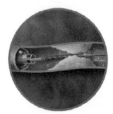

The guidewire is advanced across the lesion and the interventional device is delivered, while the vessel is protected.

Aspirate

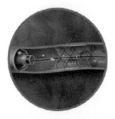

Fluid and embolic debris are aspirated from the vessel.

Restore

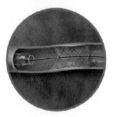

Balloon is deflated and antegrade blood flow is restored.

FIGURE 17-16. Steps in utilizing the Proxis system. (Courtesy of St. Jude Medical, St. Paul, Minnesota.) (See color insert.)

significant opportunity for improved protection against distal embolization and no-reflow in this high-risk population (Fig. 17-18). Use of EPD in STEMI has been disappointing, with no significant benefit demonstrated. For this reason, no recommendations regarding use of EPD in PCI for native coronary artery acute infarction have been offered.

Thrombus Aspiration Systems

Since EPDs have not demonstrated efficacy in the setting of PCI for acute MI involving native coronary lesions, the technique of IC thrombectomy by aspiration has developed. The equipment to accomplish this can be classified into two broad categories: (1) simple aspiration catheters or (2) disruption plus aspiration devices (see Table 17-4). Manual thrombectomy with simple aspiration catheters improves myocardial perfusion as reflected by blush score and ST-resolution (40–42) (Fig. 17-19). This has translated into a decreased risk of major adverse cardiac events and death at 1 year in those who received upfront thrombus aspiration before

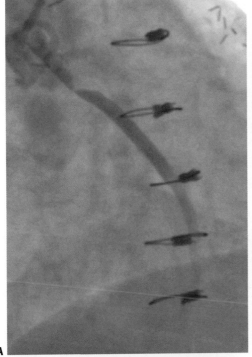

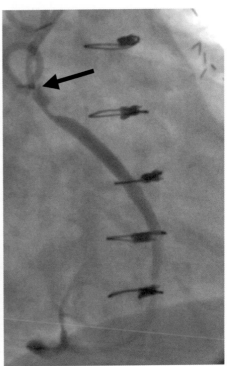

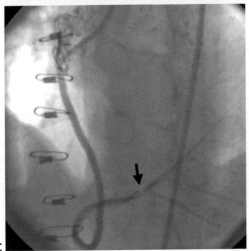

FIGURE 17-17. (A) Severe proximal lesion in saphenous vein graft to the right coronary artery. **(B)** Proxis system balloon (*black arrow*) inflated in the very proximal graft, occluding distal flow. **(C)** After stenting of the proximal lesion and deflation of the Proxis system balloon, there is no residual stenosis and TIMI 3 flow. However, there is a severe lesion at the distal anastomosis. Stent shafts are not long enough to reach the distal lesion due to the additional length of the Proxis system. (*continued*)

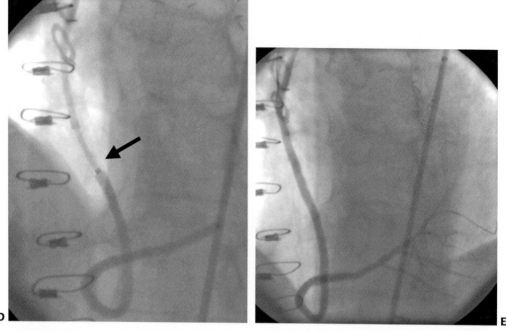

FIGURE 17-17. (*Continued*) (**D**) The Proxis system is advanced part way down the graft, through the proximal stent just deployed, and the occlusion balloon is inflated in this position. This allows the second stent to reach the distal anastomotic lesion. (**E**) Final result with both proximal and distal lesions successfully stented, TIMI 3 flow, and no distal embolization.

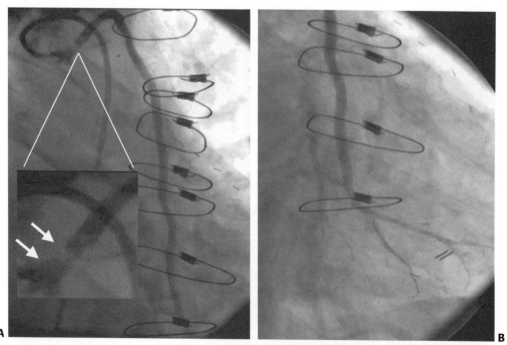

FIGURE 17-18. (**A**) A very proximal lesion due to in-stent restenosis in a saphenous vein graft to the obtuse marginal system. The magnified view of the lesion demonstrates a critical lesion followed by a filling defect just beyond the obstruction. (**B**) The subtended marginal system. (*continued*)

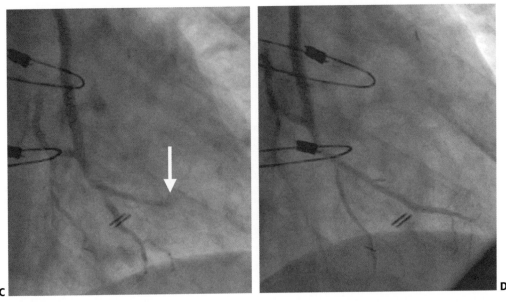

FIGURE 17-18. *(Continued)* **(C)** Distinct cutoff (*white arrow*) of the upper branch of the obtuse marginal due to distal embolization during stenting of the ostial lesion without embolic protection. **(D)** Restoration of flow after balloon angioplasty of the cutoff site.

stenting (48). These findings are reflected in the 2009 ACC/AHA guidelines for STEMI/PCI, in which aspiration thrombectomy received a class IIa recommendation. The distinction between simple aspiration and disruption plus aspiration systems should be noted when interpreting these guidelines. Although effective at removing thrombus burden, the disruption plus aspiration devices have not demonstrated consistent favorable effects on myocardial perfusion or

cardiac outcomes. In the AiMI trial, adjunctive AngioJet during primary PCI did not reduce infarct size or improve TIMI flow grade, blush score, ST-segment resolution, or 30-day major adverse cardiac events (39).

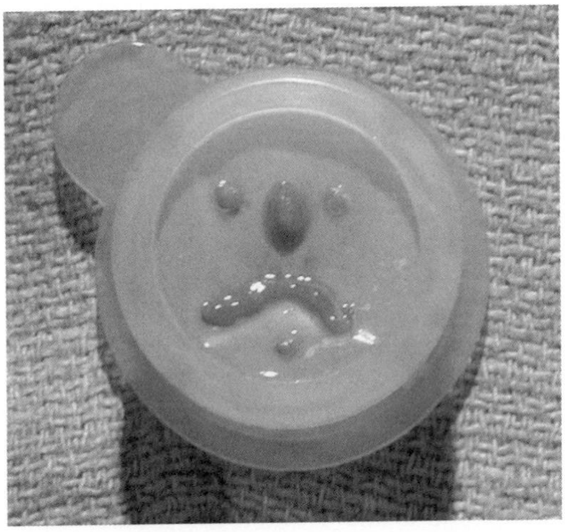

■ MANAGEMENT AND BAILOUT TECHNIQUES

Pharmacologic Management

An arsenal of pharmacologic therapies is available to reverse no-reflow when it occurs despite diligent preventive efforts (Table 17-5). The best results are obtained when these therapies are applied with consideration of the probable pathophysiology involved in each individual case (Fig. 17-20).

Adenosine

Adenosine is an endogenously made purine nucleoside that has properties of a potent arterial vasodilator. Adenosine also has been shown to limit ischemia and reperfusion-mediated injury by inhibiting neutrophil adhesion to endothelial cells and platelet activation (62–63). Adenosine can be administered via an intravenous or IC route, and due to its short half-life, the duration of any adverse effect is limited. The intravenous route of administration has been studied in the

FIGURE 17-19. Thrombus extracted during percutaneous intervention for an acute coronary syndrome.

TABLE 17-5   **Strategies for the Pharmacologic Management of No-Reflow**

Mechanism	Drug (Route)	General Dose Regimen	Adverse Effects	Key Literature
Purine nucleoside/ vasodilator	Adenosine (IV)	70 μg/kg/min for 3 h	Transient heart block, hypotension, bronchospasm	Ross[49]
	Adenosine (IC)	12–36 μg boluses or 4 mg over 1 minute		Barcin[50] Marzilli[51]
Direct NO donor/vasodilator	Nitroprusside (IC)	50–200 μg boluses	Hypotension, rare bradycardia	Pasceri[52] Hillegass[53]
Direct vasodilator	Papaverine (IC)	8–12 mg single bolus	QT prolongation, ventricular dysrhythmias	Wilson[54] Ishihara[55]
K$^+$ channel activator/ vasodilator	Nicorandil (IV)	4 mg bolus IV followed by 6–8 mg/h infusion (24 hours)		Ono[56] Ito[57]
Calcium channel blocker/ vasodilator	Verapamil (IC)	50–250 μg boluses	Heart block, bradycardia, hypotension	Piana[13] Kaplan[58]
	Diltiazem (IC)	2.5 mg over 1 minute	Bradycardia, hypotension	McIvor[59]
	Nicardipine (IC)	100–200 μg boluses	Hypotension, less bradycardia	Huang[60]
Inhibition of platelet aggregation	Abciximab (IV)	0.25 mg/kg bolus followed by 0.125 mcg/kg/min over 12 hours	Bleeding, rare thrombocytopenia	Neumann[61]

IC, intracoronary; IV, intravenous.

Acute Myocardial Infarction Study of Adenosine (AMISTAD) series of trials. AMISTAD-I showed a significant relative reduction (33%) in infarct size when adenosine was infused for 3 hours following thrombolytic therapy (64). The subsequent AMISTAD-II trial included patients receiving either fibrinolytic or mechanical revascularization for STEMI and again showed a decrease in infarct size in the adenosine arm compared with placebo, although clinical outcome was not improved (49). IC adenosine has also demonstrated efficacy in reversing angiographic no-reflow in primary PCI for acute MI and in SVG interventions (51,65).

Calcium Channel Blockers

CCBs have been hypothesized to relieve the vasospastic component of no-reflow through a direct effect promoting relaxation of vascular smooth muscle (13). Certain CCBs (such as verapamil) may also have ancillary effects to limit infarct size by lowering myocardial oxygen demand

and improving global oxygen supply–demand mismatch (66). Verapamil IC improves TIMI flow grade and angina and ST-segment elevation in a significant majority of no-reflow cases (13,58). Compared with IC nitroglycerin, IC verapamil is more effective in reversing no-reflow in SVGs (58). The adverse effects of IC verapamil include AV block, negative inotropy, and hypotension. Other CCBs shown to be effective in no-reflow management include IC nicardipine and IC diltiazem (59,60).

Nitric Oxide-Dependent Vasodilators

Nitroglycerine and nitroprusside promote vasodilatation via endogenous NO pathways. Nitroprusside has the advantage of being a direct NO donor and hence does not require intracellular metabolism. IC bolus doses of 200 μg nitroprusside have been shown to improve no-reflow without significant adverse effects (53). Nitroprusside has also been shown in a randomized, placebo-controlled

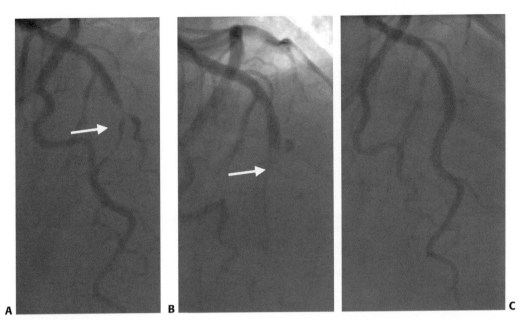

FIGURE 17-20. (**A**) Left anterior oblique cranial view of a bifurcation lesion in the mid-left anterior descending artery followed by a long segment of diffuse disease. (**B**) After successful stenting, the lesion is resolved but there is no-reflow with TIMI 0 flow. (**C**) After intracoronary vasodilators, there is resolution of no-reflow and restoration of TIMI 3 flow.

trial, to improve 6-month clinical combined outcome of death, target vessel revascularization, and MI (67). By contrast, nitroglycerin requires intracellular metabolism to generate NO. Unfortunately, the coronary microcirculation at baseline lacks a robust capability for enzymatic conversion of nitroglycerin to NO (68–69), and this pathway is further impaired in the setting of ischemia–reperfusion (70). Nitroglycerin therefore demonstrates very limited efficacy in reversing no-reflow.

Direct Vasodilators

Papaverine is an opiate derivative that produces arterial vasodilatation via direct arteriolar smooth muscle relaxation. It has been shown to cause maximal coronary vasodilatation when given in doses of 8 to 12 mg by an IC route of administration (54). In the setting of no-reflow as a consequence of PTCA, Ishihara et al. (55) showed that a single 10 mg dose of IC papaverine significantly improved TIMI frame count. Adverse effects of papaverine include QT prolongation and risk of ventricular dysrhythmias (71).

Glycoprotein IIb/IIIa Inhibitors

The use of antiplatelet therapy in no-reflow makes teleological sense given the role of activated platelets in thrombus propagation and as suppliers of vasoactive substances. The use of Gp IIb/IIIa inhibitors is intended to prevent embolization of platelet aggregates into the microcirculation and hence prevent a cascade of platelet activation, platelet–leukocyte interaction, and release of vasoactive mediators. Investigations using intravenous abciximab have shown greater preservation of microcirculation integrity following PCI for MI and greater ST-segment resolution following PCI (61,72). Some data have suggested that IC abciximab is superior to intravenous administration with more early ST-resolution (73). Tirofiban has been also shown to decrease no-reflow and limit infarct size in nonthrombotic canine coronary occlusion model (74). These data support the concept that platelet activation is an important component of RNR, and the use of platelet antagonism may have beneficial effects on the integrity of the microcirculation during MI. However, the use of intracoronary Gp IIb/IIIa inhibitors to treat PNR has not been studied, and it should be noted that Gp IIb/IIIa inhibitors have not demonstrated clinical benefit in SVG intervention, one of the highest-risk scenarios for PNR.

Potassium Channel Activators

Nicorandil is a potassium channel activator that also possesses nitrate-like vasodilating properties.

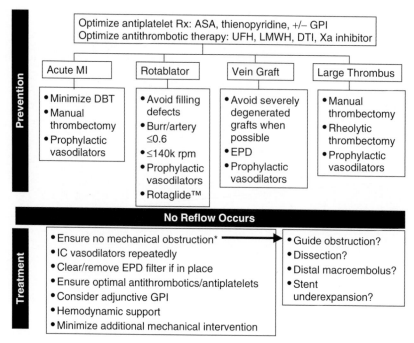

FIGURE 17-21. Suggested algorithm for the differentiation and management of no-reflow based on pathophysiology and mechanisms involved. ASA, aspirin; GPI, glycoprotein IIb/IIIa inhibitor; UFH, unfractionated heparin; LMWH, low-molecular-weight heparin; DTI, direct thrombin inhibitor; DBT, door-to-balloon time; EPD, embolic protection device; IC, intracoronary; MI, myocardial infarction.

It has not reached routine clinical use for no-reflow, but in several randomized trials, it has shown promise as a treatment for impaired microcirculatory function following PCI. Nicorandil limits infarct size, improves angiographic outcome, and preserves left ventricular function when compared with placebo (56,57).

■ CONCLUSION

No-reflow is a consequence of impaired microcirculatory function due to distal embolization, vasoconstriction, and cellular damage from ischemia–reperfusion injury.

It is most often seen in the setting of reperfusion therapy for MI ("reperfusion related no-reflow") and also can occur as "primary no-reflow" during non-MI coronary interventions. No-reflow is important because it portends a worse prognosis. Understanding the pathophysiology enables the interventionalist to anticipate and prevent no-reflow in many cases and to institute immediate therapeutic measures when no-reflow complicates PCI (Fig. 17-21).

References

1. Kloner R, Ganote C, Jennings R. The "no reflow" phenomenon after temporary coronary occlusion in the dog. *J Clin Invest.* 1974;54:1496–1508.
2. Krug A, Rochmont DM, Korb G. Blood supply of the myocardium after temporary coronary occlusion. *Circ Res.* 1966;19:57–62.
3. Eeckhout E, Kern MJ. The coronary no-reflow phenomenon: a review of mechanisms and therapies. *Eur Heart J.* 2001;22:729–739.
4. Schofer J, Montz R, Mathey D. Scintigraphic evidence of the "no reflow" phenomenon in human beings after coronary thrombolysis. *J Am Coll Cardiol.* 1985;5:593–598.
5. Wilson R, Laxson D, Lesser J, White C. Intense microvascular constriction after angioplasty of acute thrombotic coronary arterial lesions. *Lancet.* 1989;1:807–811.
6. Reffelmann T, Kloner RA. The no-reflow phenomenon: a basic mechanism of myocardial ischemia and reperfusion. *Basic Res Cardiol.* 2006; 101:359–372.
7. Kotani J, Nanto S, Mintz GS, et al. Plaque gruel of atheromatous coronary lesion may contribute to

the no-reflow phenomenon in patients with acute coronary syndrome. *Circulation.* 2002;106: 1672–1677.

8. Hori M, Inoue M, Kitakaze M, et al. Role of adenosine in hyperemic response of coronary blood flow in microembolization. *Am J Physiol.* 1986;250:H509–H518.

9. Chesebro J, Knatterud G, Roberts R. Thrombolysis in Myocardial Infarction (TIMI) Trial, Phase I: a comparison between intravenous tissue plasminogen activator and intravenous streptokinase: clinical findings through hospital discharge. *Circulation.* 1987;76:142–154.

10. vant Hof AW, Liem A, Suryapranata H, Hoorntje JC, de Boer MJ, Zijlstra F. Angiographic assessment of myocardial reperfusion in patients treated with primary angioplasty for acute myocardial infarction: myocardial blush grade. Zwolle Myocardial Infarction Study Group. *Circulation.* 1998;97:2302–2306.

11. Iwakura K, Ito H, Takiuchi S, et al. Alternation in the coronary blood flow velocity pattern in patients with no reflow and reperfused acute myocardial infarction. *Circulation.* 1996;94:1269–1275.

12. Morishima I, Sone T, Okumura K, et al. Angiographic no-reflow phenomenon as a predictor of adverse long-term outcome in patients treated with percutaneous transluminal coronary angioplasty for first acute myocardial infarction. *J Am Coll Cardiol.* 2000;36:1202–1209.

13. Piana RN, Paik GY, Moscucci M, et al. Incidence and treatment of "no-reflow" after percutaneous coronary intervention. *Circulation.* 1994;89: 2514–2518.

14. Mehta RH, Harjai KJ, Cox D, et al. Clinical and angiographic correlates and outcomes of suboptimal coronary flow inpatients with acute myocardial infarction undergoing primary percutaneous coronary intervention. *J Am Coll Cardiol.* 2003;42:1739–1746.

15. Stone GW, Grines CL, Cox DA, et al. Comparison of angioplasty with stenting, with or without abciximab, in acute myocardial infarction. *N Engl J Med.* 2002;346:957–966.

16. Dibra A, Mehilli J, Dirschinger J, et al. Thrombolysis in myocardial infarction myocardial perfusion grade in angiography correlates with myocardial salvage in patients with acute myocardial infarction treated with stenting or thrombolysis. *J Am Coll Cardiol.* 2003;41:925–929.

17. Ito H, Okamura A, Iwakura K, et al. Myocardial perfusion patterns related to thrombolysis in myocardial infarction perfusion grades after coronary angioplasty in patients with acute anterior wall myocardial infarction. *Circulation.* 1996;93:1993–1999.

18. Tarantini G, Cacciavillani L, Corbetti F, et al. Duration of ischemia is a major determinant of transmurality and severe microvascular obstruction after primary angioplasty: a study performed with contrast-enhanced magnetic resonance. *J Am Coll Cardiol.* 2005;46:1229–1235.

19. Abbo KM, Dooris M, Glazier S, et al. Features and outcome of no-reflow after percutaneous coronary intervention. *Am J Cardiol.* 1995;75:778–782.

20. Mattichak SJ, Dixon SR, Shannon F, Boura JA, Safian RD. Failed percutaneous coronary intervention: a decade of experience in 21,000 patients. *Catheter Cardiovasc Interv.* 2008;71: 131–137.

21. Ishihara M, Kojima S, Sakamoto T, et al. Acute hyperglycemia is associated with adverse outcome after acute myocardial infarction in the coronary intervention era. *Am Heart J.* 2005;150: 814–820.

22. Brosh D, Assali AR, Mager A, et al. Effect of no-reflow during primary percutaneous coronary intervention for acute myocardial infarction on six-month mortality. *Am J Cardiol.* 2007;99: 442–445.

23. Celik T, Iyisoy A, Yuksel CU, et al. Impact of admission glomerular filtration rate on the development of poor myocardial perfusion after primary percutaneous intervention in patients with acute myocardial infarction. *Coron Artery Dis.* 2008;19:543–549.

24. Hong YJ, Jeong MH, Choi YH, et al. Predictors of no-reflow after percutaneous coronary intervention for culprit lesion with plaque rupture in infarct-related artery in patients with acute myocardial infarction. *J Cardiol.* 2009;54:36–44.

25. Huczek Z, Kochman J, Filipiak KJ, et al. Mean platelet volume on admission predicts impaired reperfusion and long-term mortality in acute myocardial infarction treated with primary percutaneous coronary intervention. *J Am Coll Cardiol.* 2005;46:284–290.

26. Niccoli G, Giubilato S, Russo E, et al. Plasma levels of thromboxane A2 on admission are associated with no-reflow after primary percutaneous coronary intervention. *Eur Heart J.* 2008;29: 1843–1850.

27. Yip HK, Chen MC, Chang HW, et al. Angiographic morphologic features of infarct-related arteries and timely reperfusion in acute myocardial infarction: predictors of slow-flow and no-reflow phenomenon. *Chest.* 2002;122:1322–1332.

28. Kirma C, Izgi A, Dundar C, et al. Clinical and procedural predictors of no-reflow phenomenon after primary percutaneous coronary interventions: experience at a single center. *Circ J.* 2008; 72:716–721.

29. Ellis SG, Popma JJ, Buchbinder M, et al. Relation of clinical presentation, stenosis morphology, and operator technique to the procedural results of rotational atherectomy and rotational atherectomy-facilitated angioplasty. *Circulation.* 1994;89: 882–892.

30. Hanna GP, Yhip P, Fujise K, et al. Intracoronary adenosine administered during rotational atherectomy of complex lesions in native coronary arteries reduces the incidence of no-reflow phenomenon. *Catheter Cardiovasc Interv.* 1999;48:275–278.

31. Safian RD, Freed M, Lichtenberg A, et al. Are residual stenoses after excimer laser angioplasty and coronary atherectomy due to inefficient or small devices? Comparison with balloon angioplasty. *J Am Coll Cardiol.* 1993;22:1628–1634.

32. Gibson CM, Cannon CP, Murphy SA, Marble SJ, Barron HV, Braunwald E. Relationship of the TIMI myocardial perfusion grades, flow grades, frame count, and percutaneous coronary intervention to long-term outcomes after thrombolytic administration in acute myocardial infarction. *Circulation.* 2002;105:1909–1913.

33. Resnic FS, Wainstein M, Lee MK, et al. No-reflow is an independent predictor of death and myocardial infarction after percutaneous coronary intervention. *Am Heart J.* 2003;145:42–46.

34. Sangiorgi G, Colombo A. Embolic protection devices. *Heart.* 2003;89:990–992.

35. Baim DS, Wahr D, George B, et al. Randomized trial of a distal embolic protection device during percutaneous intervention of saphenous vein aorto-coronary bypass grafts. *Circulation.* 2002; 105:1285–1290.

36. Gick M, Jander N, Bestehorn HP, et al. Randomized evaluation of the effects of filter-based distal protection on myocardial perfusion and infarct size after primary percutaneous catheter intervention in myocardial infarction with and without ST-segment elevation. *Circulation.* 2005;112:1462–1469.

37. Kelbaek H, Terkelsen CJ, Helqvist S, et al. Randomized comparison of distal protection versus conventional treatment in primary percutaneous coronary intervention: the drug elution and distal protection in ST-elevation myocardial infarction (DEDICATION) trial. *J Am Coll Cardiol.* 2008; 51:899–905.

38. Stone GW, Webb J, Cox DA, et al. Distal microcirculatory protection during percutaneous coronary intervention in acute ST-segment elevation myocardial infarction: a randomized controlled trial. *JAMA.* 2005;293:1063–1072.

39. Ali A, Cox D, Dib N, et al. Rheolytic thrombectomy with percutaneous coronary intervention for infarct size reduction in acute myocardial infarction: 30-day results from a multicenter randomized study. *J Am Coll Cardiol.* 2006;48:244–252.

40. Burzotta F, Trani C, Romagnoli E, et al. Manual thrombus-aspiration improves myocardial reperfusion: the randomized evaluation of the effect of mechanical reduction of distal embolization by thrombus-aspiration in primary and rescue angioplasty (REMEDIA) trial. *J Am Coll Cardiol.* 2005;46:371–376.

41. Svilaas T, Vlaar PJ, van der Horst IC, et al. Thrombus aspiration during primary percutaneous coronary intervention. *N Engl J Med.* 2008;358:557–567.

42. De Luca G, Dudek D, Sardella G, Marino P, Chevalier B, Zijlstra F. Adjunctive manual thrombectomy improves myocardial perfusion and mortality in patients undergoing primary percutaneous coronary intervention for ST-elevation myocardial infarction: a meta-analysis of randomized trials. *Eur Heart J.* 2008;29:3002–3010.

43. Laufs U, La Fata V, Plutzky J, Liao JK. Upregulation of endothelial nitric oxide synthase by HMG CoA reductase inhibitors. *Circulation.* 1998;97: 1129-1135.

44. Zhao JL, Yang YJ, Cui CJ, You SJ, Gao RL. Pretreatment with simvastatin reduces myocardial no-reflow by opening mitochondrial K(ATP) channel. *Br J Pharmacol.* 2006;149:243–249.

45. Stone GW, Rogers C, Hermiller J, et al. Randomized comparison of distal protection with a filter-based catheter and a balloon occlusion and aspiration system during percutaneous intervention of diseased saphenous vein aorto-coronary bypass grafts. *Circulation.* 2003;108:548–553.

46. Mauri L, Cox D, Hermiller J, et al. The PROXIMAL trial: proximal protection during saphenous vein graft intervention using the Proxis Embolic Protection System: a randomized, prospective, multicenter clinical trial. *J Am Coll Cardiol.* 2007;50:1442–1449.

47. Mehta SK, Frutkin AD, Milford-Beland S, et al. Utilization of distal embolic protection in saphenous vein graft interventions (an analysis of 19,546 patients in the American College of Cardiology-National Cardiovascular Data Registry). *Am J Cardiol.* 2007;100:1114–1118.

48. Vlaar PJ, Svilaas T, van der Horst IC, et al. Cardiac death and reinfarction after 1 year in the Thrombus Aspiration during Percutaneous coronary intervention in Acute myocardial infarction Study (TAPAS): a 1-year follow-up study. *Lancet.* 2008;371:1915–1920.

49. Ross AM, Gibbons RJ, Stone GW, Kloner RA, Alexander RW. A randomized, double-blinded, placebo-controlled multicenter trial of adenosine as an adjunct to reperfusion in the treatment of acute myocardial infarction (AMISTAD-II). *J Am Coll Cardiol.* 2005;45:1775–1780.

50. Barcin C, Denktas AE, Lennon RJ, et al. Comparison of combination therapy of adenosine and nitroprusside with adenosine alone in the treatment of angiographic no-reflow phenomenon. *Catheter Cardiovasc Interv.* 2004;61:484–491.

51. Marzilli M, Orsini E, Marraccini P, Testa R. Beneficial effects of intracoronary adenosine as an adjunct to primary angioplasty in acute myocardial infarction. *Circulation.* 2000;101:2154–2159.

52. Pasceri V, Pristipino C, Pelliccia F, et al. Effects of the nitric oxide donor nitroprusside on no-reflow phenomenon during coronary interventions for acute myocardial infarction. *Am J Cardiol.* 2005;95:1358–1361.

53. Hillegass WB, Dean NA, Liao L, Rhinehart RG, Myers PR. Treatment of no-reflow and impaired flow with the nitric oxide donor nitroprusside following percutaneous coronary interventions: initial human clinical experience. *J Am Coll Cardiol.* 2001;37:1335–1343.

54. Wilson RF, White CW. Intracoronary papaverine: an ideal coronary vasodilator for studies of the coronary circulation in conscious humans. *Circulation.* 1986;73:444–451.

55. Ishihara M, Sato H, Tateishi H, et al. Attenuation of the no-reflow phenomenon after coronary angioplasty for acute myocardial infarction with intracoronary papaverine. *Am Heart J.* 1996;132:959–963.

56. Ono H, Osanai T, Ishizaka H, et al. Nicorandil improves cardiac function and clinical outcome in patients with acute myocardial infarction undergoing primary percutaneous coronary intervention: role of inhibitory effect on reactive oxygen species formation. *Am Heart J.* 2004;148:E15.

57. Ito H, Taniyama Y, Iwakura K, et al. Intravenous nicorandil can preserve microvascular integrity and myocardial viability in patients with reperfused anterior wall myocardial infarction. *J Am Coll Cardiol.* 1999;33:654–660.

58. Kaplan BM, Benzuly KH, Kinn JW, et al. Treatment of no-reflow in degenerated saphenous vein graft interventions: comparison of intracoronary verapamil and nitroglycerin. *Cathet Cardiovasc Diagn.* 1996;39:113–118.

59. McIvor ME, Undemir C, Lawson J, Reddinger J. Clinical effects and utility of intracoronary diltiazem. *Cathet Cardiovasc Diagn.* 1995;35:287–291, discussion 92–93.

60. Huang RI, Patel P, Walinsky P, et al. Efficacy of intracoronary nicardipine in the treatment of no-reflow during percutaneous coronary intervention. *Catheter Cardiovasc Interv.* 2006;68:671–676.

61. Neumann FJ, Blasini R, Schmitt C, et al. Effect of glycoprotein IIb/IIIa receptor blockade on recovery of coronary flow and left ventricular function after the placement of coronary-artery stents in acute myocardial infarction. *Circulation.* 1998;98:2695–2701.

62. Olafsson B, Forman MB, Puett DW, et al. Reduction of reperfusion injury in the canine preparation by intracoronary adenosine: importance of the endothelium and the no-reflow phenomenon. *Circulation.* 1987;76:1135–1145.

63. Rezkalla SH, Kloner RA. Coronary no-reflow phenomenon: from the experimental laboratory to the cardiac catheterization laboratory. *Catheter Cardiovasc Interv.* 2008;72:950–957.

64. Mahaffey KW, Puma JA, Barbagelata NA, et al. Adenosine as an adjunct to thrombolytic therapy for acute myocardial infarction: results of a multicenter, randomized, placebo-controlled trial: the Acute Myocardial Infarction STudy of ADenosine (AMISTAD) trial. *J Am Coll Cardiol.* 1999;34:1711–1720.

65. Fischell TA, Carter AJ, Foster MT, et al. Reversal of "no reflow" during vein graft stenting using high velocity boluses of intracoronary adenosine. *Cathet Cardiovasc Diagn.* 1998;45:360–365.

66. Campbell CA, Kloner RA, Alker KJ, Braunwald E. Effect of verapamil on infarct size in dogs subjected to coronary artery occlusion with transient reperfusion. *J Am Coll Cardiol.* 1986;8:1169–1174.

67. Amit G, Cafri C, Yaroslavtsev S, et al. Intracoronary nitroprusside for the prevention of the no-reflow

phenomenon after primary percutaneous coronary intervention in acute myocardial infarction: a randomized, double-blind, placebo-controlled clinical trial. *Am Heart J.* 2006;152:887 e9–e14.

68. Kurz MA, Lamping KG, Bates JN, Eastham CL, Marcus ML, Harrison DG. Mechanisms responsible for the heterogeneous coronary microvascular response to nitroglycerin. *Circ Res.* 1991;68:847–855.

69. Sellke FW, Myers PR, Bates JN, Harrison DG. Influence of vessel size on the sensitivity of porcine coronary microvessels to nitroglycerin. *Am J Physiol.* 1990;258:H515–H20.

70. Vural KM, Oz MC. Endothelial adhesivity, pulmonary hemodynamics and nitric oxide synthesis in ischemia-reperfusion. *Eur J Cardiothorac Surg.* 2000;18:348–352.

71. Wilson RF, White CW. Serious ventricular dysrhythmias after intracoronary papaverine. *Am J Cardiol.* 1988;62:1301–1302.

72. Petronio AS, De Carlo M, Ciabatti N, et al. Left ventricular remodeling after primary coronary angioplasty in patients treated with abciximab or intracoronary adenosine. *Am Heart J.* 2005;150:1015.

73. Thiele H, Schindler K, Friedenberger J, et al. Intracoronary compared with intravenous bolus abciximab application in patients with ST-elevation myocardial infarction undergoing primary percutaneous coronary intervention: the randomized Leipzig immediate percutaneous coronary intervention abciximab IV versus IC in ST-elevation myocardial infarction trial. *Circulation.* 2008;118:49–57.

74. Kunichika H, Ben-Yehuda O, Lafitte S, Kunichika N, Peters B, DeMaria AN. Effects of glycoprotein IIb/IIIa inhibition on microvascular flow after coronary reperfusion: a quantitative myocardial contrast echocardiography study. *J Am Coll Cardiol.* 2004;43:276–283.

18

Retained Devices: Embolization, Guidewire Fracture, and Device Entrapment

KYUNG J. CHO AND JAMES J. SHIELDS

etained devices are devices or portions of devices or nonmetabolizable residuals that remain in an unintended site within the body after some medical intervention. Examples include materials deployed during or abandoned after vascular catheterization and intervention or organ access procedures. These may have been inadvertently released or deliberately released or injected during the procedure. Occasionally, the product is not released but is still entrapped by a percutaneous catheter or device and is resistant to removal or planned deployment. In that there was no deliberate intent to place or abandon these products, strong consideration should be given to their removal.

The increased use of endovascular interventions has resulted in a growing number of complications of "retained devices" from embolization, guidewire and catheter fracture, dislocated or fractured vena cava filters, and device entrapment (including snares, filters, retrieval devices) (1–3). These complications may arise during the procedure due to technical error or device failure or at the follow-up. While often asymptomatic, the retained devices may cause infection, thrombosis, and perforation. Most intravascular and intracardiac devices are potentially retrievable with percutaneous transcatheter techniques. Before beginning to undertake a retrieval attempt, the risks of retrieval must be weighed against the risks of abandoning the product. Retrieval risks include hemorrhage, vascular or organ

damage, further breakup of the product, and migration of the product into an even less desired position within the body. Prolonged fluoroscopy also may have undesired effects. Risks of abandoning the product include local thrombotic effects, infection, interference with normal organ function, product decay and fragmentation, and migration to other, often remote sites. Examples of retained devices are listed in Table 18-1.

In this chapter, the complications of retained devices related to endovascular procedures and principles in bailout techniques are discussed with emphasis on how to minimize the risk of retained devices.

■ RECOVERY OF RETAINED DEVICES

When one considers removing a retained device, it is useful to first review the literature to learn from the experiences of others. Usually, one finds that others have reported on similar problems. A well-stocked inventory of various sizes of intravascular sheaths and several basket and snare devices and intravascular forceps should be immediately at hand.

Before removal of the retained device, the procedure should be explained in detail to patients. They should be fully informed, including information about the benefits, risks, alternative therapeutic procedures, and the complications that can occur. They should also be apprised that various techniques including nonstandard techniques

TABLE 18-1	Examples of Retained Devices

Vascular catheter fragments

Swan–Ganz catheter

Dilator and sheath fragment

Guidewire fragments

Needles or portions

Biopsy localization wires

Pacemaker leads or fragments

Misplaced venous filters

Misplaced intravascular coils

Angioplasty balloon fragments

Vascular stents

Embolic agents or particles

Intravascular biopsy devices or fragments

Fragments of artificial heart valve

Laser probe

Retained IVUS catheter

IVUS, intravascular ultrasound.

might be needed, including the possible need for more than one access and even surgical intervention during or after the procedure. During the procedure, vigilant monitoring of the patient is often needed. Retrievals can stimulate arrhythmias. Coagulation status should be as close to ideal as possible. Ideally, unusual retrievals are best performed during the regular work day, as sometimes backup help from another physician might be unexpectedly needed.

If the retrieved product was defective, this needs to be reported internally within the hospital, to the vendor or manufacturer, and to the U.S. Food and Drug Administration. If the initial deployment was due to operator error, this should be openly discussed at a protected peer review conference so that others may learn. Finally, thorough documentation in the permanent medical record is essential. Consideration should be given to reporting unusual events to the hospital's risk management office.

■ RETRIEVAL TECHNIQUE

Removal of retained devices arisen from the endovascular procedure is most often done exclusively by the percutaneous transcatheter technique. Successful retrieval of the retained device depends on selection of the proper retrieval equipment and development of a facile catheterization technique. A variety of methods and instruments have been used for retrieving foreign bodies. They depend on the differing experience and the location and type of the retained device. The veins that have been used for removing venous foreign bodies have been the femoral, jugular, and brachial veins. Of these, the femoral approach is usually the most preferable. Similarly, the femoral arterial approach is used for removing the arterial foreign body. The necessary equipment consists of a tip deflecting wire, a pigtail catheter, a sheath, a guiding catheter, a snare, a basket, and a grasping forceps.

When the puncture site is selected, selection of the proper sheath is essential and should depend on the diameter of the foreign body to be removed. Diagnostic angiography should be performed to visualize the vessel and foreign body. For the venous retrieval, the catheter and guidewire must be passed through the retained device and contrast medium injected proximally. The injection is made at least in two projections to demonstrate the free end of the foreign body.

The Amplatz Goose Neck snare (ev3, Plymouth, Minnesota) is most commonly used in the retrieval of foreign bodies from the vascular system (2,4,5). The snare loop opens at 90 degree from the delivery catheter to help in capturing the foreign body (Fig. 18-1A). Snare loops with varying diameter ranging 2 to 35 mm are available. The delivery catheter diameter ranges from 2.3F to 6F. It provides excellent torque control, excellent grasping capability, and radiopacity. The loop snare is effective and safe in retrieving fractured catheters, sheath fragments, wire fragments, pacemaker leads, and dislocated endovascular stents (5,6). The snare technique is to advance the catheter near the catheter fragment. The snare loop is opened and advanced to encircle the catheter fragment, and the loop is tightened by advancing the catheter. The En Snare (Merit Medical Systems, Inc. South Jordan, Utah) consists of three interlaced nitinol preformed loops (Fig. 18-1B). It is designed to provide broader vessel coverage that increases the likelihood of encircling and retrieving the retained devices.

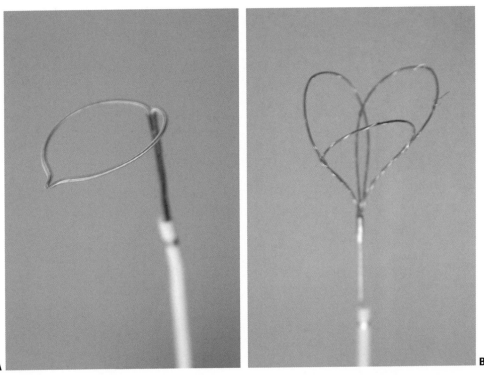

A   **B**

FIGURE 18-1. Loop snares for foreign body retrieval. **(A)** Amplatz Goose Neck snare (ev3, Plymouth, Minnesota). It consists of nitinol cable and a gold-plated tungsten loop. The 90 degree snare loop facilitates capturing the foreign body. **(B)** En Snare (Merit Medical Systems, Inc. South Jordan, Utah) consists of three loop snares that provide larger capturing area for retrieval efficiency.

The Dormia basket retrieval device consists of a set of helically arranged loops that can be expanded and collapsed (Fig. 18-2). This is originally designed to remove ureteral and biliary stones. The use of the guiding catheter and Dormia basket is an effective and safe technique for the removal of various intravascular foreign bodies including stents, coils, guidewires, and small foreign bodies such as intravascular bullets, bullet fragments, and pellets (7). They should not be used in cardiac chambers because of the risk of injuring the trabeculae or valves.

Vascular retrievable forceps consist of a handle, stainless steel shaft, and forceps with grasping jaws (Fig. 18-3A). It is useful in retrieving lost coils. It is not steerable and should not be used for retrieval of foreign body from the cardiac chambers. It is introduced through a diagnostic catheter, a sheath, or a guiding catheter and is advanced to the foreign body. The jaw of the forceps is opened to engage the foreign body and closed to capture it for removal. Biopsy forceps (Cook Medical, Bloomington, Indiana) (Fig. 18-3B) are available in three different forceps

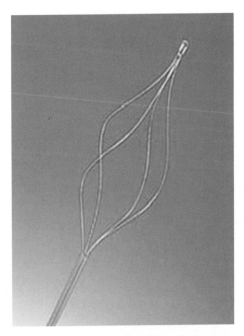

FIGURE 18-2. Retrieval basket. The helically arranged loops can be expanded to capture the foreign body and collapse to retrieve a variety of objects. The basket was most commonly utilized as a retrieval device before the advent of the Goose Neck and En Snare devices.

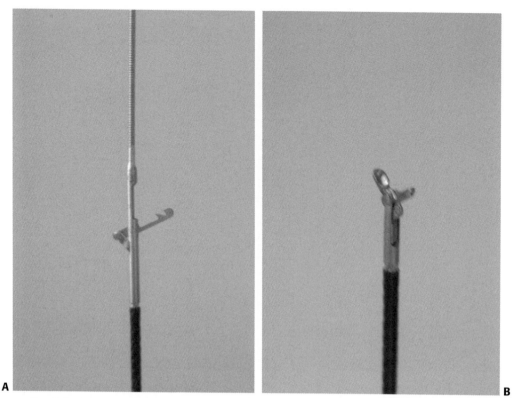

FIGURE 18-3. (**A**) Vascular retrieval forceps (Cook Medical, Bloomington, Indiana). The forceps is advanced through a sheath or a guiding catheter to the foreign body. The button on the handle is pushed forward to open the jaw of the forceps and advanced toward the foreign body to capture it. Once the foreign body has been engaged, the jaws should be closed firmly, and the forceps and foreign body are removed through the sheath. (**B**) Forceps (Cook Medical, Bloomington, Indiana). The forceps are available in three different forceps cup volume (3.0F and 5.2F shaft). The forceps are designed for myocardial tissue biopsy, but it can be used for retrieval of a foreign body embedded in the wall or located in a small vessel.

cup volume (3.0F and 5.2F shaft). The forceps were designed for myocardial tissue biopsy, but it can be used for retrieval of a foreign body embedded in the wall or located in a small vessel.

A pigtail catheter and a tip deflecting wire (manipulator) (Fig. 18-4) are used to dislocate the catheter fragment into the favorable location for removal. If the catheter extends from a peripheral vein to the heart or pulmonary artery, the catheter should be pulled toward the inferior vena cava by using a pigtail catheter or a tip deflector. The pigtail is advanced over a guidewire beyond the catheter and is pulled down to engage the catheter fragment, allowing retraction of the catheter toward the operator. When a manipulator is to be used, a Cobra-shaped catheter is passed beyond the catheter to be snared, the manipulating guidewire is then introduced into the new catheter and a bend is

made and retracted to catch the catheter to be retrieved. While the manipulator wire is held steady, the manipulator wire and catheter are pulled toward the operator to dislocate the catheter fragment. The manipulator wire is also useful to release the catheter tangled in the vena cava filter (Fig. 18-5). If the catheter fragment to be retrieved has no free end because its tip is embedded into the vessel wall, the tip must be freed before snaring by looping the catheter fragment with a Glide wire and then should be pulled. A tip deflector is useful in releasing the embedded catheter tip.

■ RETRIEVAL OF SPECIFIC RETAINED DEVICES

Catheter Fragment

Central venous access is essential in modern patient care of acute and chronically ill patients.

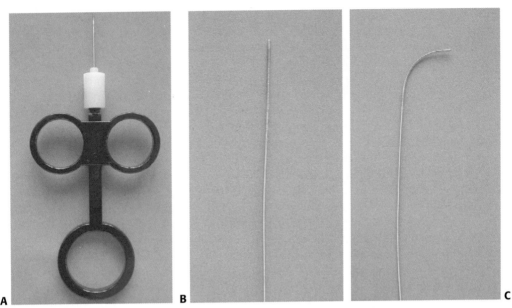

FIGURE 18-4. Reuter Tip Deflecting Wire Guides and Handle (Cook Medical, Bloomington, Indiana). (**A**) The handle is used for curving or deflecting catheter tips to pull or change the position of the foreign body to favorable position for snaring. (**B**) Before deflection, the wire is straight. (**C**) After deflection, the tip of the wire is curved.

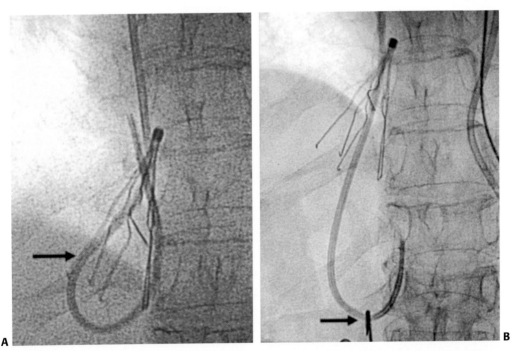

FIGURE 18-5. Use of the manipulator instrument disengages the central venous catheter entangled by the vena cava filter. (**A**) The central venous catheter is entangled by the vena cava filter placed in the suprarenal IVC (*arrow*). (**B**) A 5F Cobra catheter was advanced from the right femoral vein into the suprarenal IVC. A manipulator guidewire (called *tip-deflecting wire*) was advanced into the catheter. A bend is made to engage the catheter loop and is being pulled caudally, disengaging the catheter from the filter (*arrow*).

Placing the tip of the catheter in the central vein allows for safe and effective administration of hypertonic fluids, chemotherapy, antibiotics, transfusion, total parenteral nutrition, and hemodialysis. A central venous catheter is commonly placed into the internal jugular, subclavian, or femoral vein, with its tip positioned in the superior vena cava or the right atrium. There are several types of central venous catheters, including temporary lines, tunneled catheters, peripherally inserted central catheter (PICC), and ports.

A tunneled catheter is inserted into the jugular or subclavian vein and tunneled under the skin to a separate exit site. It is held in place by a Dacron cuff underneath the skin at the exit site in the chest. Implanted port is similar to a tunneled catheter but is left in place in the subcuta-neous pocket. A PICC line is a central venous catheter inserted into a vein (usually basilic or cephalic vein).

Central venous catheters may cause a variety of complications, including myocardial infarction, arrhythmia, valvular perforation, cardiac perforation, venous perforation, pulmonary embolism, infections, and catheter fracture and embolization. Catheter fragments may be embolized into the cardiac chamber and pulmonary artery, and embolized catheter fragments may cause infection, thrombosis, and perforation. Therefore, the fractured catheter fragment must be retrieved by percutaneous method by using the snare technique (Fig. 18-6). The "pinch-off syndrome" is a potentially serious complication of implantable subclavian

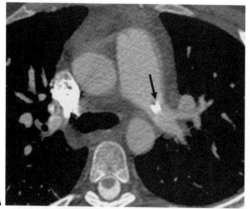

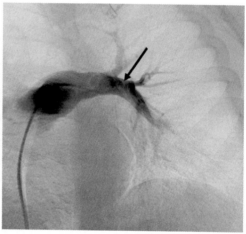

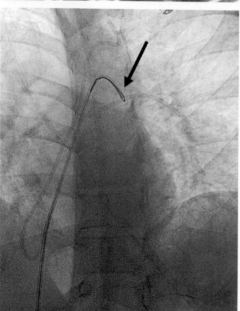

FIGURE 18-6. Retrieval of a catheter fragment from the pulmonary artery. (**A**) Computed tomography of the chest shows the proximal free end of the catheter fragment in the central left pulmonary artery (*arrow*). (**B**) Left pulmonary digital subtraction angiography (DSA) in left anterior oblique projection from the right femoral vein shows the free end of the catheter fragment in the left descending pulmonary artery (*arrow*). (**C**) The catheter fragment was snared using a 20-mm Amplatz Goose Neck snare and removed through a 12F vascular sheath.

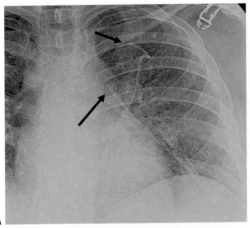

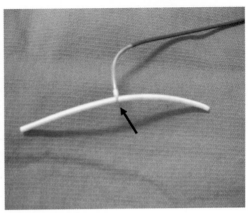

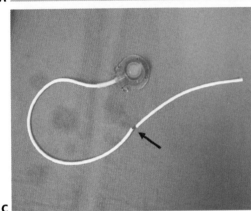

FIGURE 18-7. Fracture of left subclavian port catheter and embolization in a woman with burning pain in the left clavicle area with port flushing. (**A**) Left subclavian port was placed 7 months ago. Chest radiograph shows fracture of the port catheter between the clavicle and first rib (*shorter arrow*) with migration of the fractured catheter fragment into the left descending pulmonary artery (*longer arrow*). (**B**) The snared catheter fragment (*arrow*). (**C**) The port with the attached catheter and the fractured catheter fragment (*arrow*). This is an example of catheter fracture and subsequent embolization complicating "pinch-off syndrome," where the subclavian catheter is compressed between the clavicle and first rib, causing catheter obstruction and fracture.

venous access devices. In this situation, the catheter is obstructed during administration of fluids or may fracture resulting in central embolization (Fig. 18-7).

Occasionally, central venous catheters (port catheter or PICC line) are left unused for many years. They are found incidentally at chest radiograph taken for other indications (Fig. 18-8). These catheters are often well incorporated within chronically thrombosed vein, precluding removal. Rarely, the vascular sheath may break, leaving the fragment in the vascular system. Retrieval of the broken sheath is achieved using a Goose Neck snare (Fig. 18-9).

Knotted Catheter

A knot formation is a rare complication but can occur when any type of catheter is introduced in the vascular system. A catheter is rarely knotted in a smaller vessel such as the innominate or subclavian vein as in this case (Fig. 18-10). Knotting has occurred with coronary catheters,

pulmonary catheters, head hunter catheters and Swan–Ganz catheters, and thermodilution catheters. A variety of techniques have been used to untie the knotted catheters, including catheter rotation; advancement of a guidewire, forceps, loop snare, and tip deflecting wire guide; and a combination of balloon catheter and Amplatz Goose Neck snare (8–10).

Wire Fragments

Guidewires can be lost into the vascular system during the insertion or catheter exchange. Rarely, they can be entangled with intravascular objects such as filter and stents or caught even in a small artery, resulting in fracture. It is known that the guidewire tip can be entangled in an obstructed segment of the coronary artery or in a small branch. Attempts at withdrawal may result in uncoiling of the spring portion of the wire or separation. Rarely, the guidewire can be entangled when the wire is pushed aggressively in the presence of venous obstruction (Fig. 18-11).

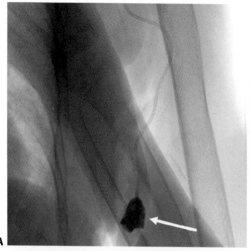

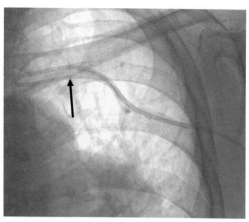

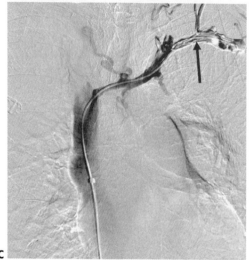

FIGURE 18-8. Retained arm port and catheter placed for chemotherapy in an 88-year-old woman with colon cancer. The port has not been used for 9 years. (**A**) Left arm radiograph shows the port (*arrow*). (**B**) Chest radiograph shows coiling of the port catheter in the left subclavian vein (*arrow*). (**C**) Left subclavian venogram from the right femoral vein shows chronic occlusion of the subclavian vein. Attempt to remove the catheter was unsuccessful.

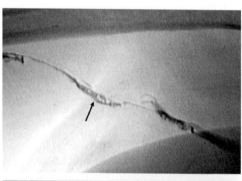

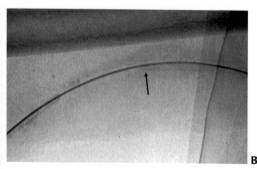

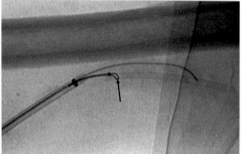

FIGURE 18-9. Retrieval of the fragment of the broken sheath in a woman with a right arm brachioaxillary arteriovenous graft. (**A**) Contrast injection into the proximal graft shows thrombosis of the AV graft (*arrow*). (**B**) The sheath fractured with a fragment during the declotting procedure. (**C**) The sheath fragment was snared using an Amplatz Goose Neck snare and removed through the sheath.

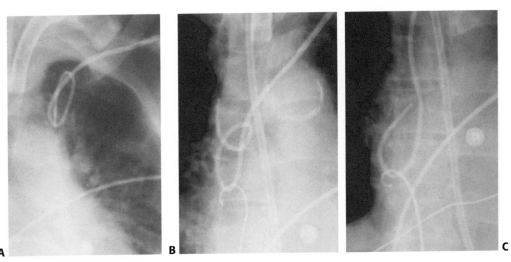

A   B   C

FIGURE 18-10. Knotted central venous catheter in left innominate vein. (**A**) Knotted central venous catheter in the left innominate vein, which was confirmed with venogram from the femoral vein. A 5F Cobra catheter was advanced through the knotted catheter and a tip deflecting wire was advanced. (**B**) The knotted catheter was engaged and pulled into the superior vena cava. (**C**) While holding the central catheter, the tip deflecting wire is being pulled toward the groin to unknot the catheter.

Intravascular Stents

With the increasing use of endovascular stents in both the arterial and venous systems, a variety of complications of "retained stents" has occurred. These include incomplete expansion, dislocation, and fracture (6,11–15).

If the stent being placed cannot be fully expanded because of the rupture of the stent-mounted balloon, contrast medium is injected forcefully exceeding the rate of contrast leak to further expand the stent. This will allow placement of a second balloon catheter for

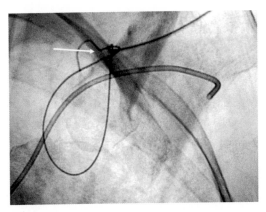

FIGURE 18-11. Entangled guidewire during insertion from the subclavian vein. The use of catheter and loop snare was successful in untangling of the wire.

additional expansion. When removing the balloon catheter from the stent, extreme care must be taken to avoid stent dislocation. While the guidewire is kept in place, the guiding catheter is advanced to the stent, and the balloon catheter should be rotated 360 degrees once or twice to free the balloon from the stent. Then the balloon catheter is withdrawn. A hydrophilic coated balloon catheter of the proper size is passed through the stent over the guidewire to further expand the stent. Alternatively, the incompletely expanded stent is retrieved. A low-profile balloon catheter is placed within the stent and snared by a loop snare and removed through the femoral sheath (16,17).

A dislocated stent in the aorta can be repositioned in the common or external iliac artery or removed. For repositioning of the stent, a balloon catheter 1 to 2 mm larger than the stent diameter is advanced over the guidewire and is inflated within the stent. The stent is then withdrawn into the common iliac artery and deployed using the proper balloon size. For retrieval of the stent, a loop snare is passed through the guiding catheter over the existing guidewire to snare the stent. If this fails, the snare is advanced beyond the stent to capture the distal end of the guidewire and then snare the stent. The stent is then compressed and drawn into the sheath for removal. Prior to stent

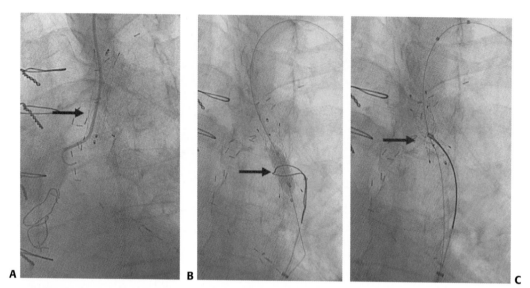

FIGURE 18-12. Misplaced subclavian nitinol stent in a patient with subclavian artery stenosis proximal to a patent left internal mammary artery to left anterior descending coronary artery bypass. (**A**) The subclavian stent was misplaced into the aorta (*arrow*). (**B**) A balloon catheter was placed within the stent that was snared by a Amplatz Goose Neck snare (*arrow*). (**C**) After removal of the balloon from the stent, the stent is constricted for removal (*arrow*). However, removal of the stent was unsuccessful.

retrieval, the properties of the stent should be considered with respect to flexibility, self-expanding or balloon-expanding stent, compressibility, and rigidity to facilitate retrieval (Fig. 18-12). Stents are frequently used for the treatment of venous stenosis of hemodialysis resistant to balloon dilatation. If the stent is too small for the vein, the stent can migrate into the chest once the blood flow is established through

the fistula (Fig. 18-13). Generally, both bare and covered stents should be oversized when stenting the venous stenosis.

Stent fracture is not an uncommon complication. The nitinol self-expanding stent has the propensity for fracture. Stent fractures have been reported following placement in the superficial femoral, popliteal, subclavian, carotid, and renal arteries, as well as the bile duct. Techniques

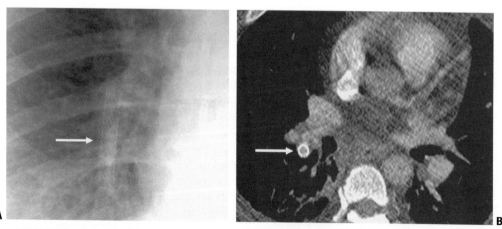

FIGURE 18-13. Stent migration into the pulmonary artery. (**A**) Computed tomography in a patient after placement of a covered stent at the stenotic venous anastomosis of the femoral AV graft. The stent is seen in the descending pulmonary artery (*arrow*). (**B**) Computed tomography of the chest confirmed the stent in the pulmonary artery (*arrow*). The stent was left in the pulmonary artery.

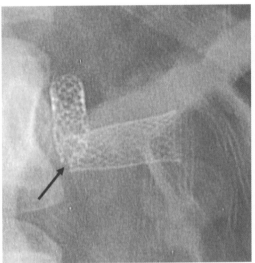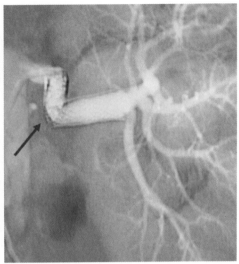

FIGURE 18-14. Maldeployed renal stents in a pediatric patient with hypertension and left renal artery stenosis. (**A**) Radiograph of the renal stent shows angulation of the left renal stents at the junction of the two stents (*arrow*). (**B**) Left renal arteriogram obtained because of recurrent hypertension shows left renal arterial deformity with in-stent restenosis (*arrow*). Subsequently, the patient underwent surgical revascularization of the left kidney.

for management of stent fracture includes placement of a second stent, bypass, and percutaneous transluminal angioplasty (Fig. 18-14).

Vena Cava Filters

Vena cava filters are used increasingly to prevent pulmonary embolism in patients with deep vein thrombosis, a contraindication to anticoagulation or complication of anticoagulation. Filters provide quite effective mechanical protection from pulmonary embolism. The reported complications include puncture site hematoma and thrombosis, migration, penetration, fracture, and vena cava/filter thrombosis. Central migration of the filter and its fragment may result in a serious complications including cardiac arrest, arrhythmia, and pericardial tamponade (Fig. 18-15) (17,18). Filters have been misplaced in the iliac, subclavian, renal, hepatic, and gonadal veins; the aorta; and the right atrium.

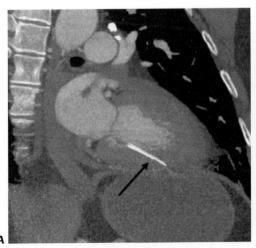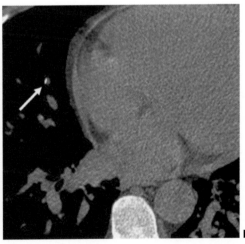

FIGURE 18-15. Filter fracture and migration of strut fragments to the chest. (**A**) Computed tomography shows the fractured filter limb in the right ventricle with pericardial penetration and pericardial tamponade (*arrow*). (**B**) Computed tomography of the chest shows a filter limb fragment in a pulmonary artery branch (*arrow*).

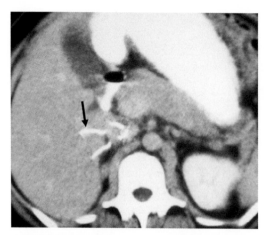

FIGURE 18-16. Filter leg penetration into the liver. Axial computed tomography scan of a vena cava filter shows penetration of filter struts into the liver. Asymptomatic caval penetration by a permanent filter does not usually require surgical intervention. If the patient is at risk of recurrent pulmonary embolism, a second filter should be placed above the filter.

Misplacement at deployment is usually due to operator error and rarely due to device failure. A variety of percutaneous methods have been used successfully in retrieving intracardiac filters, eliminating the need for open heart surgery. If a filter is misplaced in the heart, it should be retrieved immediately because of the potential complication of arrhythmia and cardiac perforation. Retrieval of temporary filters is easier that of permanent filters. Penetration of the filter struts into the pericaval tissue is usually asymptomatic. Penetration has been reported to occur into the liver, kidney, bowel, and aorta (Fig. 18-16). Rarely, the filter may fail to open due to vena caval thrombosis or device failure (Fig. 18-17).

Retrieval of vena cava filters is usually straightforward and safe when retrieval is attempted within the recommended dwell time. The OptEase filter is retrieved from the femoral approach and has the shortest recommended dwell time of 2 weeks. If the filter has been placed for more than 1 month, retrieval may be difficult. Recovery and G-2 Express filters have much longer recommended dwell-times, and retrieval may be possible after a year of placement. Prolonged dwell time and increasing patient age influence the retrievability of these filters. Potential adverse events associated with retrieval include caval injury, caval stenosis, pul-

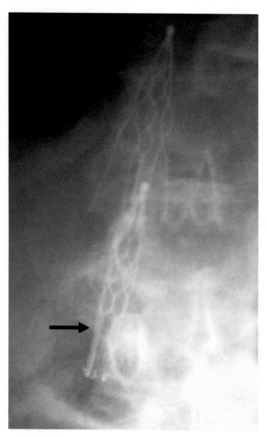

FIGURE 18-17. Failure of the filter to open. The filter failed to open upon release into the inferior vena cava (*arrow*). A second filter was placed above the first filter from the internal jugular vein.

monary embolism, deep vein thrombosis, filter fracture, migration, retrieval site bleeding, and contrast extravasation.

Nonopaque Objects

Most vascular foreign bodies such as guidewires, catheter fragments, and pacing wires are radiopaque and, therefore, can be demonstrated by plain radiographs. Nonopaque foreign bodies can be difficult to demonstrate. However, they can be identified by using contrast injection, ultrasound, intravascular ultrasound, and CO_2 injection. The inferior free end of the nonradiopaque objects should be visualized with the injection of contrast medium for loop snare retrieval (19–21).

Retained Pacemaker Leads

The most common complications of pacemaker and leads are infection, malfunction, fracture, and cardiac perforation. When these complications occur, the pacing and defibrillator leads should be removed. Because of fixation of the chronically implanted leads to the myocardium by fibrous tissue, extraction can be difficult and may result in fracture of the lead. A variety of techniques have been utilized to extract the adhered lead including transvenous approach using locking stylets, sheaths, snares, retrieval baskets, and recently laser lead extraction (22,23).

Foreign Material: Bullets, Pellets

Intravascular bullets, bullet fragments, or shotgun pellets can be retrieved using the percutaneous technique (24,25). Intravenous bullets usually migrate into the heart or pulmonary arteries, whereas intra-arterial bullets usually migrate peripherally. Since the bullet may migrate during retrieval, it must be trapped by an occlusion balloon catheter. Most bullets can be retrieved by a basket.

Coils

Coils are the most frequently used permanent occlusive device for embolization of large vessels (arteries and veins), aneurysm, and arteriovenous fistula. These are available in various sizes and configuration. Misplacement and migration are the most common complications of coil embolization. If the coils are too small for an arteriovenous fistula, inadvertent migration will likely occur, resulting in pulmonary embolism. Coil migration during embolization of pulmonary arteriovenous malformation results in arterial embolization. Rarely, the deployed coils can be displaced during surgery. For example, if coils are placed close to the origin of the renal artery, they may be displaced into the aorta or into the contralateral renal artery during ipsilateral nephrectomy, resulting in acute renal failure. Mazer et al. (26) reported a case in which the coils were displaced into the contralateral renal artery after nephrectomy.

Inadvertent coil migration into the bile duct can occur after coil embolization of hepatic artery pseudoaneurysm, causing hemobilia (Fig. 18-18). Therefore, coils should be placed immediately distal and proximal to the pseudoaneurysm instead of placing at the pseudoaneurysm. Similarly coil migration into the renal pelvis can occur following coil

embolization of a renal artery pseudoaneurysm associated with hematuria. The availability of detachable coils, such as Interlock coil (Boston Scientific, Natick, Massachusetts) and Hydrocoil (Terumo, Inc., Somerset, New Jersey) and Amplatzer vascular plugs (AGA Medical Corp, Plymouth, Minnesota), has reduced the risk of coil migration and misplacement.

Retrieval of the misplaced or lost coils is simple and easy with the use of the current retrieval devices such as Amplatz Goose Neck, En Snare, grasping forceps, and Dormia basket. With any of these methods, most coils misplaced in a large artery can be retrieved without difficulty. The loop diameter of the snare should be similar to the diameter of vessels with the coil. The retrieval technique is as follows: When femoral arterial access is present, the existing sheath is replaced for a 9F sheath through which a catheter is advanced over a guidewire beyond the misplaced coil. Over the guidewire, a 5F sheath or guiding catheter is advanced before the coil, and the snare is opened. It is then advanced to snare the coil and grasped by advancing the sheath or the guiding catheter and then removed through the sheath.

Misplaced and Retained Embolic Materials, and Cement Pulmonary Embolism

Embolization therapy has been used to control hemorrhage, to occlude arteriovenous malformations or fistulae, to devascularize tumors, to occlude the gonadal vein, to occlude hypogastric artery prior to endovascular aneurysm repair (EVAR), and to treat type 2 endoleak. The availability of hydrophilic coated catheters, torque guidewires, and 3Fr coaxial catheter systems have facilitated superselective catheterization of the arteries and veins for endovascular therapy, minimizing complications of the procedure. Selection of the embolic agent depends on the desired level of occlusion, pathovascular anatomy, and potential complications. The embolic agents in current use can be grouped into particulate (Gelfoam and polyvinyl alcohol particles), mechanical occluding devices (coils and Amplatzer vascular plug) and liquid agents (ethyl alcohol, N-butylcyanoacrylate [nBCA], Onyx, thrombin, and Sotradecol).

Embolization therapy has the potential complication of retained embolic agents whenever it is utilized. The complication may arise from

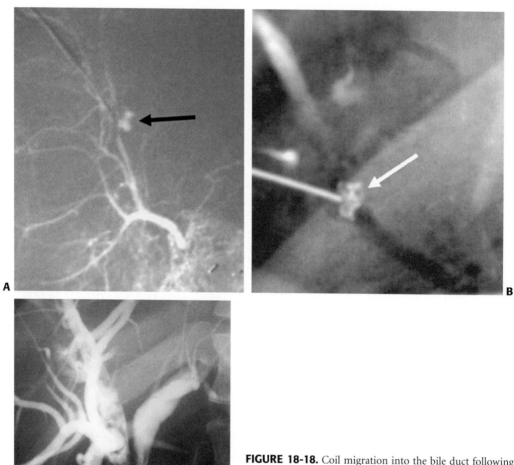

FIGURE 18-18. Coil migration into the bile duct following hepatic artery embolization for hemobilia. (**A**) Celiac and superior mesenteric angiograms showed occlusion of the hepatic artery. The intrahepatic artery branches filled through collateral vessels showing a pseudoaneurysm (*arrow*). (**B**) Percutaneous coil embolization was performed and stopped hemobilia (*arrow*). (**C**) Three months later, percutaneous transhepatic cholangiogram showed migration of the coils into the bile duct causing obstructive jaundice and cholangitis (*arrow*).

reflux, misplacement, or migration of the embolic agent.

Particulate agents such as gelatin sponge (Gelfoam) and polyvinyl alcohol (PVA) are frequently used embolic materials for various disorders. When injecting any particulate occluding agent into arteries, extreme care must be taken to prevent inadvertent embolization. During diastole, the emboli may move in a retrograde manner when blood flow has been slowed in the vessels being embolized. The refluxing emboli may occlude other arterial branches with the potential for ischemia or infarction. Inadvertent embolization can be avoided by injecting only a small amount of embolic agent as close to the lesion as possible and by stopping embolization when the target artery is occluded.

N-butylcyanoacrylate (Trufill, Cordis, Bridgewater, New Jersey) is a liquid embolic agent that rapidly polymerizes into solid material upon contact to body fluid or tissue. This glue is currently used as an embolic agent for a variety of vascular disorders including cerebral and peripheral arteriovenous malformations, gastrointestinal bleeding, pseudoaneurysm, varicocele, varices, and endoleak. The microcatheter is flushed with dextrose 5%, and following injection, the syringe is aspirated and rapidly withdrawn. The glue is

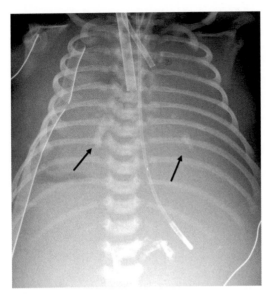

FIGURE 18-19. Pulmonary glue embolism following embolization of a large hepatic arteriovenous malformation in a pediatric patient. Chest radiograph 5 days after embolization of the hepatic AVM with glue (*N*-butyl cyanoacrylate, Cordis) shows radiopaque emboli in both right and left pulmonary arteries (*arrows*). Radiopaque glue is seen in the liver.

mixed with lipiodol to prolong the polymerization time. Excessive nBCA injection cause reflux, resulting in embolization of unintended vessels. Another rare complication of glue embolization is the migration of glue into the bile duct secondary to rupture of hepatic artery pseudoaneurysm and escape of glue into the venous circulation resulting in pulmonary embolism when injected into a high-flow arteriovenous malformation (Fig. 18-19).

Polymethylmethacrylate is cement used in vertebroplasty for the treatment of compression fractures. Leakage of the cement into the perivertebral veins results in pulmonary embolism (27). The cement in the pulmonary artery can be seen as radiopaque density on chest radiographs, computed tomography, and echocardiography (Fig. 18-20) (28,29). Surgical removal should be considered for symptomatic central cement embolism. Anticoagulation is recommended for asymptomatic central or peripheral cement emboli.

Calcified catheter "cast" masquerades a retained catheter fragment after removal of an

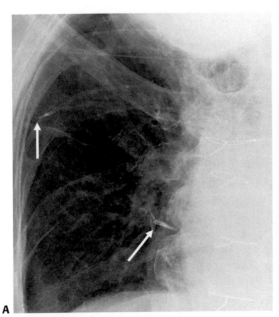
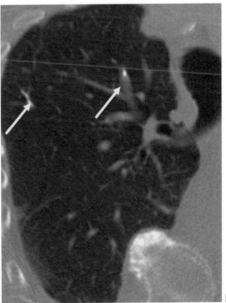

FIGURE 18-20. Cement pulmonary embolism complicating vertebroplasy in a patient with acute shortness of breath. (**A**) Chest radiograph shows multiple small radiopaque cement emboli (*arrows*). (**B**) Computed tomography of chest without contrast injection shows multiple radiopaque cement emboli (*arrows*). Bird Nest filter was placed in the inferior vena cava to capture intracaval extension of the cement from the vetebral body.

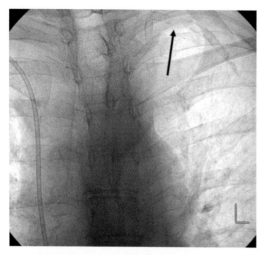

FIGURE 18-21. Calcified catheter "cast" masquerading as a retained catheter fragment after removal of a venous access device. There is a tubular calcification along the tract of the previous tunneled subclavian catheter (*arrow*).

implanted venous access device (Fig. 18-21). This likely represents calcification of thrombus along the tract that occurred after removal of the catheter.

■ DEVICE ENTRAPMENT

Filter Entrapment

Guidewire entrapment by vena cava filters occurs with J-tipped wires during a central venous catheter placement (30,31). Both clinical and experimental studies have shown that J-tipped wires can be entrapped in the Greenfield filter, Vena Tech filter, and Trapease (Fig. 18-22). Vigorous manipulation and traction can lead to dislodgement of the filter. If the filter has been pulled into the innominate vein or jugular vein, the filter may be left in place after removal of the wire (Fig. 18-23).

Removal of the entrapped guidewire from the filter is done by advancing a catheter or a guiding catheter over the guidewire from the jugular approach to the apex of the entrapped filter. Then the catheter and wire are advanced toward the filter hooks to release the entangled wire from the filter.

This complication can be avoided by limiting the distance that a guidewire is advanced during the insertion of a central venous catheter or by inserting the straight end of the guidewire.

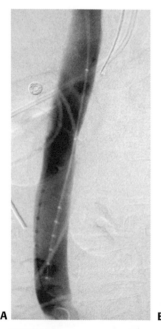
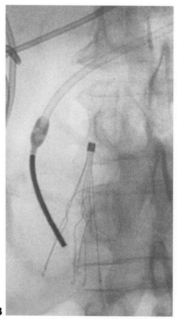
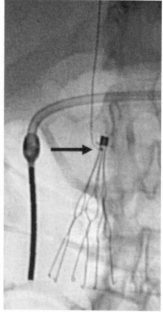

A   B   C

FIGURE 18-22. Entanglement of a J-tipped guidewire by the IVC filter during placement of a central venous catheter from the internal jugular vein. (**A**) The inferior vena cavogram (DSA technique) taken before filter insertion shows a normal vena cava in a patient with pulmonary embolism and a contraindication to anticoagulation. (**B**) A Greenfield filter was placed. (**C**) One week later, a J-tipped guidewire was entrapped by the filter during placement of a central venous catheter (*arrow*). The filter was dislocated into the right innominate vein where the filter was left following disengagement of the wire from the filter by advancing a catheter toward the filter hooks.

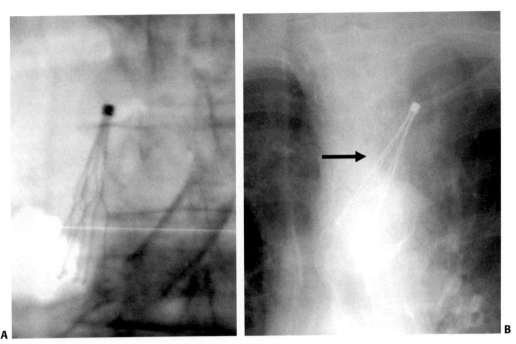

A   B

FIGURE 18-23. Filter dislocation secondary to entrapment of the guidewire by the IVC filter. (**A**) The IVC filter was in a good position after placement. (**B**) During placement of a central venous catheter from the left subclavian vein without the use of fluoroscopy, the guidewire was entangled by the IVC filter and the filter was pulled into the left innominate vein (*arrow*).

If a filter is present in the superior vena cava, fluoroscopy should be used when carefully inserting a central venous catheter. Fluoroscopy should also be used when a Swan–Ganz catheter is inserted from the femoral approach in the presence of a filter in the IVC.

Stent Ensnarement

Various interventional techniques are used to treat in-stent stenosis, thrombosed stents, and thrombosed hemodialysis graft with stent in place. Devices used for intervention such as the Arrow-Trerotola PTD (Teleflex Medical, Triangle Park, North Carolina) can ensnare the stent in the graft being treated. For example, Trerotola PTD basket can be ensnared by the existing stent (Fig. 18-24). If the Trerotola basket is ensnared in the stent, the activation switch must be turned off immediately and the device cable should be rotated counterclockwise until the basket is disengaged from the stent. When the device is ensnared in the stent, an audible change in pitch becomes apparent. Another potential complication with the use of this device is separation of the distal tip from the basket or separation of the basket from the cable if the distal tip is held stationary while the basket is activated.

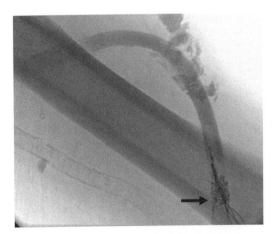

FIGURE 18-24. Stent ensnarement by Trerotola PTD device in brachial artery–axillary vein AV graft. The patient had undergone unsuccessful declotting of the thrombosed AV graft with PTA and stent placement. The stent in the venous outflow was inadvertently snared by the Arrow-Trerotola PTD device (*arrow*), which required surgical cut-down for removal.

■ AVOIDING RETAINED DEVICES

Complications of "retained devices" can occur whenever intravascular devices are utilized. It is important to have a thorough understanding of how a product has been designed and constructed and its intended use, limitations, and manufacturer's recommendations and instructions for safe use. Thorough training with the device should be obtained before attempting use in patients. The manufacturer may have specific recommendations as to what constitutes this training, and occasionally may, in fact, certify that a practitioner has been trained. For some devices, credentialing and specific privileging by a hospital is appropriate, desirable, and required.

Before using a new device, the operator should review the literature to understand the problems that others have encountered. The operator should consider alternatives that might be applicable. Practice in an in vitro setting or animal laboratory can be useful. A thorough knowledge of the particular patient's vascular anatomy and angiograms of good quality are essential. Careful and meticulous technique must always be consistently applied. Normally, each step should be fluoroscopically visualized, and key steps should be documented. Absolutely sterile technique must be used when any foreign object is introduced intravascularly. The device must be inspected before its use. If a device appears damaged, it should not be used.

■ CONCLUSION

The common use of central venous catheterization and endovascular interventions using various devices has resulted in complications "retained devices." These may take the form of entire device or device fragment knowingly or unknowingly left behind, stent dislocation and fracture, filter migration and fracture, filter entrapment of guidewires, stent ensnarement, retained embolic devices and material, and intravascular bullets. Since retained devices may cause central migration into the heart and lung, infection, thrombosis, or perforation, percutaneous retrieval should be done. Selection of the proper device, thorough understanding of endovascular equipments, and development of a facile endovascular technique are essential in achieving a successful retrieval. It is important to be aware of the potential complications of

retained devices and learn how to prevent such complications through understanding of the devices and good endovascular technique. Retained devices must be recorded in medical records. The patients should be informed of retained devices. All adverse events involving medical devices and retained device fragments should be reported to the manufacturers and the Food and Drug Administration.

References

1. Wolf F, Schoder M, Stadler A. Endovascular management of lost or misplaced intravascular objects: experiences of 12 years. *Cardiovas Intervent Radiol.* 2008;31:563–568.
2. Cekirge S, Weiss JP, Foster RG, et al. Percutaneous retrieval of foreign bodies: experience with the nitinol Goose Neck snare. *J Vasc Interv Radiol.* 1993;4:805–810.
3. Dondelinger RF, Lepoutre B, Kurdziel JC. Percutaneous vascular foreign body retrieval: experience of an 11-year period. *Eur J Radiol.* 1991;12:4–10.
4. Yedlicka JW Jr, Carson JE, Hunter DW, et al. Nitinol Goose Neck snare for removal of foreign bodies: experimental study and clinical evaluation. *Radiology.* 1991;178:691.
5. Koseoglu K, Parildar M, Oran I, et al. Retrieval of intravascular foreign bodies with Goose Neck snare. *Eur J Radiol.* 2004;49:281.
6. Gabelmann A, Kramer SC, Tomczak R, et al. Percutaneous techniques for managing maldeployed or migrated stents. *J Endovas Therapy.* 2001;8:291.
7. Sheth R, Someshwar V, Warawdekar G. Percutaneous retrieval of misplaced intravascular foreign objects with the Dormia basket: an effective solution. *Cardiovasc Intervent Radiol.* 2007;30:48–53.
8. Bhatti WA, Sinha S, Rowlands P. Percutaneous untying of a knot in a retained Swan-Ganz catheter. *Cardiovasc Intervent Radiol.* 2000;23:224–225.
9. Hirabayashi Y, Saitoh K, Fukuda H, et al. A knotty problem of a central venous catheter. *J Anesth.* 1995;9:85–86.
10. Tanner MA, Ward D. Percutaneous technique for the reduction of knotted coronary catheters. *Heart.* 2003;89:1132–1133.
11. Hartnell GG, Jordan SJ. Percutaneous removal of a misplaced Palmaz stent with a coaxial snare technique. *J Vasc Interv Radiol.* 1995;6:799–801.

12. Veldhuijzen FL, Bonnier HJ, Michels HR, et al. Retrieval of undeployed stents from the right coronary artery: report of two cases. *Cathet Cardiovasc Diagn.* 1993;30:245–248.

13. Grosso M, Spalluto F, Muratore P, et al. Palmaz stent dislodgement into the left pulmonary artery complicating TIPS: percutaneous retrieval and extraction after venotomy. *Cardiovasc Interv Radiol.* 1995;18:106–108.

14. Elsner M, Pefifer A, Kasper W. Intracoronary loss of balloon-mounted stents: successful retrieval with a 2 mm "Microsnare" device. *Cathet Cardiovasc Diagn.* 1996;39:271–276.

15. Bolte J, Neumann U, Pfafferott C, et al. Incidence, management, and outcome of stent loss during intracoronary stenting. *Am J Cardiol.* 2001;88: 565–567.

16. Seong CK, Kim YJ, Chung JW, et al. Tubular foreign body or stent: safe retrieval or repositioning using the coaxial snare technique. *Korean J Radiol.* 2002;3:30–37.

17. Saeed I, Garcia M, McNicholas K. Right ventricular migration of a Recovery IVC Filter's fractured wire with subsequent pericardial tamponade. *Cardiovasc Intervent Radiol.* 2006;29:685–686.

18. Goertzen TC, McCowan TC, Garvin KL, et al. An unopened titanium Greenfield IVC filter: intravascular ultrasound to reveal associated thrombus and aid in filter opening. *Cardiovasc Intervent Radiol.* 1993;16:251–253.

19. Morse SS, Strauss EB, Hashim SW, et al. Percutaneous retrieval of an unusually large, nonopaque intravascular foreign body. *AJR Am J Roentgenol.* 1986;146:863–864.

20. Moreno AJ, Fredericks P, Pan P, et al. Ultrasonic localisation of a non-opaque intravascular catheter fragment. *Br J Radiol.* 1987;60:91–92.

21. Woo V, Gerber AM, Scheible W, et al. Real-time ultrasound guidance for percutaneous transluminal retrieval of nonopaque intravascular catheter fragment. *AJR Am J Roentgenol.* 1979;133:760–761.

22. Smith MC, Love CJ. Extraction of transvenous pacing and ICD leads. *Pacing Clin Electrophysiol.* 2008;31:736–752.

23. Bongiomi MG, Zucchelli SE, Di Cori A, et al. Transvenous removal of pacing and implantable cardiac defibrillating leads using single sheath mechanical dilatation and multiple venous approaches: high success rate and safety in more than 2000 leads. *Eur Heart J.* 2008;29:2886–2893.

24. Rehm C, Alspaugh JP, Sherman R. Bullet embolus to the right hepatic vein after a gunshot wound to the heart and its percutaneous retrieval. *J Trauma.* 1988;28:719–720.

25. Sclafani SJA, Shatzkes D, Scalea T. The removal of intravascular bullets by interventional radiology: the prevention of central migration by balloon occlusion: case report. *J Trauma.* 1991;31:1423–1425.

26. Mazer JM, Baltaxe HA, Wolf GL. Therapeutic embolization of the renal artery with Gianturco coils: limitations and technical pitfalls. *Radiology.* 1981;138:37–46.

27. Kim YJ, Lee JW, Park KW, et al. Pulmonary cement embolism after percutaneous vertebroplasty in osteoporotic vertebral compression fractures: incidence, characteristics, and risk factors. *Radiology.* 2009;251:250–259.

28. Choe DH, Marom EM, Ahrar K, et al. Pulmonary embolism of polymethyl methacrylate during percutaneous vertebroplasty and kyphoplasty. *AJR Am J Roentgenol.* 2004;183:1097–1102.

29. Cadeddu C, Nocco S, Secci E, et al. Echocardiographic accidental finding of asymptomatic cardiac and pulmonary embolism caused by cement leakage after percutaneous vertebroplasty. *Eur J Echocardiogr.* 2009;10:590–592.

30. Andrews RT, Geshwind JFH, Savader SJ, et al. Entrapment of J-tip guidewires by venatech and stainless steel Greenfield vena cava filters during central venous catheter placement: percutaneous management in four patients. *Cardiovasc Intervent Radiol.* 1998;21:424–428.

31. Loehr SP, Hamilton C, Dyer R. Retrieval of entrapped guide wire in an IVC filter facilitated with use of a myocardial biopsy forceps and snare device. *J Vasc Interv Radiol.* 2001;12:1116–1119.

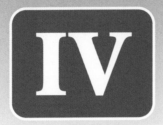

SECTION

IV

Specific Complications of Noncoronary Cardiac Interventions

Transseptal Catheterization, Atrial Septostomy, and Left Ventricular Apical Puncture

CLAUDIA A. MARTINEZ AND MAURO MOSCUCCI

■ TRANSSEPTAL PUNCTURE

Transseptal (TS) heart catheterization was introduced in the late 1950s to perform hemodynamic evaluations by direct accessing the left atrium (LA) (1,2). Subsequently, with the advent of indirect hemodynamic measurements, there was a decline in the initial enthusiasm for performing TS catheterizations. However, during the last two decades, an exponential increase in the number of TS procedures has occurred because of emerging electrophysiologic and structural interventions (3,4). Table 19-1 presents the current indications for TS puncture (TSP).

The original TS technique underwent minor modifications and equipment refinements to prevent earlier complications (5–8). Nevertheless, this procedure continues to intimidate most operators who have not been trained in the technique or who do not perform TSP regularly. More recently, the availability of adjuvant, intraprocedure imaging tools has and will continue to improve the learning curve for TS procedures (3,9).

The volume of procedures that will require TSP is expected to increase. Therefore, current interventional operators should acquire a thorough understanding of the anatomy and techniques involved in TSP, as well as of how to prevent and manage complications.

■ ANATOMIC FACTORS

Before engaging into any procedure, it is imperative to have a three-dimensional (3D) understanding of the cardiac structures, particularly of the interatrial septum (IAS) and its anatomical landmarks (Fig. 19-1). In normal hearts, the IAS results from the fusion of the embryological septum secundum on the right atrial side with the thin septum primum of the LA. Their junction constitutes a fibrous adhesion known as the *limbus*, beneath which lies a thin depression called the *fossa ovalis* (FO) in the posterior and mid to lower right atrium (RA). The FO is the only true interatrial structure. It constitutes approximately 28% of the IAS and is approximately 2 cm in diameter (10,11). Because of its location, thickness (approximately 1.8 mm), and the fact that it has less vasculature than the rest of the septum, the FO is the safest place to puncture. It is also worth noting that the walls of the LA vary in thickness, the posterior wall, roof, and atrial appendage, being one of the thinnest sections (less than 2 mm thick) (12,13).

A significant number of patients requiring TSP have distorted anatomy due to chamber enlargement, valvular disease, congenital abnormalities and prior surgical repair, scars from previous TSP, or the presence of extrinsic factors (14). Clinical reports have indicated that the majority of complications during TSP occur in

TABLE 19-1	Indications for Transseptal Puncture

Direct hemodynamic evaluation of the left heart

Mitral and aortic valvuloplasty

Percutaneous mitral valve repairs and percutaneous aortic valve implantation

Pulmonary veins evaluation and interventions

Inaccessible left ventricle (mechanical aortic valve, peripheral vascular disease)

Long tunnel patent foramen ovale ± interatrial septal aneurysm

Paravalvular leak closure

Left atrial appendage closure device

Atrial fenestration in Fontan circulation

Percutaneous left ventricular assist device (TandemHeart)

Electrophysiology procedures

Atrial septostomy

superior and anterior because the septum is more vertical. On the other hand, in the presence of left atrial enlargement, the septum lies horizontally and the FO is displaced inferiorly and posterior in the septum. In addition, the presence of an enlarged RA imposes a challenge and requires the TS needle to have a greater curvature to reach the septum. The presence of an aneurysmal IAS is also problematic due to the difficulty in localizing the FO, the risk of dissecting the thin walls, and the potential instability of the sheath once in the LA. Table 19-2 lists other anatomical factors that may complicate TSP.

Patients with kyphoscoliosis, severe rotational anomalies of the heart and great vessels, marked dilatation of the ascending aorta, and dilatation of the coronary sinus have increased risks during TSP procedures. Furthermore, previous aortic root surgery or thoracic surgery can increase the risks during TSP. Simultaneous echocardiographic imaging (intracardiac or transesophageal echo) is necessary when performing TSP in these cases (14,15).

Patients with congenital heart anomalies, especially those with complex anatomies, baffles, patches, and percutaneous devices, also pose challenging circumstances during TSP procedures. Therefore, these cases are associated with an increased risk of complications (6). A preprocedure multi-image evaluation of the anatomical

patients with distorted anatomy (6,7). Therefore, it is essential to be aware of potential distortions of anatomy associated with different conditions. In patients with aortic valve disease and aortic root distortion, the FO is displaced

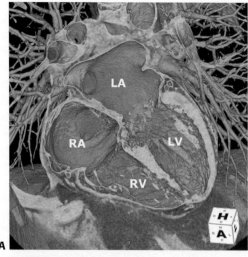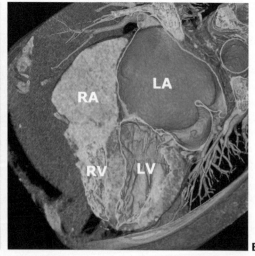

FIGURE 19-1. (A) Normal intracardiac anatomy. **(B)** Enlarged left atrium demonstrating the variations in the landmarks of the interatrial septum, by volume-rendered computed tomography angiography. RA, right atrium; LA, left atrium; RV, right ventricle; LV, left ventricle. (Courtesy of Dr. Carlos E. Ruiz, MD and Dr. Vladimir Jelnin, MD, Department of Interventional and Structural Heart Disease, Lenox Hill Institute, New York, New York.)

TABLE 19-2	Relative High-Risk Contraindications during Transseptal Puncture

Kyphoscoliosis or previous spine surgeries

Severe rotational anomalies of the heart or great vessels

Dilatation of the ascending aorta or aortic root surgery

Dilatation of the coronary sinus

Thoracic surgery

Congenital anomalies with unusual IAS orientation

Baffles, patches, and percutaneous devices

Undegenerated septum primum

Lipomatose interatrial septum

Inability to lie flat

Left atrial myxoma or thrombus

Obstruction of the IVC

Systemic anticoagulation

IAS, interatrial septum; IVC, inferior vena cava.

structures is fundamental when planning TSP in these situations to prevent inadvertent puncture of inappropriate structures (16).

IMAGING TECHNIQUES

Fluoroscopy

Traditionally, TSP has been performed under fluoroscopic guidance using the spine, the cardiac silhouette and the aorta (identified by placing a pigtail catheter retrograde into the ascending aorta), or the coronary sinus catheter (when performing electrophysiological studies) to localize the anatomical landmarks. Ideally, TSP is performed with biplane fluoroscopy (anteroposterior, left and/or right anterior oblique at 30–40 degrees) (Fig. 19-2). Intrinsic anatomical factors, including scoliosis, enlarged chambers, or previous thoracic surgeries, may distort the relationship of the IAS with these fixed anatomical landmarks. In these circumstances, fluoroscopy alone might be inadequate in identifying the site of puncture.

Transesophageal Echocardiography

Intraprocedure transesophageal echocardiography (TEE) is valuable during cardiac interventions in patients with structural heart diseases, especially with the addition of 3D-TEE. However, during TSP, TEE has the disadvantage of requiring intubation of the esophagus, and the probe sometimes interferes with the fluoroscopy view of the IAS (17,18). In addition, TEE requires a second operator and heavier sedation. There is additional risk of coughing or movements that can result in inadvertent perforation of an unintended structure. Because of these considerations, most operators prefer prophylactic airway intubation with anesthesia when using TEE, which further increases the complexity of the procedure.

Intracardiac Echocardiography

Intracardiac echocardiography (ICE) is currently the most common imaging method used during interventional procedures. Currently, there are three commercially available catheters (one rotational and two that are phased array) (15). The use of ICE has eliminated the previous contraindication when performing TS procedures in challenging patient groups (Table 19-2), and it has contributed to a faster learning curve for TSP (9,11). ICE is also useful for localizing the site-specific puncture, based on the indications for the procedure as shown in Table 19-3.

TABLE 19-3	Site-Specific Puncture during Transseptal Puncture

Complex CHD

Hypoplastic left heart syndromes

Fontan

PFO long-tunnel

Specific ablation

LAA exclusion

Pulmonary vein procedures

Percutaneous mitral valve repair

Inoue balloon mitral valvuloplasty

Double-balloon valvuloplasty

Paravalvular leak repair

CHD, congenital heart disease; PFO, patent foramen ovale; LAA, left atrial appendage.

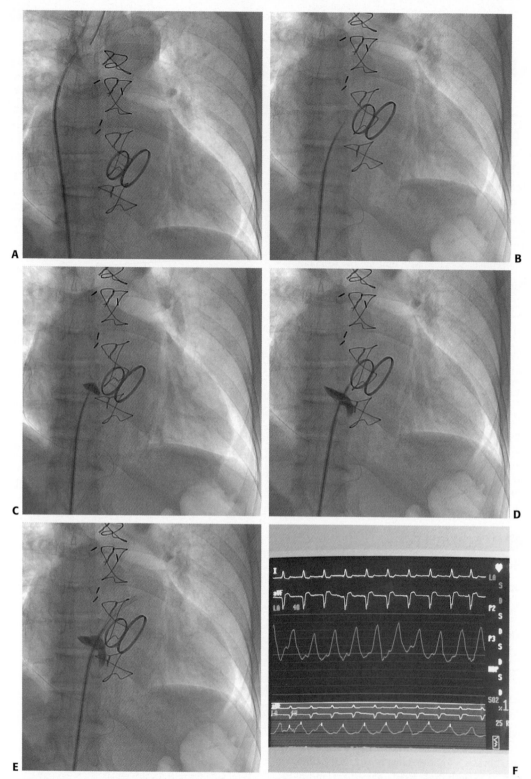

FIGURE 19-2. Steps of transseptal puncture as seen with fluoroscopy using common anatomical landmarks (spine, cardiac silhouette, left bronchus) and in this case prosthetic valves. (**A**) Transseptal (TS) kit in the superior vena cava. (**B**) Descent of the TS kit into the *fossa ovalis*. (**C**) Staining of the interatrial septum. (**D**) TS puncture and advancement into the left atrium (LA). (**E**) Advancement of the TS sheath into the LA. (**F**) Hemodynamic tracing of LA pressure. (Courtesy of Dr. Ruiz and Dr. Jelnin, Department of Interventional and Structural Heart Disease, Lenox Hill Institute, New York, New York.)

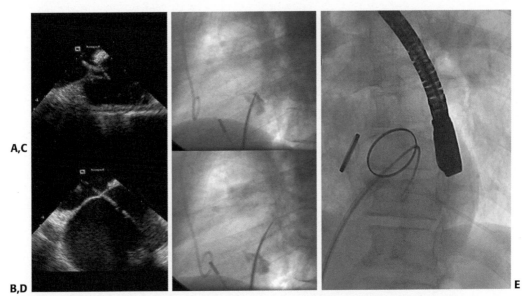

FIGURE 19-3. Anatomical landmarks using real-time intraprocedure imaging modalities. Interatrial septum as visualized using two-dimensional-intracardiac echo (ICE) with TS sheath and introducer tenting the septum confirming position prior to puncture As seen by ICE before (**A**) and after (**B**) puncture. Fluoroscopy demonstrating the staining of the septum and needle at the time of the puncture (**C**) and after puncture (**D**). (**E**) Fluoroscopic image of a TEE probe in relation to the interatrial septum at the time of the TS procedure in a lateral view. (Courtesy of Dr. Ruiz and Dr. Jelnin, Department of Interventional and Structural Heart Disease, Lenox Hill Institute, New York, New York.)

When using ICE, the anatomical landmarks including the characteristics of the septum (thickened or aneurysmal) should be evaluated, and the presence of any thrombus should be excluded. The FO is then identified and if patent, the catheter can sometimes be advanced directly through the patent foramen, thus avoiding the puncture (19). Visualization of "tenting" of the septum by the introducer is used to identify the correct puncture site (Fig. 19-3). The distance from the tip of the tenting to the free wall of the LA should be assessed to prevent perforation. Once the sheath is in the LA, ICE can help in assessing whether the position of the sheath is in a safe location (15,20).

In addition to providing anatomic guidance, ICE provides real-time monitoring of potential complications, such as the development of pericardial effusions, which can occur during the procedure. A new system is now available that can supply 3D ICE reconstructions that can be merged with 3D computed tomography (CT) images to provide real-time anatomic information (20).

Other Imaging Modalities

Presently, the availability of multimodality imaging tools has further increased the safety of TSP in complex anatomic settings. Electroanatomic mapping and image integration with CT or magnetic resonance imaging (MRI) has been widely used in electrophysiology for 3D reconstruction of the cardiac chambers. For instance, 3D CT has been used to tag the FO (21) and superimpose it onto fluoroscopy to guide the puncture location; however, this method may be replaced by intraprocedural 3D angiography in the near future (15) (Fig. 19-4).

Invasive MRI (22) and coupled imaging techniques with interventional devices are currently under development. Ultimately, the selection of the imaging tool to guide TSP will depend on the specific indications for which the procedure is being performed.

■ PROCEDURE DESCRIPTION

There is currently a wide range of equipment designed for various applications based on the specific indication for the TS procedure (Fig. 19-5). In general, the TS kit consists of a sheath

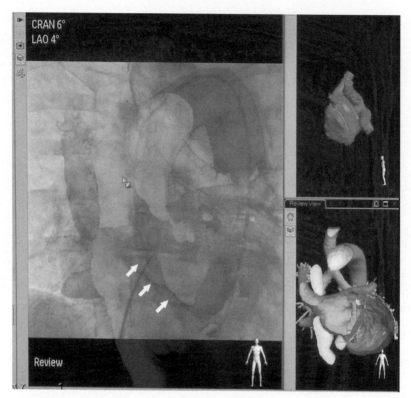

FIGURE 19-4. Newest imaging techniques superimposition of fluoroscopy and computed tomography angiography (CTA) to guide transept puncture. "Prototype" software package (Philips, Inc). *White arrows* pointing at the transatrial septum easily visualized on CTA and superimposed with fluoroscopy, transseptal needle advanced through the septum to guide procedure. (Courtesy of Dr. Ruiz and Dr. Jelnin, Department of Interventional and Structural Heart Disease, Lenox Hill Institute, New York, New York.) (See color insert.)

with an introducer and a needle. The traditional Mullins sheath (6F, 7F, 8F sheath: 59 cm and dilator: 67 cm long) paired with the Brokenbrough needle (18 gauge that tapers to 21 gauge at the tip, 71 cm long) have been the standard tools for interventional cardiologists treating adult patients. Longer or shorter kits, depending on the size and age of the patient, and different shapes depending on the indications for the procedure are also available (Fig. 19-6).

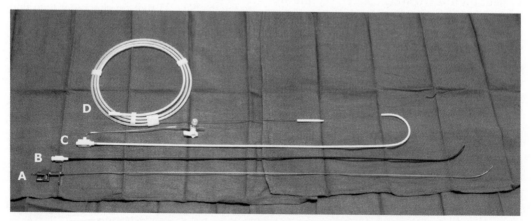

FIGURE 19-5. Transseptal kit. (**A**) Transseptal needle. (**B**) Introducer. (**C**) Sheath. (**D**) 0.32-in. J-tip wire. (Courtesy of Dr. Ruiz and Dr. Jelnin, Department of Interventional and Structural Heart Disease, Lenox Hill Institute, New York, New York.)

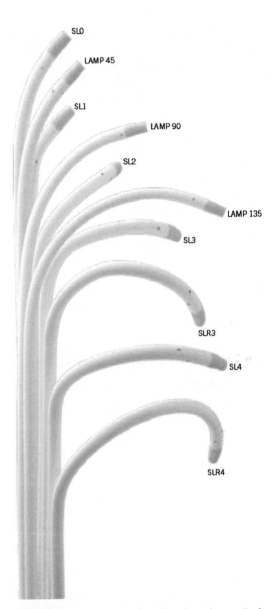

SLO

LAMP 45

SL1

LAMP 90

SL2

LAMP 135

SL3

SLR3

SL4

SLR4

FIGURE 19-6. Transseptal guiding introducers. Each shape has been designed to direct the catheter toward specific regions within the left atrium. (Courtesy of St. Jude Medical, Inc. St Paul, MN, USA.)

The operator should first inspect the tools to ensure that the needle is intact and well aligned. The curvature at the distal part of the needle can be adjusted on the basis of the anatomy of each patient (more angulation for a dilated RA and straightened for a larger LA). After flushing the catheters and needle, the operator should identify the direction of the curvature of the sheath in relation to the proximal hub and then assemble the introducer inside of the sheath making sure that they are carefully aligned. Failure to

align the introducer and sheath correctly may result in an inadvertent prolapse of the sheath when the introducer is removed from the LA. The distance between the hubs of the sheath, introducer, and needle must be measured in relation to one another prior to the insertion in the patient. A pigtail should be positioned retrograde in the ascending aorta to identify the aortic valve and monitor arterial pressure.

The traditional TSP is performed through the right femoral vein (RFV). Access through the left femoral vein (LFV) carries a higher risk of perforation and pain, due to its more angulated and tortuous trajectory into the pelvis. Nevertheless, TSP may be performed through the LFV if there is a careful advancement of the catheter. When using the LFV approach, the shoulders of the patient should be rotated toward the right and the needle angle should be increased (23).

The superior vena cava (SVC) can be accessed either from the subclavian or from the right jugular veins, particularly when there is a structural or functional absence of the inferior vena cava (IVC) or when a specific site puncture is required. A transhepatic approach with subsequent coil embolization of the tract has also been used.

When TSP is performed from the RFV, the TS sheath and introducer are advanced over a 0.032-in. J tip-wire and positioned at the junction of the SVC-innominate trunk. After removing the wire, it must be confirmed that the sheath and introducer are freely in the SVC and not engaged into any structure by gently rotating them side-to-side. Once they are placed at the junction of the SVC and RA, the TS needle is advanced inside the sheath. The TS needle should be advanced with a stylet inside, which protrudes 2 mm from the needle tip. The stylet provides more support during its trajectory through the pelvis and it prevents perforation of the sheath. The needle can be connected directly to a manifold and introduced into the sheath while flushing (to prevent air embolism), and the system can be used to monitor pressure from the needle tip. Once the needle is introduced in the sheath, it should be allowed to rotate freely without pushing, until it is close to the tip of the introducer and sheath. Once the needle is inside the sheath, the unit should be carefully handled together to prevent the needle from exteriorizing beyond the introducer and puncturing the SVC. This can be accomplished by keeping the hub of the needle approximately two fingers width back from the hub of the sheath.

Once the TS sheath and needle are at the junction of the SVC and RA, the sheath, introducer, and needle are rotated as a unit 45 degrees posteromedially (4–5 o'clock where the ceiling is 12 o'clock). The rotation is performed slowly under fluoroscopy (anteroposterior projection and ideally biplane with a lateral view). First, a lateral movement is observed from SVC to RA. Then, a second subtle movement is detected as the unit descends past the aorta. Last and most important, a lateral movement will be detected when passing over the limbic portion and engaging medially into the depression of the FO. If the anatomy is distorted, an RA angiogram can also be performed to visualize the septum, or the operator can use different imaging tools simultaneously. Once engaged in the FO, a small stain in the septum can be used to confirm the tenting of the FO, or the engagement can be visualized using ICE or TEE. The fluoroscopy should then be changed to an orthogonal view (LAO 40 or RAO 40) or to the lateral view if biplane is being used, to confirm the position of the sheath in relation to the aorta and spine. Once the correct position has been confirmed, where the needle points posterior and away from the aorta, the needle is advanced. When a tactile jump is felt, the pressure waveform should immediately change from dampened to LA pressure. At this point, the needle is slightly rotated counterclockwise to 3 o'clock to prevent perforation of the posterior LA wall. The needle position in the LA should be confirmed by injecting a small puff of contrast in the LA and observing the distance between the needle and the free LA wall. Care must be taken not to advance the needle beyond the silhouette of the left mainstem bronchus. At this point, the introduction of a 0.014-in. wire through the needle into the LA can be used to prevent perforation of the LA wall while advancing the needle and introducer (24). If the needle is inserted in the pericardium or the aorta, it should be removed, and the procedure can be restarted from the beginning, while monitoring the hemodynamic status. However, if the dilator and sheath have been advanced, they should not be removed until surgical backup is available to manage the perforation.

Once the tip of the needle is confirmed to be in the LA, the needle and introducer should be advanced carefully allowing only 2 to 3 mm of the tip of the needle to enter the LA. The introducer is advanced further over the needle in the LA, and the sheath is then advanced over the introducer to enter into a pulmonary vein or preferably the left ventricle (LV), while avoiding entry into the left atrial appendage (LAA) because of the risk of perforation.

The introducer and needle should be removed slowly, and ideally, the removal should occur at a level lower than that of the LA to prevent negative air suction leading to systemic air embolism. Then the sheath should be flushed using standard technique to ensure that there is no air or thrombus. This is a crucial step to prevent any major embolic complications. At this stage, anticoagulation with heparin should be instituted, and it should be continued throughout the procedure.

■ TIPS AND TROUBLESHOOTING

- When in doubt about the anatomy, consider imaging preprocedure to evaluate for any relevant structural abnormalities and to discard the possibility of thrombus.
- RA and pulmonary capillary wedge pressure should be assessed to estimate LA pressure prior to the TSP.
- When the sheath and needle do not engage the FO after the first descent, the needle should be removed. Then the wire should be advanced to reposition the sheath and dilator at the junction of the SVC-RA to prevent perforation of the RA with the stiff introducer. An "anterior staircase maneuver" has also been described, where the sheath containing the needle is readvanced carefully with side-to-side movements from 2 to 10 o'clock until the unit is repositioned in the SVC without a wire exchange (25). However, there are limited data to support that this technique is safe enough; therefore, it is still recommended to reposition the sheath by using the wire.
- The size of the LA and the distance from the "tenting" of the septum to the free LA wall should be visualized when using ICE or TEE, and adjustments should be made to maximize this distance to prevent perforation.
- Sudden loss of pressure from the sheath after removing the needle and introducer from the LA can occur if there is thrombus in the

sheath, if the sheath prolapses back into the RA or when the sheath is against the wall of an underfilled LA. This can also occur when the sheath is in a false lumen like in the tunnel of a patent FO or in the septum primum. Therefore, confirmation of the appropriate position of the needle in the LA by a contrast puff should be routinely done, and only when the LA pressure waveform is present.

- An arterial waveform will indicate puncture into the ascending or the descending aorta. No further advancement of the sheath should be done at this point. Reverse anticoagulation if appropriate and monitor hemodynamic status. If the advancement of the sheath is inadvertently done into the aorta, do not remove the sheath and call the surgeon for emergency repair.
- Simultaneous arterial pressure monitoring should be mandatory. Occasionally, vagal reactions during septal puncture can result in hypotension.
- Repeated TSP can be difficult in up to 30% of the patients due to scar or distorted anatomical landmarks. The septum may be calcified in chronic renal insufficiency, or it may thicken in the presence of an atrial patch. Exerting a forward force carries a greater risk of needle fracture or of perforation of the posterior LA wall secondary to sudden forward "jump" of the needle in the LA. To prevent these two complications, radiofrequency energy can be applied to the TS needle. Once the dilator is engaged in the FO and confirmed by ICE visualization of the tenting, the needle can be advanced almost to the tip of the dilator without exteriorizing the needle. Electrocautery (15–20 W) is then applied to the proximal part of the needle using 1 to 2 second pulses of cut-mode cautery while advancing the tip of the needle beyond the dilator. The cautery should be stopped as soon as the needle is pushed out fully. Initiating the cautery when the needle is still inside of the sheath minimizes the power required to puncture. Newer radiofrequency perforating catheters are being used specifically in children (26,27).

■ COMPLICATIONS

TSP remains a challenging procedure. Because of its nature, the most threatening complication is the perforation of surrounding structures.

Complications tend to be rare (<2%), but they can be serious and life-threatening (death in <0.5%) even in experienced hands (6,28). Complications of TSP are listed in Tables 19-4 and 19-5 and illustrated in Figures 19-7 and 19-8.

TABLE 19-4	Complications of Transseptal Puncture

Perforation: • Roof of the LA • Posterior LA wall • LAA
Perforation of the SVC or IVC
Aortic perforation
Arrhythmias
Puncture or dissection of coronary sinus
Embolization
From: • Layered thrombus in the LA wall • LA myxoma • Air
To: • Brain • Coronaries • Systemic
Pulmonary vein perforation
Instrumental fracture due to breakage of the 21-gauge needle tip at its junction with the 18-gauge
Bezold–Jarisch-like vasovagal response: ST-segment elevation in the inferior leads without chest pain, associated with hypotension, bradycardia, and normal coronary arteries and reversed by atropine
Transient migraine
Thrombophlebitis and pulmonary embolism after complicated venous access
Pericarditis after injection of dye in the pericardium
Serious bleeding into posterior pericardial space
Inferior ST elevation
Residual atrial septal shunt
Hemothorax
Puncturing of the posterior RA creating a stitch phenomena by reentering the LA
Atrial–aorto fistula

LA, left atrium; SVC, superior vena cava; IVC, inferior vena cava; RA, right atrium.

TABLE 19-5 Incidence of Transseptal Puncture Complications

	Braunwald et al. (6) (1968)	Roelke et al. (28) (1994)	De Ponti et al. (3) (1992–2002)	De Ponti et al. (3) (2003)
No. of patients	1,765	1,279	3,756	1,764
Cardiac perforation, %	2.4	1.2	0.07	0.17
Tamponade, %	1.2	1.2	0.07	0.11
Major complications, %	3.4	1.3	0.74	0.79
Death, %	0.2	0.08	0.02	…
Embolism, %	0.3	0.08	0.07	0.05

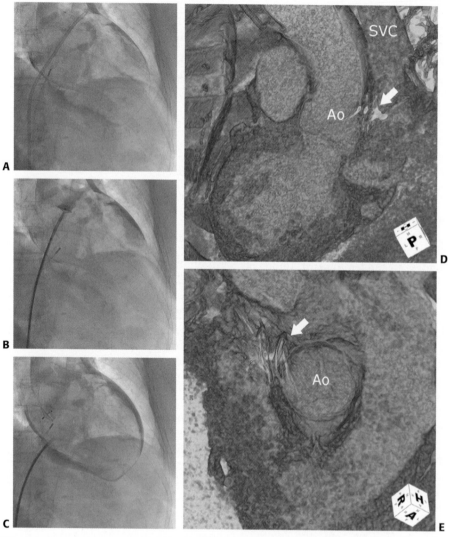

FIGURE 19-7. Transseptal needle perforating right atrial wall with contrast filling the pericardium. Amplatzer device was placed to close the right atrium perforation. Computed tomography angiography (CTA) confirmed the position of the device. (**A–C**) Step-by-step perforation closure with an Amplatzer device. (**D–E**) CTA images confirming the position of the Amplatzer device closing the perforation. (A–C, From Chiam PT, Schneider LM, Ruiz CE. Cardiac perforation during patent foramen ovale closure sealed with an amplatzer PFO occluder. *J Invasive Cardiol.* 2008;20:665–668. D–E, Courtesy of Dr. Ruiz and Dr. Jelnin, Department of Interventional and Structural Heart Disease, Lenox Hill Institute, New York, New York.) (See color insert.)

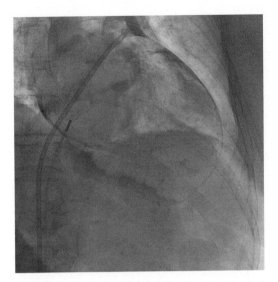

FIGURE 19-8. Pericardial staining from inadvertent perforation with the transseptal needle. (Courtesy of Dr. Ruiz and Dr. Jelnin, Department of Interventional and Structural Heart Disease, Lenox Hill Institute, New York, New York.)

During TSP, the nature of each complication dictates its management. The specific chamber affected with an injury or perforation will determine the outcome. The operator performing the procedure must be familiar with recognition of complications and with bailout techniques for their management.

Perforation

Perforation of the RA or LA should be managed by immediate pericardiocentesis, followed by surgical management if needed. Closure of the perforation by using a percutaneous closure device between the chamber and the pericardium has also been described (29). In cases where there is an inadvertent puncture of the roof of the RA, a "parallel wire" technique can be used by advancing an 0.018-in. wire through the laceration into the pericardium to maintain access while delivering a closure device through the same transseptal (TS) sheath until the stability of the device is confirmed (29) (see Fig. 19-6). Anecdotal placement of closure devices in a perforation of the free LA wall has also been performed without any available long-term data.

Perforation of the IVC is rare, but it can occur while advancing the introducer or the needle. These perforations can result in life-threatening retroperitoneal hematomas. Early recognition is mandatory, and management is required with balloon occlusion or surgical repair.

Perforation of the coronary sinus is also rare, and it can result in refractory hemorrhage and tamponade requiring surgical repair.

Pericardial Effusion and Tamponade

The possibility of a new pericardial effusion and tamponade should always be considered, especially if the patient complains of pain during the TS procedure. The presentation will depend on multiple factors including the characteristics of the device that caused the injury, the structure perforated, pericardial properties, hemodynamic state at the time of the perforation, and coagulation status (30). For example, a puncture with a 21-gauge needle does not usually lead to tamponade unless further advancement of the sheath is performed.

The same intraprocedural real-time image or a transthoracic echo should be used when there is a suspicion of perforation, even before the hemodynamic findings are evident. The presence of new septal shift by echo, indicating ventricular interdependence, should prompt the operator to discontinue the intervention and reverse the anticoagulation. Straightening and immobility of the left heart border and an epicardial halo may be observed under fluoroscopy together with hemodynamic deterioration (Fig. 19-8). Pericardiocentesis should be performed as soon as there is objective evidence of mild hemodynamic compromise like pulsus paradoxus. Occasionally, surgery is required if there is a cardiac tear and no hemodynamic improvement is obtained with catheter drainage.

■ EMERGING TRANSSEPTAL TECHNOLOGIES

- Further development of real-time, 3D image tools like coupled image devices and the 3D or 4D ICE (20) will improve the anatomical guidance during TSP.
- Newer technologies are being used to increase the safety of TSP, including the following:
  - Use of wire needle puncture (SafeSept, Pressure Products, Inc., San Pedro, California) (Figs. 19-9 and 19-10)

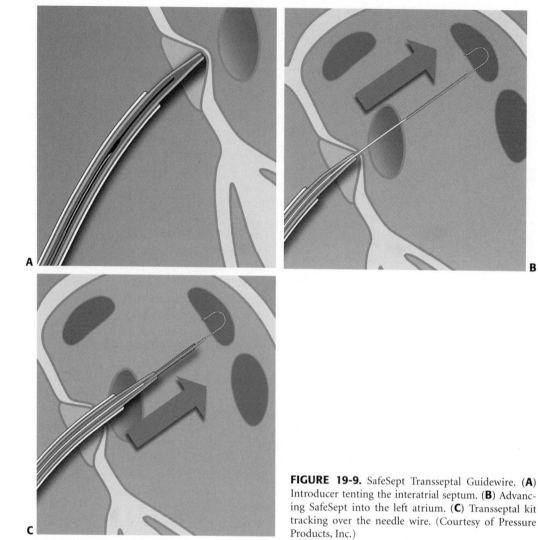

FIGURE 19-9. SafeSept Transseptal Guidewire. (**A**) Introducer tenting the interatrial septum. (**B**) Advancing SafeSept into the left atrium. (**C**) Transseptal kit tracking over the needle wire. (Courtesy of Pressure Products, Inc.)

- Using of radiofrequency energy systems instead of the needle to perforate the atrial septum (27)
- Potential use of the excimer laser catheter to perforate the septum with real-time MRI lasers (31)
- Systems design for superior access through the internal jugular veins

ATRIAL SEPTOSTOMY

Balloon atrial septostomy (AS) is a technique used to create an artificial shunt through the IAS. AS was first introduced by Rashkind and Miller in 1966 to palliate a range of congenital abnormalities in children (32). Nowadays, AS has gained wide acceptance also in the management of patients with severe pulmonary artery hypertension (PAH) refractory to medical therapy and as a therapeutic alternative in locations where economical burdens do not permit medical therapy for PAH (33,34) (see Table 19-6 for current indications).

AS is currently recommended for PAH in the setting of advanced NYHA class III/IV, patients with recurrent syncope or right heart failure despite optimal medical therapy, as a palliation or as a bridge to transplantation. The benefits are thought to be related to reduced right filling pressures and to an increase in LV filling, resulting in increased cardiac output and oxygen delivery. AS has also been used to vent the LV and to

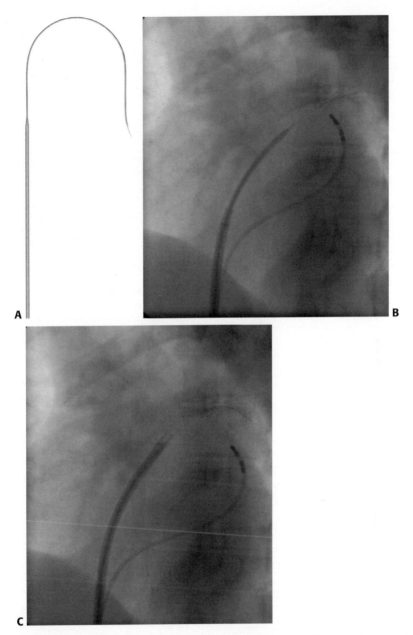

FIGURE 19-10. (**A**) SafeSept Transseptal Guidewire. (**B**) Fluoroscopy showing SafeSept wire across the septum in the left atrium. (**C**) Advancement of the sheath over guidewire. (Courtesy of Pressure Products, Inc.)

manage or prevent pulmonary hemorrhages in patients on extracorporeal circulation (see Chapter 24, circulatory support).

In a recent report of the global experience of patients treated with AS, the majority of patients were women with idiopathic pulmonary artery hypertension. Other patients treated with AS had PAH after corrected congenital heart disease or collagen vascular disease, or they were nonsurgical candidates with chronic thromboembolic pulmonary hypertension (35).

■ PROCEDURE DESCRIPTION

Several techniques for AS have been described (Figs. 19-11 and 19-12).

TABLE 19-6	Indications for Atrial Septostomy

Pulmonary hypertension despite maximal medical therapy with:
    Recurrent syncope
    Right ventricular failure
    Bridge to transplant
    Palliative

Complex congenital heart disease
    Transposition of the great vessel with intact
        atrial septum
    Mitral, tricuspid, or pulmonary atresia
    Total anomalous pulmonary venous return
    Double-outlet right ventricle
    Univentricular heart and unilateral restrictive
        atrioventricular valve
    Failing Fontan circulation

Venting of the left ventricle/pulmonary hemorrhage in patients on bypass support

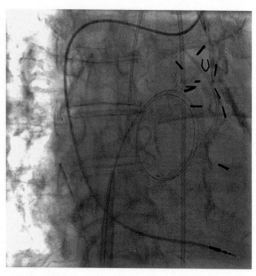

FIGURE 19-11. Atrial septostomy as seen by fluoroscopy. Anteroposterior projection demonstrating a 14F dilator cannula over an Inoue wire before dilating the interatrial septum. (Courtesy of Dr. Londono, Mount Sinai, Miami Beach, Florida.)

Balloon Dilatation

Balloon dilatation is the most commonly used AS technique (36,37). Right and left heart catheterizations are always performed first for hemodynamic evaluations. Transseptal sheath and needle are used to perform a standard TSP, as described previously, and an Inoue or an Amplatz extra stiff wire is then advanced into the LA. Several balloons have been used depending on the technique including, the Miller catheter (Edwards-Baxter Healthcare Co., Santa Ana, California), the Rashkind balloon catheter (USCI-CR Bard, Inc., Billerica, Massachusetts), the Fogarty (Paul) balloon (Edwards-Baxter Healthcare), the Z-5 septostomy catheter (NuMED, Inc., Hopkinton, New York), and other peripheral balloons. Regardless of the technique, it is crucial to appropriately position the balloon prior to inflation and to avoid the left atrial appendage, pulmonary veins, and mitral valve. In the original technique, the appropriate balloon is inflated in the LA and rapidly pulled back into the RA, and then it is deflated and reintroduced into the LA to repeat the procedure until adequate communication is achieved (32). Another common technique nowadays has been to progressively dilate the septum with different sizes balloons until the desired shunt has been created (36). Other balloon techniques described

include static balloon atrial dilatation, which is performed until the waist of the balloon disappears, and cutting balloon AS, which is performed more commonly in small children.

Independent of the technique used, the operator must simultaneously assess changes in RV and LV end-diastolic pressure (LVEDP) and systemic arterial saturation, as well as visualize the shunt by TEE or ICE (see Fig. 19-12). It is recommended that arterial saturation be maintained at a level higher than 75% and LVEDP should be less than 18 mmHg.

Blade Balloon AS

Blade balloon AS has been available since 1978 (38,39), but it is less frequently performed currently because of the risk of laceration. After performing the TSP and introducing the sheath in the LA, a 9.4-, 13.4-, or 20-mm blade catheter can be advanced through the sheath into the LA. The sheath is then withdrawn to the level of the IVC. The blade is directed inferiorly and then withdrawn, and the sheath is repositioned into the LA. Subsequently, several orthogonal blade incisions can be performed, or instead further postdilation can be performed with a balloon. The blade technique is preferred in cases where there is a thick fibrotic septum or after repeated procedures. In addition, it is thought

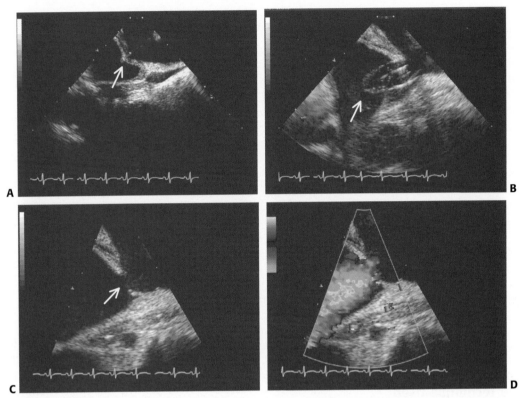

FIGURE 19-12. Atrial septostomy in a patient with end-stage pulmonary hypertension performed using ICE. **(A)** Typical tenting of the fossa ovalis from the transseptal needle. **(B)** Balloon inflation. **(C)** Atrial septal defect at the septostomy site. **(D)** Doppler color flow through the atrial septal defect. (From Moscucci M, Dairywala IT, Chetcuti S, et al. Balloon atrial septostomy in end-stage pulmonary hypertension guided by a novel intracardiac echocardiographic transducer. *Catheter Cardiovasc Interv.* 2001;52:530–534.) (See color insert.)

to reocclude less often than with the balloon technique (38).

Similar hemodynamic and clinical results have been described with balloon and blade techniques, but balloon-only techniques pose a lower procedure-related risk (37).

No further dilatation should be performed if oxygen saturation decreases by more than 10% or LVEDP increases to greater than 18 mmHg. After uncomplicated septostomies the defect size is approximately 8 mm, and this has been thought to increase cardiac output by 25% (35). After blade septostomy, spontaneous closure rates have been reported in 3% of cases, whereas for balloon septostomy, spontaneous closures occur in 15% to 17% of patients. Both balloon septostomy and blade technique may require repeated procedures (33,34) but a lower procedure-related mortality is associated with balloon septostomy than with the blade technique (40).

Other techniques, such as stenting the atrial septum, deploying custom-made fenestrated Amplatzer devices or butterfly stents (41,42) are promising alternative techniques that have been used more recently but require further studies.

■ COMPLICATIONS

In addition to the TSP complications that have already been mentioned, AS is usually performed in fragile patients who have very little cardiopulmonary reserve. The prognosis after AS depends on the functional status of the right ventricle. The procedure-related mortality is currently approximately 16%, but it has been reported to range between 5% and 50% in small studies and in extremely ill patients (34,35,37) Therefore, AS should be performed only in the appropriate centers by experienced hands (36).

Recommendations to minimize procedure-related mortality during AS have included optimization of pre- and postprocedure cardiac function and oxygen delivery. Contraindications for performing AS continue to be severe right ventricular failure on cardiorespiratory support, mean RA pressure higher than 20 mmHg, pulmonary vascular resistance index greater than 55 U/m^2, resting oxygen saturation less than 90% on room air, and the LVEDP higher than 18 mmHg (35).

Deaths related to the procedure are usually a consequence of the creation of a large defect with refractory hypoxemia due to massive right to left shunting, which can occur if the initial RAP is greater than 20 mmHg (36). This is the reason why a progressive step-up approach is recommended in conjunction with Doppler echocardiography monitoring of the shunt size using TEE or ICE (see Fig. 19-12). In the setting of refractory hypoxemia, inhaled iloprost has been used (43).

Complications of AS According to the Technique Used

- Balloon septostomy:
  - Perforation after balloon inflation, especially of the LAA
  - Balloon rupture and fragment embolization requiring retrieval or surgical removal
  - Nondeflatable balloon. In this situation, the balloon must be ruptured either with a wire or by injecting contrast under pressure
- Blade septostomy:
  - Laceration of the left atrial wall or perforation of the right ventricular outflow tract with the blade.
  - Failure to retract the blade into the catheter, requiring surgical removal
- Stenting the IAS:
  - Thrombus on the stent placed with risk of embolization
  - Stent erosions, which can be avoided by using the shortest possible stent
  - Stent migration, which can be avoided by flaring both ends of the stents

See Table 19-7 for a full list of complications.

▮ LV APICAL PUNCTURE

Percutaneous direct LV puncture has been performed since the late 1940s (6,45) for direct

TABLE 19-7	Complications of Atrial Septostomy
Laceration
Death
Neurological events including CVA and seizures
Bleeding
Defective catheter or equipment malfunction
Interatrial groove tear
Severe hypoxemia due to an oversize defect
Acute LV failure
Arrhythmias
Pulmonary arterial vasospasm

LV, left ventricle; CVA, cerebrovascular accident.

hemodynamic evaluation. With the subsequent introduction of the Seldinger technique and the development of specific catheters, peripheral vascular access became the most common approach for percutaneous cardiac procedures. Nevertheless, there are several clinical circumstances where direct LV access continues to be useful for diagnostic or interventional indications (see Table 19-8 for indications). In addition, recently there has been an increase in the use of the transthoracic direct LV access methods due to the rapid expansion of percutaneous transapical aortic valve program (46). It is therefore important in our time to be familiar with direct transapical LV access techniques and potential complications.

TABLE 19-8	Indications for Direct Transapical Access
LV access in the setting of double mechanical valves
Inaccessible percutaneous paravalvular leak repair
Complex congenital heart disease
Inaccessible carotid or coronary interventions
Percutaneous valve implantation
Inaccessible LV in the setting of severe peripheral vascular disease

LV, left ventricle.

ANATOMIC FACTORS

The normal LV is the thickest heart chamber (approximately 10 mm thick). The LV apex is directed downward, forward, and to the left. It is the lowest superficial part of the heart, and occasionally, it is overlapped by the left lung and pleura. In relation to the chest wall, the apex is usually behind the fifth intercostal space and is located 8 cm to the left from the midsternal line. This location can be displaced laterally due to right ventricular enlargement and may vary in cases with rotated hearts or congenital abnormalities.

The pericardium covers the heart from the lower SVC to the apex. It consists of two layers, a fibrous, parietal, noncompliant layer (<2 mm thick) and a visceral segment, separated by a small volume of fluid (20–50 cc). After cardiac surgery, the pericardium may be absent or adherent but localized effusion can still occur. The left anterior descending artery (LAD) runs through the interventricular groove and usually tapers into three different patterns: an LAD that does not reach the apex, and gives rise only to small distal branches, a bifurcating apical LAD that forms two branches, and the most common pattern, which is a single apical LAD that is medial to the apex and extends into the posterior interventricular groove.

The relatively easy access to the LV apex via the thoracic wall and the close distance from the apex to the left side valve structures makes this technique a very attractive approach in specific situations. It is an alternative in cases of peripheral vascular disease and in patients with small femoral arteries. In addition, it has been commonly used in the hemodynamic evaluation of patients with dual mechanical valves in mitral and aortic position.

IMAGING TECHNIQUES

The site of the apical impulse can be located by palpation and confirmed by transthoracic echo separated by a small volume (47). A radiopaque marker can be placed to identify the location of the LV apex and serve as a guide to the puncture site using fluoroscopy. Ideally, the location of the apical LAD in relation to the puncture should be known, and in the majority of cases, it tapers medially from the apex. This can be confirmed by simultaneous coronary angiography (via the radial or femoral approach) at the time of the apical puncture. During the direct transthoracic LV apical puncture, diluted contrast should be injected while advancing the needle forward through the chest wall under fluoroscopy. This can allow the identification of the passage of the needle tip across any coronary artery.

Apical epicardial echocardiography and TEE are useful tools for determining the best site to insert the needle and sheaths. In addition, these imaging modalities can be used to make sure that the needle and the sheath are appropriately lined up with the specific working structures, depending on the indications of the procedure. For example, the insertion axis should be lined up with the aortic valve for a transcatheter aortic valve implantation or for a paravalvular leak engagement.

More recently, 3D and 4D CTA reconstructions have been very helpful in identifying the anatomical landmarks surrounding the apex, the location and pattern of the coronaries, and the distance between the lungs and pleura. 3D rotational angiography is another attractive technique for evaluating the relationship between the apex and chest wall at the time of the puncture (Fig. 19-13).

PROCEDURE DESCRIPTION

Direct LV apical puncture has been routinely performed in the catheterization laboratories under fluoroscopy. More recently, with the advent of transapical aortic valve implantations, a hybrid room with fluoroscopy, echocardiography imaging, and backup cardiorespiratory support has become the ideal environment for direct LV apical puncture. The need for respiratory support will depend on the specific indications of the procedure.

Direct Transthoracic Percutaneous LV Apical Puncture

Once the puncture site has been identified, the skin and subcutaneous tissue are anesthetized. Caution should be taken not to injure the neurovascular bundle that runs underneath the ribs. A 21-gauge micropuncture needle and kit can be used to access the LV directly from the chest wall under fluoroscopic guidance while injecting diluted contrast. Once the needle is in the LV cavity, the needle and dilator are exchanged over

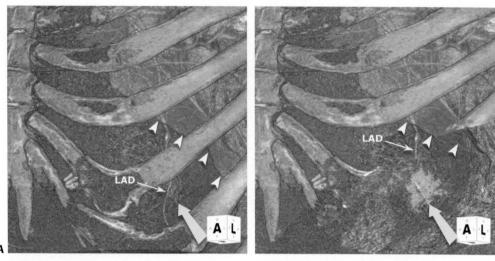

FIGURE 19-13. (**A**) Anatomical landmarks using three-dimensional-computed tomography angiography reconstruction (volume-rendered technique) demonstrating the left ventricle (LV) apex in relation to the ribs and the left anterior descending coronary artery. *White arrow* indicates edge of the lung. *Broad arrow* indicates LV apex. (**B**) Oblique cut plane removing tissue and exposing LV cavity to delineate the path of the transapical puncture. LAD, left anterior descending. (Courtesy of Dr. Ruiz and Dr. Jelnin, Department of Interventional and Structural Heart Disease, Lenox Hill Institute, New York, New York.) (See color insert.)

a J-tip wire for the specific sheath size required for the intended procedure. It is important to note that the most frequent time of bleeding is during catheter exchange. Once the sheath is in place, direct LV pressure will confirm the location, and the specific procedure can then be performed. Anticoagulation must be administered at this time (Figs. 19-14 and 19-15).

Hemostasis at the end of the procedure will be obtained depending on the size of the sheath inserted. Small sheaths can be manually pulled without major complications and bigger sheaths,

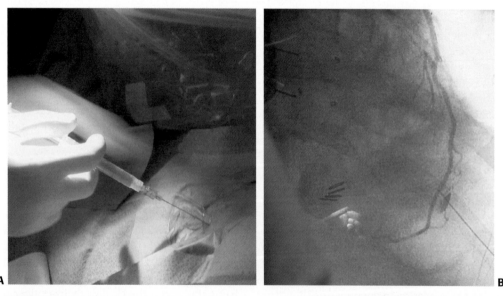

FIGURE 19-14. (**A**) Position of the micropuncture needle through the chest wall. (**B**) Fluoroscopic guidance using simultaneous coronary angiography to identify the location of the left anterior descending artery in relation to the puncture. Forward injection of contrast during left ventricle needle puncture. (Courtesy of Dr. Ruiz and Dr. Jelnin, Department of Interventional and Structural Heart Disease, Lenox Hill Institute, New York, New York.)

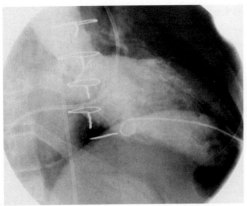 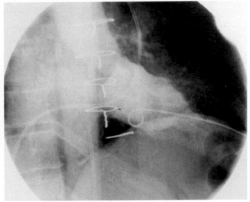

FIGURE 19-15. Left ventriculography via the left ventricular apical approach in a patient with mechanical valves in mitral and aortic position. **A.** Pigtail in the left ventricle during diastole. **B.** Pigtail in the left ventricle during systole. (Courtesy of Mauro Moscucci, University of Miami, Miami, Florida.)

up to 9F, have been removed by using off-label ventricular closure devices at the ventriculostomy site separated by a small volume (48). When this fails, open minithoracotomy may be required to close or patch the puncture site.

Direct LV Access through a Minithoracotomy

When the sheaths required for transapical access are large, as in the case of a percutaneous valve implantation, transapical access is performed under general anesthesia by a team of cardiac surgeons, cardiologist, and anesthesiologist. An anterolateral fifth or sixth intercostal space minithoracotomy is performed to expose the LV apex. The pericardium is dissected longitudinally, and access to the LV is obtained by a needle puncturing lateral to the apex. The ventriculostomy is dilated to insert larger sheaths, and at the end of the procedure, it is repaired with preinserted pledged sutures. A short burst of rapid ventricular pacing to decrease the LV systolic pressure is helpful during the repair (50). Caution should be taken when performing a direct LV puncture in cases with chest wall deformities, compromised respiratory function, or the presence of LV abnormalities such as thrombus.

■ COMPLICATIONS

The most feared complication of direct LV puncture is the perforation of surrounding structures leading to tamponade, pneumothorax,

or coronary artery laceration. These complications can be avoided by the use of adjuvant imaging tools during the puncture to evade injury of surrounding structures.

The larger the size of the sheaths used, the higher the risk of complications. In view of this, when larger sheaths (20F–30F) are required, direct LV access through the minithoracotomy is currently the safest method. The risk of lung injury, pneumothorax, or pleural bleeding with direct exposure of the apex has been reported to be low in case series of percutaneous valves replacement (51); however, chest wall discomfort and the associated potential for respiratory compromise and prolonged ventilation is still a serious concern.

Additional complications when performing direct LV puncture can occur when removing the sheaths. Unfortunately, there is no approved closure device currently available for safe percutaneous hemostasis. The risk of bleeding depends on the size of the sheath introduced and the LV pressure. Postprocedure bleeding from the access may result in tamponade or hemothorax, requiring further repair and chest tube placement, whereas management of a large tear may require cardiopulmonary support.

When sutures have been placed at the ventriculostomy site, a friable repair or suture dehiscence can lead to persistent bleeding. The formation of a pseudoaneurysm at the site of the puncture has been reported weeks to months after percutaneous direct LV procedures separated by a

TABLE 19-9 Incidence of Complications from Direct Left Ventricle Access			
	Braunwald et al. (6) (1968)	Morgan et al. (53) (1989)	Havranek et al. (49) (1995)
No. of procedures	260	112	1,167
Major complications, %	3.1	3	1.4–2.7

small volume (51). For a list and incidence of reported complications, see Tables 19-9 and 19-10.

■ CONCLUSION

The recent advancements in electrophysiology and in the percutaneous management of structural heart diseases have resulted in a resurgence of TS cardiac catheterization, AS, and direct LV apical puncture. Thorough knowledge of cardiac anatomy and of anatomical landmarks, identification of patient's characteristics leading to increase complexity, and the use of different imaging modalities can increase the safety of these procedures.

TABLE 19-10 Complications during Transapical Left Ventricle (LV) Access
Bleeding and tamponade
Pain: precordial and pleuritic
Pleural effusion and hemothorax
Pneumothorax
Intramural LV hematoma
Postpericardiotomy syndrome
Ventricular arrhythmias
Pneumonia
Coronary laceration
Reflex hypotension from vagal stimulation
Fistula
Infarction
Sepsis
Embolization
LV pseudoaneurysm
Delayed rupture of the apex

References

1. Ross J Jr, Braunwald E, Morrow AG. Transseptal left atrial puncture: new technique for the measurement of left atrial pressure in man. *Am J Cardiol.* 1959;3:653–655.
2. Cope C. Technique for transseptal catheterization of the left atrium: preliminary report. *J Thorac Surg.* 1959;37:482–486.
3. De Ponti R, Casari A, Salerno JA, et al. [Radiofrequency transcatheter ablation of anomalous left atrioventricular pathways: the role of the transseptal approach]. *G Ital Cardiol.* 1992;22:1255–1264.
4. Babaliaros VC, Green JT, Lerakis S, et al. Emerging applications for transseptal left heart catheterization old techniques for new procedures. *J Am Coll Cardiol.* 2008;51:2116–2122.
5. Ross J Jr. Considerations regarding the technique for transseptal left heart catheterization. *Circulation.* 1966;34:391–399.
6. Braunwald E. Cooperative study on cardiac catheterization: transseptal left heart catheterization. *Circulation.* 1968;37:III74–III79.
7. Brockenbrough EC, Braunwald E, Ross J Jr. Transseptal left heart catheterization: a review of 450 studies and description of an improved technic. *Circulation.* 1962;25:15–21.
8. Mullins CE. Transseptal left heart catheterization: experience with a new technique in 520 pediatric and adult patients. *Pediatr Cardiol.* 1983;4:239–245.
9. Villacastin J, Castellano NP, Moreno J, et al. [Learning process for transseptal puncture guided by intracardiac echocardiography]. *Rev Esp Cardiol.* 2004;57:359–362.
10. Sweeney LJ, Rosenquist GC. The normal anatomy of the atrial septum in the human heart. *Am Heart J.* 1979;98:194–199.
11. Daoud EG, Kalbfleisch SJ, Hummel JD. Intracardiac echocardiography to guide transseptal left heart catheterization for radiofrequency catheter ablation. *J Cardiovasc Electrophysiol.* 1999;10:358–363.

12. Schwinger ME, Gindea AJ, Freedberg RS, et al. The anatomy of the interatrial septum: a transesophageal echocardiographic study. *Am Heart J.* 1990;119:1401–1405.

13. Sokolov VV, Brezhnev FF, Kharlamov EV. [Sources of the vascularization of the human interatrial septum of the heart with different variants of the atrial blood supply]. *Arkh Anat Gistol Embriol.* 1986;91:29–34.

14. Hung JS, Fu M, Yeh KH, et al. Usefulness of intracardiac echocardiography in complex transseptal catheterization during percutaneous transvenous mitral commissurotomy. *Mayo Clin Proc.* 1996; 71:134–140.

15. Kim SS, Hijazi ZM, Lang RM, et al. The use of intracardiac echocardiography and other intracardiac imaging tools to guide noncoronary cardiac interventions. *J Am Coll Cardiol.* 2009;53: 2117–2128.

16. El-Said HG, Ing FF, Grifka RG, et al. 18-year experience with transseptal procedures through baffles, conduits, and other intra-atrial patches. *Catheter Cardiovasc Interv.* 2000;50:434–439, discussion 440.

17. Hellenbrand WE, Fahey JT, McGowan FX, et al. Transesophageal echocardiographic guidance of transcatheter closure of atrial septal defect. *Am J Cardiol.* 1990;66:207–213.

18. Hijazi Z, Wang Z, Cao Q, et al. Transcatheter closure of atrial septal defects and patent foramen ovale under intracardiac echocardiographic guidance: feasibility and comparison with transesophageal echocardiography. *Catheter Cardiovasc Interv.* 2001;52:194–199.

19. Knecht S, Wright M, Lellouche N, et al. Impact of a patent foramen ovale on paroxysmal atrial fibrillation ablation. *J Cardiovasc Electrophysiol.* 2008;19:1236–1241.

20. Hijazi ZM, Shivkumar K, Sahn DJ. Intracardiac echocardiography during interventional and electrophysiological cardiac catheterization. *Circulation.* 2009;119:587–596.

21. Graham LN, Melton IC, MacDonald S, et al. Value of CT localization of the fossa ovalis prior to transseptal left heart catheterization for left atrial ablation. *Europace.* 2007;9:417–423.

22. Nazarian S, Kolandaivelu A, Zviman MM, et al. Feasibility of real-time magnetic resonance imaging for catheter guidance in electrophysiology studies. *Circulation.* 2008;118:223–229.

23. Clugston R, Lau FY, Ruiz C. Transseptal catheterization update 1992. *Cathet Cardiovasc Diagn.* 1992;26:266–274.

24. Hildick-Smith D, McCready J, de Giovanni J. Transseptal puncture: use of an angioplasty guidewire for enhanced safety. *Catheter Cardiovasc Interv.* 2007;69:519–521.

25. Shaw TR. Anterior staircase manoeuvre for atrial transseptal puncture. *Br Heart J.* 1994;71:297–301.

26. McWilliams MJ, Tchou P. The use of a standard radiofrequency energy delivery system to facilitate transseptal puncture. *J Cardiovasc Electrophysiol.* 2009;20:238–240.

27. Sherman W, Lee P, Hartley A, et al. Transatrial septal catheterization using a new radiofrequency probe. *Catheter Cardiovasc Interv.* 2005;66:14–17.

28. Roelke M, Smith AJ, Palacios IF. The technique and safety of transseptal left heart catheterization: the Massachusetts General Hospital experience with 1,279 procedures. *Cathet Cardiovasc Diagn.* 1994;32:332–339.

29. Chiam PT, Schneider LM, Ruiz CE. Cardiac perforation during patent foramen ovale closure sealed with an Amplatzer PFO occluder. *J Invasive Cardiol.* 2008;20:665–668.

30. Holmes DR Jr, Nishimura R, Fountain R, et al. Iatrogenic pericardial effusion and tamponade in the percutaneous intracardiac intervention era. *JACC Cardiovasc Interv.* 2009;2:705–717.

31. Elagha AA, Kim AH, Kocaturk O, et al. Blunt atrial transseptal puncture using excimer laser in swine. *Catheter Cardiovasc Interv.* 2007;70: 585–590.

32. Rashkind WJ, Miller WW. Creation of an atrial septal defect without thoracotomy: a palliative approach to complete transposition of the great arteries. *JAMA.* 1966;196:991–992.

33. Nihill MR, O'Laughlin MP, Mullins CE. Effects of atrial septostomy in patients with terminal cor pulmonale due to pulmonary vascular disease. *Cathet Cardiovasc Diagn.* 1991;24:166–172.

34. Kerstein D, Levy PS, Hsu DT, et al. Blade balloon atrial septostomy in patients with severe primary pulmonary hypertension. *Circulation.* 1995;91: 2028–2035.

35. Keogh AM, Mayer E, Benza RL, et al. Interventional and surgical modalities of treatment in pulmonary hypertension. *J Am Coll Cardiol.* 2009; 54:S67–S77.

36. Sandoval J, Rothman A, Pulido T. Atrial septostomy for pulmonary hypertension. *Clin Chest Med.* 2001;22:547–560.

37. Klepetko W, Mayer E, Sandoval J, et al. Interventional and surgical modalities of treatment for

pulmonary arterial hypertension. *J Am Coll Cardiol.* 2004;43:73S–80S.

38. Park SC, Neches WH, Zuberbuhler JR, et al. Clinical use of blade atrial septostomy. *Circulation.* 1978;58:600–606.

39. Park SC, Neches WH, Mullins CE, et al. Blade atrial septostomy: collaborative study. *Circulation.* 1982;66:258–266.

40. Micheletti A, Hislop AA, Lammers A, et al. Role of atrial septostomy in the treatment of children with pulmonary arterial hypertension. *Heart.* 2006;92:969–972.

41. Prieto LR, Latson LA, Jennings C. Atrial septostomy using a butterfly stent in a patient with severe pulmonary arterial hypertension. *Catheter Cardiovasc Interv.* 2006;68:642–647.

42. O'Loughlin AJ, Keogh A, Muller DW. Insertion of a fenestrated Amplatzer atrial septostomy device for severe pulmonary hypertension. *Heart Lung Circ.* 2006;15:275–277.

43. Kurzyna M, Dabrowski M, Bielecki D, et al. Atrial septostomy in treatment of end-stage right heart failure in patients with pulmonary hypertension. *Chest.* 2007;131:977–983.

44. Moscucci M, Dairywala IT, Chetcuti S, et al. Balloon atrial septostomy in end-stage pulmonary hypertension guided by a novel intracardiac echocardiographic transducer. *Catheter Cardiovasc Interv.* 2001;52:530–534.

45. Buchbinder WC, Katz LN. Intraventricular pressure curves of the human heart obtained by direct transthoracic puncture. *Proc Soc Exp Biol Med.* 1949;71:673–675.

46. Walther T, Simon P, Dewey T, et al. Transapical minimally invasive aortic valve implantation: multicenter experience. *Circulation.* 2007;116: I240–I245.

47. Vignola PA, Swaye PS, Gosselin AJ. Safe transthoracic left ventricular puncture performed with echocardiographic guidance. *Cathet Cardiovasc Diagn.* 1980;6:317–324.

48. Pawelec-Wojtalik M, von Segesser LK, Liang M, et al. Closure of left ventricle perforation with the use of muscular VSD occluder. *Eur J Cardiothorac Surg.* 2005;27:714–716.

49. Havranek EP, Sherry PD. Left heart catheterization by direct puncture with two-dimensional echocardiographic guidance: a case report. *Cathet Cardiovasc Diagn.* 1995;35:358–361.

50. Masson JB, Kovac J, Schuler G, et al. Transcatheter aortic valve implantation: review of the nature, management, and avoidance of procedural complications. *JACC Cardiovasc Interv.* 2009; 2:811–820.

51. Webb JG, Altwegg L, Boone RH, et al. Transcatheter aortic valve implantation: impact on clinical and valve-related outcomes. *Circulation.* 2009;119:3009–3016.

52. Turgut T, Deeb M, Moscucci M. Left ventricular apical puncture: a procedure surviving well in the new millennium. *Catheter Cardiovasc Interv.* 2000;49:68–73.

53. Morgan JM, Gray HH, Gelder C, et al. Left heart catheterization by direct ventricular puncture: withstanding the test of time. *Cathet Cardiovasc Diagn.* 1989;16:87–90.

20 Valvuloplasty

MICHAEL S. KIM AND JOHN D. CARROLL

Since being performed to treat congenital pulmonary valve stenosis in 1979 (1), percutaneous balloon valvuloplasty (PBV) has emerged as a mainstay for the treatment of congenital aortic and pulmonic valve stenosis and of rheumatic mitral stenosis (MS). Although surgical valve replacement is likely to remain the standard of care for the foreseeable future for most patients with symptomatic valvular heart disease, with the advent of newer valve replacement therapies and in the evolving era of novel stent-mounted replacement valves for patients with aortic and pulmonic valve disease, PBV has enjoyed a clinical renaissance in interventional cardiology. In addition, despite the eradication of rheumatic fever in developed countries, rheumatic heart disease (specifically rheumatic MS) remains an important valvular pathology not only in developing countries but also in developed cultures where immigration is prominent. Although PBV currently remains as a relative niche among only a subgroup of structural cardiologists who possess the training and skills needed to integrate their knowledge of valve pathology with both two-dimensional (2D) and novel three-dimensional (3D) imaging modalities, the reality remains that within the next decade, PBV may extend beyond being a niche procedure being performed by the selective few to one being performed by the masses. As the incidence of PBV being performed worldwide continues to rise, knowledge of the potential complications that may arise during these specialized procedures must be disseminated to maximize both patient safety and clinical outcomes.

Balloon valvuloplasty of aortic, mitral, and pulmonic valves and the potential complications of each procedure are discussed in the following sections. Tricuspid valvuloplasty at the present time, however, is rarely performed and thus is not discussed.

■ PERCUTANEOUS AORTIC BALLOON VALVULOPLASTY

The etiology of aortic stenosis may be congenital, rheumatic, or calcific/degenerative. While the incidence of congenital aortic stenosis has remained relatively stable and that of rheumatic aortic stenosis continues to decline, the incidence of calcific aortic stenosis continues to rise. In fact, recent data suggest that calcific aortic stenosis affects up to 4% of adults older than 65 years in the United States alone (2–4). Although surgical aortic valve replacement remains the mainstay therapy, the procedure is associated with high mortality, with in-hospital death rates approaching 9% to 13% in patients older than 65 years. Furthermore, a recent study reported that nearly 33% of patients older than 75 years with severe aortic stenosis were deemed too high-risk for surgical valve replacement and were subsequently left untreated (5,6).

First described in 1985 by Cribier (7), percutaneous aortic balloon valvuloplasty (PABV) offered a nonsurgical option in managing unstable and critically ill patients with aortic stenosis and refractory heart failure or cardiogenic shock. Relatively high complication (20% to 25% acute complication rate within 24 hours of PABV) and restenosis rates (approximately 80% at 1 year) (8–11), however, limited the use of PABV in patients who were deemed acceptable candidates for surgical aortic valve replacement (3). Instead, PABV was offered to patients in whom surgical valve replacement could not be performed secondary to serious comorbid conditions or for use as a bridge to definitive surgical valve replacement and in younger patients with noncalcific aortic valve stenosis. In the era of novel stent-mounted aortic valve replacements, however, the incidence of PABV procedures continues to grow (i.e., as the initial first step in "preparing" the calcific valve for the stent implant) as patients once thought to have no

TABLE 20-1 Reported Procedural and Acute Complications of Percutaneous Aortic Balloon Valvuloplasty[a]

Complication	Rate, %
Death	3
Hemodynamic: **prolonged hypotension, cardiopulmonary resuscitation, pulmonary edema, cardiac tamponade, intra-aortic balloon pump use,** acute valvular insufficiency, cardiogenic shock	1–8
Neurologic: vasovagal reaction, seizure, transient loss of consciousness, **focal neurologic event**	0.6–5
Respiratory: intubation	4
Arrhythmia: persistent bundle branch block, **atrioventricular (AV) block requiring pacing,** ventricular fibrillation (VF) or ventricular tachycardia (VT) requiring defibrillation	3–5 (*10% required treatment*)
Vascular: significant hematoma, surgical vascular repair, systemic embolic event	2–7 (*20% required transfusion*)
Ischemic: prolonged angina, acute myocardial infarction	1
Balloon rupture	17
Other: fever, pulmonary artery perforation, emergency PCI, cardiac surgery, acute tubular necrosis, transient confusion, pneumonia, nonsustained ventricular tachycardia, gastrointestinal bleeding	0.3–1
Patients with any severe complication	25

[a]Bold indicates a severe complication.
(Adapted from Percutaneous balloon aortic valvuloplasty: acute and 30-day follow-up results in 674 patients from the NHLBI Balloon Valvuloplasty Registry. *Circulation.* 1991;84:2383–2397.)

therapeutic hope can now be offered a viable invasive treatment alternative.

Potential Complications of PABV

A comprehensive list of potential complications and a detailed explanation of the most common complications encountered in PABV are shown in Tables 20-1 and 20-2, respectively. Based on procedural data reported in the National Heart Lung and Blood Institute (NHLBI) Registry and the Mansfield Scientific Aortic Valvuloplasty Registry, the most com-

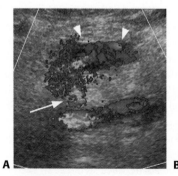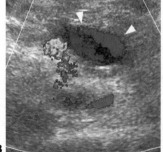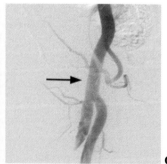

A   **B**   **C**

FIGURE 20-1. Common femoral artery (CFA) pseudoaneurysm formation following percutaneous aortic balloon valvuloplasty. (**A**) Vascular ultrasound demonstrating a large CFA pseudoaneurysm (*arrowhead*) and connecting neck (*arrow*). (**B**) Vascular ultrasound illustrating the "Yin and Yang" sign (*arrowheads*) indicating swirling blood flow within the pseudoaneurysm. (**C**) Digital subtraction angiography of the right CFA following pseudoaneurysm repair with thrombin injection demonstrating no evidence of a residual pseudoaneurysm (*arrow* indicates original arteriotomy site). (See color insert.)

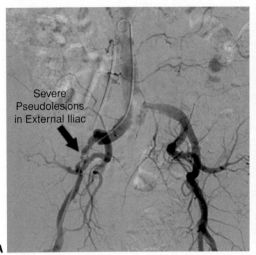
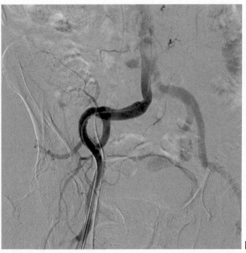

A Severe Pseudolesions in External Iliac

B

FIGURE 20-2. Digital subtraction angiography showing iliac tortuosity in a patient undergoing percutaneous aortic balloon valvuloplasty. (**A**) Development of severe pseudolesions from a rigid catheter. (**B**) Resolution of pseudolesions with placement of a more flexible catheter.

mon acute complication of PABV is trauma at the vascular entry site (Fig. 20-1) resulting in either blood loss necessitating transfusion (up to 23% of cases) or surgical vascular repair (5%–8% of cases) (8,11,12). The elevated risk of vascular injury, however, is somewhat expected given the advanced age of most patients undergoing PABV, preexisting peripheral arterial disease (Figs. 20-2 and 20-3), and the large diameter balloons and sheaths (12F–14F) inserted into the femoral artery during the procedure. Although some newer balloon technologies allow for smaller (i.e., 10F) sheath sizes, the risk of vascular injury remains palpable. More contemporary studies (13–15) have demonstrated reduced vascular complication rates (0%–9%) and mortality (<3%) in patients undergoing PABV, however, suggesting that improved imaging modalities and the use of suture-mediated closure devices may play a major role in improving the clinical outcomes of patients undergoing PABV.

Other severe complications, with relatively low reported incidences (<5% risk based on registry data), include embolic events from showering of calcific debris from either the aortic valve or aorta, myocardial infarction, ventricular arrhythmias requiring therapy, persistent hypotension or cardiogenic shock from ineffective or excessive balloon dilations, vasovagal reactions and persistent hypoten-

sion resulting from rapid ventricular pacing, and ventricular perforation leading to tamponade. Despite the preexisting comorbid conditions of patients undergoing PABV, the overall reported mortality from the procedure remains low (3%–5%).

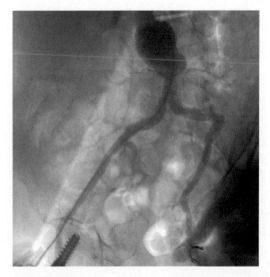

FIGURE 20-3. Aortography in an elderly woman with severe aortic stenosis. An abdominal aortic aneurysm, bilateral ostial iliac narrowing, and a relatively small diameter of the iliofemoral conduit are all risk factors for vascular complications from percutaneous aortic balloon valvuloplasty.

TABLE 20-2 Complications of Percutaneous Aortic Balloon Valvuloplasty

Complication	Cause	Prevention	Recognition	Treatment
Death	*Intraprocedure:* • Cardiogenic shock from acute LV decompensation • Intractable ventricular fibrillation • Major vascular-related hemorrhage • Tamponade from perforation *Postprocedure:* • Sequelae of vascular complication	• Prevent or immediately treat vasovagal episodes • Inflations must be rapid but effective with withdrawal of balloon catheter into aorta as soon as possible • Have defibrillation pads placed on everyone? • Meticulous attention to keeping straight wires and catheters out of apex	Continuous monitoring of hemodynamic state and rhythm	Per specific cause
Aortic dissection	Balloon inflation mediated	Do not oversize balloons	Chest pain, aortography/ultrasound	Depends on location, degree, candidacy for surgery, availability of stent graft
Aortic regurgitation	Balloon inflation mediated	Do not oversize balloon	Acute elevation of left ventricular end diastolic pressure (LVEDP), fall in aortic systolic pressure, and aortography/ultrasound	• Depends on severity and candidacy for surgery • Nitroprusside
Left bundle branch block (LBBB)	Balloon inflation mediated	Probably cannot prevent but being aware of preexisting right bundle branch block (RBBB) is key	LBBB on monitor or complete heart block with preexisting RBBB	• If only LBBB, no treatment necessary • If complete heart block, then temporary followed by permanent pacemaker
Iliofemoral dissection and/or occlusion	Large sheath size or wire trauma	• Assess vascular entry sites and use best side • Consider anterograde (i.e., transseptal) approach in those with severe peripheral vascular disease (PVD)	Loss of pulses	• Angiography to ascertain location and cause to direct treatment • Expertise in vascular intervention should be available
Femoral artery hemorrhage	Large sheath, failed closure, torn femoral artery	• Assess vascular entry sites and use best side • Predeployment of suture-based closure • Meticulous attention to careful vascular technique and avoiding trauma	Hematoma	Compression, reversal of anti-coagulation, assessment by angiography/ultrasound if persists
Stroke	• Atheroembolism from catheter trauma • Thromboembolism from equipment	Anticoagulation, minimize manipulations in arch, identify those with shaggy aortas, and consider anterograde approach.	Neurological findings	Immediate CTA to rule out intracranial hemorrhage and then treatment dictated by cause and availability of neurointerventional resources

CTA, computed tomography angiography.

TABLE 20-3   **Wilkins Echocardiographic Score**[a]

Grade	Mobility	Subvalvular Thickening	Thickening	Calcification
1	Highly mobile valve with only leaflet tip restriction	Minimal thickening just below the leaflets	Leaflets near normal thickness (4–5 mm)	Single area of calcification
2	Normal mobility of mid and base leaflet segments	Thickening of chordal structures extending up to 1/3 of chordal length	Mid leaflets normal; moderate to severe thickening (5–8 mm) of leaflet margins	Scattered areas of calcification confined to leaflet margins
3	Valve moves forward in diastole, mainly from the base	Thickening extends to distal 1/3 of chords	Moderate to severe thickening (5–8 mm) of the entire leaflet	Calcification extends to mid leaflets
4	No or minimal forward movement during diastole	Extensive thickening and shortening of all chordal structures extending to papillary muscles	Severe thickening (>8–10 mm) of the entire leaflet	Extensive calcification throughout leaflets

(Adapted with permission from Wilkins GT, Weyman AE, Abascal VM, Block PC, Palacios IF. Percutaneous balloon dilatation of the mitral valve: an analysis of echocardiographic variables related to outcome and the mechanism of dilatation. *Br Heart J.* 1988;60:299–308. [a]Wilkins score >9 predictive of suboptimal results from percutaneous mitral balloon valvuloplasty.)

■ PERCUTANEOUS MITRAL BALLOON VALVULOPLASTY

MS typically manifests clinically during adulthood and is most commonly a consequence of childhood rheumatic carditis (occurring in 60%–90% of cases of rheumatic fever). Although the incidence of rheumatic MS remains highest in both developing countries and the South Pacific (16), immigration to the United States and other industrialized countries has brought with it a resurgence of patients suffering from rheumatic MS in developed countries (17).

In the last three decades, the invasive treatment of MS has dramatically evolved, first with the introduction of percutaneous mitral balloon valvuloplasty (PMBV) in the mid 1980s (18,19), and subsequently with the Food and Drug Administration–approval of PMBV using the Inoue balloon catheter in 1994. Since then, PMBV has proven to be a safe and cost-effective means by which to provide symptomatic and hemodynamic relief in patients suffering from severe MS. While the immediate results of PMBV are favorable, often with near doubling of the critically stenotic valve area, the long-term results of PMBV heavily depend on several factors including, but not limited to, baseline patient characteristics, Wilkins echocardiographic score (20) (Table 20-3), and New York Heart Association functional class (21–24).

Potential Complications of PMBV

A comprehensive list of both minor and major complications of PMBV is shown is Table 20-4 (25) and detailed descriptions of the most common serious complications during PMBV is given in Table 20-5. The majority of complications relevant to PMBV are intraprocedural and are related to transseptal catheterization, manipulation of the Inoue balloon catheter in the left atrium, or commissurotomy of the mitral valve (16). One of the most common complications of transseptal puncture is penetration of the needle into an adjacent, nonatrial space (i.e., ascending aorta, posterior atrial pericardial space) (Figs. 20-4 and 20-5). In the era of advanced 2D and 3D imaging to guide transseptal catheterization (Figs. 20-6 and 20-7), however, the overall risk of unintended needle penetration into an adjoining space remains low. Nonetheless, when it occurs, hemodynamically significant hemopericardium or rupture into the space surrounding the aortic root may develop in up to 2% of cases, necessitating emergent pericardiocentesis (Fig. 20-8) and immediate reversal of anticoagulation with protamine sulfate to promote hemostasis.

Minor Procedural Complication	Rate, %
Hemodynamic: prolonged hypotension, pericardial effusion requiring pericardiocentesis, cardiopulmonary resuscitation, intra-aortic balloon pump use	0.9–6.7
Neurologic: vasovagal reaction, seizure	2.5–6.9
Respiratory: intubation	3.8
Arrhythmia: persistent bundle branch block, AV block requiring pacing, VF or VT requiring defibrillation	0.5–1 (*9.6% required treatment*)
Vascular: significant hematoma, surgical vascular repair	0.4–0.5 (*8.5% required transfusion*)
Ischemic: prolonged angina, acute myocardial infarction	0.1–0.5
Balloon rupture	0.4 (*with sequelae*) 4.5 (*without sequelae*)
Other: left-to-right shunt, drug reaction, acute tubular necrosis	0.1–9.9

Major Procedural Complication	Rate, %
Death	1
Hemodynamic: emergency cardiac surgery, cardiac perforation, cardiac tamponade, acute MR, pulmonary edema, cardiogenic shock	1–4
Neurologic: cerebrovascular accident	2
Respiratory: pulmonary embolus	0.1
Ischemic: myocardial infarction	0.5

In-Hospital Complication > 24 Hours Postprocedure	Rate, %
Death	1.6
Hemodynamic: cardiac decompensation requiring surgery, cardiogenic shock, cardiac tamponade	0–1.6
Neurologic: cerebrovascular accident	0.4
Vascular: systemic thromboembolic event, pulmonary embolus, vascular injury requiring surgery, amputation	0.1–0.7 (*0.5% required transfusion*)
Ischemic: myocardial infarction	0.4
Other: acute tubular necrosis	0.3

MR, mitral regurgitation; AV, atrioventricular; VF, ventricular fibrillation; VT, ventricular tachycardia.
(Adapted from complications and mortality of percutaneous balloon mitral commissurotomy. A report from the National Heart, Lung, and Blood Institute Balloon Valvuloplasty Registry. *Circulation.* 1992;85:2014–2024.)

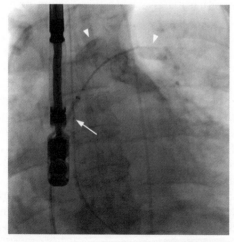

FIGURE 20-4. Anteriorly directed transseptal puncture and advancement of the transseptal sheath (*arrow*) into the pulmonary artery (*arrowheads*).

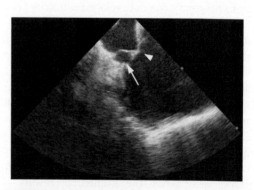

FIGURE 20-5. Presence of tenting (*arrowhead*) from the transseptal sheath and dilator against the interatrial septum immediately adjacent to the coronary sinus (*arrow*). The transseptal device was repositioned using echocardiographic and fluoroscopic guidance, and the patient underwent successful and uncomplicated transseptal catheterization.

TABLE 20-5 Complications of Percutaneous Mitral Balloon Valvuloplasty

Complication	Cause	Prevention	Recognition	Treatment
Severe mitral regurgitation (MR)	Typically tearing of leaflet	• Stepwise inflation of Inoue balloon • Avoidance of catheter entrapment in chordal apparatus • Proper alignment of catheter to valve • Exclude patients with baseline moderate MR	• Acute increase in left atrial (LA) pressure with large regurgitant wave and fall in system pressure association with echo/Doppler signs of severe MR • Consider left ventriculogram	Immediate treatment with nitroprusside followed by intraaortic balloon pump (IABP) and emergency mitral valve replacement (MVR) if hemodynamically compromised
Cardiac tamponade	Transseptal puncture improperly placed	• Experience with transseptal technique • Echocardiographic guidance	Acute drop on blood pressure, vasovagal, appearance of pericardial effusion, rise in right atrial (RA) pressure, loss of pulsations of cardiac silhouette, pericardial pain	• Pericardiocentesis with placement of catheter drain • Reversal of anticoagulation • Consideration of surgery if catheter drain can not be placed or persistent high volume of blood drainage from catheter
Systemic embolism	Dislodgment of thrombus from left atrium vs. formation of thrombus on equipment	• Full anticoagulation while in left atrium • Good catheter technique with flushing and avoidance of catheter tip against LA wall • Preprocedure transesophageal echocardiography (TEE) to exclude left atrial appendage (LAA) thrombus	Acute change in neurologic status, acute limb ischemia, acute abdominal pain	Immediate assessment for other causes of clinical status change, immediate consultation with stroke team to consider catheter-based diagnosis and treatment of stroke
Atrial fibrillation	Catheter induced premature atrial contractions in atrial fibrillation–prone patient	• Careful catheter technique • Maintain persistent medical treatment the day of the procedure	ECG rhythm change. Rapid ventricular rhythm in mitral stenosis may cause acute hemodynamic collapse	Rate control vs. immediate cardioversion depending on clinical state
Atrial septal defect	Transseptal procedure combined with excessive catheter manipulation, inadvertent withdraw of unslenderized Inoue catheter or thin fragile septal tissue	• Careful technique • Identification of patients with thin septal tissue. • Placement of transseptal puncture at appropriate site	• Immediate Doppler assessment of septal after removal of Inoue catheter • Hypoexemia may immediately occur when right/left atrial pressure gradient results in right to left shunting	• Follow-up with serial echocardiographic assessment with most atrial septal defects (ASD) closing by 6 months. • Percutaneous ASD device closure if defect appears too large to close spontaneously or right-to-left shunting occurs with hypoxemia.

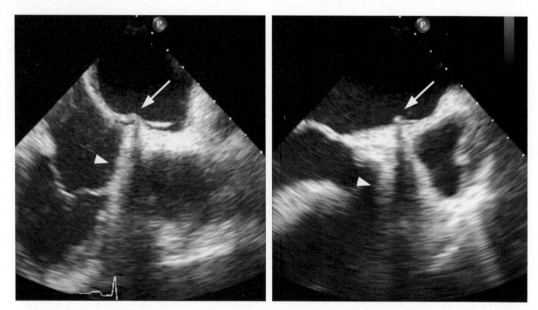

FIGURE 20-6. Two-dimensional transesophageal echocardiogram images illustrating tenting (*arrow*) of the transseptal sheath/dilator (*arrowhead*) near the fossa ovalis in two, simultaneously displayed orthogonal views.

Manipulation of the Inoue balloon catheter within the left atrium may result in perforation of the left atrial appendage, pulmonary veins, or left ventricular apex (4% of cases based on NHLBI registry data). Although very rare, such complications may also result in hemodynamically significant and potentially life-threatening hemopericardium as described earlier. Furthermore, embolic events (2% of cases) may occur, as undetected microthrombi in the left atrium or left atrial appendage (Fig. 20-9) are dislodged during either catheter or wire manipulation in the left atrium.

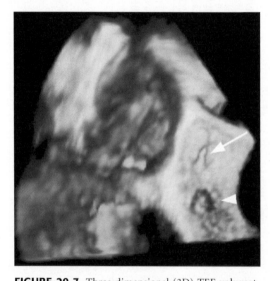

FIGURE 20-7. Three-dimensional (3D) TEE volumetric reconstruction demonstrating tenting of the transseptal sheath/dilator (*arrow*) superior to the fossa ovalis (*arrowhead*). The transseptal device was subsequently repositioned against the fossa ovalis using 3D TEE guidance, and the patient underwent successful and uncomplicated transseptal catheterization. (See color insert.)

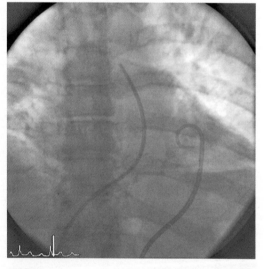

FIGURE 20-8. Percutaneous mitral balloon valvuloplasty complicated by cardiac tamponade necessitating emergent pericardiocentesis and placement of a pericardial drain.

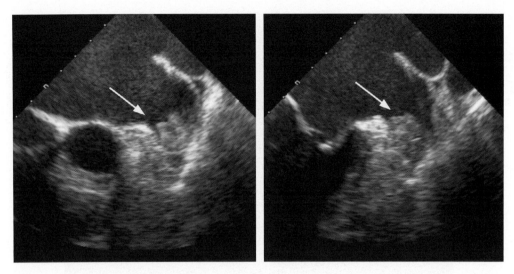

FIGURE 20-9. Pre–percutaneous mitral balloon valvuloplasty transesophageal echocardiogram demonstrating a large left atrial thrombus (*arrow*).

Perhaps, the most serious complication of PMBV is resultant severe mitral regurgitation (MR). In most cases, severe MR following balloon inflation typically results from tearing or shearing of the mitral valve leaflets (Fig. 20-10). Severe acute MR (Fig. 20-11) remains a relatively uncommon complication with reported incidences of 1.4% to 9.4% (and approximately 3% by NHLBI registry data), and fortunately only a small percentage of such patients (<4%) require emergent cardiac surgery with mitral valve replacement.

Finally, creation of a persistent left-to-right shunt at the interatrial septum following Inoue

balloon catheter removal occurs in up to 10% of cases (Fig. 20-12). The presence of a thin interatrial septum at baseline (Fig. 20-13) likely increases the risk of residual septal defect following Inoue balloon removal. Fortunately, the majority (≥90%) of residual defects are usually small, are not hemodynamically significant, and spontaneously close after several months. In rare instances, a residual right-to-left shunt may occur following Inoue balloon catheter removal and typically will occur in patients with underlying elevated right heart filling pressure due to pulmonary hypertension or cor pulmonale (Fig. 20-14A). In such instances, profound desaturation often excludes the option of waiting for spontaneous closure, thereby necessitating defect repair with a commercially available closure device (Fig. 20-14B).

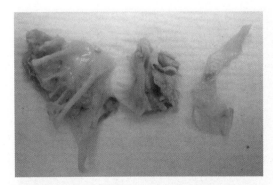

FIGURE 20-10. Surgically removed specimen of a sheared and torn rheumatic mitral valve from a patient who underwent percutaneous mitral balloon valvuloplasty complicated by severe mitral regurgitation necessitating emergent surgical valve replacement.

■ PERCUTANEOUS PULMONIC BALLOON VALVULOPLASTY

Congenital pulmonic stenosis (PS) accounts for up to 9% of all congenital heart defects. While in the past, surgical valvotomy was the preferred treatment, more recently, percutaneous pulmonic balloon valvuloplasty (PPBV), first described in the 1950s (26) and then again in 1979 (1), has emerged as the first option in the management of most cases of congenital PS (27). PPBV is primarily employed in children with congenital PS, although while infrequently employed in

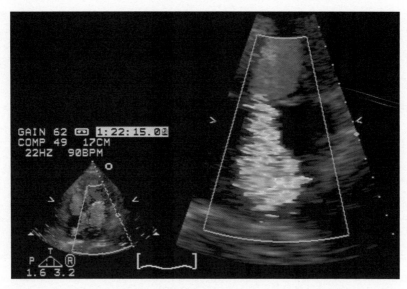

FIGURE 20-11. Percutaneous mitral balloon valvuloplasty complicated by the development of severe eccentric mitral regurgitation. Given the absence of immediate hemodynamic compromise, the patient underwent elective surgical valve replacement 1 week postprocedure. (See color insert.)

adults, it remains the treatment of choice for adult patients suffering from PS with impressive immediate- and mid-term clinical results (28–31). Long-term follow-up of patients undergoing PPBV remains scarce, although does suggest a low (1%–2%) late recurrence of PS or development of hemodynamically significant pulmonary insufficiency (PI) and need for subsequent surgical therapy (5%) (27,32).

Potential Complications of PPBV

A comprehensive list of potential complications is shown in Table 20-6. Overall, PPBV remains a remarkably safe procedure, with reported death and major complications rates of 0.24% and 0.35%, respectively (33). The most common minor complications include transient hypotension, bradycardia, and premature ventricular contractions during balloon inflation. Utilization of both a double balloon technique and shorter durations of balloon inflations successfully mitigate these adverse effects. Blood loss requiring transfusion and/or femoral venous occlusion at follow-up have also been reported but have been dramatically reduced in the era of improved catheter systems and sheaths.

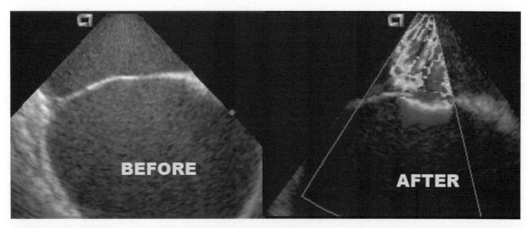

FIGURE 20-12. Intracardiac echocardiography showing residual atrial septal defect with predominant left-to-right shunting following removal of the Inoue balloon catheter.

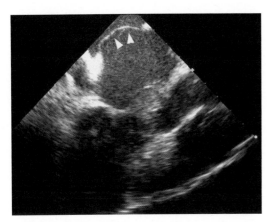

FIGURE 20-13. Thin interatrial septum (*arrowhead*) that likely increases the risk of forming a persistent atrial septal defect following Inoue balloon catheter removal.

The development of severe infundibular obstruction and hemodynamically significant PI are perhaps the two most common long-term complications of PPBV, both of which may ultimately require surgical intervention. Infundibular gradients have been reported to occur in up to 30% of patients who have undergone PPBV (34). Advanced age (likely due to long-standing right ventricular hypertrophy) and a higher severity of PS correlate with a higher likelihood of patients developing subsequent infundibular obstruction (35). Typically, when the infundibular gradient is in excess of 50 mmHg, therapy with oral β-blockers is recommended and, in the vast majority of cases, the obstruction

TABLE 20-6	Reported Complications of Percutaneous Pulmonic Balloon Valvuloplasty

Death

Vascular
    Blood loss requiring transfusion
    Femoral venous occlusion or stenosis

Neurologic
    Seizure
    Stroke

Arrhythmia
    Transient bradycardia
    Transient or permanent heart block
    Transient prolongation of the QTc
    PVC, nonsustained, or sustained ventricular
      arrhythmia
    Complete right bundle branch block

Hemodynamic
    Transient hypotension
    Severe infundibular obstruction
    Severe pulmonic insufficiency

Mechanical
    Tricuspid valve papillary muscle rupture
    Tear of the pulmonary artery

regresses dramatically over time, thereby avoiding the need for surgical intervention (34).

As many as 90% of patients undergoing PPBV will be noted to have some degree of PI at follow-up, with the majority being in the range of mild to moderate. In these cases, right ventricular

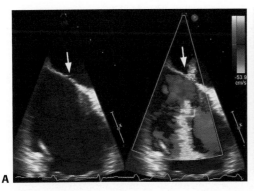
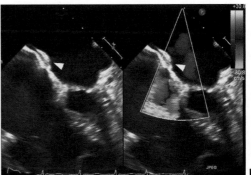

FIGURE 20-14. Percutaneous mitral balloon valvuloplasty complicated by the formation of a small atrial septal defect with right-to-left shunting. (**A**) Two-dimensional TEE demonstrating a small atrial septal defect with predominant right-to-left shunting (*arrow*) associated with profound, irreversible hypoxemia postprocedure. (**B**) Successful closure of the defect with a 6-mm Amplatzer Septal Occluder (AGA Medical Corporation, Plymouth, Minnesota) device (*arrowhead*) and resolution of the right-to-left shunt and systemic desaturation. (See color insert.)

volume overload necessitating surgical intervention rarely, if ever occurs (36). The development of severe PI, however, has been noted in up to 17% of patients at late follow-up and has been correlated to the following factors: young age, high degrees of obstruction, large balloon:annulus ratio, use of noncompliant balloons, and low postdilation peak-to-peak systolic pressure gradients (37). Other smaller studies have subsequently supported these findings (38,39).

■ SUMMARY

Since being introduced in the late 1970s, PBV has emerged as a mainstay in the realm of interventional cardiology. While utilized primarily in the invasive treatment of rheumatic MS through the 1980s and 1990s, PBV has experienced a recent renaissance in the treatment of both congenital pulmonic valve stenosis and calcific aortic stenosis with the advent of percutaneous valve replacement therapy. In most areas of the world, PBV remains limited as a niche procedure to a subgroup of structural interventional cardiologists. Yet, in light of the current evolution of structural heart interventions and novel technologies being developed and utilized worldwide, PBV is poised to expand beyond its niche market and become a procedure performed by the masses. As is the case with any specialized procedure on the brink of widespread adoption, information on the wide array of potential complications that may arise during these unique procedures must be disseminated in order to maximize both patient safety and clinical outcomes.

References

1. Semb BK, Tjonneland S, Stake G, Aabyholm G. "Balloon valvulotomy" of congenital pulmonary valve stenosis with tricuspid valve insufficiency. *Cardiovasc Radiol.* 1979;2:239–241.

2. Bonow RO, Carabello BA, Chatterjee K, et al. 2008 Focused update incorporated into the ACC/AHA 2006 guidelines for the management of patients with valvular heart disease: a report of the American College of Cardiology/American Heart Association Task Force on Practice Guidelines (Writing Committee to Revise the 1998 Guidelines for the Management of Patients With Valvular Heart Disease): endorsed by the Society of Cardiovascular Anesthesiologists, Society for Cardiovascular Angiography and Interventions, and Society of Thoracic Surgeons. *Circulation.* 2008;118:e523–e661.

3. Bonow RO, Carabello BA, Kanu C, et al. ACC/AHA 2006 guidelines for the management of patients with valvular heart disease: a report of the American College of Cardiology/American Heart Association Task Force on Practice Guidelines (writing committee to revise the 1998 Guidelines for the Management of Patients With Valvular Heart Disease): developed in collaboration with the Society of Cardiovascular Anesthesiologists: endorsed by the Society for Cardiovascular Angiography and Interventions and the Society of Thoracic Surgeons. *Circulation.* 2006;114:e84–e231.

4. Freeman RV, Otto CM. Spectrum of calcific aortic valve disease: pathogenesis, disease progression, and treatment strategies. *Circulation.* 2005; 111:3316–3326.

5. Iung B, Cachier A, Baron G, et al. Decision-making in elderly patients with severe aortic stenosis: why are so many denied surgery? *Eur Heart J.* 2005;26:2714–2720.

6. Singh IM, Shishehbor MH, Christofferson RD, Tuzcu EM, Kapadia SR. Percutaneous treatment of aortic valve stenosis. *Cleve Clin J Med.* 2008; 75:805–812.

7. Cribier A, Savin T, Saoudi N, Rocha P, Berland J, Letac B. Percutaneous transluminal valvuloplasty of acquired aortic stenosis in elderly patients: an alternative to valve replacement? *Lancet.* 1986; 1:63–67.

8. Percutaneous balloon aortic valvuloplasty: acute and 30-day follow-up results in 674 patients from the NHLBI Balloon Valvuloplasty Registry. *Circulation.* 1991;84:2383–2397.

9. Hara H, Pedersen WR, Ladich E, et al. Percutaneous balloon aortic valvuloplasty revisited: time for a renaissance? *Circulation.* 2007;115:e334–e338.

10. Jabbour RJ, Dick R, Walton AS. Aortic balloon valvuloplasty—review and case series. *Heart Lung Circ.* 2008;17(suppl 4):S73–S81.

11. McKay RG. The Mansfield Scientific Aortic Valvuloplasty Registry: overview of acute hemodynamic results and procedural complications. *J Am Coll Cardiol.* 1991;17:485–491.

12. Feldman T. Core curriculum for interventional cardiology: percutaneous valvuloplasty. *Catheter Cardiovasc Interv.* 2003;60:48–56.

13. O'Keefe JH Jr, Vlietstra RE, Bailey KR, Holmes DR Jr. Natural history of candidates for balloon aortic valvuloplasty. *Mayo Clin Proc.* 1987;62:986–991.

14. Eltchaninoff H, Cribier A, Tron C, et al. Balloon aortic valvuloplasty in elderly patients at high risk for surgery, or inoperable: immediate and mid-term results. *Eur Heart J.* 1995;16:1079–1084.

15. Shareghi S, Rasouli L, Shavelle DM, Burstein S, Matthews RV. Current results of balloon aortic valvuloplasty in high-risk patients. *J Invasive Cardiol.* 2007;19:1–5.

16. Nobuyoshi M, Arita T, Shirai S, et al. Percutaneous balloon mitral valvuloplasty: a review. *Circulation.* 2009;119:e211–e219.

17. Carroll JD, Feldman T. Percutaneous mitral balloon valvotomy and the new demographics of mitral stenosis. *JAMA.* 1993;270:1731–1736.

18. Inoue K, Owaki T, Nakamura T, Kitamura F, Miyamoto N. Clinical application of transvenous mitral commissurotomy by a new balloon catheter. *J Thorac Cardiovasc Surg.* 1984;87:394–402.

19. Lock JE, Khalilullah M, Shrivastava S, Bahl V, Keane JF. Percutaneous catheter commissurotomy in rheumatic mitral stenosis. *N Engl J Med.* 1985;313:1515–1518.

20. Wilkins GT, Weyman AE, Abascal VM, Block PC, Palacios IF. Percutaneous balloon dilatation of the mitral valve: an analysis of echocardiographic variables related to outcome and the mechanism of dilatation. *Br Heart J.* 1988;60:299–308.

21. Palacios IF, Block PC, Wilkins GT, Weyman AE. Follow-up of patients undergoing percutaneous mitral balloon valvotomy: analysis of factors determining restenosis. *Circulation.* 1989;79:573–579.

22. Ben-Farhat M, Betbout F, Gamra H, et al. Predictors of long-term event-free survival and of freedom from restenosis after percutaneous balloon mitral commissurotomy. *Am Heart J.* 2001;142:1072–1079.

23. Palacios IF, Sanchez PL, Harrell LC, Weyman AE, Block PC. Which patients benefit from percutaneous mitral balloon valvuloplasty? Prevalvuloplasty and postvalvuloplasty variables that predict long-term outcome. *Circulation.* 2002;105:1465–1471.

24. Cohen DJ, Kuntz RE, Gordon SP, et al. Predictors of long-term outcome after percutaneous balloon mitral valvuloplasty. *N Engl J Med.* 1992; 327:1329–1335.

25. Complications and mortality of percutaneous balloon mitral commissurotomy. a report from the National Heart, Lung, and Blood Institute Balloon Valvuloplasty Registry. *Circulation.* 1992; 85:2014–2024.

26. Rubio-Alvarez V Lason RL, Soni J. Valvulotomias intracardiacas por medio de un cateter. *Arch Inst Cardiol Mex.* 1952;23:183–192.

27. Rao PS. Percutaneous balloon pulmonary valvuloplasty: state of the art. *Catheter Cardiovasc Interv.* 2007;69:747–763.

28. Rao PS. Influence of balloon size on short-term and long-term results of balloon pulmonary valvuloplasty. *Tex Heart Inst J.* 1987;14:57–61.

29. Rao PS. Indications for balloon pulmonary valvuloplasty. *Am Heart J.* 1988;116:1661–1662.

30. Rao PS. Balloon pulmonary valvuloplasty: a review. *Clin Cardiol.* 1989;12:55–74.

31. Rao PS. Right ventricular filling following balloon pulmonary valvuloplasty. *Am Heart J.* 1992; 123:1084–1086.

32. Rao PS, Fawzy ME, Solymar L, Mardini MK. Long-term results of balloon pulmonary valvuloplasty of valvar pulmonic stenosis. *Am Heart J.* 1988;115:1291–1296.

33. Stanger P, Cassidy SC, Girod DA, Kan JS, Lababidi Z, Shapiro SR. Balloon pulmonary valvuloplasty: results of the Valvuloplasty and Angioplasty of Congenital Anomalies Registry. *Am J Cardiol.* 1990;65:775–783.

34. Fontes VF, Esteves CA, Sousa JE, Silva MV, Bembom MC. Regression of infundibular hypertrophy after pulmonary valvuloplasty for pulmonic stenosis. *Am J Cardiol.* 1988;62:977–979.

35. Thapar MK, Rao PS. Significance of infundibular obstruction following balloon valvuloplasty for valvar pulmonic stenosis. *Am Heart J.* 1989;118:99–103.

36. Rao PS, Galal O, Patnana M, Buck SH, Wilson AD. Results of three to 10 year follow up of balloon dilatation of the pulmonary valve. *Heart.* 1998;80:591–595.

37. Berman W Jr, Fripp RR, Raisher BD, Yabek SM. Significant pulmonary valve incompetence following oversize balloon pulmonary valveplasty in small infants: a long-term follow-up study. *Catheter Cardiovasc Interv.* 1999;48:61–65, discussion 66.

38. Abu Haweleh A, Hakim F. Balloon pulmonary valvuloplasty in children: Jordanian experience. *Saudi Heart J.* 2003;15:31–34.

39. Garty Y, Veldtman G, Lee K, Benson L. Late outcomes after pulmonary valve balloon dilatation in neonates, infants and children. *J Invasive Cardiol.* 2005;17:318–322.

21 Balloon Aortic Valvuloplasty and Transcatheter Aortic Valve Implantation

ALAN W. HELDMAN AND WILLIAM W. O'NEILL

I n 1982, Dr. Jean Kan and her team at Johns Hopkins first performed balloon valvuloplasty for congenital pulmonic valve stenosis (1), and Dr. Zuhdi Lababidi and colleagues at the University of Missouri performed balloon valvuloplasty for congenital aortic stenosis (AS) (2). Soon Lababidi described dilating the aortic valve in a series of 23 patients with isolated AS, ages 2 to 17 (3). Using balloons 10 to 20 mm in diameter, the mean baseline gradient of 113 Hg was reduced to 32 mm Hg. Since that time, valvuloplasty expanded beyond congenital lesions to the treatment of acquired mitral and aortic stenosis, and investigators reported technical considerations, challenges, and complications for each advance. As we now know, of course, the dramatic results achieved in pediatric patients would not be equaled in acquired AS until an entirely new class of devices was invented.

The recent advent of transcatheter implantable valve prostheses is now revolutionizing the field again. The implantation of these devices and the management of patients receiving them are substantially more complex than for balloon valvuloplasty. Complications associated with the new devices include all of those seen during the preceding 20 years of valvuloplasty, plus some new and even unexpected issues. In this chapter, we will review the complications of balloon aortic valvuloplasty (BAV) and transcatheter aortic valve implantation (TAVI) in adults with acquired AS.

In 1986, Dr. Alain Cribier and colleagues from Hospital Charles Nicolle in Rouen reported valvuloplasty in adult calcific AS, using 8-, 10-, and 12-mm diameter balloons, with significant reduction of the gradient (4). It was soon recognized that, compared with the congenitally fused valves, where balloon dilation was a major advance with long-lasting benefits, senile calcific AS was rather refractory to balloon valvuloplasty. The reasons were identified early in the history of the endeavor. In 1986, McKay and colleagues at the Beth Israel Hospital, Boston, studied the effects of balloon dilation of calcific AS in postmortem hearts and in intraoperative hearts, identifying two mechanisms of valvuloplasty: (1) fracture of leaflet nodular calcification, and (2) displacement and increased mobility of rigid valve cusps (5).

Efforts followed to improve the dilating efficacy of the balloon. After Dorros described the use of two balloons at once (6), Midei and colleagues at Johns Hopkins compared single- versus double-balloon technique in 21 patients. A maximum single-balloon diameter of 19.4 ± 1.4 mm was selected to match the echocardiographically determined annulus dimension. Twelve patients went on to have double-balloon dilation using two 15- to 20-mm balloons with a combined diameter of 36.3 ± 3.9 mm, or 156 ± 21% oversized compared to the annulus. The valve area increased 28% with the single balloon versus 71% with the double balloon (7). However, despite these efforts to develop technical solutions including double balloons, Trefoil (triple) (8) balloons, and double (9) or triple (10) balloons oversized beyond the annulus, and in distinction from the more amenable congenital valve lesions, the therapeutic gain from dilating calcific AS was generally modest, and marked by a propensity for short- or mid-term restenosis. Robicsek and Harbold photographed intraoperative valves before and after double-balloon dilation, and found minimal or at most moderate increase in the measured orifice of the valve (11). BAV has remained decidedly inferior to surgical aortic valve replacement (AVR), and the intervention does carry significant risk, so that in most centers it is reserved for poor surgical candidates with deteriorating clinical situations, or in an attempt to improve the condition of patients being readied for noncardiac surgery (12,13).

■ VALVULOPLASTY OUTCOMES, PATHOPHYSIOLOGY, AND COMPLICATIONS

As the field of balloon aortic valvuloplasty developed, interventionalists recognized a number of opportunities to investigate cardiac physiology in the beating heart under extreme loading conditions. These pathophysiologic insights in turn can inform clinicians about many of the expected complications of both BAV and TAVI.

One theoretical advantage postulated for the double-balloon technique was that two balloons would be less occlusive of left ventricular (LV) ejection than a single balloon. In swine undergoing single- or double-balloon inflation, left anterior descending (LAD) coronary artery blood flow was 15% of baseline (single balloon) or 64% of baseline (double balloon). Pulmonary blood flow and systemic pressure were similarly less affected by double balloon inflation, and coronary blood flow normalized more quickly with double- (4.8 seconds) than with single (23.2 seconds)-balloon inflation (14). In patients with ventricular hypertrophy and dysfunction, coronary atherosclerosis, and nearly fixed AS, it is not surprising that interventions upon the valve (or even merely crossing the valve with a catheter) can precipitate rapid hemodynamic deterioration with coronary ischemia, myocardial depression, and low cardiac output, from which it may be difficult

to recover. As we will describe, maneuvers to prevent such decompensation are central to the safe performance both of BAV and of TAVI.

The series of clinical trials of BAV can generally be summarized by the finding of significant short-term hemodynamic and clinical benefits, important potential complications, and mid- and long-term survival similar to the untreated disease (15). However, when BAV is used as a bridge to definitive therapy by valve replacement, long-term survival can be achieved. Several large registries collected during the 1980s illustrate the outcomes with BAV; these include a number of single center series, the Mansfield registry, and the subsequent National Heart Lung and Blood Institute (NHLBI) registry. The report of 30-day outcomes from the NHLBI registry indicates declining rate of enrollment over the course of the trial, reflecting "waning enthusiasm for the procedure."

Some fortunate recipients of valvuloplasty do have a medium-term sustained improvement, and in this group, functional status and LV systolic (16) and diastolic (17,18) function may improve significantly. In a carefully done hemodynamic study of 17 patients (19), LV pressure–volume loops and wall stress were studied before, immediately following, and 6 months after BAV. Ejection fraction increased after BAV, mostly as a result of decreased afterload, but at 6 months had largely returned to baseline; the LV changes reflected changing loading conditions, and not intrinsic changes in myocardial performance.

From the various registry series of BAV, the frequency of serious complications was defined (Table 21-1). Twenty-five patients underwent BAV at the Thoraxcenter in 1986 to 1987 (20); procedural mortality was 8%, and 4% suffered a stroke. Vascular access site complications occurred in 28%. At St. Luke's Hospital in Milwaukee during the period 1986 to 1988, 125 cases (using multiple-balloon technique in 95%) had a 10% incidence of in-hospital mortality. The 12-month survival was 62% (21), and in a later report of 149 patients treated with the double-balloon technique, 24-month survival was 52% (22).

The Mansfield registry enrolled 492 patients at 27 centers in 1986 and 1987 (23). The retrograde femoral approach was used in 452, the brachial approach in 30, and the transseptal antegrade approach in 10 cases. From this large series, complications included vascular injuries (11%), moderate or severe increase in aortic regurgitation

TABLE 21-1 Major Complications of Balloon Aortic Valvuloplasty (BAV) in Single Center and Multicenter Registries

	Mortality (%)	Stroke/Embolism (%)	Vascular Complications (%)
Thoraxcenter ($n = 25$)	8	4	28
Milwaukee ($n = 125$)	10	3	4[a]
Mansfield Registry ($n = 492$)	7.5	2.2	11
National Heart Lung and Blood Institute Registry ($n = 674$)	10.2	3	7[a]
Beth Israel Hospital ($n = 170$)	3.5	0	10

[a]Defined as arterial repair.

(2.1%), embolic complications (2.2%), cardiac perforation and tamponade (1.8%), and overall 7.5% in-hospital mortality (24), with higher risk of in-hospital death related to procedural complications, lower initial LV systolic pressure, smaller final valve area, and lower baseline cardiac output.

The 7-month mortality in the Mansfield registry was 23% (25), and 1-year mortality was 36%; 1-year, event-free (of valve replacement or repeat valvuloplasty) survival was 43%. Risk factors associated with mortality included previous myocardial infarction (MI: 2% of survivors vs. 6% of nonsurvivors), and severe LV dysfunction (22% vs. 48%) (26). LV systolic pressure was higher in survivors (208 mm Hg vs. 188 mm Hg), and pulmonary artery pressure was lower in survivors (systolic, mean: 43, 28 mm Hg vs. 54, 36 mm Hg.) Both initial and final cardiac outputs were higher in those who survived. In decreasing order of significance, survival was greater in patients with higher initial LV systolic pressure, absence of coronary artery disease (CAD), higher initial cardiac output, better functional class, lower LVEDP (left ventricular end-diastolic pressure), greater final valve area, younger age, and fewer balloon inflations performed. From these findings, a formula was generated to predict risk of mortality.

Discriminate score = 0.612 + 0.020 (age in years) + 0.023 (LVEDP in mm Hg) + 0.881 (coronary angiography*) + 3.371 (initial NYHA class) + 0.014 (LV systolic pressure in mm Hg) 2 0.782 (postprocedure AVA),

On the basis of this score, ranging from −2.75 to +3.20, risk of death at 1 year could be predicted, with the lowest risk quintile (≤20% mortality) having a score of −0.80 or lower, and the highest risk quintile (≥80% mortality) having a score of 0.96 or higher. Final severity of AS did predict survival. However, more inflations done in an attempt to achieve a greater final valve area was associated with worse survival.

In the Mansfield registry, 6.3% of patients suffered acute catastrophic complications (27), including ventricular perforation (1.8%; seven women and two men) which was fatal in six of nine. The perforations were found at autopsy to involve the base of the lateral free wall. Pericardiocentesis was done in five, and three survived—two with operative repair and one without.

Acute severe aortic regurgitation occurred rarely (four, 0.8%, all women.) Three of four had emergency valve replacement and survived. Cardiac arrest occurred in 13 (2.6%), including cardiogenic shock and refractory ventricular arrhythmias. Fatal stroke occurred in two (0.4%), limb amputation in three (0.6%).

Following the Mansfield registry, the NHLBI Registry enrolled patients during 1987 to 1989, at 24 sites (Table 21-2). For 674 patients undergoing initial aortic valvuloplasty, a single balloon was used in 89%, with 20-mm (53%) and 23-mm (37%) diameter balloons being most common; 18-mm (2%) and 25-mm (5%) balloons were also used (28). Double-balloon technique was used in 11%, and the mean diameter of the pair was 35 ± 4 mm (e.g., 15 mm + 20 mm balloons). Aortic valve area (AVA) increased

---

*where 1 = CAD present; 0 = CAD absent.

TABLE 21-2 Complications of Aortic Valvuloplasty in the National Heart Lung and Blood Institute (NHLBI) Registry (674 Patients)

Deaths[a]	17 (3%)
Number of patients with any severe complication[a]	167 (25%)
Hemodynamic complications	
Prolonged hypotension[a]	51 (8%)
CPR required[a]	26 (4%)
Pulmonary edema[a]	19 (3%)
Cardiac tamponade[a]	10 (1%)
Intra-aortic balloon pump use[a]	11 (2%)
Acute valvular insufficiency[a]	
Aortic	6 (1%)
Mitral	1 (0.1%)
Cardiogenic shock[a]	15 (2%)
Neurologic complications	
Vasovagal reaction	36 (5%)
Seizure[a]	15 (2%)
Transient loss of consciousness	4 (0.6%)
Focal neurological event[a]	13 (2%)
Respiratory complications	
Intubation[a]	28 (4%)
Arrhythmia	
Arrhythmia requiring treatment	64 (10%)
Persisting bundle branch block	34 (5%)
AV block requiring pacing[a]	30 (4%)
VF or VT requiring countershock[a]	18 (3%)
Vascular complications	
Significant hematoma	44 (7%)
Vascular surgery performed[a]	35 (5%)
Systemic embolic event[a]	11 (2%)
Transfusion required	135 (20%)
Ischemic complications	
Prolonged angina	9 (1%)
Acute myocardial infarction[a]	10 (1%)
Other complications	
Protamine reaction	2 (0.3%)
Fever	2 (0.3%)
Pulmonary artery perforation[a]	1 (0.1%)
Balloon rupture	111 (17%)
Emergency PTCA	2 (0.3%)
Cardiac surgery[a]	6 (1%)
Acute tubular necrosis[a]	1 (0.1%)
Transient confusion	1 (0.1%)
Pneumonia	1 (0.1%)
Nonsustained VT	1 (0.1%)
Gastrointestinal bleeding	1 (0.1%)

CPR, cardiopulmonary resuscitation; AV, atrioventricular; VF, ventricular fibrillation; VT, ventricular tachycardia; PTCA, percutaneous transluminal coronary artery angioplasty.

[a]Complications considered severe. Some patients suffered more than one severe complication.

(From Percutaneous balloon aortic valvuloplasty: acute and 30-day follow-up results in 674 patients from the NHLBI Balloon Valvuloplasty Registry. *Circulation*. 1991;84:2383–2397.)

from 0.5 ± 0.2 cm^2 to 0.8 ± 0.3 cm^2. Gain in valve area with a single-balloon (0.32 ± 0.22 cm^2) was not significantly greater than that after a double-balloon procedure (0.26 ± 0.17 cm^2), although double balloon often was used after failure of single-balloon technique, and thus presumably in more refractory cases.

Acute (24 hour) complications in the NHLBI registry were common—at least one acute complication occurred in 57% of subjects, and at least one severe acute complication in 25%. These included in-lab death in 17 (3%), cardiogenic shock in 12, and 1 death each associated with LV perforation, pulmonary artery rupture attributed to a Swan Ganz catheter, arrhythmia, sudden death, and myocardial infarction. Perforation with tamponade and pericardiocentesis was reported in 10 subjects, prolonged hypotension in 8%, and cardiopulmonary resuscitation (CPR) in 4%. Intra-aortic balloon pump (IABP) counterpulsation was used rarely, in only 2% of cases. Acute focal neurologic deficits and other systemic embolization occurred occasionally (2% each). Arrhythmias required treatment in 10%, including atrioventricular block (4%), ventricular tachycardia or ventricular fibrillation (3%). Blood transfusion was frequently used (20%), with significant hematoma developing in 7%, and vascular surgery in 5% (some cases electively operated for sheath removal).

Balloon rupture was common (17%), but caused sequelae in only three patients (0.5%). Severe aortic insufficiency (AI) was rare, occurring in six patients, two of whom died and four went to surgery. Overall, cardiac surgery was performed in 1%. At least one in-hospital complication occurred in 61%, and a significant in-hospital complication in 211 (31%), including in-hospital death (10%).

The hospital length of stay in the NHLBI registry was 12 days. Despite difficult hospitalizations, at discharge, cardiovascular symptoms were improved in 68%, and overall functional status improved in 55%. In 20% there was no improvement in cardiovascular symptoms, and in 33% no improvement in overall functional status. Except for deaths, only two (0.3%) were worse as regards cardiovascular status, and eight (1%) were worse overall.

Twenty three more patients died between discharge and 30 days, resulting in a cumulative 30-day mortality rate of 14%. Predictors of 30-day mortality included history of myocardial infarction, liver disease, BUN (blood urea nitrogen) greater than 30 mg/dL, reduced LV function by echo, cardiac output (CO) less than or equal to 3.0 l/min, baseline AVA of less than or equal to 0.5 cm^2, and pulmonary wedge pressure greater than 20 mm Hg. An especially high-risk group was of those with Class IV heart failure symptoms and systolic blood pressure less than 100 mm Hg; for these patients, 30-day mortality was 49% (odds ratio = 4.4). The need for an antiarrhythmic agent conferred an odds ratio for 30-day mortality of 2.9. An aortic valve gradient greater than 50 mm Hg was associated with lower 30-day mortality (9% vs. 19% for those ?50 mm Hg.) At least one New York Heart Association (NYHA) functional class improvement was gained by 75% at 30 days.

Embolic Complications

In a prospective series of aortic and mitral valvuloplasty at Duke (29), investigators actively surveyed subjects for signs of embolization. Using brain computed tomography and fundoscopy, they recognized that cerebral embolic events could be asymptomatic. Clinical stroke is rare.

Complications Related to the Native Valve

It is rare to cause severe aortic valve insufficiency with BAV, but when it occurs it can be devastating. Two patients of the 73 BAVs reported by the Texas Heart Institute (1986 to 1989) developed acute severe aortic insufficiency (AI) and underwent emergency surgery (30). One had a calcified bicuspid valve with a midline longitudinal tear in the posterior leaflet, extending to but not involving the annulus. The other patient had a calcified tricuspid aortic valve, with perforation and nearly complete avulsion of the left coronary leaflet. In one case from the Brigham and Women's Hospital (31), fatal AI after BAV proved to have been caused by leaflet entrapment by a fractured nodule in the noncoronary cusp, with resulting eversion of the leaflet. This was easily reduced in postmortem examination, suggesting the possibility that some such cases might be treated by catheter manipulation of the cusp. There is also a report of oversized dilation causing transient severe AI that resolved within 24 hrs (32). However, disruption of the annulus related to balloon oversizing is to be feared; aortic rupture from BAV was first described in 1987 by the Emory group (33), after serial dilation with increasing balloon size in a relatively small and heavily calcified aorta. There was rupture below the right and noncoronary cusps, with acute and fatal hemopericardium. After 2 of 100 patients had annulus disruption at St. Luke's Medical Center, Milwaukee, a ratio for the areas of balloon-to-aortic annulus by echo of less than 1.2:1 was recommended (34).

Mitral Valve Complications of Aortic Valvuloplasty

Whether the retrograde or antegrade approach is taken to the aortic valve, it is possible to interfere with the mitral apparatus. Mitral cord rupture has been described causing death after retrograde BAV, where the balloon encountered an aberrant cord crossing below the aortic valve from mitral to the septum (35). Laceration of the mitral anterior leaflet during retrograde aortic valvuloplasty has also been reported by de Ubago, et al. (36), who suggested that in retrospect, balloon entrapment in the chordae tendinae might have been recognized by indentation of the balloon at that level, and that stretching of the chords lacerated the valve. It seems likely, however, that the antegrade approach to aortic valvuloplasty may be more likely to interfere with the mitral valve, particularly related to a guidewire looped in the LV and externalized.

■ EVOLUTION OF TECHNIQUES FOR AORTIC VALVULOPLASTY

The past decades have been characterized by a trend toward decreasing complication rates over time. In a series from the University of California, San Francisco, from 1989 to 2005, 78 patients underwent 83 BAV procedures (37). A retrograde one- or two-balloon approach was used, resulting in acute increase in the valve area from 0.63 ± 0.21 to 1.01 ± 0.36 cm^2. Complications occurred in 22%, including death, myocardial infarction, and stroke in 1% each. Femoral bleeding occurred in 13%, and vascular surgery was required in 7%. Vascular surgery was performed in no patient in whom suture-mediated arteriotomy closure with a Perclose® device had been attempted, but surgery was performed in

12% of those for whom closure was not attempted. Overall, the complication rate fell during three intervals: 1989 to 1993 ($n = 36$, 31%), 1994 to 1999 ($n = 20$, 25%), and 2000 to 2005 ($n = 22$, 9%). However, the progress at avoiding complications was not matched by any real change in procedural efficacy. The median survival after BAV was 6.6 months, and survival at 1, 2, 3, and 5 years was 38%, 32%, 20%, and 14%, respectively. Vascular complications decreased since adopting suture-mediated femoral closure in 1999. Surgical valve replacement was performed in 22%, being mostly younger patients "bridged" to surgery (average 36 days after BAV), and for these patients, the median survival was 6.2 years.

More recently, the antegrade approach, the use of rapid pacing, and evolutions in vascular access and vascular closure have resulted in improvement in acute success rates and reduced complications.

Antegrade Approach

While the vast majority of valvuloplasties in these trials were performed by a retrograde, transfemoral approach, the antegrade, transseptal approach has proponents and potential advantages. In patients with rheumatic mitral and aortic stenosis, this approach even allowed the treatment of both valves antegrade using the Inoue balloon (38). Eisenhauer has proposed that the dumbbell-shaped Inoue balloon may yield a more effective dilation of the aortic valve. Comparing a series of antegrade Mansfield balloon dilations versus a series of antegrade Inoue balloon dilations in calcific AS, the mean change in AVA was 0.19 versus 0.43 (39). It is hypothesized that the larger diameter of the distal part of the Inoue balloon may compress the leaflets deeper into the sinuses for a given diameter at the annulus.

Sakata and colleagues from Evanston Hospital also compared antegrade versus retrograde (40) outcomes using a series of 31 retrograde (1998 to 2000) procedures versus 40 antegrade (2001 to 2004) procedures. The valve area increased from 0.6 ± 0.2 to 1.0 ± 0.3 cm^2 (retrograde) versus 0.6 ± 0.2 to 1.2 ± 0.5 cm^2 (antegrade Inoue balloon.) Maximum balloon size was greater with the Inoue balloon (20 mm vs. 24 mm). One advantage proposed for the Inoue balloon is the potentially lower risk of vascular access complications with a

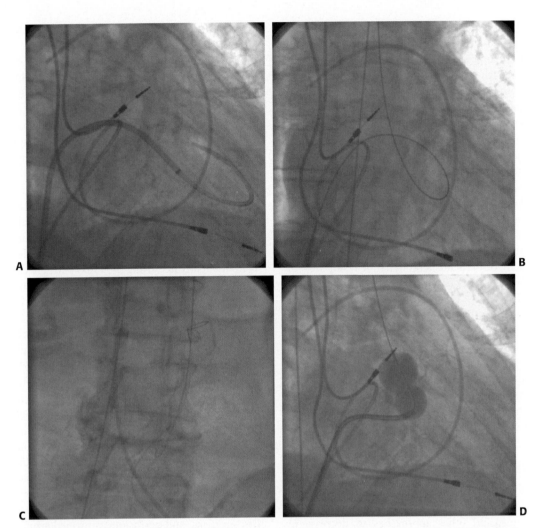

FIGURE 21-1. Balloon aortic valvuloplasty using the antegrade Inoue balloon technique. (**A**) A Mullins sheath has been passed through the left atrium across the mitral valve. The tip marker can be seen in the left ventricular inflow. Through the Mullins sheath, a 7F single-lumen balloon catheter has been advanced into the left ventricle and looped in the apex to point upward toward the aortic valve. The silhouette of the inflated balloon at the tip of the catheter can be noted just within the curve of the pulmonary artery catheter. (**B**) A wire has been passed through the 7F balloon tip catheter, traversing the left ventricle and passing into the aortic arch and then the descending aorta. Please note the loop in the left ventricle. (**C**) The proximal part of a 0.032-in wire can be seen passing through a 14F sheath in the inferior vena cava (*left*). The J curve of the wire can be seen in the descending aorta (*right*). A microsnare has been passed over the distal end of the wire in the descending aorta. The snare will be anchored on the wire and left in place in the descending aorta to stabilize the wire for balloon passage through the left ventricle into the aortic valve. (**D**) The inflated Inoue balloon is seen in the calcified aortic valve leaflets. The wire loop has been straightened in the left ventricle during inflation. After balloon deflation, the balloon will be pulled back into the left atrium and the loop reestablished in the left ventricle. (From Baim DS. *Grossman's cardiac catheterization, angiography, and intervention.* 7th ed. Philadelphia, PA: Lippincott Williams & Wilkins, 2006.)

venous approach. The Inoue balloon positions itself by the nature of its multiphase inflation profile, and has a relatively rapid inflation/deflation cycle. However, the antegrade approach requires transseptal catheterization and generally also requires guidewire snaring and externalization, so is a more complex procedure. The transseptal/LV/Ao/externalized guidewire requires the creation of a loop in the left ventricle, and from this loop arise risks both of mitral valve and of LV complications (Fig. 21-1). In Sakata's report, two patients could not tolerate the LV loop.

Given the frequency of vascular access site complications with the retrograde femoral artery approach, the advantage of the antegrade approach may be clinically significant. In another comparison of antegrade versus retrograde approaches to aortic valvuloplasty, Block and Palacios at Massachusetts General Hospital noted that among 55 patients with severe AS, 30 had antegrade transseptal valvuloplasty, and 25 had retrograde valvuloplasty (41). The same 18- to 20-mm balloons were used for either approach. Hematomas, vascular surgery, thrombectomy, and transfusion were more common in the retrograde group, while there was no difference in the number of strokes (two each), deaths (one each), or the acute hemodynamic result. In a follow-up report 22 years later of the same hospital's series (2000 to 2006), 157 patients underwent BAV: 46 (29%) antegrade (of which 59% were Inoue balloons) and 111 (71%) retrograde. The patients had similar EuroSCOREs, baseline and postprocedural valve areas. The antegrade approach was associated with fewer vascular complications (2% vs. 19%, $P = 0.005$). The 2-year mortality in this series was 81% antegrade and 69% retrograde ($P = 0.16$) (42).

Rapid Pacing

Other technical changes in the evolving approach to BAV have included the rapid pacing technique, and other approaches to decrease LV ejection during balloon inflation. Early in the history of BAV, Bittl and colleagues at the Brigham and Women's Hospital recorded the peak LV pressure developed during balloon inflation, and this ranged from 150 ± 5 to 386 ± 22 mm Hg. Peak LV pressure during inflation correlated closely with echocardiographic LV ejection fraction and with the LV mass/volume ratio (43). The results of increased LV wall stress caused by transient obstruction of ejection include the release of atrial natriuretic peptide and vasopressin (44,45). At the same time, decreased coronary blood flow produces myocardial ischemia. In a study using coronary sinus catheter samples during BAV, Rousseau and colleagues at the Saint-Luc University Hospital in Brussels found that during acute balloon obstruction of LV outflow, coronary blood flow fell, with rapid alteration to anaerobic myocardial metabolism (46). Mitral regurgitation during balloon occlusion may partially relieve the LV hypertension (47).

The use of rapid ventricular pacing to decrease LV ejection against the inflated/occlusive balloon thus has a number of theoretical benefits: (1) to reduce movement of the inflated balloon during cardiac ejection, (2) to allow more stable and perhaps more effective dilation, and (3) to decrease the tremendous LV wall stress induced by the peak developed pressure of the ventricle's contraction against near-infinite afterload. For these and perhaps other reasons, the rapid pacing technique has been associated with reduced complications from BAV. A modern BAV series from Rouen (2002 to 2005) included 141 patients treated using the rapid pacing technique, with 4% mortality and 6% nonfatal complications including transient stroke, vascular complications, and five cases of heart block (48).

Other approaches used to decrease LV ejection temporarily for aortic or cardiac interventions have included the TandemHeart® percutaneous left ventricular assist device (LVAD), a pump with a transseptal left atrial inflow cannula that can nearly empty the left heart (49), adenosine infusion (which has also been used for aortic stent grafting (50) and congenital cardiac interventions) (51), and induction of ventricular fibrillation (52). Of course, full cardiopulmonary bypass support is also possible for the hybrid teams of interventionalists, surgeons, and perfusionists formed around transcatheter valve implantation programs. However, because of its relative simplicity, rapid pacing is the most frequently used approach for BAV as well as for transcatheter aortic valve implantation (TAVI) today. With the advent of percutaneous valves, rapid pacing has been adopted as necessary, particularly because of the critical importance of positioning the valve right the first time (53). Pacing is initiated and tested prior to valvuloplasty. The balloon is inflated only when the systemic pressure and pulse pressure have fallen; pacing is continued until the balloon is deflated. A similar sequence is followed for valve implantation, and it is important that the operating team get the sequence and timing of these steps correctly to minimize the chance of malposition or embolization. Rapid pacing has also been used for a variety of congenital heart interventions (54), to reduce coronary stent movement during deployment (55,56), and for rotational angiography with three-dimensional reconstruction (57).

Vascular Access and Vascular Closure

For femoral artery catheterization of any size, it is always best to puncture the common femoral artery (CFA), but this is particularly so with the large sheaths required for valvuloplasty (12 to 14 French) or for percutaneous transfemoral AVR (18 to 28 French). The importance of good vascular access was noted early in the history of valvuloplasty and efforts made to confirm sheath position in the CFA before upsizing for a valvuloplasty sheath (58). Some operators evolved to a planned vascular repair approach; others to a planned cut-down approach. Those who performed vascular surgical repairs only when problems arose often found that superficial femoral puncture, side wall puncture, or through-and-through puncture underlay the complication (59). For these reasons, we use real-time, two-dimensional femoral ultrasound imaging guidance with a needle guide on the probe to ensure that the arterial puncture site is on the anterior surface of the CFA.

The use of suture-mediated closure devices to predeliver one or more sutures around the arteriotomy before it is upsized (the "preclose" technique) (60) appears to reduce complications. Solomon, et al. reported successful preclosure in 27/31 (87%), with four failures converted to manual compression. No patient required vascular surgery. Compared with 39 consecutive prior patients who had manual compression, the length of stay was shorter (2.3 vs. 5.3 days) and fewer patients required transfusion (0% vs. 29%) (61). We and others (62) have successfully utilized the preclose technique for the even larger sheaths used for TAVI. Our approach is to use two or more ProGlide® devices; others prefer the 10 French ProStar® device. Success is favored by a perfect arterial puncture into the anterior wall of the CFA, ideally avoiding areas of heavy calcification or plaque, and ultrasound imaging guidance of the puncture is thus invaluable.

It is not surprising that hematomas, pseudoaneurysms, and other bleeding complications are common with BAV and TAVI, as our patients often have many of the well-known risk factors for access site complications, including advanced age, small stature/frailty, renal dysfunction, heart failure, a large sheath, and concomitant femoral venous access. Patients with AS may also have acquired von Willebrand syndrome, with platelet dysfunction resulting from high shear flow across the valve (63).

■ EVOLUTION OF TRANSCATHETER VALVES AND THEIR COMPLICATIONS

Ten years after Kan's first report of a balloon valvuloplasty, Anderson published a preclinical description of a transcatheter aortic valve (64) encompassing many of the features that have come forward to the devices we use today. By intent and design of the clinical trials and protocols for their use, percutaneous valves have been reserved for patients at high or prohibitive risk for conventional valve surgery, because of advanced age, LV dysfunction, and severe comorbidities (65). The frequency of complications seen in these series certainly has as much to do with the high-risk patients as with the technology itself.

Two transcatheter valves have significant current use; others are in various stages of development. The Edwards SAPIEN valve is a balloon-expandable device with a stainless steel frame and a fabric skirt; inside the device are three leaflets made of bovine pericardium, treated to prevent calcification (Fig. 21-2). The 23-mm diameter valve requires a 22 French sheath, while the 26-mm diameter valve requires a 24 French sheath. The next generation Sapien-XT valve uses a cobalt–chromium frame, and will require a smaller sheath.

The CoreValve is a self-expanding nitinol frame with a trileaflet valve of porcine pericardial tissue (Figs. 21-3 and 21-4). The frame contains three distinct zones: (1) subannular, (2) across the native valve leaflets, and (3) above the coronary sinuses. The total length of the expanded device is 45 mm. The inflow segment of the frame has an additional piece of porcine pericardium as a skirt. The device is compressed and loaded into a delivery catheter system, which requires (for the third-generation CoreValve) an 18 French arterial sheath.

Since the first report by Cribier and colleagues of percutaneous implantation of an

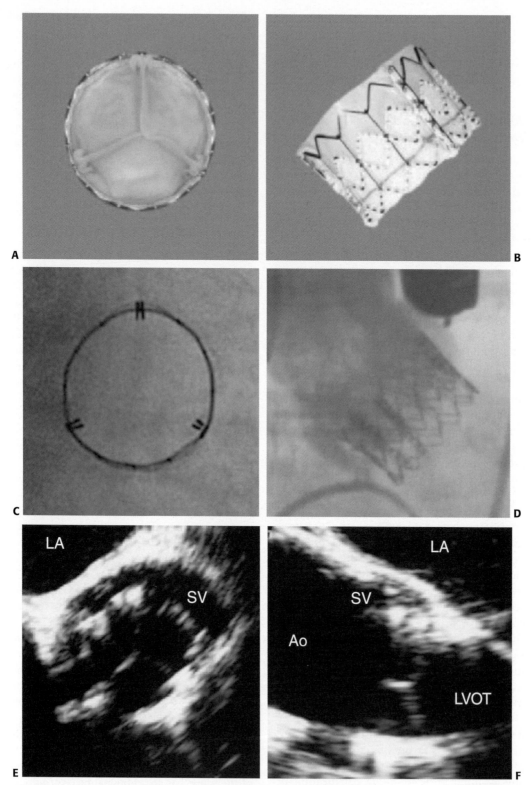

FIGURE 21-2. Balloon-expandable stent photographed from the aortic aspect, (**A**) showing leaflets in the closed position and from the side and (**B**) showing the fabric sealing cuff. (**C**) Fluoroscopic image of the implanted and fully expanded valve as seen from the aortic aspect. (**D**) The aortic angiogram shows the valve securely fixed in the annulus. The left main coronary artery can be seen to originate from the sinotubular junction above the valve, adjacent to a transesophageal echo probe. Transesophageal echocardiography performed on the (**E**) short axis and (**F**) long axis . Ao indicates aorta; LA, left atrium; LVOT, left ventricular outflow tract; and SV, sinus of Valsalva. (From Webb JG, Pasupati S, Humphries K, et al. Percutaneous transarterial aortic valve replacement in selected high-risk patients with aortic stenosis. *Circulation.* 2007;116:755–763.)

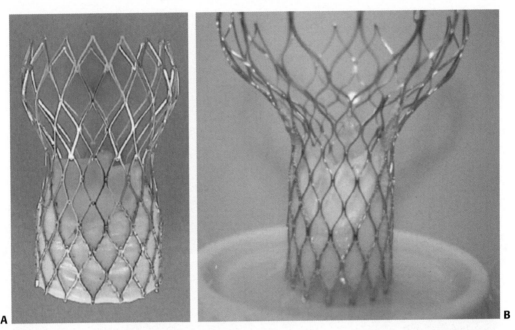

FIGURE 21-3. The CoreValve bioprosthesis: (**A**) first generation and (**B**) second generation. (From Grube E, Laborde JC, Gerckens U, et al. Percutaneous implantation of the CoreValve self-expanding valve prosthesis in high-risk patients with aortic valve disease: The Siegburg First-in-Man Study. *Circulation.* 2006;114:1616–1624.)

aortic valve prosthesis (2002) (66), approximately 4,000 cases have been performed worldwide as of mid 2009. For the first six cases, the antegrade transseptal approach was used. Results in these six included one distal valve migration, and mild (in three of six) or severe (in two of six) paravalvular regurgitation (67).

Paravalvular Regurgitation

The feasibility of retrograde TAVI was first demonstrated in a human subject treated with a balloon expandable device, the Paniagua valve (68). Hanzel, et al. from the William Beaumont Hospital reported an attempt at antegrade delivery of an early generation percutaneous heart valve (69). The transseptal guidewire was snared in the contralateral iliac artery and externalized, thus straightening the loop in the left ventricle, and causing severe mitral regurgitation followed by pulseless electrical activity. After resuscitation, the procedure was converted to a retrograde approach and the device delivered on a conventional 22 mm × 3 cm valvuloplasty balloon; this was the first report of a technically successful retrograde implantation of the Edwards valve. The valve functioned normally; new moderate

mitral regurgitation was present, and the patient deteriorated over several days and expired. At postmortem examination, there was laceration of the anterior mitral leaflet (70), as well as free space between the prosthesis and the right–left commissure. This and other early experience suggested that paravalvular regurgitation could be anticipated with the balloon-expandable device. In Webb's first series of 18 transfemoral Edwards valves, AI was seen in all but one patient, and was angiographic grade 1.6 ± 0.5 pre, and 1.8 ± 0.6 post valve implantation. At least three potential mechanisms of paravalvular regurgitation can be postulated: (1) potential gaps in the commissures of the native valve, (2) noncircular geometry of the aortic annulus around a circular device, and (3) extrinsic interference with device expansion caused by calcified disease of the native valve and annulus.

Predictors of this complication may include larger annulus diameter and greater patient height. Treatment options for paravalvular regurgitation include redilation, which may seat the valve's skirt more deeply into the commissures but may also risk valve displacement or intravalvular dysfunction,

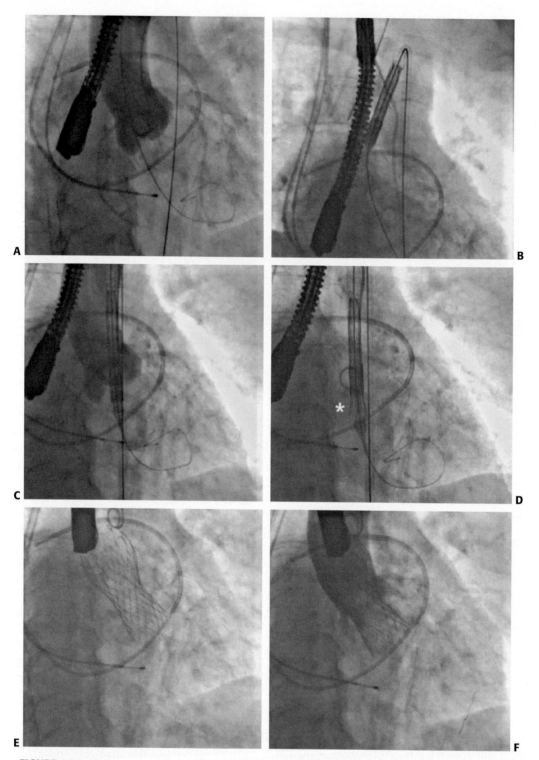

FIGURE 21-4. Case example. (**A**) Baseline supra-aortic angiogram. (**B**), Advancement of the first-generation prosthesis over the aortic arch. (**C**) The device is positioned across the native valve, with the correct position confirmed by transesophageal echocardiography. (**D**) Pullback of the outer sheath and deployment of the self-expanding prosthesis (*asterisk*). (**E**) Fully expanded valve prosthesis. (**F**) Final aortogram demonstrates no evidence of aortic regurgitation. (From Grube E, Laborde JC, Gerckens U, et al. Percutaneous implantation of the CoreValve self-expanding valve prosthesis in high-risk patients with aortic valve disease: The Siegburg First-in-Man Study. *Circulation.* 2006;114:1616–1624.)

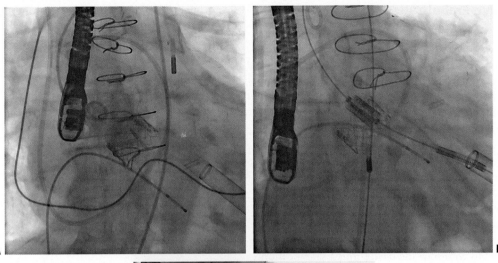

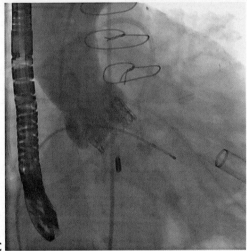

FIGURE 21-5. The patient was an 84-year-old man with aortic stenosis, prior coronary bypass, left ventricular dysfunction, and heart failure. Transapical transcatheter aortic valve implantation was done with a 23-mm Edwards SAPIEN valve (**A**). There was moderate-to-severe aortic valve regurgitation, thought to be related to native leaflet overhang (*arrow*) interference with the prosthetic leaflets. A second valve (valve-in-valve) was deployed in a slightly more aortic position (**B**). After the second valve implant, the overhanging leaflet was stented open (*arrow*) and there was no aortic regurgitation (**C**).

and sometimes requires a second "valve-in-valve" implant (Fig. 21-5).

Surgical revision of a percutaneous prosthesis because of paravalvular regurgitation was first described by the Rouen University Hospital team. The patient had a 20-mm annulus, and underwent transfemoral implantation of a 23-mm Cribier–Edwards percutaneous heart valve. There was hypotension requiring pressors, and severe AI. Postdilation was done with a 23-mm balloon resulting in cardiac arrest. At operation, there was a gap between the stent and the commissure of the right–left and right cusps, and a

smaller gap between the stent and the commissure of the left and noncoronary cusps. The valve was removed by simply pulling it out, and a 23-mm Carpentier–Edwards Perimount valve was implanted surgically. After a 30-day hospitalization, the patient was alive at 1-year follow-up (71). While this was not the course that was intended, it does raise the possibility of percutaneous AVR as a bridge to surgical valve replacement.

Central valvular regurgitation may also occur, and it might be due to interference with the new valve by an overhanging native leaflet.

Valve Embolization

In 2 of 18 patients in the early transfemoral series of Webb and colleagues at St. Paul's Hospital, British Columbia, valve embolization occurred immediately upon deflation of the delivery balloon. Factors hypothesized to contribute to embolization included native annulus/prosthesis size mismatch, aggressive predilation of the native valve, and excessively high positioning of the prosthesis. In one case, the prosthesis and its still-inflated delivery balloon were ejected by a hyperdynamic left ventricle upon termination of rapid pacing. In both cases, the delivery balloon was readvanced through the prosthesis, partially inflated, and used to withdraw the device into a safe location in the descending or transverse aorta.

Mitral Valve Complications

Since the retrograde approach to percutaneous aortic valve implantation became the standard, mitral valve complications have been rare. However, infective endocarditis, with mitral valve injury and perforation, has been reported late (11 months) after aortic valve implantation, possibly resulting from contact between the valve frame and the anterior mitral leaflet (72).

Vascular Complications

Femoral–iliac complications are among the most easily predicted complications of this approach, and can be largely mitigated by careful screening for adequate femoral vessel dimensions and freedom from severe calcific atherosclerosis. In Webb's description of 18 patients treated with retrograde delivery of the Cribier–Edwards Valve, there were vascular access site complications in the first 2, but not the subsequent 16 subjects (73). There was one visual deficit and two deaths in the first month. Avulsion of the iliac artery has also been described.

Myocardial Complications

Rapid ventricular pacing to produce hypotension, and device expansion obstructing LV outflow, if brief and well-timed, are usually remarkably well-tolerated. In most cases, LV ejection recovers within a few beats. Occasionally, defibrillation or demand pacing is required to restore a rhythm. Particularly in cases with

severe myocardial disease, either systolic dysfunction or profound hypertrophy, there is some risk that the heart will not resume ejection—the "stone heart." If anticipated, mechanical hemodynamic support might be provided in advance.

In cases where the coronary circulation depends upon aortocoronary or mammary–coronary grafts, even transient hypotension can initiate a cycle of coronary hypoperfusion and refractory LV stunning, ventricular arrhythmias, or pump failure. Prophylactic intra-aortic balloon pumping (IABP) has proved valuable in a number of such cases. Vogel and colleagues from University of Maryland reported the use of full cardiopulmonary support (CPS) to permit aortic valvuloplasty in sicker patients (74).

The TandemHeart® percutaneous LVAD empties the left atrium and returns the blood to the arterial circulation; depending on the pump flow settings, native aortic valve opening can be eliminated by complete emptying of the left heart, with conversion to nonpulsatile arterial flow. While this device requires transseptal catheterization with a large (21 French) cannula and a large (15 to 17 French) arterial return cannula, it may offer some particular advantages to certain cases for BAV or for percutaneous AVR. Tanaka and colleagues from the University of California, Los Angeles, reported using the TandemHeart? for support during BAV, both for retrograde and antegrade approaches to valve dilation. Rapid ventricular pacing was not done, yet balloon expansion was maintained in position for up to 45 seconds without LV ejection (75).

Left ventricular perforation is a rare but anticipatable complication of both valvuloplasty and transcatheter valve implantation. Prompt pericardiocentesis will almost certainly be required for a true LV perforation. Surgical decompression and repair is required in approximately 20% of cases of all types of iatrogenic cardiac perforation (76), but an LV perforation may be more serious than (for example) an atrial perforation from an electrophysiology procedure. If the catheter/wire system remains across the perforation, repair with a septal occluder device is a possible bail-out solution (77).

Conduction and Rhythm Complications

In dogs, balloon dilation at the aortic annulus caused contraction band necrosis of the cells of the left bundle branch (78). In humans, it may be surprising that heart block is not more frequent; in a series of 207 patients undergoing mitral or aortic valvuloplasty at Massachusetts General Hospital, 18% had a new intraventricular conduction defect (IVCD) on surface electrocardiography after the intervention (79). These investigators also performed His bundle recording in 19 valvuloplasty patients. Neither the AH interval nor AV node ERP changed with valvuloplasty, but the HV interval was transiently and modestly prolonged. The QRS duration was significantly prolonged (95±28 milliseconds increased to 112 ± 28 milliseconds) by inflations, and remained so 24 hours later. New IVCD or bundle branch block appearing with valvuloplasty was usually permanent. Transient or (less commonly) permanent (80) heart block may also follow BAV.

Of 106 patients receiving the balloon expandable Edwards valve and who did not already have a pacemaker, the St. Paul's team reported 6.6% developed complete AV block immediately upon valve implantation, and 5.7% developed new left bundle branch block (LBBB) (81).

The frequency of complete heart block seems to be higher with the longer, self-expanding CoreValve, presumably because of the compression of conduction tissue in the septum by the anchoring subannular segment of the device. Among 40 patients receiving the CoreValve at the Thoraxcenter between 2005 and 2008 (82), LBBB increased from 15% before, to 55% after device implantation, and was 48% at 1-month follow-up. The only two patients with preexisting right bundle branch block both required pacing, and in all 18% required a permanent pacemaker. The distance from the bottom of the noncoronary cusp to the bottom (ventricular) edge of the device was highly predictive of effects on conduction, suggesting that the depth of the device within the LV outflow tract may determine the extent of conduction tissue dysfunction. Among those developing LBBB, this valve depth distance was 10.3 ± 2.7 mm, whereas in those who did not develop LBBB, this measured 5.5 ± 3.4 mm ($P = 0.005$), and no patients developed LBBB when the valve was positioned such that this measurement was less than 6.7 mm.

A somewhat different model was generated by the investigators at Glenfield Hospital,

Leicester. Of 34 patients receiving a CoreValve, 10 required a new pacemaker (83). The presence of at least one of the following—(1) LBBB with LAD (2) diastolic septal thickness greater than 17 mm by transthoracic echo; (3) noncoronary cusp thickness greater than 8 mm—predicted the need for a pacemaker with 75% sensitivity and 100% specificity. Taken together, these two studies suggest that the ventricular component of the CoreValve's frame compresses the left bundle branch tissue below the right and noncoronary cusps and that this mechanism may be responsible for most heart block with this device. Deeper (ventricular) implantation, septal hypertrophy, and a bulkier noncoronary cusp all contribute to greater mechanical compression. Compression of the bundle of His by a localized hematoma in the interventricular septum at the site of expansion of the implanted valve has also been proposed as a mechanism for the development of AV block following TAVI (Fig. 21-6).

Coronary Obstruction

By design, the Edwards valve is positioned below the coronary ostia, but struts of the stent may extend over the coronaries; interference with coronary perfusion is rare. When it has occurred, coronary obstruction has sometimes resulted from displacement of a native leaflet that is particularly long or affected by a bulky nodule. Bail-out left coronary dilation and stenting has been lifesaving, and may be facilitated by mechanical hemodynamic support (84). In an ex vivo pig heart preparation, coronary flow embarrassment by a balloon-expandable stent valve was associated with displacement of the native leaflets; removal of the native leaflets beforehand eliminated this effect (85). Webb has proposed that coronary impingement with a percutaneous AVR may occur because of a low-lying coronary ostium, bulky native leaflets, and a narrow aortic root with little space in the sinuses of Valsalva for the displaced native leaflets (86).

The CoreValve design is quite different, and its self-expanding frame extends above the coronary ostia. Nonetheless, interference with the coronaries is uncommon; percutaneous coronary intervention has been described through the frame (87).

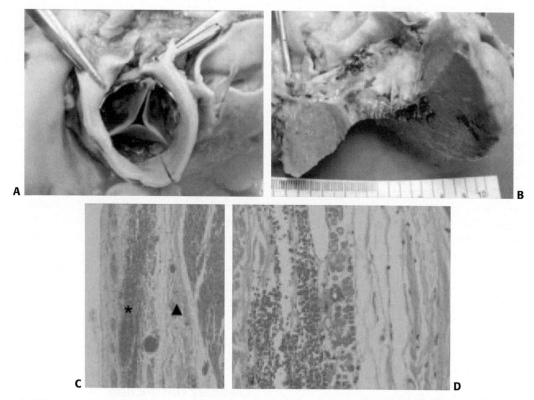

FIGURE 21-6. Potential mechanism of heart block following transcatheter aortic valve implantation. (**A**) View of the aortic root. The Edwards SAPIEN prosthetic valve is correctly implanted. The path of one of the coronary arteries is shown. (**B**) As the prosthesis was removed from the aortic outflow tract, some hemorrhagic lesions were observed, as well as calcifications of native aortic valves and severe calcification of the mitral valve, which appears as a yellowish nodule. In the upper interventricular septum, a subendocardiac hemorrhage is patent. (**C**) From an anatomopathological point of view, we can observe (*from left to right*) the endocardium, a hemorrhagic band next to the bundle of His (*asterisk*), an amyloid deposit, and myocardial fibers (') (hematoxylin and eosin, 10). (**D**) In an enlarged image, we can see conduction tissue fibers made up of specialized myocytes with central glycogen deposits that produce a myocardial fiber displacement to the periphery. Hematic extravasation next to those fibers is evident (hematoxylin and eosin). (From Moreno R, Dobarro D, López de Sá E, et al. Cause of complete atrioventricular block after percutaneous aortic valve implantation: insights from a necropsy study. *Circulation.* 2009;120:e29–e30.) (See color insert.)

Overall Complications Rates

In 2007, Webb and colleagues published a series of 50 subjects treated with retrograde transfemoral implantation of the Cribier–Edwards valve (88) (Table 21-3). Procedural success was 86%. Among seven failures were inability to pass the iliac artery (*n* = 1), inability to cross the native valve (*n* = 3), device defect (*n* = 1), and malpositioning of the device above the native annulus (*n* = 2). A learning curve effect was noted, leading to further improvement in procedural success.

In a more recent series from Webb and colleagues (89), 25 patients were treated with retrograde transfemoral implantation of bal-loon-expandable SAPIEN or SAPIEN-XT valves using a RetroFlex 2 delivery system. STS-predicted mortality for surgical valve replacement was 8.9%, and logistic EuroSCORE predicted mortality was 21%. There was 100% procedural success and 0% mortality at 30 days. There were two strokes (8%) in this cohort. 64% of cases had percutaneous closure of the vascular access with the Perclose technique. One patient each required IABP and femoral-to-femoral cardiopulmonary bypass support. Transfusion of greater than or equal to 3 units of blood was required in 12%. There was no more than mild valvular regurgitation, and 1/25 had moderate paravalvular regurgitation.

TABLE 21-3 Outcome After Percutaneous Aortic Valve Replacement (AVR) in 50 High-Risk Patients—Edwards Valve

Characteristic	
Procedural success	43 (86%)
Stroke	2 (4%)
Myocardial infarction	1 (2%)
Ventricular fibrillation	2 (4%)
Heart block, new and sustained	2 (4%)
Tamponade[a]	1 (2%)
Transfusion > 3 U	9 (18%)
Emergent cardiac surgery	0 (0%)
Endocarditis	0 (0%)
Death, intraprocedural	1 (2%)
Death, 30d	6 (12%)
Death, stroke, or myocardial infarction at 30d	8 (16%)

[a] Complication of postprocedural implantation of a permanent pacemaker.
(From Webb JG, Pasupati S, Humphries K, et al. Percutaneous transarterial aortic valve replacement in selected high-risk patients with aortic stenosis. *Circulation.* 2007;116(7):755–763.)

In a registry of 646 patients (90) receiving the third-generation CoreValve, procedural success was 97% (Table 21-4). Procedural mortality was 1.5% and 30-day mortality was 8%. Vascular complications were reported in 1.9% in this series; preclosure with the 10F ProStar device was routinely used. Balloon dilation of the device after deployment was performed in 21.2%, and a second "valve-in-valve" was implanted in 2.6%. Post procedure AI was mostly grade 0 to 1, and was grade less than or equal to 2 in 100%. There were no cases of coronary impairment. Aortic dissection or perforation occurred in 0.6%, and ventricular perforation in 1.7%. At 30 days, 9.3% required a permanent pacemaker. 30-day stroke rate was 1.9%.

Taramasso and colleagues from Milan used a CoreValve for the treatment of native aortic valve insufficiency, with resulting severe prosthetic regurgitation. After a valve-in-valve deployment of an Edwards SAPIEN valve, there was minor residual regurgitation and clinical improvement (91).

EMERGING VALVES AND TECHNIQUES

It may be hoped that refinements of the devices will overcome some of the current limitations of percutaneous aortic valve

implantation. The Ventor Embracer valve (92) is a self-expanding nitinol device with arms designed to anchor in the sinuses, and bovine pericardial leaflets within a polyester fabric sleeve. It is hypothesized that the anchoring arms may provide improved centering, fixation, and orientation. Other devices in development include the Direct Flow Medical valve and the Sadra Lotus valve.

At this point in the experience with transcatheter valve prostheses, resection of the native valves seems usually not to be necessary in order to achieve a safe and effective relief of obstruction to LV outflow. However, endovascular resection of the leaflets has been attempted in models and may be a feasible approach to improve the fit of the prosthesis in the annulus, perhaps reducing paravalvular regurgitation and providing a larger orifice (93–95). Endoluminal demineralization of calcified valves is another strategy in development (96,97).

Transapical Approach

The transapical antegrade approach to TAVI was developed (98) to address the limitation of vascular access defined by the relatively large caliber

TABLE 21-4 Procedural Outcomes following Transcatheter Aortic Valve Implantation—Third-Generation CoreValve ReValving System Registry Experience

Procedure-related death	10 (1.5%)
Cardiovascular death	11 (1.7%)
Balloon inflation after valve implantation	137 (21.2%)
Valve-in-valve implantation	17 (2.6%)
Myocardial infarction	3 (0.5%)
Neurological event	4 (0.6%)
Transient ischemic attack	0
Stroke	4 (0.6%)
Combined events: death, stroke, and myocardial infarction	16 (2.5%)
Coronary artery flow impairment	0 (0%)
Aortic root dissection or perforation	4 (0.6%)
Left ventricular or right ventricular perforation	11 (1.7%)
Cardiac tamponade	9 (1.4%)
Vascular access site complications	12 (1.9%)
Conversion to surgery	3 (0.5%)

(Adapted from Vahanian A, Alfieri O, Al-Attar N, et al. Transcatheter valve implantation for patients with aortic stenosis: a position statement from the European Association of Cardio-Thoracic Surgery (EACTS) and the European Society of Cardiology (ESC), in collaboration with the European Association of Percutaneous Cardiovascular Interventions (EAPCI). *EuroIntervention.* 2008;4:193–199.)

early generation catheters used in the Edwards system. The early experience in the first 26 patients in Vancouver (99) included 23% mortality at 30 days. Among those surviving 30 days, the 12-month survival was 85%, with a Kaplan–Meier modeled 1-year survival of 65% ± 10%. Complications of this approach include conduction system abnormalities, ventricular fibrillation, entanglement in the mitral apparatus, traumatic ventricular septal defect, early dehiscence of the apical ventriculotomy, and later development of apical pseudoaneurysm (100).

Just as with transfemoral implantation, positioning and fixation of the valve is critical. Even with perfect fluoroscopic positioning of the device, valve movement during deployment can occur. In 26 patients at the Hospital of the Johann Wolfgang Goethe University, Frankfurt, early in the development of the transapical procedure, 30-day mortality was 15% (101). In two cases, there was partial obstruction of the left coronary

orifice by displacement of the native valve, and these were treated with coronary stenting. Valve embolization occurred in one case during a second-balloon inflation intended to address severe paravalvular regurgitation. Two cases were converted to open surgery because of valve embolization or dissection of the ascending aorta after valvuloplasty. Both planned and provisional cardiopulmonary bypass supports were used.

Besides longitudinal valve movement and embolization, postimplant rotation of the device has also been reported to contribute to its displacement (102). Other reported complications from the transapical approach have included guidewire puncture of the ventricular septum and perforation of the pulmonary artery (103), and late valve embolization into the ventricle (104).

The conduction system might be differently affected by transapical procedures. Among 33 patients receiving transapical implantation of the Edwards SAPIEN valve at the Quebec Heart and

Lung Institute, LBBB increased in frequency from 9% before to 27% after the procedure. Left anterior hemiblock (LAHB) increased from 3% to 36%. A more ventricular position of implantation predicted LBBB; a greater valve prosthesis to native aortic annulus ratio predicted the development of LAHB (105). The conduction abnormalities frequently resolved within 1 month.

In programs which can perform both, the ability to offer transfemoral or transapical approaches increases the potentially treatable population and might reduce complications. Himbert and the team from Bichat–Claude Bernard Hospital, Paris, reported their process of evaluating 160 high-risk patients (mean logistic EuroScore 26 ± 13; mean STS-predicted mortality 16 ± 7) referred for TAVI with the Edwards SAPIEN device (106). Of these, 28% were too frail or ill for intervention; 13% had an annulus too large, a bicuspid valve, or intracardiac thrombus. Of the remaining 94 who did not have a contraindication to a transcatheter implant, 43 (46%) had a contraindication to the transfemoral approach because of inadequate iliac arteries or aortic disease, while the rest had a transfemoral procedure. Of the 43 who could not have a transfemoral approach, 19 (44%) also had a contraindication to transapical valve implantation, mostly severe pulmonary disease. In sum, out of 160 patients, 51 (32%) had transfemoral and 24 (15%) had transapical valve implantation. Twenty three (14%) had conventional AVR, and 62 (39%) were treated medically. Differences between transfemoral and transapical outcomes were for implantation success (90% vs. 100%) and length of stay in intensive care unit (2.5 vs. 5 days). One-year survival was 78% ± 6% for the entire cohort treated with a transcatheter valve. There was a learning curve effect with 1-year survival of 60% ± 10% among the first 25 patients and 93% ± 4% for the last 50.

Besides transfemoral and transapical, there are other potential routes of access for transcatheter delivery of an aortic valve prosthesis, including the axillary/subclavian, the carotid (with a shunt), and the ascending aorta.

■ CONCLUSION

From the beginning of the era of percutaneous transcatheter valve interventions in 1982, to the beginning of the transcatheter valve implanta-tion era in 2002, to the present use of two transcatheter aortic valves in several thousand patients, we have seen that these interventional procedures are the most complex and frequently complicated of any performed in the modern catheterization laboratory. Inserting larger catheters into older, sicker patients will challenge interventionalists, and intervening upon the aortic valve in patients with limited cardiovascular reserve is an especially serious undertaking. Awareness of the potential complications and some approaches to avoid or treat them may make these procedures a bit safer for our patients.

References

1. Kan JS, White RI, Mitchell SE, Gardener TJ. Percutaneous balloon valvuloplasty: a new method for treating congenital pulmonary valve stenosis. *N Engl J Med.* 1982;307:540–542.
2. Lababidi Z. Aortic balloon valvuloplasty. *Am Heart J.* 1983;106:751–752.
3. Lababidi Z, Wu JR, Walls JT. Percutaneous balloon aortic valvuloplasty: results in 23 patients. *Am J Cardiol.* 1984;53(1):194–197.
4. Cribier A, Savin T, Saoudi N, et al. Percutaneous transluminal valvuloplasty of acquired aortic stenosis in elderly patients: an alternative to valve replacement? *Lancet.* 1986;1(8472):63–67.
5. McKay RG, Safian RD, Lock JE, et al. Balloon dilatation of calcific aortic stenosis in elderly patients: Postmortem, intraoperative, and percutaneous valvuloplasty studies. *Circulation.* 1986;74(1):119–125.
6. Dorros G, Lewin RF, King JF, Janke LM. Percutaneous transluminal valvuloplasty in calcific aortic stenosis: the double balloon technique. *Cathet Cardiovasc Diagn.* 1987;13(3):151–156.
7. Midei MG, Brennan M, Walford GD, et al. Double vs single balloon technique for aortic balloon valvuloplasty. *Chest.* 1988;94(2):245–250.
8. Meier B, Friedli B, Oberhaensli I, et al. Trefoil balloon for percutaneous valvuloplasty. *Cathet Cardiovasc Diagn.* 1986;12(4):277–281.
9. Voudris V, Drobinski G, L'Epine Y, et al. Results of percutaneous valvuloplasty for calcific aortic stenosis with different balloon catheters. *Cathet Cardiovasc Diagn.* 1989;17(2):80–83.
10. Rocha P, Baron B, Lacombe P, et al. Aortic percutaneous transluminal valvuloplasty in elderly

patients by balloon larger than aortic anulus. *Cathet Cardiovasc Diagn.* 1988;15(2):81–88.

11. Robicsek F, Harbold NB Jr. Limited value of balloon dilatation in calcified aortic stenosis in adults: direct observations during open heart surgery. *Am J Cardiol.* 1987;60(10):857–864.

12. Roth RB, Palacios IF, Block PC. Percutaneous aortic balloon valvuloplasty: its role in the management of patients with aortic stenosis requiring major noncardiac surgery. *J Am Coll Cardiol.* 1989;13(5):1039–1041 .

13. Hayes SN, Holmes DR Jr, Nishimura RA, Reeder GS. Palliative percutaneous aortic balloon valvuloplasty before noncardiac operations and invasive diagnostic procedures. *Mayo Clin Proc.* 1989;64(7):753–757 .

14. Moore JW, Slack MC, Kirby WC, Graeber GM. Hemodynamics and coronary blood flow during experimental aortic valvuloplasty: comparison of the dual versus the single catheter methods. *Am Heart J.* 1990;119(1):136–142.

15. Lieberman EB, Bashore TM, Hermiller JB, et al. Balloon aortic valvuloplasty in adults: failure of procedure to improve long-term survival. *J Am Coll Cardiol.* 1995;26(6):1522–1528.

16. Berland J, Cribier A, Savin T, et al. Percutaneous balloon valvuloplasty in patients with severe aortic stenosis and low ejection fraction. Immediate results and 1-year follow-up. *Circulation.* 1989;79(6):1189–1196.

17. Stoddard MF, Vandormael MG, Pearson AC, et al. Immediate and short-term effects of aortic balloon valvuloplasty on left ventricular diastolic function and filling in humans. *J Am Coll Cardiol.* 1989;14(5):1218–1228.

18. Sheikh KH, Davidson CJ, Honan MB, et al. Changes in left ventricular diastolic performance after aortic balloon valvuloplasty: Acute and late effects. *J Am Coll Cardiol.* 1990;16(4): 795–803.

19. Harpole DH, Davidson CJ, Skelton TN, et al. Early and late changes in left ventricular systolic performance after percutaneous aortic balloon valvuloplasty. *Am J Cardiol.* 1990;66(3):327–332.

20. Serruys PW, Luijten HE, Beatt KJ, et al. Percutaneous balloon valvuloplasty for calcific aortic stenosis: a treatment "sine cure"? *Eur Heart J.* 1988;9(7):782–794.

21. Lewin RF, Dorros G, King JF, Mathiak L. Percutaneous transluminal aortic valvuloplasty: acute outcome and follow-up of 125 patients. *J Am Coll Cardiol.* 1989;14(5):1210–1217.

22. Dorros G, Lewin RF, Stertzer SH, et al. Percutaneous transluminal aortic valvuloplasty—the acute outcome and follow-up of 149 patients who underwent the double balloon technique. *Eur Heart J.* 1990;11(5):429–440.

23. McKay RG. The Mansfield Scientific Aortic Valvuloplasty Registry: overview of acute hemodynamic results and procedural complications. *J Am Coll Cardiol.* 1991;17(2):485–491.

24. Holmes DR Jr, Nishimura RA, Reeder GS. In-hospital mortality after balloon aortic valvuloplasty: frequency and associated factors. *J Am Coll Cardiol.* 1991;17(1):189–192.

25. Reeder GS, Nishimura RA, Holmes DR Jr (for the The Mansfield Scientific Aortic Valvuloplasty Registry Investigators). Patient age and results of balloon aortic valvuloplasty: The Mansfield Scientific Registry experience. *J Am Coll Cardiol.* 1991;17(4):909–913.

26. O'Neill WW. Predictors of long-term survival after percutaneous aortic valvuloplasty: report of the Mansfield Scientific Balloon Aortic Valvuloplasty Registry. *J Am Coll Cardiol.* 1991;17(1): 193–198.

27. Isner JM (for the Mansfield Scientific Aortic Valvuloplasty Registry Investigators). Acute catastrophic complications of balloon aortic valvuloplasty. *J Am Coll Cardiol.* 1991;17(6):1436–1444.

28. NHLBI Balloon Valvuloplasty Registry Participants. Percutaneous balloon aortic valvuloplasty. Acute and 30-day follow-up results in 674 patients from the NHLBI Balloon Valvuloplasty Registry. *Circulation.* 1991;84(6):2383–2397.

29. Davidson CJ, Skelton TN, Kisslo KB, et al. The risk for systemic embolization associated with percutaneous balloon valvuloplasty in adults: a prospective comprehensive evaluation. *Ann Intern Med.* 1988;108(4):557–560.

30. Ferguson JJ III, Riuli EP, Massumi A. et al. Balloon aortic valvuloplasty: The Texas Heart Institute experience. *Tex Heart Inst J.* 1990;17(1):23–30.

31. Treasure CB, Schoen FJ, Treseler PA, Bittl JA. Leaflet entrapment causing acute severe aortic insufficiency during balloon aortic valvuloplasty. *Clin Cardiol.* 1989;12(7):405–408.

32. Sadaniantz A, Malhotra R, Korr KS. Transient acute severe aortic regurgitation complicating balloon aortic valvuloplasty. *Cathet Cardiovasc Diagn.* 1989;17(3):186–189.

33. Lembo NJ, King SB III, Roubin GS, Hammami A, Niederman AL. Fatal aortic rupture during

percutaneous balloon valvuloplasty for valvular aortic stenosis. *Am J Cardiol.* 1987;60(8): 733–736.

34. Lewin RF, Dorros G, King JF, et al. Aortic annular tear after valvuloplasty: the role of aortic annulus echocardiographic measurement. *Cathet Cardiovasc Diagn.* 1989;16(2):123–129.

35. Baudouy PY, Masquet C, Eiferman C, et al. Une complication exceptionnelle de la valvuloplastie aortique percutanée: la rupture d'un cordage mitral aberrant. [An unusual complication of percutaneous aortic valvuloplasty: rupture of an aberrant mitral chorda] *Arch Mal Coeur Vaiss.* 1988;81(2):227–230.

36. de Ubago JL, Vazquez de Prada JA, Moujir F, et al. Mitral valve rupture during percutaneous dilation of aortic valve stenosis. *Cathet Cardiovasc Diagn.* 1989;16(2):115–118.

37. Klein A, Lee K, Gera A, Ports TA, Michaels AD. Long-term mortality, cause of death, and temporal trends in complications after percutaneous aortic balloon valvuloplasty for calcific aortic stenosis. *J Interv Cardiol.* 2006;19(3):269–275.

38. Bahl VK, Chandra S, Goswami KC. Combined mitral and aortic valvuloplasty by antegrade transseptal approach using Inoue balloon catheter. *Intl J Cardiol.* 1998;63:313–315.

39. Eisenhauer AC, Hadjipetrou P, Piemonte TC. Balloon aortic valvuloplasty revisited: the role of the inoue balloon and transseptal antegrade approach. *Catheter Cardiovasc Interv.* 2000;50(4): 484–491.

40. Sakata Y, Syed Z, Salinger MH, Feldman T. Percutaneous balloon aortic valvuloplasty: antegrade transseptal vs. conventional retrograde transarterial approach. *Catheter Cardiovasc Interv.* 2005; 64(3):314–321.

41. Block PC, Palacios IF. Comparison of hemodynamic results of anterograde versus retrograde percutaneous balloon aortic valvuloplasty. *Am J Cardiol.* 1987;60(8):659–662.

42. Cubeddu RJ, Jneid H, Don CW, et al. Retrograde versus antegrade percutaneous aortic balloon valvuloplasty: immediate, short- and long-term outcome at 2 years. *Catheter Cardiovasc Interv.* 2009;74(2):225–231.

43. Bittl JA, Bhatia SJ, Plappert T, et al. Peak left ventricular pressure during percutaneous aortic balloon valvuloplasty: clinical and echocardiographic correlations. *J Am Coll Cardiol.* 1989;14(1):135–142.

44. Lewin RF, Raff H, Findling JW, et al. Stimulation of atrial natriuretic peptide and vasopressin during percutaneous transluminal aortic valvuloplasty. *Am Heart J.* 1989;118(2):292–298.

45. Suárez de Lezo J, Montilla P, Pan M, et al. Abrupt homeostatic responses to transient intracardiac occlusion during balloon valvuloplasty. *Am J Cardiol.* 1989;64(8):491–497.

46. Rousseau MF, Wyns W, Hammer F, et al. Changes in coronary blood flow and myocardial metabolism during aortic balloon valvuloplasty. *Am J Cardiol.* 1988;61(13):1080–1084.

47. Suárez De Lezo J, Pan M, Romero M, Sancho M, Carrasco JL. Physiopathology of transient ventricular occlusion during balloon valvuloplasty for pulmonic or aortic stenosis. *Am J Cardiol.* 1988;61(6):436–440.

48. Agatiello C, Eltchaninoff H, Tron C, et al. Balloon aortic valvuloplasty in the adult. Immediate results and in-hospital complications in the latest series of 141 consecutive patients at the University Hospital of Rouen (2002–2005). *Arch Mal Coeur Vaiss.* 2006;99(3):195–200.

49. Rajdev S, Irani A, Sharma S, Kini A. Clinical utility of TandemHeart for high-risk tandem procedures: percutaneous balloon aortic valvuloplasty followed by complex PCI. *J Invasive Cardiol.* 2007;19(11):E346–E349.

50. Dorros G, Cohn JM. Adenosine-induced transient cardiac asystole enhances precise deployment of stent-grafts in the thoracic or abdominal aorta. *J Endovasc Surg.* 1996;3(3):270–272.

51. De Giovanni JV, Edgar RA, Cranston A. Adenosine induced transient cardiac standstill in catheter interventional procedures for congenital heart disease. *Heart.* 1998;80:330–333.

52. Kahn RA, Marin ML, Hollier L, Parsons R, Griepp R. Induction of ventricular fibrillation to facilitate endovascular stent graft repair of thoracic aortic aneurysms. *Anesthesiology.* 1998; 88(2):534–536.

53. Webb JG, Pasupati S, Achtem L, Thompson CR. Rapid pacing to facilitate transcatheter prosthetic heart valve implantation. *Catheter Cardiovasc Interv.* 2006;68(2):199–204.

54. Daehnert I, Rotzsch C, Wiener M, Schneider P. Rapid right ventricular pacing is an alternative to adenosine in catheter interventional procedures for congenital heart disease. *Heart.* 2004; 90(9):1047–1050.

55. Okamura A, Ito H, Iwakura K, et al. Rapid ventricular pacing can reduce heart motion and facilitate stent deployment to the optimal

position during coronary artery stenting: initial experience. *EuroIntervention.* 2007;3:239–242.

56. O'Brien DG, Smith WH, Henderson RA.. Stabilisation of coronary stents using rapid right ventricular pacing. *EuroIntervention.* 2007;3:235–238.

57. Noble S, Miró J, Yong G, et al. Rapid pacing rotational angiography with three-dimensional reconstruction: use and benefits in structural heart disease interventions. *EuroIntervention.* 2009;5: 244–249.

58. Cole PL, Krone RJ. Approach to reduction of vascular complications of percutaneous valvuloplasty. *Cathet Cardiovasc Diagn.* 1987;13(5):331–332.

59. Skillman JJ, Kim D, Baim DS. Vascular complications of percutaneous femoral cardiac interventions. Incidence and operative repair. *Arch Surg.* 1988;123(10):1207–1212.

60. Marchant D, Schwartz R, Chepurko L, Katz S. Access site management after aortic valvuloplasty using a suture mediated closure device: clinical experience in 4 cases. *J Invasive Cardiol.* 2000;12(9):474–477.

61. Solomon LW, Fusman B, Jolly N, Kim A, Feldman T. Percutaneous suture closure for management of large french size arterial puncture in aortic valvuloplasty. *J Invasive Cardiol.* 2001; 13(8):592–596.

62. Kahlert P, Eggebrecht H, Erbel R, Sack S. A modified "preclosure" technique after percutaneous aortic valve replacement. *Catheter Cardiovasc Interv.* 2008;72(6):877–884.

63. Vincentelli A, Susen S, Le Tourneau T, et al. Acquired von willebrand syndrome in aortic stenosis. *N Engl J Med.* 2003;349:343–349.

64. Andersen HR, Knudsen LL, Hasenkam JM. Transluminal implantation of artificial heart valves: description of a new expandable aortic valve and initial results with implantation by catheter technique in closed chest pigs. *Eur Heart J.* 1992;13:704–708.

65. Patel JH, Mathew ST, Hennebry TA. Transcatheter aortic valve replacement: a potential option for the nonsurgical patient. *Clin Cardiol.* 2009;32(6):296–301.

66. Cribier A, Eltchaninoff H, Bash A, et al. Percutaneous transcatheter implantation of an aortic valve prosthesis for calcific aortic stenosis: first human case description. *Circulation.* 2002; 106(24):3006–3008.

67. Cribier A, Eltchaninoff H, Tron C, et al. Early experience with percutaneous transcatheter implantation of heart valve prosthesis for the treatment of end-stage inoperable patients with calcific aortic stenosis. *J Am Coll Cardiol.* 2004; 43(4):698–703.

68. Paniagua D, Condado JA, Besso J, et al. First human case of retrograde transcatheter implantation of an aortic valve prosthesis. *Tex Heart Inst J.* 2005;32(3):393–398.

69. Hanzel GS, Harrity PH, Schreiber TL, O'Neill WO. Retrograde percutaneous aortic valve implantation for critical aortic stenosis. *Cathet Cardiovasc Interv.* 2005;64:322–326.

70. Hanzel GS, O'Neill WW. Complications of percutaneous aortic valve replacement: experience with the Cribier-Edwards percutaneous heart valve. *EuroIntervention Supplements.* 2006; 1(Suppl A):A3–A8.

71. Litzler PY, Cribier A, Zajarias A, et al. Surgical aortic valve replacement after percutaneous aortic valve implantation: What have we learned? *J Thorac Cardiovasc Surg.* 136(3):697–701.

72. Wong DR, Boone RH, Thompson CR, et al. Mitral valve injury late after transcatheter aortic valve implantation. *J Thorac Cardiovasc Surg.* 2009;137(6):1547–1549.

73. Webb JG, Chandavimol M, Thompson CR, et al. Percutaneous Aortic Valve Implantation Retrograde From the Femoral Artery. *Circulation.* 2006;113:842–850.

74. Vogel RA. The Maryland experience: angioplasty and valvuloplasty using percutaneous cardiopulmonary support. *Am J Cardiol.* 1988; 62(18):11K–14K.

75. Tanaka K, Rangarajan K, Azarbal B, Tobis JM. Percutaneous ventricular assist during aortic valvuloplasty: potential application to the deployment of aortic stent-valves. *Tex Heart Inst J.* 2007;34(1):36–40.

76. Tsang TS, Freeman WK, Barnes ME, et al. Rescue echocardiographically guided pericardiocentesis for cardiac perforation complicating catheter-based procedures. The Mayo Clinic experience. *J Am Coll Cardiol.* 1998;32(5):1345–1350.

77. Vogel R, Windecker S, Meier B. Transcatheter repair of iatrogenic left ventricular free-wall perforation. *Catheter Cardiovasc Interv.* 2006; 68(6):829–831.

78. Plack RH, Hutchins CM, Brinker JA. Aortic valvuloplasty causes conduction system injury in dogs [abstract]. *Chest* 1988;94(suppl)79S.

79. Carlson MD, Palacios I, Thomas JD, et al. Cardiac conduction abnormalities during

percutaneous balloon mitral or aortic valvotomy. *Circulation.* 1989;79(6):1197–1203.

80. Plack RH, Porterfield JK, Brinker JA. Complete heart block developing during aortic valvuloplasty. *Chest.* 1989;96(5):1201–1203.

81. Sinhal A, Altwegg L, Pasupati S, et al. Atrioventricular block after transcatheter balloon expandable aortic valve implantation. *J Am Coll Cardiol Intv.* 2008;1:305–309.

82. Piazza N, Onuma Y, Jesserun E, et al. Early and persistent intraventricular conduction abnormalities and requirements for pacemaking after percutaneous replacement of the aortic valve. *J Am Coll Cardiol Intv.* 2008 1: 310–316.

83. Jilaihawi H, Chin D, Vasa-Nicotera M, et al. Predictors for permanent pacemaker requirement after transcatheter aortic valve implantation with the CoreValve bioprosthesis. *Am Heart J.* 2009;157(5):860–866.

84. Kapadia SR, Svensson L, Tuzcu EM. Successful percutaneous management of left main trunk occlusion during percutaneous aortic valve replacement. *Catheter Cardiovasc Interv.* 2009; 73(7):966–972.

85. Flecher EM, Curry JW, Joudinaud TM, et al. Coronary flow obstruction in percutaneous aortic valve replacement. An in vitro study. *Eur J Cardiothorac Surg.* 2007;32(2):291–294.

86. Webb JG. Coronary obstruction due to transcatheter valve implantation. *Catheter Cardiovasc Interv.* 2009;73(7):973.

87. Geist V, Sherif MA, Khattab AA. Successful percutaneous coronary intervention after implantation of a CoreValve percutaneous aortic valve. *Catheter Cardiovasc Interv.* 2009;73(1):61–67.

88. Webb JG, Pasupati S, Humphries K, et al. Percutaneous transarterial aortic valve replacement in selected high-risk patients with aortic stenosis. *Circulation.* 2007;116(7):755–763.

89. Webb JG, Altwegg L, Masson JB, et al. A new transcatheter aortic valve and percutaneous valve delivery system. *J Am Coll Cardiol.* 2009;53(20): 1855–1858.

90. Piazza N, Grube E, Gerckens U, et al. Procedural and 30-day outcomes following transcatheter aortic valve implantation using the third generation (18 Fr CoreValve ReValving System: results from the multicentre, expanded evaluation registry 1-year following CE mark approval). *Eurointervention.* 2008;4:242–249.

91. Taramasso M, Sharp AS, Maisano F. First-in-man case report of the use of an Edwards-Sapien valve to treat a regurgitant CoreValve aortic valve prosthesis. *Catheter Cardiovasc Interv.* 2010; 75(1):51–55.

92. Falk V, Schwammenthal EE, Kempfert J, et al. New anatomically oriented transapical aortic valve implantation. *Ann Thorac Surg.* 2009;87(3): 925–926.

93. Quaden R, Attmann T, Schünke M, et al. Percutaneous aortic valve replacement: endovascular resection of human aortic valves in situ. *J Thorac Cardiovasc Surg.* 2008;135(5):1081–1086.

94. Bombien R, Hümme T, Schünke M, Lutter G. Percutaneous aortic valve replacement: computed tomography scan after valved stent implantation in human cadaver hearts. *Eur J Cardiothorac Surg.* 2009;36(3):592–594.

95. Wendt D, Stuhle S, Wendt H, et al. Cutting precision in a novel aortic valve resection tool. Research in progress. *Interact Cardiovasc Thorac Surg.* 2009;9(4):672–676.

96. Lima RC, Wimmer-Greinecker G, Costa MG, et al. Chemical demineralization of the aortic valve: a potential application and preliminary clinical experience. *Rev Bras Cir Cardiovasc.* [online] 2006;21(2):194–197.

97. Ohashi KL, Culkar J, Riebman JB, et al. Hemodynamic characterization of calcified stenotic human aortic valves before and after treatment with a novel aortic valve repair system. *J Heart Valve Dis.* 2004;13(4):582–592.

98. Ye J, Cheung A, Lichtenstein SV, et al. Transapical aortic valve implantation in humans. *J Thorac Cardiovasc Surg* 2006;131(5):1194–1196.

99. Ye J, Cheung A, Lichtenstein SV, Altwegg LA, et al. Transapical transcatheter aortic valve implantation: 1-year outcome in 26 patients. *J Thorac Cardiovasc Surg.* 2009;137(1):167–173.

100. Al-Attar N, Ghodbane W, Himbert D, et al. Unexpected complications of transapical aortic valve implantation. *Ann Thorac Surg.* 2009; 88(1):90–94.

101. Zierer A, Wimmer-Greinecker G, Martens S, Moritz A, Doss M. The transapical approach for aortic valve implantation. *J Thorac Cardiovasc Surg.* 2008;136(4):948–953.

102. de Isla LP, Rodriguez E, Zamorano J. Transapical aortic prosthesis misplacement. *J Am Coll Cardiol.* 2008;52(24):2043.

103. Strauch JT, Kuhn E, Haldenwang PL, Wahlers T. Pulmonary trunk perforation during transapical minimal invasive aortic valve replacement. *Eur J Cardiothorac Surg.* 2009;35:1094–1095.

104. Clavel MA, Dumont E, Pibarot P, et al. Severe valvular regurgitation and late prosthesis embolization after percutaneous aortic valve implantation. *Ann Thorac Surg.* 2009;87(2):618–621.

105. Gutiérrez M, Rodés-Cabau J, Bagur R, et al. Electrocardiographic changes and clinical outcomes after transapical aortic valve implantation. *Am Heart J.* 2009;158(2):302–308.

106. Himbert D, Descoutures F, Al-Attar N, et al. Results of transfemoral or transapical aortic valve implantation following a uniform assessment in high-risk patients with aortic stenosis. *J Am Coll Cardiol.* 2009;54(4):303–311.

Transcatheter Closure of Atrial Septal Defects and Patent Foramen Ovale

MAMATA M. ALWARSHETTY, QI-LING CAO, CLIFFORD J. KAVINSKY, AND ZIYAD M. HIJAZI

Transcatheter closure has now become an accepted treatment modality for most patients with secundum type atrial septal defects (ASD). Transcatheter closure of patent foramen ovale (PFO) is feasible; however, currently there are no approved devices to close PFOs. Therefore, many devices are widely used off-label. The results of randomized trials comparing medical therapy to device closure of PFOs are pending at the time of writing of this chapter. Transcatheter closure of ASDs and PFOs is safe and carries very little risk (1,2). However, there are potential complications that one needs to be aware of, if embarking on device closure of atrial communications.

There are various devices (approved & investigational) that can be used to close such defects. Full knowledge of the engineering aspects of the devices, techniques involved, and results and outcomes are essential to avoid and manage complications encountered during or after device closure. In this chapter, we will discuss the various devices used, the protocol of deployment, and the potential complications involved and their management.

■ DEVICES

Amplatzer Septal Occluder

The Amplatzer Septal Occluder (ASO) (AGA Medical Corp, Plymouth, MN) is a self-expandable, self-centering double disk device made of a nitinol wire mesh. It was the first device to be approved by the United States FDA for clinical use in 2001. It has three parts: a left atrial disc, right atrial disc, and a connecting waist. The device is made of a 0.004 to 0.0075″ nitinol wire mesh woven into two flat discs. The two discs extend radially from the central connecting waist that provides secure anchorage. Polyester fabric fills all three components. The length of the connecting waist corresponds to the thickness of the interatrial septum and is 3 to 4 mm. The device size denotes the diameter of the waist. The ASO comes in various sizes ranging from 4 to 40 mm [the 40 mm is not approved in the US] (1-mm increments for 4–20 mm size and then 2-mm increments for sizes 20–40 mm). As patients with an ASD usually have left to right shunt, the left atrial disc is larger than the right atrial disc. A stainless steel sleeve is welded to the right atrial disk and is used to screw the device to the delivery cable. The entire nitinol device is stretched into a linear form and placed inside a sheath for delivery. Upon delivery the device regains its original shape. A 6- to 14-Fr delivery system is used for deployment depending on the size of the ASO (3–5).

Amplatzer Cribriform Device

The Amplatzer Cribriform Device is similar to all Amplatzer family of devices; the Cribriform device is made of nitinol wire mesh. This device was approved for multifenestrated ASDs. The connecting waist is thin and 3 mm in length. The left and right atrial disks are equal in size.

Starflex and CardioSEAL Devices

The Starflex (SF) and CardioSEAL devices (NMT Medical Corp., Boston, MA) are improved versions of the original Clamshell device. They consist of two square umbrellas connected to each other in the center. The SF has a self-centering mechanism made of a nitinol microspring, which is attached to alternating sides of the umbrella arm tips and provides a self-adjusting positioning mechanism that assists to centrally locate the implant within the defect. This increases apposition of the implant arms to the septal wall. They are available in sizes from 23 to 40 mm and require 11- to 14-Fr sheath for delivery (6).

Helex Device

The Helex device (WL Gore, Flagstaff, AZ) is a double disk made of two opposing spirals made of 0.012″ nitinol wire frame covered with hydrophilic ePTFE. The two spirals sit on either side of the septum when deployed. It has a pre-assembled delivery system (rapid exchange) and requires an 11-Fr short venous introducer sheath for delivery. It is available in sizes ranging from 15 to 35 mm, with 5-mm increments.

BioSTAR

BioSTAR is the world's first bioabsorbable septal repair implant manufactured by NMT. It is not yet approved in the United States (7).

Amplatzer PFO Occluder

The Amplatzer PFO Occluder is similar to the ASD ASO occluder except that it has a thin waist and the right atrial disk is larger than the left disk. It is available in three sizes: 18/18 mm, 18/25 mm, and 25/35 mm.

Other Devices

A few other devices are used for closure of the atrial communications. The predominant ones are as follows:

- The Figulla-Occlutech device is manufactured by Occlutech (Occlutech GmbH, Jena,

Germany) and is similar to the Amplatzer but has no microscrew in the left atrial disk and uses a different attachment mechanism to the delivery cable.
- The Solysafe device manufactured by Swissimplant (Switzerland) is made of Cobalt wire with two disks attached.
- The Cardia Atrisept device is made by Cardia Medical (Minnesota).

■ PATIENT SELECTION

Patients with secundum type ASD that meet the following criteria are eligible for device closure:

- Size less than 40 mm by balloon sizing, depending on the size of the patient and the length of the atrial septum. Generally, a defect: septal length ratio of less than or equal to 50% is acceptable.
- Presence of sufficient rims of about 7 mm all around the defect, except in the anterior aspect is required. Therefore, the superior, inferior, and posterior rims have to be about 5 to 7 mm. However, there have been cases that underwent successful device closure with insufficient rims (8).
- The patient has to be of appropriate weight, that is, greater than 8 kg. However, lower weight patients have undergone successful device closure (9).

Contraindications for device closure of ASDs include the following:

- Sinus venosus defect
- Primum ASD
- Associated anomalous pulmonary venous drainage
- Deficient rims
- Pulmonary vascular resistance greater than 8 Wood units
- Contraindication to antiplatelet therapy
- Other planned cardiac surgery

Currently, there is no approved device to close a PFO. However, the off-label use has been practiced and generally any patient who sustained a transient ischemic attack, stroke, or peripheral embolism with a PFO and right to left shunt is eligible for device closure. The use of PFO devices in the United States is limited to the randomized trials. (i) CLOSURE: This randomized trial is now completed and is awaiting results. The randomization is between medical therapy and the CardioSEAL device; (ii) RESPECT: This trial is enrolling patients and randomizing patients between medical therapy and the Amplatzer PFO device; (iii) REDUCE trial: Still enrolling and randomizing patients between medical therapy and the Gore Helex device.

■ PREOPERATIVE EVALUATION

Assessing the type, size, rims, and number of ASDs prior to catheterization is key to planning device closure. Transthoracic echocardiography (TTE), transesophageal echocardiography (TEE) will help to define the anterior, posterior, inferior, and superior rims.

3D echocardiography is being used more frequently to guide device closure of ASDs. Real-time 3D TEE in addition to assisting with sizing of the defect has the added advantage of en face visualization of the ASD, allowing precise assessment of complex shaped ASDs (10).

Intracardiac echocardiography (ICE) is now the preferred imaging modality to guide device closure of PFOs and ASDs in many cardiac centers. It offers the major advantage of not requiring anesthesia. The images obtained compare very favorably to those obtained by TEE (11).

The catheter being used most commonly is the AcuNav (Siemens Medical Systems) and is available in two sizes: the 8- and 11-Fr. We use the 8-Fr exclusively in our center. Images obtained using the 8-Fr are comparable to those obtained using the 11-Fr (12).

■ SURGICAL PROCEDURE

While there are slight variations in the actual technique for the various devices, the basic requirements are similar across techniques.

The procedure can be done in a monoplane imaging laboratory. Some operators prefer to use biplane catheter laboratory imaging system. We use monoplane for all ASDs and PFOs without any problem.

Required equipment and personnel include the following:

- TEE or ICE.
- Appropriate sizing balloons (AGA, NuMED, or Meditech), devices, and delivery and rescue catheters. The AGA and NuMED sizing balloons are used for stationary sizing, and the Meditech balloons are used for the pull technique.
- Multipurpose catheter to engage the defect and left upper PV.
- 0.035 exchange length super-stiff wire with a floppy tip.
- Interventional and noninvasive cardiologists, anesthesiologist, nurse, catheterization laboratory technicians, in-house back-up cardiovascular surgeon.

The patient is given 81 mg of aspirin 48 hours prior to the procedure. Antiplatelet therapy continues for at least 6 months post procedure.

Transcatheter Closure Technique

The right femoral vein is accessed percutaneously. If ICE is used and the patient's weight is more than 35 kg, we puncture the femoral vein few millimeters below the first puncture. However, in patients weighing less than 35 kg, ICE is introduced in the contralateral femoral vein. For the diagnostic/interventional part of the procedure, a 7- to 8-Fr short sheath is used. For the ICE, as indicated earlier, we use the 8-Fr catheter. If the femoral vein is not feasible, transhepatic access is the next best option for large ASDs and perhaps the right internal jugular vein if for PFO. After the venous access is secured, we administer heparin in a dose of 3000 to 5000 units for adults (50–100 units/kg for children) to keep the activated clotting time (ACT) greater than 200 seconds at the time of device deployment.

An echocardiogram, either TEE or ICE is performed after the hemodynamic assessment. The purpose of the echocardiogram is to assess the suitability of the defect for device closure. Particular attention is paid to the defect size and the size of the surrounding rims. As mentioned above, all except the anterior rim should be at least 5 mm in length. Echocardiography is essential when measuring the "stop-flow" diameter of the defect using a balloon. The balloon is positioned across the defect over a wire positioned in the left upper pulmonary vein. The balloon is inflated until there is cessation of shunt. Once there is cessation of flow, the echocardiographer freezes the frame and measures the diameter of the balloon. For the ASO, the device size chosen should be ±1 mm of that size.

For an ASD closure, some operators perform an angiogram in the right upper pulmonary vein in the four-chamber view to profile the atrial septum. When the device is deployed across the defect, prior to release of the device, fluoroscopy is performed in the same view as the angiogram. A good device position is manifested by parallel disks to the atrial septum. If the device position is good by echocardiography, a gentle tug/push on the device (Minnesota wiggle) is performed. A stable device position is assured by the lack of device movement. Once the device position is ascertained, the device is released by counterclockwise rotation of the delivery cable using the pin vise provided with the cable.

Device Selection

ASO

Generally, a device sized $+/-$ 1 mm of the balloon stretched diameter (stop-flow) is chosen if all rims are adequate. If the anterior/superior rim is deficient we recommend the use of a device 2 mm larger than the stop-flow diameter.

Starflex

A 2:1 ratio between the device and balloon-stretched diameter is generally used.

Helex

The recommended device to defect size ratio is 1.8 to 2:1 and the largest defect that can be closed with this device is 18 mm in diameter.

Amplatzer PFO Occluder

We generally do not perform balloon sizing and rely heavily on the measurement of the distance between the aortic wall and the tip of septum secundum in short axis and the entry of the SVC and the tip of the superior rim in bicaval view. The instruction for use provided with the device highlights these measurements.

Large Atrial Septal Defects

Transcatheter closure of large ASDs is challenging. There are different techniques used to align the left disk to the atrial septum. Such techniques include the following:

■ The use of the Hausdorf sheath. This sheath is available in sizes 10-, 11-, and 12-Fr. It has specially designed curves at the tip to allow

positioning of the left atrial disk to be parallel to the atrial septum.
■ Deployment of the left disk in either the left or right upper pulmonary veins. One has to be careful performing this technique.
■ Use of the dilator-assisted technique (13).
■ Use of the balloon-assisted technique (14).

■ RESULTS

In one case series, implantation of the device was successful in 100 of 106 patients attempted, for a 94% procedural success rate. In five of the remaining patients, the ASD was too large or had inadequate tissue rims for stable implantation of the device. These patients had uncomplicated procedures and went on to surgical closure (15).

■ COMPLICATIONS AND BAILOUT TECHNIQUES

The safety of device closure of ASD has been evaluated in many studies, and comparison with open heart surgery demonstrated that device closure is safer than open heart surgery. In the study that led to the approval of the ASO in the United States, device closure had 7.2% incidence of complications compared to 24% by open heart surgery (1).

Device Migration "Embolization"

This is a rare complication and is reported in less than 1% (0.55%) of cases, regardless of ASD size, device size, or the physician's expertise (16,17). The reported sites of embolization include the right ventricle, pulmonary artery, left ventricle, arch of aorta, and peripheral vessels. Of the 33 cases of ASO embolization that have been reported in the literature, percutaneous retrieval was successful in 17 (about 50%): 4 from the right atrium, 2 from the right ventricle, 4 from the pulmonary artery, 4 from the left atrium, 2 from the aorta, and one from the left ventricle (18).

Deficient rims are the most common cause for device migration. This usually does not cause acute hemodynamic collapse and clinical decline. Embolization to the left ventricle can cause ventricular arrhythmias as well as damage to the mitral or aortic valve during the retrieval process. Percutaneous retrieval of the embolized device is possible in about 50% of cases, and several techniques have been used.

The sheath should be upsized by at least 2-Fr greater than the delivery sheath to snare and retrieve the migrated device. A gooseneck snare (ev3, Plymouth, MN), ENSNARE, or bioptomes (2) can be used to capture the device. The device can also be retrieved using the femoral artery approach to reach the left ventricle. Surgical intervention may be necessary if the operator does not have the proper equipment or if the device cannot be caught in the proper place (microscrew). To snare an embolized device, the operator has to use a long sheath (at least 2-F sizes larger than the delivery sheath) and position this sheath as close as possible to the device. The snare catheter is then introduced inside the sheath. We usually use the 10-mm snare for small devices and the 15 to 25 mm for the larger devices. Capture the microscrew of the right atrial disk with the snare and bring the snared device inside the delivery sheath. We recommend not pulling a snared device through valves or vessels; this may result in injury to these structures. We always pull the snared device inside the long sheath. On occasions, the microscrew of the right atrial disk is facing in a direction opposite to that of the snare. In such situations, we manipulate the device with a catheter to flip the disks so that the right atrial microscrew is facing the snare (Fig. 22-1).

Air Embolism

Meticulous attention to details can prevent this complication. When advancing the delivery sheath to the left upper pulmonary vein, at the right atrial-IVC junction, the dilator is removed and the sheath is advanced over the guidewire while flushing the side arm of the sheath. Once the guidewire is removed, position the sheath between the patient's legs and lower it below the level of the left atrium to allow free flowing of blood from the pulmonary vein to the sheath. Air can go to the left circulation, usually to the left ventricle or coronary arteries resulting in ischemic changes in the electrocardiogram. Air can also go to the brain causing a stroke. If an air embolism is detected, the patient is placed on 100% oxygen. If there is air that can be seen in the coronaries, one can attempt to flush the coronaries with saline. If there is air in the left ventricle, one can attempt to advance a catheter into the left ventricle and aspirate blood.

Transient Ischemic Attack or Stroke

This rare complication occurs in less than 1% of the patients. Again, meticulous attention to details is of paramount importance to prevent this from happening. Embolization of small clots that form on the sheath or device may be the culprit. Keeping the ACT greater than 200 seconds at the time of device deployment is

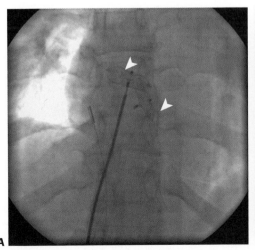
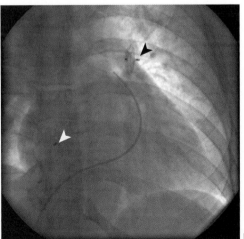

FIGURE 22-1. This patient had an ASD (white arrowheads) closed with two ASOs. One of the devices embolized to the LPA (black arrowhead). The location of the embolized ASO was confirmed by pulmonary angiography.

important. Further, all patients should receive antiplatelet therapy commencing 48 hours prior to and continue for at least a 6-month post device closure. In adult patients, we add Clopidogrel to the aspirin for 2 to 3 months. If one diagnoses a stroke, a neurology consult must be done ASAP and further work-up is begun including a MRI/CT of the head. On rare occasions, cerebral angiography is done, and if a clot is seen rt-PA is administered.

Thrombus Formation

The incidence of thrombus formation is 1.2% in ASD patients and 2.5% in PFO patients in a study of 1000 patients who underwent percutaneous device closure (19) Postprocedure atrial fibrillation and persistent atrial septal aneurysm were significant predictors of thrombus formation. The Amplatzer device with nitinol wire covered with ePTFE fabric is less thrombogenic than CardioSEAL and StarFLEX devices, which have a metallic framework with Dacron fabric. Patients should get a follow up TTE/TEE 4 to 6 months after implantation. Patients generally are on antiplatelet therapy, aspirin (81 mg per day) for 6 months, and Clopidogrel (75 mg per day) for 1 month post implantation. Heparin dosed to keep the ACT more than 200 seconds is

important to prevent this complication. Additionally, antiplatelet therapy as above is essential to prevent clots from forming. Patients with thrombus seen on the device can be managed with anticoagulation for 6 months to 1 year. A repeat TEE to confirm resolution of the thrombus is essential prior to discontinuing the therapy (Fig. 22-2).

Erosion, Pericardial Effusion, Tamponade, and Death

This is the most feared complication. Cardiac perforation is a very rare, life-threatening complication of transcatheter ASD and PFO closure. The incidence of cardiac perforation after the placement of an ASO is approximately 0.1% (20). Cardiac perforation due to an Amplatzer PFO occluder is even rarer, reported in only three patients in the literature (20,21). Cardiac erosion/perforation of an ASO occurred predominantly in the anterosuperior atrial walls and/or adjacent aortic root. It has been hypothesized that the ASO transmits deformative forces at the point of contact between the device, the anterosuperior atrial wall, and the aorta, which may result in cardiac perforation (20).

Patients with device-related cardiac perforation present with sudden death or hemoperi-

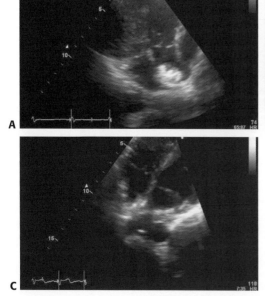

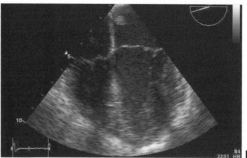

FIGURE 22-2. (**A**) Thrombus seen on the left atrial side of an Amplatzer PFO occluder greater than 6 months after closure. (**B**) TEE image of thrombus. (**C**) The patient was treated with heparin initially and oral anticoagulation with warfarin and showed resolution of thrombus at 1 month.

cardium/pericardial effusion and cardiovascular collapse. Late erosions occurred in 66.6%; 25% presented weeks later (longest, three years); three deaths were reported (22). The registry review by Amin et al. suggests a relationship between device oversizing, deficient anterosuperior rims, and cardiac perforation (20). On rare occasions, perforation can occur due to wire/catheter manipulation. Obviously, meticulous technique can avoid such complications. We believe appropriate sizing and device selection is important to avoid this complication. Therefore, we recommend performing balloon sizing to measure the "stop-flow" diameter and to choose a device no more than 2 mm larger than this diameter.

Defects with deficient anterior–superior rim are at risk of developing erosions. To minimize this, we recommend appropriate sizing. If the size of the device chosen is more than 40% of the 2D echocardiographic diameter of the defect, we recommend repeat balloon sizing. In general, if the device size is no more 35% larger than the 2D diameter of the defect, we believe the risk of erosion is extremely rare.

We recommend keeping all patients overnight. The following morning a repeat TTE is done to look for device position and presence or absence of pericardial effusion. If there is a new pericardial effusion, we recommend keeping the patient inhouse to repeat a TTE in 12 hours to see if the effusion is enlarging. Further, all patients who receive devices should be instructed about sudden onset of new, unusual symptoms such as shortness of breath, chest tightness, dizziness, and chest pain. Should they encounter such sudden symptoms, they should seek immediate help. The first test that should be done is a TTE to look for pericardial effusion. If the diagnosis is made, obviously, management depends on the extent of fluid collection in the pericardium and the patient's symptoms.

Arrhythmias, Conduction Abnormalities, and Complete Heart Block

Approximately 5% of patients may develop rhythm disturbances ranging from premature atrial contractions to supraventricular tachycardia and atrial fibrillation. Supraventricular ectopy is the most common electrical disturbance noted in up to 63% in one of the case series (23). If the patient develops atrial fibrillation, we recommend medical management, unless the patient is unstable. If unstable, cardioversion is recommended but attention to device position is important. In one of our patients, who developed atrial fibrillation immediately after the device was released, cardioversion with 200 joules resulted in device migration. Short episodes of supraventricular tachycardia can be treated with beta-blockers for 3 to 6 months. Usually, such episodes resolve in a few months. Heart block is extremely rare after device closure of ASD. We recommend that if complete heart block occurs, treatment with high-dose steroids and high-dose aspirin for few days be done. If the rhythm is not restored to sinus, we recommend surgical removal of the device and closure of the defect surgically.

Endocarditis

This is an extremely rare complication. We recommend giving antibiotic prophylaxis during the procedure and two more doses. If the patient has a history of endocarditis in the past 6 months, they should not undergo device closure and instead wait for at least 6 months prior to device implantation.

Headaches/Migraines

Up to 10% of patients may experience unusual headaches/migraines. The exact etiology is not known. Treatment with Clopidogrel for 2 to 3 months after device closure has minimized this complication.

Device Fracture

This has been reported with the cardioSEAL and also less frequently with the SF. This is more likely with larger devices and clinically a fracture is less likely to be of significance than erosion/perforation due to a chamber being unable to accommodate a device umbrella. Since a 2:1 device to defect sizing ratio is used, it is generally not recommended to be used in a defect larger than 20 mm. The Helex device has very rare incidence of fracture. Fracture of the wireframe occurred in 6.4% of HELEX devices implanted and was most common in large devices. Residual defects following the wire frame fracture became completely occluded or remained clinically insignificant. There were no clinical sequelae reported and the fracture did not alter the function of the HELEX (24).

■ CONCLUSION

Although percutaneous closure of ASD and PFO is a relatively safe procedure, major complications can still occur. Careful patient selection and a meticulous approach to device selection and procedure strategy are mandatory to minimize the risk of complications associated with this procedure.

References

1. Du ZD, Hijazi ZM, Kleinman CS, Amplatzer Investigators, et al. Comparison between transcatheter and surgical closure of secundum atrial septal defect in children and adults: results of a multicenter nonrandomized trial. *J Am Coll Cardiol.* 2002;39(11):1836–1844.
2. Marie Valente A, Rhodes JF. Current indications and contraindications for transcatheter atrial septal defect and patent foramen ovale device closure. *Am Heart J.* 2007;153(4 suppl):81–84.
3. Fu YC, Cao QL, Hijazi ZM. Closure of atrial septal defect using the amplatzer septal occluder. In: Sievert H, Qureshi SA, Wilson N, Hijazi Z, eds. *Percutaneous Interventions in Congenital Heart Disease.* Oxford, UK: Informa Health Care; 2007: 265–275.
4. Masura J, Gavora P, Formanek A, et al. Transcatheter closure of secundum atrial septal defects using the new self-centering amplatzer septal occluder: initial human experience. *Cathet Cardiovasc Diagn.* 1997;42(4):388–393.
5. Omeish A, Hijazi ZM. Transcatheter closure of atrial septal defects in children and adults using the Amplatzer Septal Occluder. *J Interv Cardiol.* 2001;14(1):37–44.
6. Kaulitz R, Paul T, Hausdorf G. Extending the limits of transcatheter closure of atrial septal defects with the double umbrella device (CardioSEAL). *Heart.* 1998;80(1):54–59.
7. Mullen MJ, Hildick-Smith D, De Giovanni JV, et al. BioSTAR evaluation STudy (BEST): a prospective, multicenter, phase I clinical trial to evaluate the feasibility, efficacy, and safety of the BioSTAR bioabsorbable septal repair implant for the closure of atrial-level shunts. *Circulation.* 2006;114(18):1962–1967.
8. Du ZD, Koenig P, Cao QL, et al. Comparison of transcatheter closure of secundum atrial septal defect using the Amplatzer Septal Occluder associated with deficient versus sufficient rims. *Am J Cardiol.* 2002;90(8):865–869.
9. Diab KA, Cao QL, Bacha EA, et al. Device closure of atrial septal defects with the Amplatzer septal occluder: safety and outcome in infants. *J Thorac Cardiovasc Surg.* 2007;134(4):960–966.
10. Lodato JA, Cao QL, Weinert L, et al. Feasibility of real-time three-dimensional transoesophageal echocardiography for guidance of percutaneous atrial septal defect closure. *Eur J Echocardiogr.* 2009;10(4):543–548.
11. Hijazi Z, Wang Z, Cao Q, et al. Transcatheter closure of atrial septal defects and patent foramen ovale under intracardiac echocardiographic guidance: feasibility and comparison with transesophageal echocardiography. *Catheter Cardiovasc Interv.* 2001;52(2):194–199.
12. Luxenberg DM, Silvestry FE, Herrmann HC, et al. Use of a new 8 french intracardiac echocardiographic catheter to guide device closure of atrial septal defects and patent foramen ovale in small children and adults: initial clinical experience. *J Invasive Cardiol.* 2005;17(10):540–545.
13. Wahab HA, Bairam AR, Cao QL, et al. Novel technique to prevent prolapse of the Amplatzer septal occluder through large atrial septal defect. *Catheter Cardiovasc Interv.* 2003;60(4):543–545.
14. Dalvi B, Pinto R, Gupta A. Device closure of large atrial septal defects requiring devices > or = 20 mm in small children weighing <20 kg. *Catheter Cardiovasc Interv.* 2008;71(5):679–686.
15. Herrmann HC, Silvestry FE, Glaser R, et al. Percutaneous patent foramen ovale and atrial septal defect closure in adults: Results and device comparison in 100 consecutive implants at a single center. *Catheter Cardiovasc Interv.* 2005;64(2): 197–203.
16. Tan CA, Levi DS, Moore JW. Embolization and transcatheter retrieval of coils and devices. *Pediatr Cardiol.* 2005;26(3):267–274.
17. Chessa M, Carminati M, Butera G, et al. Early and late complications associated with transcatheter occlusion of secundum atrial septal defect. *J Am Coll Cardiol.* 2002;39(6):1061–1065.
18. Balbi M, Pongiglione G, Bezante GP. Percutaneous rescue of left ventricular embolized Amplatzer septal occluder device. *Catheter Cardiovasc Interv.* 2008;72(4):559–562.

19. Krumsdorf U, Ostermayer S, Billinger K, et al. Incidence and clinical course of thrombus formation on atrial septal defect and patient foramen ovale closure devices in 1,000 consecutive patients. *J Am Coll Cardiol.* 2004;43(2):302–309.

20. Amin Z, Hijazi ZM, Bass JL, et al. Erosion of Amplatzer septal occluder device after closure of secundum atrial septal defects: review of registry of complications and recommendations to minimize future risk. *Catheter Cardiovasc Interv.* 2004;63(4):496–502.

21. Trepels T, Zeplin H, Sievert H, et al. Cardiac perforation following transcatheter PFO closure. *Catheter Cardiovasc Interv.* 2003;58(1):111–113.

22. Divekar A, Gaamangwe T, Shaikh N, et al. Cardiac perforation after device closure of atrial septal defects with the Amplatzer septal occluder. *J Am Coll Cardiol.* 2005;45(8):1213–1218.

23. Hill SL, Berul CI, Patel HT, et al. Early ECG abnormalities associated with transcatheter closure of atrial septal defects using the Amplatzer septal occluder. *J Interv Card Electrophysiol.* 2000; 4(3):469–474.

24. Fagan T, Dreher D, Cutright W, et al; for the Gore HELEX Septal Occluder Working Group. Fracture of the Gore HELEX septal occluder: associated factors and clinical outcomes. *Catheter Cardiovasc Interv.* 2009;73(7):941–948.

23

Pericardiocentesis and Pericardiotomy

SOLOMON SAGER AND MAURO MOSCUCCI

Drainage of pericardial effusions is a relatively uncommon cardiac procedure that is usually performed emergently in the setting of cardiac tamponade. There are multiple catheter-based techniques for draining pericardial effusions: echocardiography-guided pericardiocentesis, fluoroscopy-guided pericardiocentesis, single-balloon pericardiotomy (SBP), double-balloon pericardiotomy, and Inoue balloon pericardiotomy. The surgical creation of a pericardial window is also an option, but it is usually reserved for recurrent effusions and/or effusions that cannot be accessed percutaneously (e.g., posterior fluid collections). Balloon pericardiotomy is increasingly being used as a less invasive alternative to surgical window creation.

Over the past two decades, the exponential increase in the performance of catheter-based cardiac interventions, including coronary interventions, ablation procedures, and other procedures for structural heart disease, has been associated with an increase in the performance of emergency pericardiocentesis for coronary artery and cardiac perforation. Therefore, it is paramount that interventional cardiologists and electrophysiologists are fully familiar with all the aspects pertaining to pericardiocentesis.

◼ PERICARDIOCENTESIS

Percutaneous pericardiocentesis for the treatment of pericardial effusion was originally described in the early 18th century (1). Prior to the introduction of echocardiographic or fluoroscopic guidance, the procedure carried a 20% risk of life-threatening complications (1). The European Society of Cardiology currently recommends echocardiographic or fluoroscopic

guidance as standard of care, adding that electrocardiogram (ECG) injury tracing alone is not an adequate safeguard (2). However, according to a recent survey from the United Kingdom, 11% of cardiologists continue to perform the procedure with no guidance or with ECG tracing only (3).

Echocardiographic Guidance

Echocardiography-guided pericardiocentesis can be performed emergently at the bedside. The ideal entry site is the point at which the distance from skin to maximal fluid accumulation is minimized, with no intervening vital organs; this can be identified echocardiographically (1). In the largest series reported (1127 patients), the ideal entry site was the chest wall in 79% of cases and the subcostal region in 18% of cases. The para-apical approach was the most common chest wall entry site (714/890, 80%). Additional chest wall entry sites included the left axillary, the left and right parasternal, and the posterolateral regions. The pericardial space was entered using a polytef-sheathed needle; upon entry in the space, the needle core was withdrawn and the sheath was advanced. Continuous visualization of the needle tip by echocardiography is unnecessary and frequently not possible. Injection of agitated saline through the sheath can be used to confirm position of the sheath in the pericardial space (Fig. 23-1), particularly when the needle aspirate is hemorrhagic. To avoid post-procedure ventricular dysfunction (see "Complications"), pericardial drainage should be performed as gradually as clinically possible until tamponade physiology has resolved. Symptomatic improvement frequently occurs after aspiration of 50 to 200 mL of

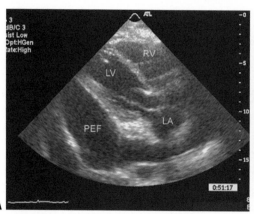 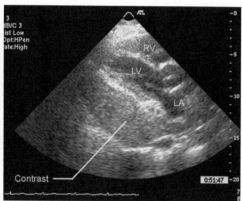

FIGURE 23-1. Parasternal long-axis echocardiogram recorded in a patient with a large posterior pericardial effusion (PEF). Pericardiocentesis is being undertaken with echocardiographic guidance. (**A**) There is a large posterior pericardial fluid collection. (**B**) Agitated saline has been injected via the pericardiocentesis needle. There is now echo contrast in the previously clear pericardial space confirming that the pericardiocentesis needle is in the pericardium. LA, left atrium; LV, left ventricle, RV, right ventricle. (From Armstrong WF, Ryan T. Feigenbaum's Echocardiography, 7th ed. Philadelphia: Lippincott Williams & Wilkins, 2010).

fluid (4). The slow removal of fluid minimizes abrupt fluctuations in loading conditions and wall stress, thus permitting adaptive changes. Extended catheter drainage should be performed on all patients, with prolonged drainage by intermittent aspiration until less than 25 mL per day is drained (2). Prolonged drainage can be performed either using dedicated pericardial drains, or via a pigtail catheter inserted through a sheath. The procedure has a 93% to 97% success rate (1,2).

Fluoroscopy Guidance

Fluoroscopy-guided pericardiocentesis is performed in the cardiac catheterization laboratory, under ECG and pressure monitoring. The subxiphoid approach is most commonly used, with a long needle with a mandrel directed towards the left shoulder at a 30 to 45 degrees angle to the skin (Fig. 23-2). As an alternative, a needle connected to a syringe filled with lidocaine is advanced toward the pericardial space. If hemorrhagic fluid is freely aspirated, injection of contrast medium under fluoroscopic observation may help confirm placement in the pericardial space. Before insertion of the dilator and drainage catheter, it is essential to check the position of the guidewire in at least two angiographic projections (2). As with echocardiography, use of extended catheter drainage is recommended.

Complications of Pericardiocentesis
Recurrence of Effusion

Pericardiocentesis without extended catheter drainage has been associated with recurrence rates of up to 55% (5). Because of this high rate, pericardial surgery was popular in the 1980s for effusion drainage (6). In 1986 Kopecky et al. demonstrated the clinical efficacy of extended catheter drainage, after which rates of catheter-based pericardial drainage increased (6,7). Indeed, Tsang et al. demonstrated that in the

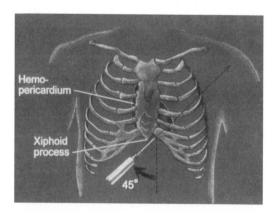

FIGURE 23-2. Schematic representation of the standard sub-xiphoid approach for pericardiocentesis. The procedure is usually performed by inserting a 20-gauge spinal needle below the xiphoid process at a 45-degree angle toward the left shoulder. (From Fleisher GR, Ludwig S, Baskin MN. Atlas of Pediatric Emergency Medicine. Philadelphia, PA: Lippincott Williams & Wilkins, 2004.)

years following the popularization of extended catheter drainage, both primary surgical treatments and recurrences following catheter-based drainage decreased significantly (1). Current estimated rates of recurrence with extended catheter drainage range from 10% to 20% (1,8).

Risk factors for recurrence include large effusion size (based upon echocardiographic assessment or if initial drainage yields > 400 mL of fluid) and malignancy with positive cytology (1,6). Use of extended pericardial catheter drainage decreases the risk of recurrence (1). Although the risk of recurrence is lower with surgical management, surgery confers a much higher morbidity risk to patients, and therefore it should be reserved for refractory effusions.

There are no guidelines for the management of recurrent effusions after extended catheter drainage. Treatment decisions should be guided clinically. Options include repeat pericardiocentesis, the creation of a pericardial window via surgery or via balloon pericardiotomy, and surgical drainage.

Complications Requiring Surgical Intervention

Complications necessitating surgical intervention include ventricular puncture, chamber lacerations, and intercostal and coronary vessel injuries (1,2,6,9). These are reported to occur in ~1% of echocardiography and fluoroscopy-guided procedures (Table 23-1) (1). Rarely, pneumothorax requiring chest tube placement can occur. The use of fluoroscopy can help in detecting the development of pneumothorax during fluoroscopy-guided procedures. Signs and symptoms of pneumothorax might be difficult to distinguish from the signs and symptoms associated with tamponade physiology, as they include agitation, respiratory distress, hypoxia, hypotension, and tachycardia; a chest x-ray post procedure is recommended.

Most cardiologists (81% in one published survey) do not believe onsite cardiothoracic surgery backup is necessary (3).

Left Ventricular Dysfunction

Transient ventricular dysfunction (most frequently left ventricular [LV] dysfunction) is a rare, well-documented, but morbid complication of pericardiocentesis (4,10–14). Each

TABLE 23-1 Major and Minor[a] Complications Following Echocardiography-Guided Pericardiocentesis in 1127 Procedures

Major Complications	14 (1.2%)
Death	1 (0.09%)
Chamber laceration requiring surgery	5 (0.44%)
Injury to intercostal vessels requiring surgery	1 (0.09%)
Pneumothorax requiring chest tube	5 (0.44%)
Ventricular tachycardia	1 (0.09%)
Bacteremia	1 (0.09%)
Minor Complications	40 (3.5%)
Chamber entry	11 (0.97%)
Small pneumothorax	8 (0.71%)
Pleuropericardial fistula	9 (0.8%)
Vasovagal reaction	2 (0.18%)
Nonsustained ventricular tachycardia	2 (0.18%)
Catheter occlusion	8 (0.71%)

[a]Complications were deemed major if intervention was required. Minor complications were those that did not require intervention.
(From Tsang TS, Enriquez-Sarano M, Freeman WK, et al. Consecutive 1127 therapeutic echocardiographically-guided pericardiocenteses: Clinical profile, practice patterns, and outcomes spanning 21 years. *Mayo Clin Proc.* 2002;77:429–436.)

reported case was associated with rapid removal of large volumes of fluid with near-immediate restoration of normal hemodynamic parameters. In one report, the patient had one liter of fluid removed with change in intrapericardial pressure from 17 mmHg to 0 mmHg (13).

The pathophysiology of LV dysfunction following pericardiocentesis is not completely understood. Animal models and one human study have shown that there is a continuous decline in coronary blood flow with increasing pericardial pressures, suggesting transient myocardial stunning as a possible etiology (15). Van Dyck et al. postulated that the LV dysfunction is a result of acute hemodynamic changes following relief of tamponade (14). Rapid drainage of a large effusion releases the compression of the right heart and produces a sudden increase in venous return. The subsequent diastolic volume overload of the left ventricle, combined with the elevated systemic vascular resistance (due to adrenergic stimulation), causes LV dysfunction.

A third hypothesis suggests that drainage of the pericardial effusion unmasks underlying LV dysfunction, which was obscured due to the high catecholamine levels produced during tamponade (13). Nearly all authors agree that rapid drainage of large amounts of fluid contributes to the development of post-pericardiocentesis LV dysfunction.

Treatment of patients with LV dysfunction and pulmonary edema following pericardiocentesis includes diuresis, vasodilator therapy, and blood pressure support as clinically indicated. With the exception of one fatal case, all case reports demonstrate complete resolution of the LV dysfunction within 10 days. The fatality occurred in a 19-year-old woman with chronic traumatic pericardial effusion who had 1.6 liters drained emergently (10).

Right Ventricular Dysfunction

Both dilation of the right ventricle (RV) and severe RV dysfunction have been reported following pericardiocentesis (16,17). Like LV dysfunction, the development of RV dysfunction has also been reported as self-limiting. However, it does carry considerable morbidity. Anguera et al. reported a patient with severe depression of RV contractility and marked dilatation resulting in cardiogenic shock. The patient needed 72 hours of high-dose inotropic drugs, but completely recovered systolic and diastolic function within 10 days (16).

The etiology of RV dilatation and failure after pericardiocentesis is not completely understood but is postulated to be similar to that of LV dysfunction. Armstrong et al. initially proposed that the abrupt increase in venous return after relief of tamponade may play a role in muscular injury (17). Anguera et al. add that the transient myocardial ischemia induced by tamponade, as discussed in the preceding text, may explain the phenomenon as well (16).

Arrhythmias

Vasovagal bradycardia is not uncommon. Ventricular tachycardia has also been reported (2).

Other Complications

Internal mammary artery fistulas, pneumopericardium (Fig. 23-3), purulent pericarditis, and pleural effusions have been reported, as well as bacteremia (2). Transient entry of the right ventricle may occur without deleterious sequelae as

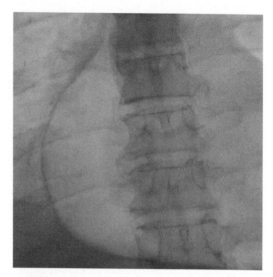

FIGURE 23-3. Pneumopericardium following pericardiocentesis.

long as it is recognized before insertion of the dilator and of the pericardial drain (6).

■ PERICARDIOTOMY

Percutaneous balloon pericardiotomy was first reported by Palacios et al. in 1991 using a single-balloon technique (18). Modification of the procedure has included dilatation at two adjacent pericardial sites, use of the Inoue balloon catheter, and the use of a double-balloon technique (19,20). Reports of multiple small series demonstrate the efficacy of the technique in treating large pericardial effusions and especially malignancy-related effusions. For nonmalignant effusions, the literature is conflicting on the safety profile. Primary management of large effusions and tamponade using balloon pericardiotomy yields similar success rates, complications, and recurrence profiles when compared with simple pericardiocentesis (21) (Table 23-2). However, there is no prospective data on the subject. Operator experience should be considered in clinical decision-making.

Single-Balloon Pericardiotomy

The SBP procedure is well described in the literature (18,20). Antibiotic prophylaxis with intravenous flucloxacillin or equivalent has been recommended (21). Using the subxiphoid approach, a pigtail pericardial drain is inserted. After draining the fluid, the pericardial space is

TABLE 23-2 **Comparison of Complication and Recurrence Rates for Pericardiocentesis and Single-Balloon Pericardiotomy in a Case Series Including 43 Patients**

	Balloon Pericardiotomy	Pericardiocentesis	P Value
Number	27/43 (63%)	14/43 (33%)	
Complications	2/27 (7.4%)	1/14 (7.1%)	0.98
Recurrences	2/27 (7.4%)[a]	2/14 (14.3%)[b]	0.48

[a]Recurrences at 61 and 166 days after initial procedure in SBP group.
[b]Recurrences at 10 and 4 days after initial procedure in pericardiocentesis group.
(Adapted from Swanson N, Mirza I, Wijesinghe N, et al. Primary percutaneous balloon pericardiotomy for malignant pericardial effusion. *Catheter Cardiovasc Interv.* 2008;71:504–507.)

delineated with contrast. A balloon angioplasty catheter (20 mm diameter, 3 to 4 cm long) is introduced into the pericardial space and inflated several times) until waisting of the balloon by the pericardium disappears (Figs. 23-4 and 23-5) (21). It is important to ensure that the proximal end of the balloon is inflated beyond the skin entry site and the subcutaneous tissues. Injection of contrast media can help in delineating the pericardial space and in

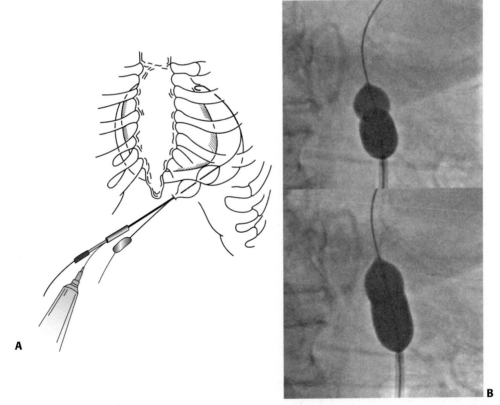

A

B

FIGURE 23-4. (**A**) Illustration of the percutaneous balloon pericardiotomy technique. After partial drainage of the pericardium using a pericardial catheter, a 0.038-inch stiff J-tip wire is introduced into the pericardial space. A 3-cm long dilating balloon is then advanced over the guidewire to straddle the parietal pericardial membrane and is manually inflated to create a rent in the pericardium. (**B**) Still frames from a percutaneous balloon pericardiotomy. (Reprinted from Ziskind AA, Pearce AC, Lemmon CC, et al. Percutaneous balloon pericardiotomy for the treatment of cardiac tamponade and large pericardial effusions: Description of technique and report of the first 50 cases. *J Am Coll Cardiol.* 1993;21:1, with permission from Elsevier.)

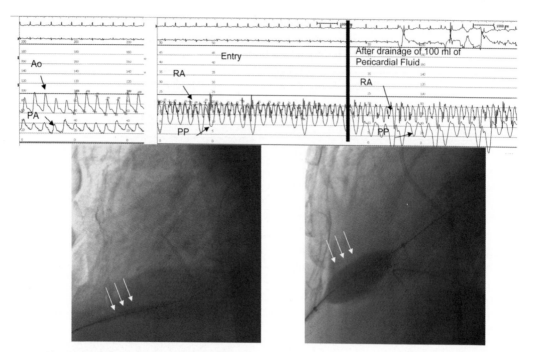

FIGURE 23-5. Patient with recurrent pericardial tamponade undergoing balloon pericardiotomy. (**Top left**) Aortic (Ao) and pulmonary artery pressure tracing showing narrow pulse pressure and a paradoxical pulse on Ao pressure tracing. (**Top middle**) Right atrial (RA) and pericardial pressure (PP) displayed simultaneously, showing an elevated PP with some separation of pericardial and right atrial pressure unlike initial tap, which showed equalization. (**Top right**) Post removal of 100 mL of bloody fluid, PP decreased significantly. At end of procedure, PP decreased further and became negative. (**Bottom left**) The pericardium and tract were dilated with a small balloon (predilation), which is often not necessary with newer low-profile peripheral balloons. (**Bottom right**) The pericardium is dilated with a larger balloon (15 × 40 mm) to achieve an adequate pericardiotomy. Balloons as large as 20 mm in diameter can be used in larger patients. (From Donald S. Baim, Grossman's Cardiac Catheterization, Angiography, and Intervention, 7th ed. Philadelphia, PA: Lippincott Williams & Wilkins, 2006.)

ensuring that the balloon is across the pericardial margin. Ziskind et al. attempted to achieve visualization of free exit of contrast from the pericardium. However, they did not find a correlation between free exit of contrast and procedure success, and therefore this is probably not necessary (20). Analgesia with intravenous opiates should be used because procedure-related pain is common. Failure of the proximal end of the balloon to expand might indicate that the pericardium is apposed to the chest wall. In this case Ziskind et al. have described a technique in which the balloon catheter is gently advanced while counter traction is applied to the skin.

Inoue Balloon Pericardiotomy

The first revision reported to the single-balloon technique was the use of the low-profile Inoue

balloon for the same technique (22–25). The Inoue balloon is unique in that inflation occurs first at the distal portion of the balloon and then at the proximal portion. Positioning of the balloon catheter at the parietal pericardium can be achieved by pulling back the catheter with the distal portion inflated until resistance is felt; this precludes the need for injecting contrast material into the pericardial cavity to outline parietal pericardium (22). Case reports in the literature have described the use of the Inoue balloon for recurrent pericardial effusion, as a substitute to surgical window. Ohke et al. suggest that because of the high cost of the Inoue balloon, the procedure should be reserved for recurrent effusions (23).

Several case reports have suggested that, there is less pain with this procedure than classic SBP, and this may be due to the ease with which the operator can position the Inoue balloon. The procedure has been performed without sedation (24), and must be performed under fluoroscopy. If being performed when a pericardial pigtail catheter is in place, the guidewire can be inserted through the catheter. Following dilation of the skin insertion site, the Inoue balloon catheter can be exchanged over the guidewire and advanced into the pericardial space. Three inflations are recommended to ensure adequate opening of the pericardium.

Double-Balloon Pericardiotomy

First described by Iaffaldano in 1995, the double-balloon technique is also a safe procedure for pericardial fluid drainage (26). Theoretically, it is more efficacious than the single-balloon technique, because the pericardium that is resistant to single-balloon dilation can successfully be dilated with two balloons (20). However, no study exists comparing the two techniques. The procedure has been described by Wang et al. (Fig. 23-6). After drainage of the pericardial fluid, two J-tip guidewires are then advanced through the same sheath; this sheath is then removed and replaced by two sheaths, one along each of the two guidewires. An 8- to 12-mm by 2-cm balloon and an 8- to 12-mm by 4-cm balloon are advanced into the pericardial space over the guidewires. The guidewires separate from each other after they enter the pericardial cavity; this separation point can be visualized under fluoroscopy and indicates the pericardial border. After partial inflation of the balloons, their locations should be adjusted to place the centers at the pericardial border. The two balloons are inflated simultaneously until their waists disappear; while holding the longer balloon still, the shorter one is pushed and pulled across the pericardium to ensure creation of an adequate window.

A chest x-ray should be performed after removal of the pigtail to evaluate for pneumothorax and pleural effusion.

Complications of Balloon Pericardiotomy

Risk Factors for Complications

Many patients undergoing balloon pericardiotomy are acutely ill and no absolute contraindications exist. However, the procedure should probably be avoided or postponed if INR is greater than 2 or platelet count is less than $50 \times 10^9/L$ (27). Most of the series in the literature have included patients with malignant pericardial effusions, and long-term outcomes

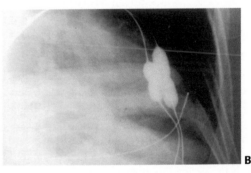

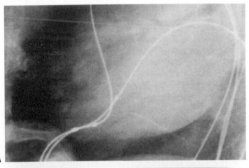

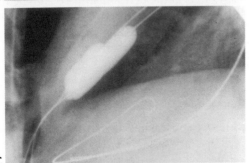

FIGURE 23-6. Double-balloon technique for balloon pericardiotomy. (**A**) The pericardial border can be defined clearly as the two guidewires in the same tract separate from each other after entering. (**B**) Double balloons were straddled over the pericardium and partially inflated, showing a central waist appearance. (**C**) Fully expanded double balloons creating a pericardial window. (From Iaffaldano BA, Jones P, Lewis BE et al. Percutaneous balloon pericardiotomy: A double-balloon technique. *Cathet Cardiovasc Diagn* 1995;36:79–81, with permission.)

TABLE 23-3 Effusion Type, Complication Rates, and Recurrences in the Four Largest Published Series of Balloon Pericardiotomy

Series	n	Type	Major Complication	Minor Complication	Recurrence
Swanson et al. (21)	27	Malignant	1 periprocedural stroke and death	1 pneumopericardium	2a
Wang et al. (19)	50	Malignant	1 broken balloon, patient needed surgical window	7 pleural effusion and PTX	5b
Del Barrio et al. (27)	11	9 malignant 1 post heart transplant 1 idiopathic	1 RV perforation requiring surgical window in idiopathic	7 pleural effusions	2c
Ziskind et al. (20)	50	44 malignant 2 idiopathic 1 uremic 1 HIV 1 viral 1 hypothyroid	1 Bleeding requiring surgery in uremic patient	8 pleural effusions	3d
TOTAL	**138**		**4**	**23**	**12**

aOne patient required repeat SBP and one required simple aspiration only.
bAll went for either repeat double-balloon pericardiotomy or surgical window.
cHeart transplant patient required surgical window; one malignant effusion had repeat SBP.
dAll three required surgical intervention.

in this patient population are not as promising as in patients with nonmalignant effusions (Table 23-3). At this time, it has been suggested that the procedure should be reserved for malignant disease.

Recurrence of Effusion

Following balloon pericardiotomy, effusions recur 5% to 10% of the time. Swanos et al. performed a retrospective comparison of balloon pericardiotomy with simple pericardiocentesis. There was a trend toward a lower recurrence rate in the pericardiotomy group when compared with the pericardiocentesis group (Table 23-2). Moreover, time to recurrence was longer in the pericardiotomy group.

Complications Requiring Surgical Intervention

Major technical complications of balloon pericardiotomy are uncommon and are similar to those described for pericardiocentesis (Table 23-3). Wang et al. reported one major complication, balloon breakage that necessitated surgical pericardiotomy for removal (19).

There are reports of RV perforation requiring surgical intervention (21), and one report of stroke and subsequent death (though whether or not the stroke was a result of the procedure is unclear) (19).

Balloon Fracture

Balloon fracture is a rare occurrence and it usually requires surgical intervention. However, Block et al. have reported one case in which a balloon fracture was successfully managed percutaneously (28). A second catheter was advanced in the pericardial space and the first guidewire was snared. A balloon catheter was then advanced over the guidewire and it was used to push the fractured portion of the balloon outside the skin entry site (Fig. 23-7).

Complications Requiring Nonsurgical Intervention

Minor complications are relatively common. New left pleural effusions develop in nearly a third of patients and may require thoracentesis. This is the result of a successful pericardial–pleural

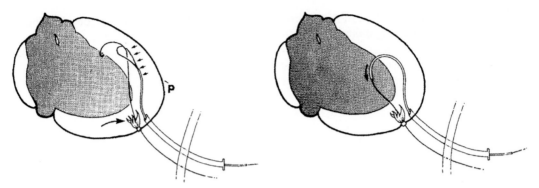

FIGURE 23-7. Percutaneous removal of a fractured balloon following balloon pericardiotomy. A second pericardial catheter has been inserted and the first guidewire has been snared. A catheter is then used to push the balloon fragment back through the pericardium and the skin. (From Block PC, Wilson MA. Hemi-balloon dislodgement during a percutaneous balloon pericardial window procedure: Removal using a second pericardial catheter. *Cathet Cardiovasc Diagn* 1993;29:289–291, with permission.)

communication from the procedure. Chest x-ray should be performed after the procedure to evaluate for pneumothorax.

■ PREVENTION OF COMPLICATIONS

Interventions aimed toward reducing the risk of complications of pericardiocentesis and balloon pericardiotomy are summarized in Tables 23-4 and 23-5. Overall, meticulous preparation, use of fluoroscopy or echo guidance, confirmation of entry of the pericardial space prior to insertion of pericardial drains or prior to balloon dilatation, and avoidance of removal of large amounts of fluid in a single session represent the mainstay to reduce the risk of complications. In general, except those instances where echo-guided procedures are performed emergently at the bedside, the cardiac catheterization suite is the best environment where all the steps needed to enhance the safety of the procedure can be easily undertaken. Continuous hemodynamic monitoring during the procedure and particularly the ability to measure pericardial pressure further increase the safety of the procedure. Measurement of pericardial pressure after entry in the pericardial space and before insertion of a larger catheter can confirm the presence of tamponade physiology and that the position of the catheter is in the pericardial space rather than in other cardiac chambers (determined by the pressure wave form). In addition, following removal of pericardial fluid, the expectation is to

---

TABLE 23-4 **Optimization of Procedure Strategy to Minimize the Risk of Complications Following Echocardiography- or Fluoroscopy-Guided Echocardiography**

- Meticulous echocardiographic assessment prior to the procedure to determine size and location of the effusion, as well echocardiographic findings consistent with tamponade physiology
- Echocardiographic or fluoroscopic guidance
- Sterile technique
- Pressure and ECG monitoring prior to insertion of dilator
- Measurement of pericardial pressure at the beginning and at the end of the procedures
- Under fluoroscopy guidance, confirm guidewire position in at least two angiographic projections
- Use of contrast to confirm position in pericardial space
- Use of agitated saline to confirm positioning of the needle in the pericardial space prior to insertion of the sheath with echocardiography-guided pericardiocentesis
- Initial drainage of only enough fluid to resolve tamponade physiology
- Use of extended catheter drainage to prevent recurrence
- Chest x-ray to rule out pneumothorax

TABLE 23-5	Optimization of Procedure Strategy to Minimize the Risk of Complications Following Balloon Pericardiotomy

- Meticulous echocardiographic assessment prior to the procedure to determine size and location of the effusion, as well echocardiographic findings consistent with tamponade physiology
- Antibiotic prophylaxis
- Sterile technique
- Fluoroscopic guidance
- Pressure and EKG monitoring prior to insertion of dilator
- Measurement of pericardial pressure at the beginning and at the end of the procedure
- Confirm placement of balloon at pericardial border prior to dilation
  - Single-balloon pericardiotomy: Contrast injection
  - Inoue: Pullback catheter with distal portion of balloon inflated
  - Single-balloon pericardiotomy: Point at which guidewires separate
- Rapid inflation of balloon 2–3 times
- Chest x-ray to rule out pneumothorax

see a reduction in pericardial pressure associated with a reduction in heart rate and an increase in systemic pressure. Observing these hemodynamic changes can be very reassuring, particularly in the setting of hemorrhagic effusions. Finally, a chest x-ray at the end of the procedure to rule out pneumothorax is recommended.

References

1. Tsang TS, Enriquez-Sarano M, Freeman WK, et al. Consecutive 1127 therapeutic echocardiographically guided pericardiocenteses: Clinical profile, practice patterns, and outcomes spanning 21 years. *Mayo Clin Proc.* 2002;77:429–436.
2. Maisch B, Seferovic PM, Ristic AD, et al. Guidelines on the diagnosis and management of pericardial diseases executive summary; the task force on the diagnosis and management of pericardial diseases of the European society of cardiology. *Eur Heart J.* 2004;25:587–610.
3. Balmain S, Hawkins NM, MacDonald MR, et al. Pericardiocentesis practice in the United Kingdom. *Int J Clinc Pract.* 2008;62:1515–1519.
4. Bernal JM, Pradhan J, Li T, et al. Acute pulmonary edema following pericardiocentesis for cardiac tamponade. *Can J Cardiol.* 2007;23:1155–1156.
5. Vaitkus PT, Herrmann HC, LeWinter MM. Treatment of malignant pericardial effusion. *JAMA.* 1994;272:59–64.
6. Tsang TS, Barnes ME, Gersh BJ, et al. Outcomes of clinically significant idiopathic pericardial effusion requiring intervention. *Am J Cardiol.* 2003;91:704–707.
7. Kopecky SL, Callahan JA, Tajik AJ, et al. Percutaneous pericardial catheter drainage: Report of 42 consecutive cases. *Am J Cardiol.* 1986;58:633–635.
8. Kabukcu M, Demircioglu F, Yanik E, et al. Pericardial tamponade and large pericardial effusions: Causal factors and efficacy of percutaneous catheter drainage in 50 patients. *Tex Heart Inst J.* 2004;31:398–403.
9. Duvernoy O, Borowiec J, Helmius G, et al. Complications of percutaneous pericardiocentesis under fluoroscopic guidance. *Acta Radiol.* 1992;33:309–313.
10. Karamichalis JM, Gursky A, Valaulikar G, et al. Acute pulmonary edema after pericardial drainage for cardiac tamponade. *Ann Thorac Surg.* 2009;88:675–677.
11. Ligero C, Leta R, Bayes-Genis A. Transient biventricular dysfunction following pericardiocentesis. *Eur J Heart Fail.* 2006;8:102–104.
12. Flores VM, Figal DA, Martinez CC, et al. Transient left ventricular dysfunction following pericardiocentesis. An unusual complication to bear in mind. *Rev Esp Cardiol.* 2009;62:1071–1072.
13. Wolfe MW, Edelman ER. Transient systolic dysfunction after relief of cardiac tamponade. *Ann Intern Med.* 1993;119:42–44.
14. Vandyke WH Jr, Cure J, Chakko CS, et al. Pulmonary edema after pericardiocentesis for cardiac tamponade. *N Engl J Med.* 1983;309:595–596.
15. Skalidis EI, Kochiadakis GE, Chrysostomakis SI, et al. Effect of pericardial pressure on human coronary circulation. *Chest.* 2000;117:910–912.

16. Anguera I, Pare C, Perez-Villa F. Severe right ventricular dysfunction following pericardiocentesis for cardiac tamponade. *Int J Cardiol.* 1997;59:212–214.

17. Armstrong WF, Feigenbaum H, Dillon JC. Acute right ventricular dilation and echo cardiographic volume overload following pericardiocentesis for relief of cardiac tamponade. *Am Heart J.* 1984;107: 1266–1270.

18. Palacios IF, Murat Tuzcu E, Ziskind AA, et al. Percutaneous balloon pericardial window for patients with malignant pericardial effusion and tamponade. *Cathet Cardiovasc Diagn.* 1991;22:244–249.

19. Wang HJ, Hsu KL, Chiang FT, et al. Technical and prognostic outcomes of double-balloon pericardiotomy for large malignancy-related pericardial effusions. *Chest.* 2002;122:893–899.

20. Ziskind AA, Pearce AC, Lemmon C, et al. Percutaneous balloon pericardiotomy for the treatment of cardiac tamponade and large pericardial effusions: Description of technique and report of the first 50 cases. *J Am Coll Cardiol.* 1993;21:1–5.

21. Swanson N, Mirza I, Wijesinghe N, et al. Primary percutaneous balloon pericardiotomy for malignant pericardial effusion. *Catheter Cardiovasc Interv.* 2008;71:504–507.

22. Chow WH, Chow TC, Cheung KL. Nonsurgical creation of a pericardial window using the Inoue balloon catheter. *Am Heart J.* 1992;124(4):1100–1102.

23. Ohke M, BesshoA, Haraoka K, et al. Percutaneous balloon pericardiotomy by the use of Inoue balloon for the management of recurrent cardiac tamponade in a patient with lung cancer. *Intern Med.* 2000;39:1071–1074.

24. Velchev V, Finkov B. Case report: Percutaneous balloon pericardiotomy using Inoue balloon for patients with massive pericardial effusion. *Int J Cardiol.* 2008;doi: 10.1016/j.ijcard.2008.06.095.

25. Chow WH, Chow TC, Yip AS, et al. Inoue balloon pericardiotomy for patients with recurrent pericardial effusion. *Angiology.* 1996;47:57–60.

26. Iaffaldano BA, Jones P, Lewis BE, et al. Percutaneous balloon pericardiotomy: A double balloon technique. *Cathet Cardiovasc Diagn.* 1995;36: 79–81.

27. Del Barrio LG, Morales JH, Delgado C, et al. Percutaneous balloon pericardial window for patients with symptomatic pericardial effusion. *Cardiovasc Intervent Radiol.* 2002;24:360–364.

28. Block PC, Wilson MA. Hemi-balloon dislodgement during a percutaneous balloon pericardial window procedure: Removal using a second pericardial catheter. *Cathet Cardiovasc Diagn* 1993;29: 289–291.

CHAPTER 24

Complications of Circulatory Support

JONATHAN W. HAFT AND MAURO MOSCUCCI

Mechanical circulatory support is used with increasing frequency for patients with cardiac dysfunction. Implantable ventricular assist devices (VADs) can restore hemodynamic stability and durably provide effective cardiac support when used either as bridge to heart transplant (1) or as destination therapy (2). However, the implantation procedure is complex and cannot be safely performed in the sickest of patients in cardiogenic shock. Temporary circulatory support can restore stability and allow time for resuscitation and determination of the patient's suitability for implantable devices. Percutaneously delivered mechanical support can restore hemodynamic stability and allow time to determine the best long-term options for each individual patient, which may include recovery after time (i.e., myocarditis) or revascularization (acute myocardial infarction), bridging to an implantable VAD or heart transplantation.

A variety of approaches are available for percutaneous mechanical circulatory assistance, including extracorporeal membrane oxygenation (ECMO), TandemHeart percutaneous VAD (Cardiac Assist, Pittsburgh, PA), and the Impella microaxial flow catheters (Abiomed Inc., Danvers, MA). Although many of the complications associated with percutaneous mechanical support are universal across any of these modalities, some are unique to each mode of support. Each of these approaches will be discussed separately; their unique features are outlined in Table 24-1.

■ EXTRACORPOREAL MEMBRANE OXYGENATION

ECMO is a modification of cardiopulmonary bypass which can allow support for days or weeks. First successfully employed in 1954 by

Gibbon (3), cardiopulmonary bypass is used to support the circulation during open heart surgery. Venous blood volume is drained into a reservoir and selectively pumped through an oxygen exchange device prior to return to the systemic arterial circulation. The venous reservoir is essential to empty the chambers of the heart and create a bloodless field for optimal intracardiac visualization. In addition, shed blood from the mediastinal surgical field can be actively returned to the reservoir, avoiding loss of the red cell mass (Fig. 24-1). Cardiopulmonary bypass is essential for intracardiac surgery; it requires high levels of anticoagulation and will cause hemolysis and white cell activation from the excessive sheer forces and the interface between blood and air (4). Although these deficiencies can be acceptable for the 1 or 2 hours necessary to complete surgical cardiac reconstruction, prolonged support using cardiopulmonary bypass is not possible. ECMO, however, is a closed system without direct blood and air interface, thus minimizing cellular blood activation and damage, and allows prolonged support with reduced anticoagulation.

There is currently no system designed, produces, and marketed specifically for ECMO. Rather, the equipment used for ECMO can be obtained separately from different manufacturers. Although many institutions differ on what constitutes their ECMO system, there are several essential basic components. Cannulae are tubes designed for insertion into the circulation either for drainage or return of blood. Flexible polyvinyl chloride tubing is used to connect these cannulae with the remainder of the circuit, typically 3/8th inch in outer diameter. A blood pump is used to generate flow and can come in a variety of types. ECMO programs are mixed in

TABLE 24-1   **Comparison of Percutaneous Mechanical Circulatory Assistance Modes**

Support Mode	Advantages	Relative Drawbacks
ECMO	Biventricular support Pulmonary support Ease of initiation	Complex care Left ventricular distension Aortic root thrombus Cerebral hypoxia
TandemHeart	Left ventricular decompression Simpler post-implant care	Expertise in insertion Univentricular support (currently) Aortic root thrombus
Impella	Left ventricular decompression Ease speed of insertion	Univentricular support (currently) Catheter malposition

terms of their choice of blood pump design (5). Roller design pumps are inexpensive, durable, and efficient, but can generate extremely high negative or positive pressure, hazarding cavitation or circuit rupture if unregulated electronically or manually (Fig. 24-2A). Centrifugal design pumps are safer than roller pumps, but are more costly and can be prone to thrombus formation (Fig. 24-2B). The last essential component of an ECMO circuit is the oxygenator: a

membrane with large surface area capable of exchanging respiratory gases. Like the blood pumps, oxygenators for ECMO come in a variety of forms. Silicone rubber oxygenators take advantage of the material's unique permeability to respiratory gases (Fig. 24-3). They are expensive, have high resistance to blood flow, and can be time consuming to prime for use, but are durable, often supporting patients for more than one week. Microporous polypropylene

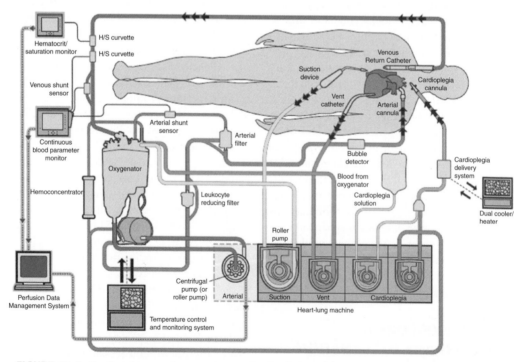

FIGURE 24-1. Cardiopulmonary bypass supports the circulation while creating a quiet and bloodless intracardiac field. The complex system is required for most cardiac surgery reconstruction, but the large air–blood interface causes significant cellular blood damage and cannot be used for more than several hours. (Courtesy of Terumo Cardiovascular Systems, Ann Arbor, MI.) (See color insert.)

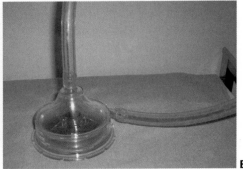

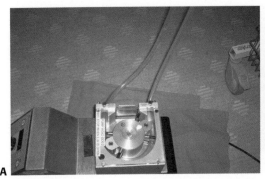

A B

FIGURE 24-2. (**A**) Traditional roller pump. Reliable and durable, and the disposable components are inexpensive. Roller pumps create very high positive and negative pressure, and must be continuously observed by trained personnel. (**B**) Centrifugal pump. Excessive positive and negative pressures can be controlled, but they are more expensive and are prone to thrombus formation in zones of stagnation around the mechanical bearings.

oxygenators are used throughout the world for cardiopulmonary bypass. Thousands of capillary sized tubes of polypropylene deliver oxygen on the inside while surrounded by blood. Gas exchange occurs through the tiny micropores within the plastic. Unlike the silicone oxygenators, they are low in resistance and easy to prime. However, they are prone to leak plasma after 24 to 48 hours of use from deposition of plasma lipids onto the membrane and reduction in the surface tension (6). The latest generation of oxy-

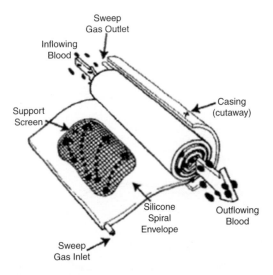

FIGURE 24-3. Silicone rubber oxygenator. An envelope of permeable thin silicone rubber is rolled tightly within an outer casing. Blood travels between the rolled layers, while oxygen is delivered inside the envelope. (Courtesy of the Extracorporeal Life Support Organization, Ann Arbor, MI.)

genators is made of polymethyl pentene. Cut into capillary tubes similar to the polypropylene fibers, they are permeable to respiratory gases without the micropores responsible for plasma leakage (Fig. 24-4). At the time of this book's publication, only one polymethyl pentene oxygenator is available in the US market: the Quadrox-D from Maquet, Inc (Rastatt, Germany).

ECMO can be provided in one of two applications: veno-venous and veno-arterial. Veno-venous ECMO involves drainage of blood from the venous system, pumping through the oxygenator, and returning back into the venous system (Fig. 24-5A). There is no hemodynamic support with veno-venous ECMO, only gas exchange, and thus is used primarily for patients with isolated respiratory failure. There has been widespread enthusiasm for ECMO related to the H1N1 outbreak (7) as well as the recently published prospective randomized trial demonstrating ECMO's superiority compared to conventional treatment of advanced acute respiratory failure (8). Veno-arterial ECMO is partial heart-lung bypass (Fig. 24-5B) and can be used to support patients in cardiogenic shock. Drainage is accomplished from a catheter placed in a large central vein or the right atrium directly. Blood then flows from the blood pump and oxygenator back into the systemic circulation.

Cannulation for ECMO can be accomplished from a variety of approaches. If patients require ECMO support for cardiac failure following open heart surgery, the cannulae for cardiopulmonary bypass can be left in place and

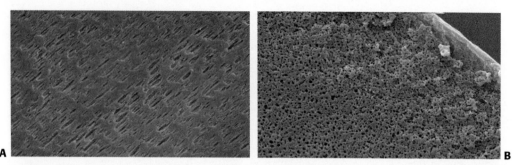

FIGURE 24-4. Images of different artificial lung membranes. (**A**) Polypropylene, with micropores prone to leak plasma after 24 to 48 hours. (**B**) Polymethyl Pentene with outer skin, eliminating plasma leakage. (Courtesy of Membrana, GmbH, Wuppertal, Germany.)

connected to the ECMO circuit. Neonates who require ECMO typically are cannulated using the carotid artery and jugular vein by surgical exposure. For adult patients that require veno-venous ECMO for isolated respiratory failure, a specially designed double-lumen catheter can be inserted percutaneously into the jugular vein and advanced into the inferior vena cava (Fig. 24-6). The 31-Fr catheter can deliver up to 5 liters per minute of flow with minimal recirculation. Alternatively, adult patients who require veno-venous ECMO for respiratory failure can be cannulated using separate drainage and infusion cannulae, typically draining from a catheter in the femoral vein, and infusing into a catheter in the jugular vein. For adult patients that require veno-arterial ECMO, the femoral

vessels are the most frequently utilized because of their accessibility. Although surgical exposure of the femoral vessels can be employed, cannulation can proceed percutaneously, with 23- to 28-Fr catheters typically used for venous drainage, and 17- to 21-Fr sizes used for arterial access. Regardless of the mode of cannulation, patients should be systemically anticoagulated, typically with a bolus of 100 IU/kg of heparin.

Complications of ECMO and Bailout Techniques

ECMO is ordinarily initiated under conditions of profound circulatory collapse or severe respiratory failure when all other measures have failed and death is nearly imminent. Not surprisingly,

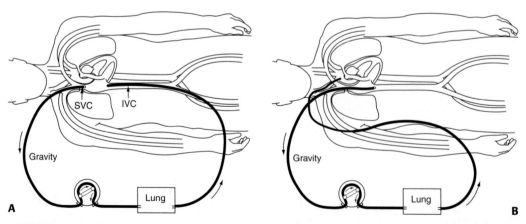

FIGURE 24-5. Configuration of ECMO support. (**A**) Veno-venous ECMO (VV). Extracorporeal gas exchange occurs in venous blood, which is then returned to the venous circulation. VV ECMO provides no direct hemodynamic support. (**B**) Veno-arterial ECMO (VA). Venous blood is actively pumped into the system circulation, effectively bypassing the cardiorespiratory system. VA ECMO is partial cardiopulmonary bypass. (Courtesy of the Extracorporeal Life Support Organization, Ann Arbor, MI.)

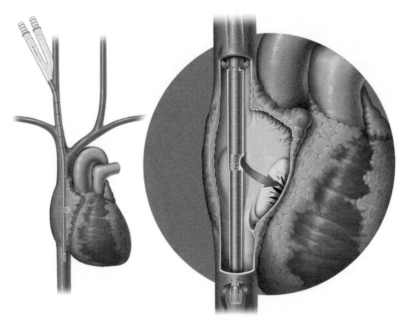

FIGURE 24-6. Double-lumen cannula created for veno-venous ECMO. The bicaval cannula is designed to minimize recirculation while providing optimal ECMO support from a single cannulation site. (Courtesy of Avalon Laboratories, LLC, Rancho Dominguez, CA.) (See color insert.)

outcomes in the adult population reflect the acuity these patients typically have, with survival rates of only 30% to 60% (9,10). Long-term survival, however, is reasonably good, assisted by heart transplantation and implantable VADs. Complications during support are common, and a thorough understanding will assist in prevention, early recognition, and treatment.

Bleeding

Bleeding is the most frequently reported complication, occurring in approximately 30% of patients on ECMO (11). Bleeding occurs not only because of the required anticoagulation, but also because of platelet dysfunction associated with extracorporeal support, as well as coagulopathy which frequently exists in this moribund patient population. Bleeding frequently occurs at sites of cannulation as well as other surgical wounds. In addition, troublesome bleeding can be seen from other instrumentation typically used in critically ill patients, including nasogastric tubes, endotracheal tubes, as well as spontaneously from mucus membranes, the brain, abdomen, and the retroperitoneum. As with any complication, the best treatment is prevention by carefully titrating anticoagulation, correction of coagulopathy and

thrombocytopenia, and meticulous technique with surgical procedures and cannulation.

Thrombocytopenia is extremely common in patients on ECMO. Stimulants of platelet activity include sheer stresses and contact activation seen with any type of extracorporeal blood flow. Newer circuits designed to reduce surface area and blood flow resistance appear to be more biocompatible, and may reduce platelet consumption associated with ECMO support (12). Nonetheless, thrombocytopenia should be aggressively corrected with transfusions, even when there are no signs of active bleeding. Many centers have adopted policies to replace platelets when counts are less than 80 to 100 K. Platelet inhibitors should be avoided unless absolutely necessary following recent percutaneous coronary interventions.

Anticoagulation is typically accomplished with a heparin infusion, although direct thrombin inhibitors such as Argatroban can be used in the setting of confirmed or suspected Heparin Induced Thrombocytopenia (HIT). Anticoagulation can be variably monitored using either activated clotting times (ACT), with a target of 180 to 220 seconds, or a partial thromboplastin time (PTT), targeting 40 to 50 seconds. These targets should be reduced in the setting of severe bleeding, and heparin can be discontinued altogether in the case of refractory life threatening hemorrhage, although the ECMO circuit must be carefully monitored for signs of thrombus formation.

Bleeding from surgical wounds should be meticulously explored for sites of reversible hemorrhage. To reduce the incidence of bleeding from percutaneous cannulation sites, the vessels should be treated gently and not overdilated. Cannulae should be inserted an adequate distance and reliably secured to the patient's leg to avoid accidental decannulation. As with intra-aortic balloon pumps, patients should also be appropriately immobilized, and when necessary sedated and restrained to avoid inadvertent self-injury. Nursing staff and other caregivers should be instructed in the care of cannulation sites, and they should alert physicians for new bleeding or hematoma formation, particularly at the arterial site. This is especially important when patients are turned during linen changes and bathing, or when they require transport throughout the hospital for further imaging or surgery. Bleeding at the cannulation sites can often be controlled with simple adjustments of the cannula position along with prolonged topical pressure.

Clotting

Thrombus formation is common within any extracorporeal life support system, despite therapeutic anticoagulation. Although surface coatings with heparin and other lipophilic substances can reduce the inflammatory response from blood exposure to artificial surfaces, they do not reduce the need for systemic anticoagulation and will not eliminate circuit clotting (13). The ECMO system should be inspected routinely and frequently to detect signs of clot, which typically occur at tubing connectors and within the oxygenator. Small adherent clots can merely be observed for growth, however when clots becomes large or appear mobile and risk embolization, the offending component should be exchanged. Although this requires temporary discontinuation of support, with preparation and experience it can usually be accomplished in seconds.

Inadequate Support

Depending upon the etiology of circulatory collapse, many patients will require full support, typically 50 to 100 cc/kg/min blood flow. To ensure the ability to meet these needs, venous access must be adequate. Flow through a venous cannula is related to its radius to the fourth power, cannula length, the number and orientation of venous side holes, as well as the intravascular position of the cannula. An undersized cannula will result in insufficient drainage, inadequate flow, and persistent cardiogenic shock. Likewise, a cannula inserted with its tip located within a peripheral vein may deliver insufficient flow, as the small vein will collapse around the cannula as suction is applied. It is ideal for the venous cannula to be advanced to the level of the right atrium (14). As with other complications, prevention is the best treatment. Understanding the flow dynamics of the available cannulae will help guide clinicians in appropriate choices. Furthermore, drainage cannulae should ideally be advanced into the right atrium when possible. Intravascular volume depletion should be corrected, but if venous drainage remains inadequate and signs of persistent tissue underperfusion are present, there should be a low threshold to insert an addition venous cannula.

Hemolysis

Despite the sheer forces within extracorporeal circuits, red cell destruction and clinically significant hemolysis should not occur when ECMO support is delivered properly. However, serum hemoglobin levels should be assessed daily, as hemolysis can be a sign of correctable problems within the circuit. An undersized arterial cannula will result in excessively high circuit pressures. These pressures should be monitored, and if levels exceed 400 to 500 mmHg, there is the potential for catastrophic circuit rupture. However, pressures of 350 to 400 mmHg can result in red cell destruction. A sudden rise in circuit pressures suggests a tubing kink or acute obstructing thrombus and warrants immediate inspection. If circuit pressures remain high and there are signs of hemolysis, flows should be decreased to avoid unnecessary renal injury. Consideration should be made for insertion of a larger or even an additional arterial cannula. Hemolysis may also be a sign of undetected thrombus within the circuit, typically in the oxygenator. If no other explanation for hemolysis can be identified, the oxygenator should be exchanged, usually resulting in normalization of serum-free hemoglobin levels.

Hemolysis can also present when there is excessive venous suction, as can occur when inappropriately using a centrifugal design blood pump. With these pumps, inlet pressure should be measured and pump RPM speed adjusted to avoid suction pressures of greater than −200 mmHg. At these levels, intermittent occlusion of the cannula tip occurs from venous or atrial collapse, manifested by "chattering" of the lines. The sheer forces from intermittent venous obstruction can cause high levels of hemolysis and should be avoided. At the extreme, suction pressures exceeding −400 mmHg can result in cavitation, or vaporization of dissolved nitrogen into gas bubbles, similar to the formation of bubbles underwater from a motor boat's propeller. These gaseous bubbles can become trapped in the oxygenator or heat exchanger when small, or can embolize into the patient when they are larger. Cavitation should be avoided at all costs by monitoring inlet pressures with centrifugal pump systems, or by servo regulation when using roller pump systems. Cavitation and air embolization are catastrophic events related to extracorporeal support and the occurrence represents a serious breech of patient safety.

Limb Ischemia

As with other procedures involving femoral arterial access, injury to the femoral artery can result in ipsilateral leg ischemia, either from dissection, thrombosis, or inadequate flow around the catheter. This is far more common with ECMO support, given the size of the indwelling catheter relative to the femoral artery. The frequency of this problem is likely exacerbated by the use of vasoconstrictor drugs typically employed when ECMO support is required. Because there may be very little arterial pulsation during ECMO support, clinically palpable pulses will invariably be absent. In addition, audible Dopplers may be unhelpful when the expected pulsatile signal is diminished. The foot should be assessed for color, warmth, and capillary refill and comparison should be made to the contralateral foot to differentiate cannulation-related ischemia from systemic hypoperfusion from shock and vasoconstrictor use. If there are signs of limb threatening ischemia, maneuvers to perfuse the extremity should be performed expeditiously. An additional cannula can be

placed antegrade down the superficial femoral artery. This can be done percutaneously, although it may be challenging given the vessel depth and lack of signals on Doppler ultrasonography (15). Another technique includes obtaining antegrade access via the common femoral artery and then place the arterial ECMO cannula using the retrograde femoral artery approach. The cannula and the antegrade sheath can then be connected using a pressure line connected to the side arm of the sheath. However, surgical exposure might be necessary. Alternatively, the posterior tibial artery is easily exposed surgically, and a small cannula can be placed in a retrograde orientation. This cannula can be connected in parallel to the arterial limb of the ECMO circuit. Flow into the extremity can be measured, and typically 100 cc/min is required to maintain leg viability.

Left Ventricular Distention and Pulmonary Hemorrhage

Although ECMO support can restore tissue perfusion and blood pressure for patients in profound cardiogenic shock, inherent in its design is its inability to decompress the left-sided circulation. Unlike cardiopulmonary bypass, where a reservoir allows complete drainage of the venous circulation, ECMO is a closed system without a reservoir. Regardless of the flow rates, ECMO is partial bypass and there will always remain some right ventricular output. This pulmonary blood flow, in addition to bronchial blood flow, will return to the left ventricle during diastole. The left ventricle may be incapable of ejecting this volume against the additional afterload of ECMO support, either because of severe systolic dysfunction or because of persistent ventricular arrhythmias. The left ventricle will progressively distend, resulting in left atrial hypertension, pulmonary venous congestion, pulmonary edema, and eventually pulmonary hemorrhage. The end result is universally fatal and must be recognized and avoided. Left ventricular distension will be exacerbated by aortic valve insufficiency, and severe aortic valvular incompetence is an absolute contraindication for ECMO.

Once ECMO support is initiated, signs of ventricular distension must be monitored. Placement of a Swan-Ganz catheter can be helpful in detecting a progressive rise in pulmonary artery pressures, suggesting left ventricular volume overload. Absence of any arterial pressure pulsation also suggests that the left ventricle is failing to eject. Frequent use of echocardiography is advisable to evaluate for aortic valve opening and ventricular size. Several interventions can help with ventricular ejection. Clearly, malignant arrhythmias must be corrected immediately with electrical cardioversion, and anti-arrhythmic agents should be used as necessary. Inotropic infusions should be continued or initiated to maximize ventricular systolic function. Systemic afterload should be reduced by minimizing vasoconstrictor agents while maintaining a mean arterial perfusion pressure of at least 60 mmHg. An intra-aortic balloon pump can be very helpful in reducing afterload and facilitating ventricular ejection, in addition to augmenting diastolic coronary perfusion.

If these maneuvers are unsuccessful at generating adequate ventricular decompression, mechanical decompression is required. This can be accomplished percutaneously by balloon atrial septostomy (Fig. 24-7), insertion of a surgically placed left atrial drainage cannula or placement of a micro-axial transaortic pump (16) as will be discussed later in this chapter. Percutaneous insertion of a left atrial cannula using the transseptal approach has also been used successfully in our institution. The left atrial cannula can then be connected to the ECMO circuit using a Y connector, allowing direct drainage in the circuit from the left atrium (Fig. 24-8). In the interim, manual chest compressions can be very effective at temporarily decompressing the distended ventricle. Ventricular distension is probably the most

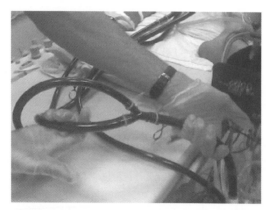

FIGURE 24-8. A cannula has been inserted in the left atrium using the percutaneous transseptal approach, and it has been connected to the ECMO circuit using a Y connector.

important and under-recognized complication of ECMO support for cardiogenic shock.

Atrial septostomy and related complications have been described in Chapter 19. Atrial septostomy in this patient population is associated with the additional challenges of ongoing anticoagulation and limited vascular access. The limitation of vascular access is due to the fact that vascular access for ECMO is often obtained using the right femoral vein and femoral artery approach. In these cases, the technique that we have developed includes obtaining venous access using the internal jugular vein approach, switching the ECMO cannula from the right femoral vein to the right internal jugular vein, and clamping the soft plastic portion of the right femoral vein cannula. A 14-Fr sheath is inserted in the right femoral cannula, and the hub of the sheath is pushed inside the soft

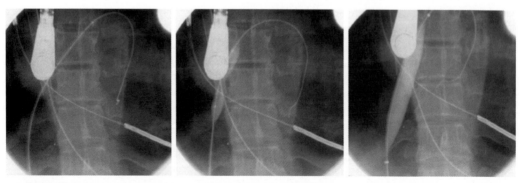

FIGURE 24-7. Atrial septostomy. After left atrial access is obtained, the interatrial septum is balloon dilated to create a septal defect and decompress the left atrium and ventricle.

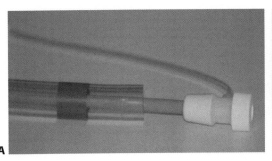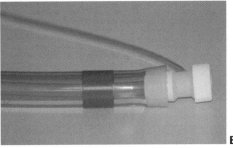

FIGURE 24-9. Right percutaneous transfemoral approach for transseptal puncture. (**A**) Use of a 14-French sheath inside the femoral vein cannula. (**B**) The 14-French sheath is advanced all the way to the hub to obtain a seal. The transseptal puncture is then performed through the 14-French sheath.

portion of the cannula until a seal is obtained. The transseptal puncture is then performed through this sheath (Fig. 24-9).

Aortic Root Thrombus

During ECMO support, blood flow from the circuit travels retrograde up the descending thoracic aorta and meets the antegrade flow ejected from the left ventricle. When there is very little left ventricular ejection, blood flow travels entirely retrograde around the aortic arch and stops at the persistently closed aortic valve, resulting in some degree of stasis. Despite continuous anticoagulation, thrombus can form in the aortic root (Fig. 24-10). Interestingly, this complication occurs infrequently with implantable VADs, despite the fact that the aortic valve commonly fails to open in this setting. This difference is likely due to the high degree of turbulence seen in the aortic root from the proximal location of the VAD outflow graft on the ascending aorta. Thrombus in the aortic root places the patient at extremely high risk of embolization resulting in catastrophic stroke. This complication is best avoided by maintaining ventricular ejection with the measures described in the preceding text. If a thrombus is detected on echocardiography, or stasis is a serious concern because the ventricle fails to eject, anticoagulation should be increased aggressively.

Cerebral Hypoxia

Another frequently overlooked complication of ECMO is unrecognized hypoxia to the brain and the coronary circulation. Although ECMO typically delivers blood with a hemoglobin oxygen saturation of 100%, this well-oxygenated circuit flow will mix with blood ejected from the left ventricle. The location of mixing depends upon the amount of native ventricular ejection. When the ventricle is only nominally functioning, mixing will occur in the aortic root and the entire circulation will benefit from extracorporeal oxygenation (Fig. 24-11). However, when the ventricle begins to recover, mixing may occur in the distal aortic arch or descending thoracic aorta. If the lungs are significantly dysfunctional, as is often the case with severe pulmonary edema after massive myocardial infarction, tissues perfused proximal to the level of mixing may be hypoxic. There is frequently the misconception that because the patient is "on bypass" the lungs are unimportant. Ventilator settings are often decreased or patients may even be extubated. Nurses commonly recognize this complication before physicians, noting a cyanotic appearing face with normal blood gases drawn from a femoral arterial line. Pulse oxymetry should always be measured in the right hand, since it

FIGURE 24-10. Thrombus within the aortic root.

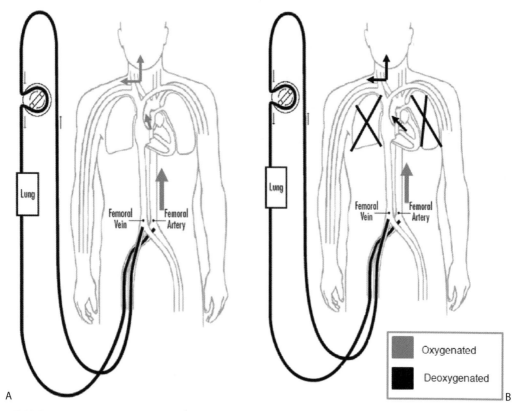

FIGURE 24-11. Cerebral hypoxia. (**A**) While on veno-arterial ECMO using the femoral artery and vein, fully saturated blood travels retrograde up the descending aorta and mixes with any residual native cardiac ejection. (**B**) If the lungs are significantly damaged, blood ejected from the native heart may be hypoxic. This cyanotic blood mixes with the fully saturated blood from the ECMO circuit. The location of mixing will determine the degree of cerebral hypoxia. If mixing occurs in the distal aortic arch, the proximal aortic branches will be hypoxic, hazarding coronary and cerebral ischemia. Arterial saturations in the right hand will best reflect cerebral and coronary oxygen content.

most accurately reflects the saturation of blood in the brain and the coronary circulation because its blood flow originates from the proximal aortic arch. Failure to recognize a differential in tissue oxygenation by measuring pulse oxymetry in different extremities can result in cerebral hypoxia and irreversible brain injury. If the right hand saturations are low, appropriate adjustments should immediately be made in the ventilator settings to optimize native lung function. If the patient remains cyanotic, additional ECMO flow can transition the mixing point more proximally towards the ascending aorta, improving global tissue oxygenation.

Decannulation

Inadvertent removal of the femoral arterial and venous cannula is a rare complication of extracorporeal circulatory support which can occur during movements or transportation of the patient. This can result in immediate death due to hemorrhagic shock, given that decannulation will result not only in bleeding from the femoral artery access site, but also in pumping blood through the extruded arterial cannula. Thus, extreme care should be taken in securing the arterial and venous cannula in multiple sites, and in immobilizing the lower extremity with leg immobilizers.

TandemHeart

The TandemHeart percutaneous ventricular assist device is provided as a complete system consisting of a blood pump, controller, tubing, and cannulae for initiation of percutaneous temporary circulatory assistance. The blood pump is a centrifugal design with novel features

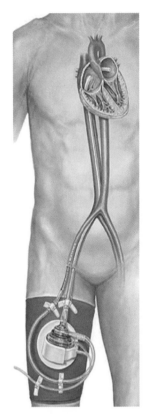

FIGURE 24-12. TandemHeart percutaneous ventricular assist device. A venous drainage cannula is inserted into the left atrium percutaneously across the interatrial septum. Blood flow is then pumped by a centrifugal pump into the systemic circulation. (Courtesy of CardiacAssist, Pittsburgh, PA.) (See color insert.)

including a magnetically actuated rotor and continuous lubrication of the single bearing. This reduces heat generation and the formation of stagnant blood clot, which has been problematic in centrifugal pumps of other designs. The other novel feature of the TandemHeart system is the proprietary venous drainage cannula designed to be placed into the left atrium across the interatrial septum from the femoral vein (Figs. 24-12 and 24-13). Blood is then returned into the systemic circulation via a cannula in the femoral artery. The TandemHeart system is capable of delivering up to 7 liters per minute blood flow, and has been used extensively in the treatment of cardiogenic shock and in support of complex percutaneous interventions (17,18). Interestingly, the obligate atrial septal defect created with cannula insertion typically closes spontaneously following catheter removal after

cardiac recovery. If it does not close, it can usually be addressed percutaneously by insertion of a plug or occluder.

Complications of TandemHeart Support and Bailout Techniques

Many of the complications associated with use of the TandemHeart are similar to those described above for ECMO, including vascular complications and leg ischemia, aortic root thrombus, hemolysis, bleeding, thrombus formation, and "decannulation." Because the left-sided circulation is actively drained, left ventricular distension is not seen, offering a unique advantage over ECMO support. However, right ventricular failure can result in persistent cardiogenic shock, as blood flow cannot be delivered through the lungs to the mechanical support system. This will manifest as low device flow despite adequate pump speed, hypotension, signs of poor tissue perfusion, and an elevated central venous pressure. Treatment should be directed at optimizing right ventricular function with inotropic agents and pulmonary vasodilators such as inhaled nitric oxide. When shock persists despite these efforts, consideration should be made to convert to ECMO by adding an additional venous cannula, along with the oxygenator and the

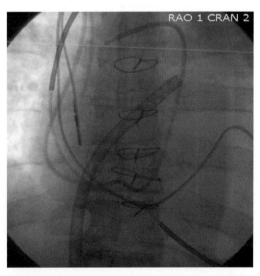

FIGURE 24-13. TandemHeart. The venous drainage cannula has been inserted into the left atrium. The added complexity to the procedure is that many patients have additional lines, pacing and ICD leads that can be displaced by and/or interfere with the transseptal puncture.

remainder of the ECMO circuit. The Tandem-Heart left atrial cannula placement can also be technically challenging. Although the techniques of transseptal puncture are well described, the skills required may not be uniform throughout the interventional cardiology community. Because of the angle of approach, access using the right femoral vein is preferable. If this site cannot be used because of thrombus, the left femoral vein or the internal jugular vein are feasible but pose additional challenges. In addition, patients with a small left atrium can present further difficulties because of the smaller target and cavity size required to maintain the catheter.

Hemolysis is rare with the TandemHeart. However, it can occur suddenly when there is excessive suction from the left atrium. As with ECMO, intermittent occlusion of the cannula tip can occur from atrial collapse, and it is manifested by "chattering" of the lines and of the TandemHeart. It should be managed immediately by reducing the RPM. Preventive interventions include monitoring filling pressure with a Swan-Ganz catheter.

Refractory hypoxemia secondary to significant right to left shunting through the residual acquired ASD is an additional delayed complication, which can occur following removal of the left atrial TandemHeart cannula. Successful percutaneous closure of the ASD using an Amplatzer septal occluder device with rapid correction of hypoxemia has been described (19) (Fig. 24-14).

■ IMPELLA CATHETERS

Impella is a miniaturized micro-axial flow catheter designed to be positioned across the aortic valve (Fig. 24-15). The internal rotor spins from 25,000 to 50,000 revolutions per minute, and can produce blood at a rate of 2.5 to 5 liters per minute. Two products are available in the United States that are designed to be inserted from the femoral artery. The Impella 2.5 is placed percutaneously via a 14-Fr sheath, whereas the Impella 5.0 requires surgical exposure of the femoral artery to admit its 22-Fr delivery system. These miniaturized ventricular assist devices are frequently used to assist complex percutaneous interventions electively in high-risk patients, or to support the circulation in patients presenting in cardiogenic shock from acute myocardial infarctions (20,21). When appropriately positioned, these catheters reliably unload the left ventricle with minimal hemolysis and thrombus.

Many of the complications from use of the Impella catheter are similar to those described in the preceding text, and are attributed to limb ischemia or other vascular injuries. Given their inherent design, left ventricular distension is not seen, offering the Impella an advantage over ECMO for treatment of cardiogenic shock. In addition, because blood is ejected into the proximal ascending aorta, thrombus formation within the aortic root would not be expected and has not been reported. In fact, Impella has been used to unload the left ventricle and prevent stasis in the

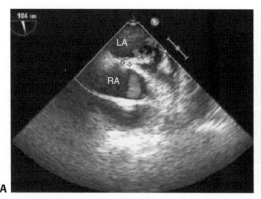 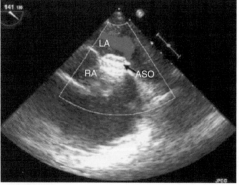

FIGURE 24-14. (A) Iatrogenic atrial septal defect with right to left shunting following removal of a Tandem-Heart left atrial cannula. **(B)** The defect has been repaired using an Amplatzer atrial septal occluder. (From Sur JP, Pagani FD, Moscucci M. Percutaneous closure of an iatrogenic atrial septal defect. *Catheter Cardiovasc Interv.* 2009;73:267–271, with permission.) (See color insert.)

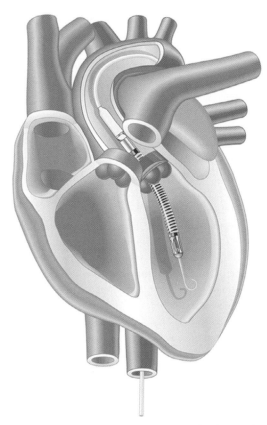

FIGURE 24-15. The Impella micro-axial catheter. The catheters can be advanced either from the femoral artery or the ascending aorta into the left ventricle. The catheter traverses the aortic valve, and the micro-axial flow pump produces 2.5 or 5.0 liters per minute, depending upon which model has been chosen. (Courtesy of Abiomed, Inc., Danvers, MA). (See color insert.)

aortic root for patients on ECMO. However, Impella in its current form is designed only for left ventricular support, limiting its use to patients with reasonable right ventricular function and a relatively stable life sustaining cardiac rhythm. In addition, catheter malposition can be challenging, particularly when used for days in the intensive care unit setting. The catheter has the tendency to migrate deep into the ventricular cavity, placing both the inflow and outflow ports within the ventricle, thus making it ineffective. More subtle changes of position can result in hemolysis from inflow occlusion by papillary muscles or mitral subvalvar chordae, or outflow occlusion from aortic valve leaflets. Catheter migration can be avoided by withdrawing any additional slack from the percutaneous lead after initiation of support under direct fluoroscopic

guidance. Despite careful attention to Impella catheter position, migration can still occur during manipulation of the patients for linen changes, transportation, or patient movement. The Impella console measures transcatheter pressure gradient, and will alert the user when pressures suggest malposition. Because of its transaortic position, the Impella catheters cannot be used if there is a heavily calcified aortic valve or mechanical prosthesis.

■ BRIDGE TO NOWHERE

Although not a complication of mechanical circulatory support per se, arguably the most frustrating scenario occurs in a patient on mechanical support with stable end organ perfusion but no destination. Temporary mechanical support is a bridge, either to recovery, implantable ventricular assistance, or heart transplantation. Because of cost and finite resources, the latter two options mandate extremely restrictive exclusion criteria. Not infrequently, a patient presents in cardiogenic shock but will never be a suitable candidate for a durable implantable VAD or heart transplantation, either because of chronic irreversible co-morbidities, psychiatric illness, or compromising social limitations. Patients who satisfy this description *and* have no hope for myocardial recovery should not be placed on any form of mechanical circulatory support. It can be extremely challenging to discontinue mechanical life support in awake and neurologically intact patients, particularly if their and their family's expectations are unrealistic. Although it is not always clear at the time of presentation, every effort should be made to avoid this scenario. A multidisciplinary approach incorporating expertise from interventional cardiology, heart failure, and cardiac surgery should be used in evaluating patients prior to initiation of temporary circulatory support, limiting this expensive and labor intensive therapy to appropriate indications.

References

1. Miller LW, Pagani FD, Russell SD, et al. Use of a continuous-flow device in patients awaiting heart transplantation. *N Engl J Med.* 2007;357:885–896.
2. Slaughter MS, Rogers JG, Milano CA, et al. Advanced heart failure treated with continuous-flow left ventricular assist device. *N Engl J Med.* 2009;361:2241–2251.

3. Gibbon JH. Maintenance of cardiorespiratory functions by extracorporeal circulation. *Circulation.* 1959;19:646–656.

4. Dobell ARC, Mitri M, Galva R, et al. Biologic evaluation of blood after prolonged recirculation through film and membrane oxygenators. *Ann Surg* 1965;161:617–622.

5. Lawson DS, Lawson AF, Walczak R, et al. North American neonatal extracorporeal membrane oxygenation (ECMO) devices and team roles: 2008 survey results of Extracorporeal Life Support Organization (ELSO) centers. *J Extracorpor Technol.* 2008;40:166–174.

6. Montoya JP, Shanley CJ, Merz SI, et al. Plasma leakage through microporous membranes. Role of phospholipids. *ASAIO J.* 1992;38:M399–M405.

7. Davies A, Jones D, Bailey M, et al. Extracorporeal membrane oxygenation for 2009 influenza A (H1N1) acute respiratory distress syndrome. *JAMA.* 2009;302:1888–1895.

8. Peek GJ, Mugford M, Tiruvoipati R, et al. Efficacy and economic assessment of conventional ventilatory support versus extracorporeal membrane oxygenation for severe adult respiratory failure (CESAR): A multicentre randomised controlled trial. *Lancet.* 2009;374:1351–1363.

9. Hemmila MR, Rowe SA, Boules TN, et al. Extracorporeal life support for severe acute respiratory distress syndrome in adults. *Ann Surg.* 2004;240: 595–605.

10. Smedira NG, Moazami N, Golding CM, et al. Clinical experience with 202 adults receiving extracorporeal membrane oxygenation for cardiac failure: Survival at five years. *J Thorac Cardiovasc Surg.* 2001;122:92–102.

11. Conrad SA, Rycus PT, Dalton H. Extracorporeal Life Support Registry Report 2004. *ASAIO J.* 2005;51:4–10.

12. Toomasian JM, Schreiner RJ, Meyer DE, et al. A polymethylpentene fiber gas exchanger for long-term extracorporeal life support. *ASAIO J.* 2005;51: 390–397.

13. Gorman RC, Ziats N, Rao AK, et al. Surface-bound heparin fails to reduce thrombin formation during clinical cardiopulmonary bypass. *J Thorac Cardiovasc Surg.* 1996;111:1–11.

14. Wenger RK, Bavaria JE, Ratcliffe MB, et al. Flow dynamics of peripheral venous catheters during extracorporeal membrane oxygenation with a centrifugal pump. *J Thorac Cardiovasc Surg.* 1988;96:478–484.

15. Madershahian N, Nagib R, Wippermann J, et al. A simple technique of distal limb perfusion during prolonged femoro-femoral cannulation. *J Cardiac Surg.* 2006;21:168–169.

16. Jouan J, Grinda JM, Bricourt MO, et al. Successful left ventricular decompression following peripheral extracorporeal membrane oxygenation by percutaneous placement of a micro-axial flow pump. *J Heart Lung Transplant.* 2010;29:135–136.

17. Thiele H, Sick P, Boudriot E, et al. Randomized comparison of intra-aortic balloon support with a percutaneous left ventricular assist device in patients with revascularized acute myocardial infarction complicated by cardiogenic shock. *Eur Heart J.* 2005;26:1276–283.

18. Bonvini RF, Hendiri T, Camenzind E, et al. High-risk left main coronary stenting supported by percutaneous left ventricular assist device. *Cath Cardiovasc Intervent.* 2005;66:209–212.

19. Sur JP, Pagani FD, Moscucci M. Percutaneous closure of an iatrogenic atrial septal defect. *Catheter Cardiovasc Interv.* 2009;73(2):267–271.

20. Burzotta F, Paloscia L, Trani C, et al. Feasibility and long-term safety of elective Impella-assisted high-risk percutaneous coronary intervention: A pilot two-centre study. *J Cardiovasc Med.* 2008;9: 1004–1010.

21. Seyfarth M, Sibbing D, Bauer I, et al. A randomized clinical trial to evaluate the safety and efficacy of a percutaneous left ventricular assist device versus intra-aortic balloon pumping for treatment of cardiogenic shock caused by myocardial infarction. *J Am Col Cardiol.* 2008;52:1584–1588.

25

Complications of Alcohol Septal Ablation for Hypertrophic Obstructive Cardiomyopathy

VALERIAN L. FERNANDES, MAURO MOSCUCCI, AND WILLIAM H. SPENCER III

Alcohol septal ablation (ASA) is a less invasive alternative to surgical myectomy for relieving medically intractable symptoms of left ventricular outflow tract (LVOT) obstruction in patients with hypertrophic obstructive cardiomyopathy (HOCM).

LVOT obstruction is produced by the combination of asymmetric septal hypertrophy and systolic anterior motion of the mitral valve and is present in two-thirds of patients with hypertrophic cardiomyopathy (1–3). Although medical therapy can be effective in relieving symptoms in a majority of patients, some patients still remain severely symptomatic or intolerant of medical therapy. For more than 40 years, the standard for treating HOCM has been surgical myectomy which involves the resection of the hypertrophied septal muscle from the outflow tract (4,5). The surgical results from experienced tertiary centers have been very good, but widespread application is associated with significant morbidity and mortality (6–8).

Transcatheter ablation of the septum with ethanol was first performed in 1994 at the Royal Brompton Hospital in London and reported by Sigwart in 1995 (9). The first patient had intractable symptoms despite good beta blockade and had a 25 mm Hg resting gradient that increased markedly with Valsalva. ASA successfully reduced both the resting and provoked gra-

dients, and the patient was asymptomatic 10 months later. Since then, many ASA procedures have been performed successfully. At this time, ASA is a well-established and readily available treatment option with good short, mid-term, and long-term results (10–15).

■ GENERAL PRINCIPLES
Patient Selection

ASA is appropriate for patients with HOCM who have symptoms that interfere with their lifestyle and are refractory to optimal medical therapy. Like surgical myectomy, there is no role for this procedure in asymptomatic patients despite any LVOT gradient. The criteria for selection of patients for ASA are shown in Table 25-1.

Procedure

Most procedures are performed via the femoral arterial approach. Two arterial accesses and a venous access for temporary pacemaker are needed. Transthoracic echocardiographic guidance is routinely used to guide the procedure (16). The procedural steps commonly used are as follows.

1. A pigtail catheter is inserted into the left ventricle (LV) to measure intraventricular pressure and simultaneous systemic

TABLE 25-1	Criteria for Selection for Alcohol Septal Ablation

Indications for alcohol septal ablation
   Symptomatic patients with HOCM despite
     optimal medical therapy
   Resting LVOT gradient > 30 mm Hg or Provoked
     gradient > 60 mm Hg (provocation is now
     done by Valsalva maneuver or exercise)
   LVOT obstruction is at the level of the outflow
     tract due to contact of the anterior mitral leaflet
     with the thickened septum
   The septal thickness is ≥ 1.6 cm with a
     septal/posterior wall ratio of ≥ 1.3:1
   Accessible septal branches
Contraindications for alcohol septal ablation
   Asymptomatic patients with HOCM
   Intrinsic mitral valve disease
   Associated aortic valve disease needing surgery
   Coronary artery disease needing bypass surgery

arterial pressure is obtained via a catheter introduced into the left main artery. A resting or provoked (Valsalva) LVOT gradient is demonstrated before proceeding with ASA.

2. The coronary and septal anatomy is evaluated with coronary angiography to assess whether the anatomy is suitable for ASA.
3. A trans-venous pacemaker is inserted in patients who have no preexisting permanent pacemaker or implantable cardioverter defibrillator (ICD).
4. Therapeutic anticoagulation is administered (i.e., heparin 100 U/kg).
5. A 0.014″ guidewire is inserted via the left anterior descending (LAD) artery into the first septal artery and a short over-the-wire (OTW) balloon is introduced into the septal artery.
6. After confirming that the balloon is well seated in the septal artery and not obstructing the LAD, the balloon is inflated to occlude the septal artery (Fig. 25-1). A significant reduction in the LVOT gradient with septal balloon inflation is a good predictor that the correct septal artery is identified.
7. The septal guidewire is removed and the position of the inflated balloon is confirmed by angiography.

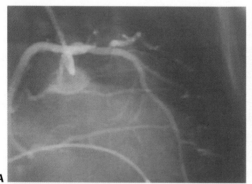
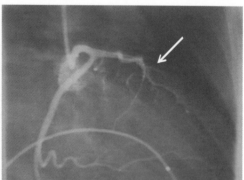
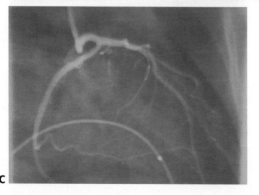

FIGURE 25-1. (**A**) Baseline coronary angiogram—left anterior descending artery (LAD). (**B**) Coronary angiogram after inflation of the balloon in the septal perforator artery. The balloon is clearly obstructing flow in the LAD (*arrow*). (**C**) Repeat coronary angiogram after repositioning of the balloon.

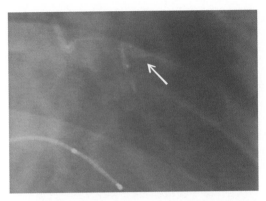

FIGURE 25-2. Contrast injection through the inflated balloon. There is extravasation of contrast in the left anterior descending (LAD) artery (*arrow*). Injection of alcohol in this case would lead to catastrophic consequences.

8. The septal anatomy is defined by angiographic contrast injection through the balloon lumen, making sure that there is no leakage of contrast into the LAD (Fig. 25-2).

9. Agitated angiographic contrast or echo contrast is injected into the occluded septal artery via the balloon lumen, and the location of the intended infarct at the mitral–septal contact site is correctly identified by transthoracic echocardiography (Figs. 25-3 and 25-4).

10. Additional narcotic analgesia is administered.

11. Finally, 1 to 3 cc absolute alcohol is injected slowly (over 2–5 min) into the septal artery via the balloon lumen to infarct the targeted area of the septum. Atrioventricular (AV) conduction is closely monitored during the alcohol injection. The rate of injection may need to be slowed significantly or stopped altogether if significant AV block occurs.

12. The balloon is left inflated for an additional 5 minutes after the alcohol administration.

13. The balloon's central lumen is then continually aspirated while the balloon is deflated and withdrawn. Continual aspiration prevents any alcohol seepage into the LAD or guiding catheter. Care must be taken during balloon withdrawal to limit the guiding catheter's tendency to telescope further into the left main and LAD and cause dissections.

14. After confirming by catheter and echo Doppler that the LVOT gradient is successfully reduced, the procedure is deemed complete.

15. A final coronary angiogram is performed to demonstrate the septal occlusion and absence of coronary complications.

If inadequate gradient reduction is achieved, then another septal artery may be injected with alcohol to reduce the gradient.

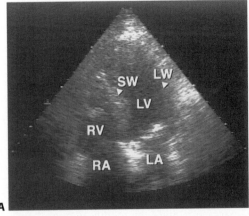
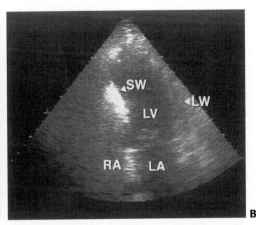

FIGURE 25-3. Apical four-chamber view of heart showing hypertrophied septum before (**A**) and after (**B**) Albumex injection into target septal branch delineating area to be infarcted. SW, septal wall; LW, lateral wall; RV, right ventricle; LV, left ventricle; RA, right atrium; and LA, left atrium. (From Lakkis NM, Nagueh SF, Kleiman NS, et al. Echocardiography-guided ethanol septal reduction for hypertrophic obstructive cardiomyopathy. *Circulation.* 1998;98:1750–1755.)

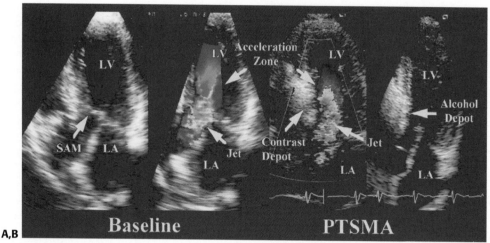

FIGURE 25-4. Intraprocedural myocardial contrast echocardiography. From left to right (**A through D**): Baseline apical four-chamber view with SAM-septum apposition (friction area). Baseline color flow mapping of LVOT with flow acceleration above and jet formation at and below friction area. Intraprocedural MCE showing complete coverage of acceleration zone and friction area by echo contrast depot. Alcohol depot after PTSMA in place of previous echo contrast depot. (From Faber L, Seggewiss H, Gleichmann U. Percutaneous transluminal septal myocardial ablation in hypertrophic obstructive cardiomyopathy: results with respect to intraprocedural myocardial contrast echocardiography. *Circulation.* 1998;98:2415–2421.) (See color insert.)

Classification of Complications of ASA

This procedure is uniquely suited for interventional cardiologists with sufficient experience in coronary procedures. However, unlike most other coronary interventions, ASA involves occluding and therapeutically infarcting a targeted area of myocardium—a diametrically opposite concept for interventional cardiologists. Over the years interventional cardiologists have become very familiar with complications occurring during revascularization procedures. Advances in technology and enhanced operator experience have resulted in a reduction in the frequency and in improved management of complications. However, the complexity of ASA and the new complications that it might introduce when compared to a standard revascularization procedure require a different skill and mindset to master the challenges of the procedure. There is a significant and steep learning curve, and the procedure is best performed by high-volume operators in high-volume centers if the results are to compare favorably against surgical myectomy.

In general, complications of ASA can be divided into two main groups—early complications and late complications. An alternative classification includes three secondary groups. The first group includes complications related to cardiac catheterization, the second group includes complications related to percutaneous coronary intervention (PCI), and the third group includes complications specific to ASA (Table 25-2). For example, because of the need of multiple vascular accesses (2 arterial and 1 venous) and therapeutic anticoagulation, the risk of local access complications is higher. Further discussion in this chapter will focus on the complications specific to ASA.

■ EARLY PERIPROCEDURAL COMPLICATIONS

Aborted Procedures

The Baylor and Medical University of South Carolina case series included 629 patients who underwent ASA between 1996 and 2007 (14). The procedure was aborted in 10 patients (Table 25-3). ASA was aborted in four cases due to coronary dissections, all of which occurred in the early experience. Since the modification of the procedure with the use of coaxial guide catheters and soft-tipped guidewires, no dissections have occurred. Two early procedures were aborted for technical reasons. It is unknown whether they

TABLE 25-2 Complications of Alcohol Septal Ablation Procedure

| | | | Related to ASA | | |
| | | | Periprocedural | | Late |
Related to Cardiac Cath	Related to PCI				
Death	Contrast Nephropathy	Dissection	Death	V Tach	V Tach
MI	Atheroembolism	Perforation	Remote MI	Mitral regurgitation	Mitral regurgitation
Stroke	Local complications	Distal embolization	High-grade block	VSD	VSD
TIA	Hematoma	MI	Hypotension	Septal hematoma	CHF
Embolic events	Pseudoaneurysm	Death	Dissection	Delayed infarction	Death
Arrhythmia	Bleeding	Stroke	Tamponade	Tako-tsubo cardiomyopathy	
Perforation	AV fistula		Alcohol leak into LAD		
Tamponade	Distal emboli				
Allergic reactions	Arterial thrombosis Infection				

AV, atrioventricular; ASA, alcohol septal ablation; Cath, catheterization; CHF, coronary heart failure; LAD, left anterior descending artery; MI, myocardial infarction; PCI, percutaneous coronary intervention; TIA, transient ischemic attack; VSD, ventricular septal defect; V tach, ventricular tachycardia.

could have been done today with the availability of lower profile balloons, coaxial guiding catheters, more choices of , and better operator's experience. ST-segment elevation associated with chest pain was noted in the inferior leads during contrast injection in one patient. This was possibly due to entry of contrast into the inferior wall and right ventricle (RV) through the septal collateral network. Overall, ASA was highly feasible with a success rate of greater than 99% in the last 400 cases.

Death

In the Baylor and Medical University of South Carolina case series, there were 6 procedure-related deaths (14). Since then, three additional deaths have occurred in our series of 850 patients. The causes of periprocedural deaths are shown in Table 25-4.

Early on in the case series, two patients died due to dissection of the left main or LAD during the procedure before the alcohol was injected. One patient died of a retroperitoneal hematoma, which was identified when the patient remained

persistently hypotensive after the procedure. The patient was emergently resuscitated with volume and blood products but died soon after. One patient with mild calcific aortic stenosis developed acute ventricular septal rupture and subsequent pulmonary edema after the procedure and died. Another patient died suddenly 10 days after the procedure, likely due to a ventricular arrhythmia. One case of late inferior wall myocardial infarction (MI) with RV infarct and cardiogenic shock occurred 10 days after ASA. The right coronary artery (RCA) was angiographically normal at ASA, and autopsy revealed fresh clot in the mid RCA and evidence of recent septal infarct and also inferior–posterior infarct. It is possible that the alcohol injected into the septal artery entered into the distal RCA via collaterals and produced this infarct. Since then, we have noted angiographic appearance of the distal RCA during angiographic imaging of the septal artery on four separate occasions. In these cases we selected a different septal artery for ASA or we recommended surgical myectomy. More recently, one patient with severe diastolic heart failure and

TABLE 25-3 **Aborted Procedures**

Cause of Failure	Outcome
LAD dissection	Died at surgery
Balloon could not be engaged in the septal perforator artery	Elective myectomy
Guide no-engagement with the left coronary ostium due to tortuosity	Medical therapy
Tamponade developing due to LV biopsy	Emergent surgery and myectomy
LAD dissection	Emergent CABG and myectomy
Septal artery dissection	Elective myectomy
Left main dissection	Died after emergent CABG and myectomy
Inadequate septal perforator arteries for ASA	Elective myectomy
Chest pain and ST-segment elevation in inferior leads before ASA	Medical therapy
Septal wire perforation with myocardial extravasation	Successful ASA later

ASA, alcohol septal ablation; CABG, coronary artery bypass graft surgery; LAD, left anterior descending artery; LV, left ventricle. (Reprinted from Fernandes VL, Nielsen C, Nagueh SF, et al. Follow-up of alcohol septal ablation for symptomatic hypertrophic obstructive cardiomyopathy. *JACC Cardiovasc Interv.* 2008; 1:561–570, with permission from Elsevier.)

elevated filling pressures developed cardiogenic shock and pulmonary edema and could not be resuscitated. The last patient in our series to die was a very anxious male with HOCM who had his beta blockade stopped before the ASA proce-

TABLE 25-4 **Causes of Procedure-Related Deaths (of 850 Patients Series Baylor–MUSC)**

LAD dissection and ventricular fibrillation during ASA; died during CABG
Retroperitoneal bleed
Acute septal perforation (VSD) with pulmonary edema
Left main dissection
Sudden death 10 days after ASA
Late inferior MI with RV infarct and cardiogenic shock (10 days post-ASA)
RV perforation and tamponade from temporary pacemaker lead
Cardiogenic shock
Stress cardiomyopathy

dure. The ASA procedure was uneventful except for the patient's high level of anxiety, which needed significantly more intravenous sedation than usual. About 30 minutes after the procedure, the patient developed hypotension with a Tako-tsubo-like ventricle and could not be resuscitated. This could have been due to stress cardiomyopathy (Tako-tsubo syndrome). Additional reported causes of death are ventricular arrhythmia, pulmonary embolism, and progressive right heart failure.

The reported early 30-day mortality for ASA ranges between 0% and 5%, with a mean of 1.5% (15).

Nontargeted Remote MI

ASA is designed to create a targeted MI in the distribution of the chosen septal artery. The site of intended infarct is the hypertrophied anterior septum at the contact site of the anterior mitral leaflet in systole (Fig. 25-4). In our series, 1.3 ± 0.5 septal arteries were injected with 2.6 ± 1.0 ml ethanol per patient (14). Creatine kinase levels are generally ~500 units per cc of alcohol injected.

Remote infarction can be due to extravasation of ethanol or to the presence of collateral circulation (Fig. 25-5). The common areas of nontargeted infarct are the anterior wall and

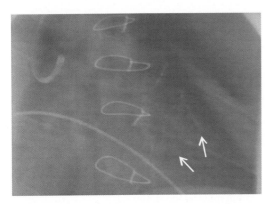

FIGURE 25-5. Injection of contrast through the inflated balloon in the septal perforator branch. There is filling of the distal LAD via septal to LAD collaterals (*arrows*).

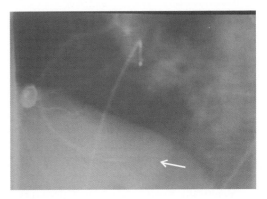

FIGURE 25-7. Coronary angiogram of the right coronary artery (RCA) after injection of alcohol in a septal perforator branch of the LAD. There is no flow in the distal RCA, likely due to extravasation of alcohol in the RCA territory through collateral flow (*arrow*).

apex from seepage of alcohol from the septal artery (Fig. 25-6) or the distal RCA territory from egress of alcohol through septal collaterals (Fig. 25-7). ASA can also result in undesirable infarction in the location of the RV free wall, LV free wall, or the papillary muscles. Echocardiographic guidance (16) with use of agitated x-ray contrast or echo contrast agents will identify inappropriate sites for alcohol injection.

ECG Changes and High-grade AV Block

ASA has been complicated by ECG changes which include QT prolongation, Q waves, right bundle branch block (RBBB, 72%), left bundle branch block (LBBB, 6%), first-degree heart block (53%), and complete heart block (CHB) (15,17,18).

The incidence of complete heart block requiring a pacemaker has been reported to be up to 40% in some early series (15). In the reported series of 629 consecutive patients, the incidence of high-grade AV block necessitating permanent pacemaker implantation in the initial 50 patients was 28% (14). The incidence of AV block decreased significantly after the procedure was modified by slower injection of smaller amounts of ethanol per septal perforator artery and the use of myocardial contrast echocardiography (MCE). It is important to note that patients referred for ASA might have previously undergone implantation of a permanent pacemaker or of an ICD. Therefore, reported case series might underestimate the true pacemaker requirement following ASA. However, in the Baylor and Medical University of South Carolina case series, after exclusion of patients with prior permanent pacemaker and ICD, the new pacemaker requirement was 9.7%. In the subsequent 579 patients,

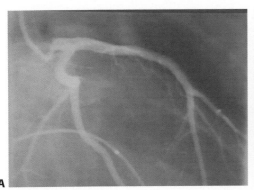
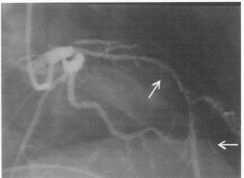

FIGURE 25-6. Leakage of alcohol in the LAD. (**A**) Baseline coronary angiogram. (**B**) Coronary angiogram obtained after injection of alcohol (*arrows*).

the pacemaker requirement rate was 6.5%, yielding a net rate of permanent pacing of 8.2% in the entire cohort of 629 patients.

There is clearly a learning curve, and the rate of new pacemaker implantation in high-volume centers is currently less than 10% (15,18). In some European centers in which patients are usually monitored for several days after ASA, or who receive steroid therapy for relief of peri-infarct edema, the incidence of new pacemaker implantation is less than 5%.

Significant predictors of new pacemaker implantation are pre-existing LBBB or first-degree heart block, injection of ethanol by bolus rather than slow infusion, lack of use of MCE, injection of more than one septal artery, and the female gender (19).

Hypotension

Mild hypotension can be seen in up to 25% of patients after ASA. The etiology of hypotension can be diverse (Table 25-5) and should be assiduously sought because the treatment can be quite different. In some cases hypotension persists for hours despite successful relief of LVOT obstruction and absence of any other obvious complication or cause. Vasomotor instability (20), which is known to occur in hypertrophic cardiomyopathy patients, could be responsible for some of the hypotensive episodes after ASA. Supportive measures include volume resuscitation with hemodynamic monitoring and use of inotropic support. IV phenylephrine is the favored agent in this situation to maintain hemodynamic stability.

TABLE 25-5 Hypotension after ASA

Cause	Treatment
Vasomotor instability	Volume resuscitation and phenylephrine
Hypovolemia	Volume resuscitation
Medications	Reversal of meds, volume
Cardiogenic shock (dissection, large infarct, alcohol spillover into LAD, RV infarct, remote infarct)	Phenylephrine, IABP
Stress cardiomyopathy	Volume, beta blockers
Tamponade	Pericardiocentesis
Bleeding	Volume and blood products
Mitral regurgitation	IABP and surgery
VSD	IABP and surgery

Coronary Artery Dissection

In the Baylor and Medical University of South Carolina case series, the procedure was complicated by coronary dissections in 8 of 629 patients (Fig. 25-8) (14). Five dissections were treated successfully by coronary stents, one spiral dissection was complicated by ventricular fibrillation and arrest (the patient expired during emergency surgery), one dissection occurred prior to alcohol injection and was referred to surgery, and one dissection did not require any additional treatment. One additional dissection

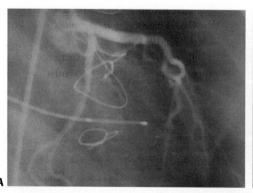 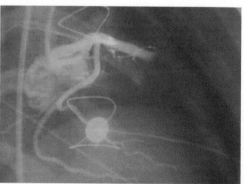

A   B

FIGURE 25-8. (**A**) Baseline coronary angiography. (**B**) Occlusive dissection in the proximal left anterior descending artery.

was treated successfully with stent implantation 10 days after the procedure, when the patient presented with chest pain. Interestingly, 7 out of 8 dissections occurred in women. This could be due to the progestational effects on the vessel wall making it more prone to dissection during instrumentation. The procedure has been modified by a focus on coaxial guide catheter position, and by the use of soft-tip guidewires. No further dissections have been noted in the last 400 patients. In addition, special care should be taken while withdrawing the deflated balloon from the septal artery after alcohol injection. The guiding catheter will tend to telescope into the left main and LAD during balloon withdrawal unless it is held back by the operator. Noncoaxial guiding catheters should not be used for ASA for the same reason.

Perforation and Tamponade

During ASA, perforation and tamponade, while rare, are usually due to temporary pacemaker leads perforating through the RV free wall. If appreciated early, the anticoagulation should be held or reversed with protamine, and immediate pericardiocentesis should be done with echocardiographic guidance when appropriate. However, most often the perforation and tamponade are noted at the end of the procedure when the patient decompensates hemodynamically. The cause of the perforation in most instances is due to inadvertent pacemaker lead manipulation. One patient in our series (14) developed tamponade during endomyocardial LV biopsy performed as part of a research protocol. In a series from the Mayo Clinic (21), there were five cases of tamponade; three were seen in elderly women and were thought to be related to the trans-septal puncture used to measure LV pressure; the other two cases were due to pacemaker lead perforation. Recommendations were made against transseptal puncture in elderly women and in support of the use of relatively less traumatic pacemaker leads to avoid this complication.

Alcohol Leak into the LAD

Alcohol leak is a potentially disastrous complication of ASA. Alcohol can leak back into the LAD either during the injection of alcohol into the septal artery or when the balloon is withdrawn from the septal artery. Alcohol is very toxic to the endothelium and produces endothelial coagulative necrosis as well as myocardial ischemic necrosis in the territory subtended by the vessel. Leakage of alcohol causes no reflow or complete occlusion of the LAD (Fig. 25-6). This may manifest as anterolateral ST elevation MI, severe chest pain, hemodynamic or electrical instability, and cardiac arrest. Alternatively the echocardiogram may reveal anterior, anterolateral, or apical wall motion abnormality, which may be an earlier indicator of this complication.

This complication can be avoided by meticulous technique, the use of a slightly oversized balloon (1.2:1 balloon:septal diameter ratio), and angiography of the LAD after injection of alcohol. Alcohol injection should be done slowly rather than as a bolus and intermittent fluoroscopy should be done to ensure that the balloon has not migrated from its position. After alcohol injection is completed, the balloon lumen may be gently flushed with a saline solution and the inflated balloon should be left in the septal artery for 5 to 10 minutes. Negative aspiration on the balloon lumen should be maintained when the balloon is withdrawn into the guiding catheter and out of the guide. After the balloon is withdrawn outside the guide, the guide should be allowed to bleed back before any contrast is injected again.

If the LAD flow is compromised, the differential diagnosis includes dissection, spasm, or LAD alcohol leak (22). This should be quickly ascertained and general supportive measures for anterior MI should be instituted. A guidewire should be placed into the LAD and intracoronary nitroglycerine should be administered. Intravascular ultrasound (IVUS) may be helpful to rule out dissection. Intracoronary agents that help no reflow like adenosine, Nipride and nicardipine, or diltiazem may help restore or improve flow. An intra-aortic balloon pump (IABP) can be used to improve coronary perfusion. IIb/IIIa inhibitors may be administered intracoronary or intravenously and adequate anticoagulation (ACT > 250 sec) should be maintained. There is no role for coronary artery bypass graft surgery or PCI in this situation and the treatment is mostly supportive.

Ventricular Arrhythmia

Ventricular arrhythmia can occur in 5% of patients during and after ASA (15). Causes of ventricular

TABLE 25-6	Causes of Ventricular Arrhythmia with ASA
Temporary pacemaker induced	
LV pigtail catheter induced	
Because of intended septal infarction	
Because of inadvertent nontargeted remote infarction	
Because of complication of the procedure	
Ventricular fibrillation	
Intractable ventricular tachycardia storm	

arrhythmia with ASA are shown in Table 25-6. Most episodes of ventricular tachycardia are short lasting and are due to catheter irritation or to the septal infarction itself. However, they can also be secondary to other acute complications of the procedure (i.e., dissection, remote infarct, perforation/tamponade, etc.). Intractable ventricular tachycardia and incessant ventricular fibrillation have been reported in a minority of patients.

If an arrhythmia is noted during alcohol injection, the rate of injection is slowed considerably or discontinued altogether. Major complication must be quickly ruled out. Patients are monitored very closely in the hospital and are considered on a case-by-case basis for an ICD implantation.

Mitral Regurgitation

In the Baylor and Medical University of South Carolina case series, periprocedural mitral regurgitation occurred in two patients who were then referred for mitral valve replacement (14). The mitral regurgitation was thought to be due to subendocardial ischemia. Acute mitral regurgitation could also result from inadvertent injection of alcohol into the papillary muscle. Rarely, papillary muscle rupture or chorda tendinea rupture can cause acute mitral regurgitation.

Acute mitral regurgitation is poorly tolerated and it can be associated with hemodynamic instability or acute pulmonary edema. Treatment involves intravenous nitroprusside and IABP support as a bridge to surgery.

Ventricular Septal Defect

In the reported series, one patient with mild calcific aortic stenosis developed acute pulmonary edema and died from an acute VSD which developed within 6 hours of ASA (14). To prevent the occurrence of this potentially lethal complication, the anterior septal wall thickness should be greater than 1.6 cm if ASA is to be considered and aortic stenosis must be excluded. Management involves an early echocardiogram or Swan-Ganz catheterization to confirm the diagnosis and rule out acute mitral regurgitation. Patients can be hemodynamically supported by intravenous nitroprusside and IABP as a bridge to surgery. More recently these VSDs have been closed percutaneously by a variety of VSD closure devices (23).

Figure 25-9 illustrates a rare case of coronary artery fistula occurring after alcohol injection.

Septal Dissection and Hematoma

Septal dissection and hematoma with extravasations of contrast into the septal myocardium have been seen during ASA. This complication occurs during guidewire manipulation in difficult septal anatomy. Presently, with the availability of a range of flexible and supportive guidewires and small caliber short-length balloons, most septal arteries can be cannulated easily without excessive guidewire manipulation. Septal dissection, hematoma, and extravasation are usually benign but may require the procedure to be aborted and performed at another time.

Delayed Infarction

Delayed myocardial infarction has also been described. One patient in our series died 10 days after ASA from inferior wall MI, right ventricular infarct, and cardiogenic shock (14). The RCA was angiographically normal during the ASA. The autopsy revealed a recent septal infarct and evidence of fresh clot in the RCA with acute inferior wall and right ventricular MI. A review of the ASA angiograms revealed extensive septal collaterals to the distal RCA and posterior descending artery, which could have contributed to the late infarct. Figure 25-5 illustrates a case of collateral flow from the septal branches to the distal LAD artery. This anatomy and the corresponding septals to RCA collateral anatomy represent an absolute contraindication to ASA.

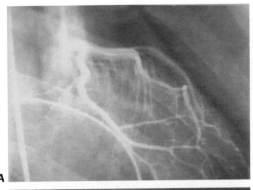
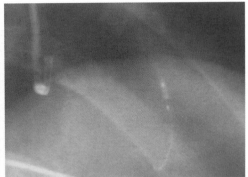
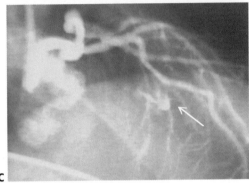

FIGURE 25-9. (**A**) Baseline coronary angiogram of the left anterior descending artery. (**B**) Contrast injection through the inflated balloon. (**C**) New coronary artery fistula (*arrow*).

Tako-tsubo Cardiomyopathy

The last death in our series was a very anxious male with HOCM who had his beta blockade stopped before the ASA procedure. The ASA procedure was uneventful except that the patient's high level of anxiety needed more than usual intravenous sedation. About 30 minutes after the procedure, the patient developed intractable hypotension with a Tako-tsubo-like ventricle with subsequent cardiac arrest, and all resuscitative measures failed. This death could have been due to acute stress cardiomyopathy (Tako-tsubo syndrome) (24). We now administer intravenous beta blockade at the end of the procedure.

■ LATE COMPLICATIONS

Complications that are observed for more than 30 days after ASA are classified as late complications.

Death

In the reported case series (14) of 629 patients, there were 51 deaths over a 10-year follow-up period (Table 25-7). Of these, 24 were cardiac deaths, 21 were noncardiac deaths, and 6 deaths were due to unknown causes. Of the 24 cardiac deaths, 6 deaths were procedure-related, and 7

were sudden cardiac deaths. Post-operative deaths occurred in 8 patients (out of 36 patients who had myectomy/mitral valve/aortic valve surgery). There were three deaths from congestive heart failure. None of the heart failure deaths were due to systolic dysfunction. A number of elderly patients had significant co-morbidities and died of noncardiac causes or from unknown causes. The mean age at death was 67 ± 14 years (range 27–88 years). At the time of death, 6 patients (12%) were less than 50 years of age, and

TABLE 25-7 **Mortality Data (51 Deaths)**

Cardiac Deaths (n = 24)	Noncardiac Deaths (n = 21)
Procedure related (n = 6)	Lung disease (n = 7)
Postoperative (n = 6)	Infection and sepsis (n = 4)
CHF (EF > 60%) (n = 5)	Cancer (n = 3)
SCD (n = 7)	CVA (n = 4) Other causes (n = 3)

CHF, congestive heart failure; CVA, cerebrovascular accident; EF, ejection fraction; SCD, sudden cardiac death. There were 6 deaths with unknown causes.

27 patients (53%) were more than 70 years of age. The older patients had significant co-morbidities.

Concern has been expressed that the septal scar resulting from ASA would create a milieu for the generation of malignant ventricular arrhythmias and resultant sudden cardiac death. Yet, the low incidence of known sudden cardiac death during the follow-up period seems to negate these concerns. The 1-year (97%), 5-year (92%), and 8-year (89%) survival is similar to the survival after surgical myectomy from Toronto General Hospital (25) (338 patients) and Mayo Clinic (26) (289 patients), which was 98%, 95% to 96%, and 83% at 1, 5, and 10 years, respectively. Reassuringly, despite the ASA patient cohort being older (53.9 ± 15 years) than the Toronto General Hospital (47 ± 14 years) or Mayo Clinic (45.3 ± 19 years) cohorts, the long-term survival was similar. No difference in survival was also observed after septal ablation when compared with surgical myectomy at 4-year follow in two age and gender-matched cohorts of patients with obstructive hypotrophic cardiomyopathy ($P = 0.18$ for ASA vs. myectomy) (Fig. 25-10). However, it is important to mention that in the Mayo Clinic cohort of patients undergoing ASA, ventricular fibrillation occurred in three patients prior to hospital discharge, and documented sustained ventricular tachycardia occurred after discharge in two other patients. Thus, it is still unclear whether ASA might have a pro-arrhythmogenic effect.

The relief of LVOT obstruction with ASA is associated with a significant regression of left ventricular hypertrophy (Fig. 25-11). The degree of hypertrophy in HOCM and severity of LVOT obstruction have been shown to be independent risk factors for cardiac death (2,3). It is likely that regression of hypertrophy and LVOT gradient reduction more than offset the putative risk due to the localized septal infarction.

Ventricular Tachycardia and Implantable Cardioverter Defibrillator Shocks

As discussed previously, there is a theoretical concern that the infarct induced by ASA could induce ventricular tachyarrhythmia in the long term. This has, however, not been substantiated in our long-term study (14). Only 7 out of 629 patients had sudden cardiac death during follow-up. The long-term survival rates too were similar to the survival rates after myectomy.

Cuoco et al. followed 123 consecutive patients with HOCM deemed to be at high risk for sudden death who underwent ASA and also received an ICD to prevent sudden cardiac death (27). During a mean follow-up period of 2.9 years, nine

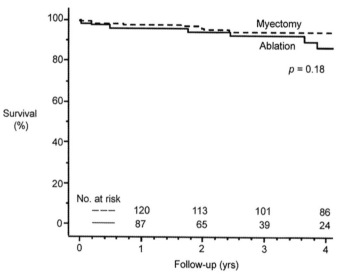

FIGURE 25-10. Comparison of survival after septal ablation with a matched cohort of surgical myectomy patients. The 4-year survival free of all mortality (including defibrillator discharge for lethal arrhythmia) among septal ablation patients was similar to that observed among age- and gender-matched patients who underwent isolated surgical myectomy. (From Sorajja P, Valeti U, Nishimura RA. Outcome of alcohol septal ablation for obstructive hypertrophic cardiomyopathy. *Circulation.* 2008;118:131–139.)

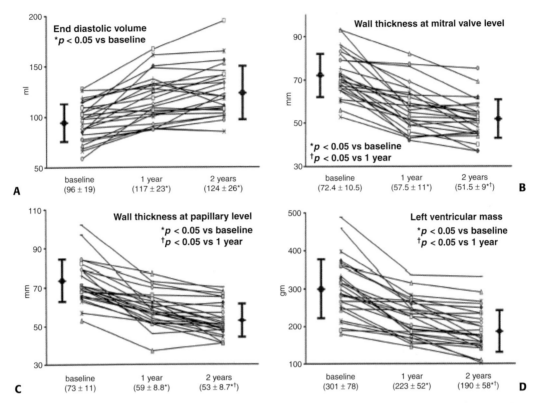

FIGURE 25-11. (**A**) Individual data points of LVEDV, (**B**) wall thickness score at mitral valve level, (**C**) wall thickness score at papillary muscle level, (**D**) and mass at baseline and 1 and 2 years after NSRT. (From Mazur W, Nagueh SF, Lakkis NM, et al. Regression of left ventricular hypertrophy after nonsurgical septal reduction therapy for hypertrophic obstructive cardiomyopathy. *Circulation.* 2001;103:1492–1496.)

appropriate defibrillator shocks were recorded. No significant differences in risk factors for sudden cardiac death were seen between patients who did and those who did not receive appropriate shocks. The estimated annual rate of appropriate ICD discharges was 2.8% over 3 years which was actually below that reported in HOCM patients with ICD but not treated with ASA. The results suggest that ASA is not pro-arrhythmic and may actually help prevent ventricular tachycardia/fibrillation by relieving outflow tract obstruction and enhancing reverse modeling.

Mitral Regurgitation

The mitral valve anatomy should be carefully assessed before ASA. Patients with intrinsic mitral valve pathology, which is independent of the systolic anterior motion of the anterior leaflet, may benefit from a surgical approach.

In the Baylor and Medical University of South Carolina case series, 7 out of 629 patients underwent mitral valve surgery during follow-up. Four patients had worsening mitral regurgitation during follow-up (2 of these 4 patients had worsening mitral regurgitation periprocedurally) (14). The other two patients needed mitral valve surgery for flail leaflets which developed during follow-up. The remaining three patients were operated elsewhere and the cause of the mitral regurgitation is unknown.

Late VSD

The infarcted septum shows an initial rapid thinning up to 3 months and then a gradual thinning over the 10-year follow-up period (Fig. 25-12). The initial rapid thinning is likely a result of the scar formation and the late slower thinning is due to ventricular remodeling due to relief of LVOT obstruction. In the case series of 629 patients no late VSDs were noted in long-term follow-up up to 10 years (14). Similar to post-myectomy, there are rare reported cases of VSD after ASA. These have been managed with surgery and patch closure and more recently

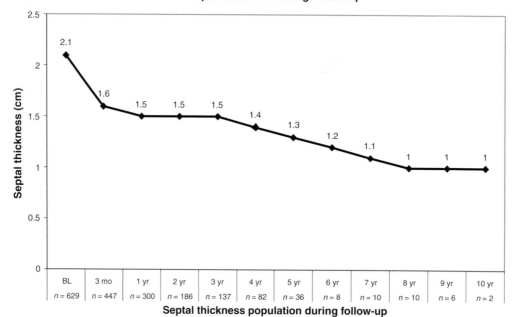

FIGURE 25-12. Septal thickness during follow-up after ASA. Changes in septal thickness after alcohol ablation are illustrated. *N*, number of individuals undergoing echocardiographic analysis to determine the septal thickness. (Reprinted from Fernandes VL, Nielsen C, Nagueh SF, et al. Follow-up of alcohol septal ablation for symptomatic hypertrophic obstructive cardiomyopathy. *JACC Cardiovasc Interv.* 2008;1:561–570, with permission from Elsevier.)

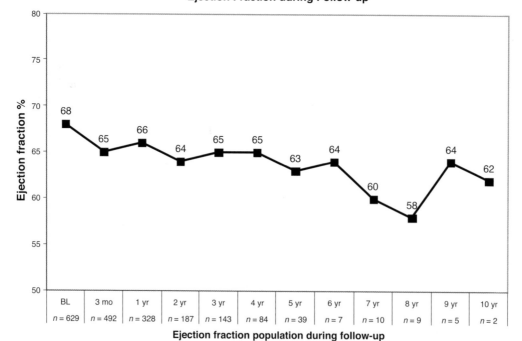

FIGURE 25-13. Ejection fraction during follow-up after ASA. Changes in LV ejection after alcohol ablation are illustrated. *N*, number of individuals undergoing echocardiographic analysis to determine the ejection fraction. (Reprinted from Fernandes VL, Nielsen C, Nagueh SF, et al. Follow-up of alcohol septal ablation for symptomatic hypertrophic obstructive cardiomyopathy. *JACC Cardiovasc Interv.* 2008;1:561–570, with permission from Elsevier.)

with percutaneous closure with VSD occluder devices (23).

Congestive Heart Failure

Both systolic and diastolic heart failure have been reported with HOCM. After ASA, most patients have significant symptomatic improvement in their dyspnea score (NYHA) and are free of symptoms. Diastolic heart failure is common because the basic "myofibrillar disarray" substrate is unchanged with ASA or myectomy; only the LVOT obstruction is relieved. Most cases of systolic dysfunction after ASA are due to coexisting coronary artery disease and ischemic cardiomyopathy.

In the Baylor and Medical University of South Carolina case series, deaths secondary to congestive heart failure (CHF) were all due to diastolic heart failure (14). During serial follow-up, the ejection fraction decreased from the hyperdynamic range to the low 60s (Fig. 25-13). Favorable ventricular remodeling, reduction in left ventric-

ular hypertrophy, and improved diastolic indices have been demonstrated after ASA (28).

Repeat ASA

Repeat procedure for persistence or recurrence of symptoms might be needed in up to 14% of patients (14). This relatively high incidence might reflect the early learning curve and subsequent conservative approach of reduced alcohol injection aimed toward reducing the incidence of AV block and the need for permanent pacemakers. Also the determinants of acute success in the laboratory are at best inexact and therefore may not always predict long-term success. Importantly, ASA can be successful in up to 94% of the repeat procedures (14).

■ CONCLUSION

ASA has been very successful in relieving LVOT obstruction in HOCM. The short, mid-term, and long-term results (Fig. 25-14) have been

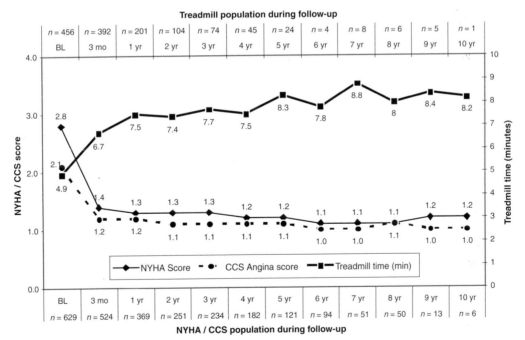

FIGURE 25-14. Subjective and objective indices of improvement during follow-up after ASA. Illustrated here is the beneficial effect of ASA on symptoms as determined by the NYHA and the CCS scores (ordinate) for heart failure symptoms and angina, respectively, and exercise tolerance as determined by the treadmill exercise time. On the lower abscissa, '*n*' indicates the number of individuals undergoing assessment for NYHA and CCS class at that follow-up period. On the upper abscissa, '*n*' indicates the number of individuals undergoing treadmill exercise testing at that follow-up period. Symptomatic (subjective) improvement occurs within the first 3 months, and is maintained for the remainder of the follow-up period. This correlates with the improved exercise tolerance (objective) at the same time points. (Reprinted from Fernandes VL, Nielsen C, Nagueh SF, et al. Follow-up of alcohol septal ablation for symptomatic hypertrophic obstructive cardiomyopathy. *JACC Cardiovasc Interv.* 2008;1:561–570, with permission from Elsevier.)

encouraging. Although the debate regarding the long-term risk of proarrhythmia due to the infarct milieu created by ASA is ongoing, the jury is still out. Hence, ASA has been eagerly adopted and is now the preferred modality for treatment of medically intractable symptoms of HOCM. However, ASA does have a steep learning curve and unique complications and is best suited for dedicated interventional cardiologists in centers, which offer comprehensive care for patients with HOCM.

References

1. Maron BJ, McKenna WJ, Danielson GK, et al. Task Force on Clinical Expert Consensus Documents. American College of Cardiology; Committee for Practice Guidelines. European Society of Cardiology. American College of Cardiology/European Society of Cardiology clinical expert consensus document on hypertrophic cardiomyopathy. A report of the American College of Cardiology Foundation Task Force on Clinical Expert Consensus Documents and the European Society of Cardiology Committee for Practice Guidelines. *J Am Coll Cardiol.* 2003;42:1687–1713.

2. Maron MS, Olivotto I, Betocchi S, et al. Effect of left ventricular outflow tract obstruction on clinical outcome in hypertrophic cardiomyopathy. *N Engl J Med.* 2003;348:295–303.

3. Maron MS, Olivotto I, Zenovich AG, et al. Hypertrophic cardiomyopathy is predominantly a disease of left ventricular outflow tract obstruction. *Circulation.* 2006;114:2232–2239.

4. Morrow AG, Reitz BA, Epstein SE, et al. Operative treatment in hypertrophic subaortic stenosis: techniques, and the results of pre and postoperative assessments in 83 patients. *Circulation.* 1975;52:88.

5. McCully RB, Nishimura RA, Tajik AJ, et al. Extent of clinical improvement after surgical treatment of hypertrophic obstructive cardiomyopathy. *Circulation.* 1996;94:467–471.

6. Schulte HD, Bircks WH, Loesse B, et al. Prognosis of patients with hypertrophic obstructive cardiomyopathy after transaortic myectomy: late results up to twenty-five years. *J Thorac Cardiovasc Surg.* 1993;106:709–717.

7. Ten Berg JM, Suttorp MJ, Knaepen PF, et al. Hypertrophic obstructive cardiomyopathy: initial results and long-term follow-up after Morrow septal myectomy. *Circulation.* 1994;90:1781–1793.

8. Heric B, Lytle BW, Miller DP, et al. Surgical management of hypertrophic obstructive cardiomyopathy: early and late results. *J Thorac Cardiovasc Surg.* 1995;110:195–206.

9. Sigwart U. Non-surgical myocardial reduction for hypertrophic obstructive cardiomyopathy. *Lancet.* 1995;346(8969):211–214.

10. Lakkis NM, Nagueh SF, Dunn JK, et al. Non-surgical septal reduction therapy for hypertrophic obstructive cardiomyopathy: one-year follow-up. *J Am Coll Cardiol.* 2000;36:852–855.

11. Gietzen FH, Leuner CJ, Raute-Kreinsen U, et al. Acute and long-term results after transcoronary ablation of septal hypertrophy (TASH): catheter interventional treatment for hypertrophic obstructive cardiomyopathy. *Eur Heart J.* 1999;20:1342–1354.

12. Fernandes VL, Nagueh SF, Wang W, et al. A prospective follow-up of alcohol septal ablation for symptomatic hypertrophic obstructive cardiomyopathy: the Baylor experience (1996–2002). *Clin Cardiol.* 2005;28:124–130.

13. Faber L, Meissner A, Ziemssen P, et al. Percutaneous transluminal septal myocardial ablation for hypertrophic obstructive cardiomyopathy: long term follow-up of the first series of 25 patients. *Heart.* 2000;83:326–331.

14. Fernandes VL, Nielsen C, Nagueh SF, et al. Follow-up of alcohol septal ablation for symptomatic hypertrophic obstructive cardiomyopathy. *JACC Cardiovasc Interv.* 2008;1:561–570

15. Alam M, Dokainish H, Lakkis N. Alcohol septal ablation for hypertrophic obstructive cardiomyopathy: a systematic review of published studies. *J Interv Cardiol.* 2006;19:319–327.

16. Lakkis NM, Nagueh SF, Kleiman NS, et al. Echocardiography-guided ethanol septal reduction for hypertrophic obstructive cardiomyopathy. *Circulation.* 1998;98:1750–1755.

17. Runquist LH, Nielsen CD, Killip D, et al. Electrocardiographic findings after alcohol septal ablation therapy for obstructive hypertrophic cardiomyopathy. *Am J Cardiol.* 2002;90:1020–1022.

18. Faber L, Welge D, Fassbender D, et al. Percutaneous septal ablation for symptomatic hypertrophic obstructive cardiomyopathy: managing the risk of procedure-related AV conduction disturbances. *Int J Cardiol.* 2007;119:163–167.

19. Chang SM, Nagueh SF, Spencer WH III, et al. Complete heart block: determinants and clinical impact in patients with hypertrophic obstructive cardiomyopathy undergoing nonsurgical septal reduction therapy. *J Am Coll Cardiol.* 2003;42:296–300.

20. Lim PO, Morris-Thurgood J, Frenneux M. Vascular mechanisms of sudden death in hypertrophic cardiomyopathy, including blood pressure responses to exercise. *Cardiol Rev.* 2002;10:15–23.

21. Sorajja P, Valeti U, Nishimura RA. Outcome of alcohol septal ablation for obstructive hypertrophic cardiomyopathy. *Circulation.* 2008;118:131–139.

22. Ziaee A, Lim M, Stewart R, Kern MJ. Coronary artery occlusion after transluminal alcohol septal ablation: differentiating dissection, spasm, and alcohol-induced no reflow. *Catheter Cardiovasc Interv.* 2005;64:204–208.

23. Aroney CN, Goh TH, Hourigan LA, et al. Ventricular septal rupture following nonsurgical septal reduction for hypertrophic cardiomyopathy: treatment with percutaneous closure. *Catheter Cardiovasc Interv.* 2004;61(3):411–414.

24. Kuhn H, Gietzen F, Leuner C. 'The abrupt no-flow': a no-reflow like phenomenon in hypertrophic cardiomyopathy. *Eur Heart J.* 2002;23(1):91–93.

25. Woo A, Williams WG, Choi R, et al. Clinical and echocardiographic determinants of long-term survival after surgical myectomy in obstructive hypertrophic cardiomyopathy. *Circulation.* 2005; 111:2033–2041.

26. Ommen SR, Maron BJ, Olivotto I, et al. Long-term effects of surgical septal myectomy on survival in patients with obstructive hypertrophic cardiomyopathy. *J Am Coll Cardiol.* 2005;46: 470–476.

27. Cuoco FA, Spencer WH III, Fernandes VL, et al. Implantable cardioverter-defibrillator therapy for primary prevention of sudden death after alcohol septal ablation of hypertrophic cardiomyopathy. *J Am Coll Cardiol.* 2008;52:1718–1723.

28. Mazur W, Nagueh SF, Lakkis NM, et al. Regression of left ventricular hypertrophy after nonsurgical septal reduction therapy for hypertrophic obstructive cardiomyopathy. *Circulation.* 2001;103: 1492–1496.

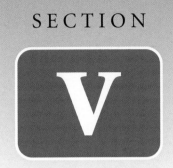

SECTION

V

Specific Complications of Peripheral Vascular Procedures

26

Complications of Carotid Stenting and Intracranial Interventions

ALEX ABOU-CHEBL, HITINDER S. GURM, AND JAY S. YADAV

arotid artery stenting (CAS) with emboli protection devices (EPDs) has now emerged as a viable technique for treatment of extracranial carotid artery (CA) disease (1,2). Similarly, intracranial interventions are increasingly being performed for the treatment of acute stroke and symptomatic intracranial atherosclerosis. This chapter focuses on common and uncommon complications and challenges that arise during these procedures and strategies to avoid these complications or to deal with them effectively once encountered.

◼ COMPLICATIONS OF EXTRACRANIAL CAROTID INTERVENTIONS

The challenges and complications related to CAS can be broadly divided into those unique to CAS and those associated with vascular access and contrast exposure. Since CA disease is often associated with increased prevalence of peripheral vascular disease, these patients are at a greater risk of access site complications and cholesterol embolization. Similarly, an increased prevalence of renal dysfunction (3) predisposes these patients to a greater risk of contrast induced acute kidney injury. The strategies to avoid or minimize these complications are listed in detail elsewhere but include appropriate case selection, meticulous vascular access technique, proper hydration protocols, and minimization of contrast dose (4,5).

Complications and Challenges Unique to Carotid Stenting

Potential risks and challenges associated with CAS include the inability to access the target site or deliver equipment, injury (dissection, perforation) of access or target vessel, neurological complications, cardiovascular complications, device malfunction, general medical complications, and mortality.

Access to Carotid Lesion

Safe CAS requires access to the common CA (CCA) in an atraumatic fashion, followed by safe crossing of the lesion and delivery of the stent with successful deployment and then retrieval of EPDs. There are challenges unique to each aspect of the process that an operator needs to be aware of. Most CAS is performed via a femoral approach, but this approach may not be feasible in patients with occlusive aortoiliac disease. Such patients can be successfully treated via a brachial or a radial approach (6). A contralateral radial approach is usually preferred although some operators prefer to approach the right CA from the right side. The usual practice for a brachial or radial approach is to cannulate the target CCA using a 5F Simmons 1 or an Amplatz L1 or R2 diagnostic catheter and wire the external CA (ECA) with an extrasupport 0.014-in. or an 0.018-in. guidewire. The catheter is then advanced into the ECA. After removing the initial guidewire, a 0.035-in. extrasupport guidewire is

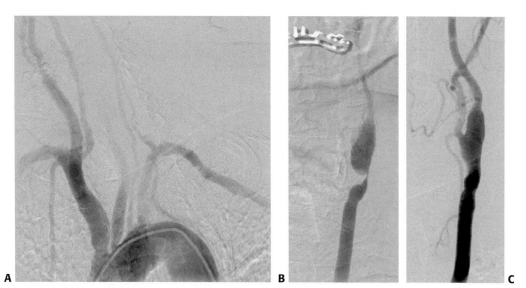

FIGURE 26-1. A 55-year-old woman with symptomatic left carotid artery stenosis 4 years after carotid endarterectomy. (**A**) A type III arch with slow flow in the left common carotid artery. The left common carotid artery (LCCA) is not fully opacified while the rest of the arch and great vessels are well visualized. (**B**) Selective LCCA injection demonstrates a severe lesion in the distal common carotid artery. No flow in the external carotid artery (ECA) is seen. Such a lesion is best approached with a guide in the arch approach. This patient was successfully treated using an AL.75 guide. (**C**) Postintervention result. Normal flow in the internal carotid artery and the ECA is evident.

advanced into the ECA, the catheter is exchanged for a 5F or 6F Shuttle sheath (Cook Medical Inc., Vandergrift Pennsylvania) and positioned in the distal CCA. The procedure is then performed per routine.

While access to common carotid arteries via a femoral approach has been well established, a particular challenge is the left CCA in patients with a bovine or type III arch. Our approach is to engage these vessels with an Amplatz Left (AL1 or AL 0.75) guiding catheter (Fig. 26-1). A 0.014-in. support wire is placed in the ECA to stabilize the guide and helps facilitate equipment delivery.

Delivery of a guiding catheter or sheath to the CCA is an unprotected procedure and has the potential to generate atheroembolism with resultant stroke not only in the ipsilateral carotid bed but also in the posterior circulation or the contralateral bed. Meticulous attention to the technique is required to avoid disruption of proximal plaque and CA dissection.

Delivery of EPDs

EPDs have played a major role in reducing the complications associated with CAS, and we do not support unprotected CAS. Currently, the choice of EPD includes distal occlusion devices, proximal occlusion devices, and filters. There are advantages and disadvantages unique to each system. Our current preference is to use a filter device except for special cases.

The Guardwire (Medtronic Inc., Minneapolis, Minnesota) has a low crossing profile and can be used to negotiate lesions in extremely tortuous vessels. Similarly, the proximal occlusion devices can be very useful in vessels with large thrombotic burden or a diffusely diseased internal CA (ICA) that prevents safe placement of a filter device. The distal and proximal occlusion devices can be used only in patients with an intact circle of Willis, and symptomatic cerebral ischemia with cessation of anterograde flow is a major limitation to their use. Furthermore, the Guardwire provides poor support, has somewhat more difficult preparation, and occasionally may not inflate to seal; the balloon can leak or the movement of the balloon can cause the seal to break and allow anterograde flow. Furthermore, a "suction shadow" below the balloon may retain debris that can potentially embolize upon balloon deflation. Finally, it limits angiographic visualization and hinders precise stent placement. The proximal occlusion devices require larger groin access and are associated with greater risk for vascular complications. Given these drawbacks, most operators prefer to use the filter devices as the preferred EPD for CAS.

One of the challenges in safe deployment of an EPD is the inability to advance the device across an extremely tight, calcified, or tortuous segment (Fig. 26-2). The choices in such cases are to cross with a 0.014-in. bare guidewire and use devices that can be delivered over such a wire (e.g., Emboshield, Spider). However, if the difficulty to cross is noticed while attempting to cross with a filter in its delivery sheath, several strategies can be used. First, if the distal wire has crossed the lesion, it should be left in place and a buddy wire advanced alongside the EPD. Usually, this is sufficient to allow the EPD to cross. If that maneuver fails, the next step is to advance a 1.5- or 2.0-mm balloon of a length sufficient to cover the entire lesion. Most operators will predilate the lesion at this point to permit the filter to be advanced, whereas some will first dotter the lesion and attempt to cross with a filter before predilating. On the basis of the author's experience, the risk of embolization from predilation with such small balloons is less, and they have not noticed any strokes in association with this maneuver. The use of an 8F guide catheter is preferred in cases of severe tortuosity or when EPD delivery is expected to be difficult since it gives more support, bounces less with every systole, and allows torque control when compared with sheaths.

Difficulty in EPD Retrieval

The placement of the stent often changes the normal mechanical properties of the artery and can make removal of the EPD difficult. This may be a particular problem when the proximal edge of the stent is at the ostium of the ICA. The capture sheath will catch at the edge of the stent and can disrupt the stent if force is used (Fig. 26-3). This problem can be minimized by ensuring that the stent is placed covering the distal CCA. Other problems occur because of transmission of tortuosity distally because of the placement of a rigid stent (e.g., Wallstent, Boston Scientific Inc.). If the capture sheath does not advance (Fig. 26-4), force must not be used and every effort must be made to ensure that the filter does not prolapse into the stent. Open filters can get entangled in the freshly deployed stent, and this can lead to loss of captured emboli or fracture and embolization of the EPD (Fig. 26-5). Usually the filter capture sheath is biased toward the stent edge and this prevents the sheath from advancing. Turning the head in a contralateral direction accompanied by neck extension is usually successful in directing the wire bias away

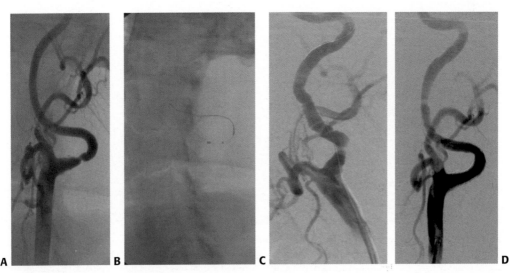

A   **B**   **C**   **D**

FIGURE 26-2. (**A**) A 67-year-old patient with asymptomatic left internal carotid artery (LICA) stenosis. (**B**) An angioguard fails to go around the bend. (**C**) Severe pseudostenosis following placement of two ironman buddy wires. An angioguard was advanced as the ironman wire was withdrawn. (**D**) The results following successful stenting.

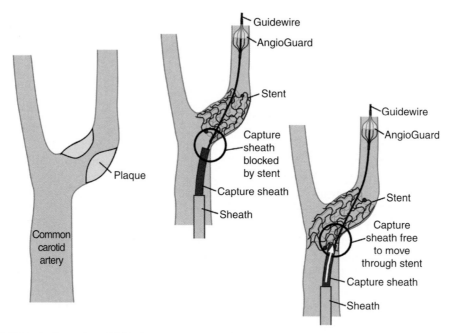

FIGURE 26-3. Illustration of difficulties in capturing emboli protection device when placing a stent at the ostium of the internal carotid artery. (From Casserly IP, Yadav JS. Carotid Artery Intervention. In: Casserly IP, Sachar R, Yadav JS, eds. *Manual of Peripheral Vascular Interventions.* Philadelphia, PA: Lippincott Williams & Wilkins; 2005).

from the stent and unraveling the distal tortuosity and typically permits the delivery of the capture sheath. Sometimes the opposite motion is needed. If the sheath still cannot be advanced and is noticed to catch on the stent edge, use of a buddy balloon or proximal balloon dilation will help change the local geometry and permit delivery of the capture sheath. In cases of severe ICA tortuosity at the bulb where filter retrieval [difficulty] is more likely, the use of a guide

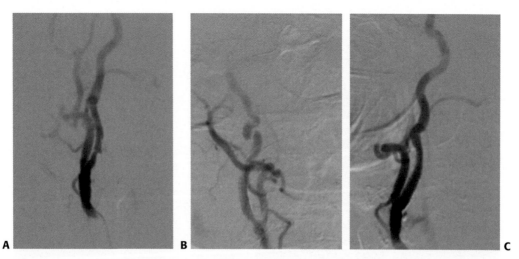

FIGURE 26-4. An 88-year-old patient with a severe asymptomatic right carotid stenosis and aortic stenosis. (**A**) Angiogram demonstrates the lesion. The lesion could not be crossed with a Maverick interceptor despite the use of a buddy wire. The lesion was crossed with a filter wire and a stent was successfully deployed. (**B**) Significant distal tortuosity and vasospasm is evident. The wire biases toward the proximal edge of the stent. The capture sheath could not be advanced, but the filter was finally removed using a long JR4 catheter. (**C**) The distal tortuosity is still evident after removal of the filter.

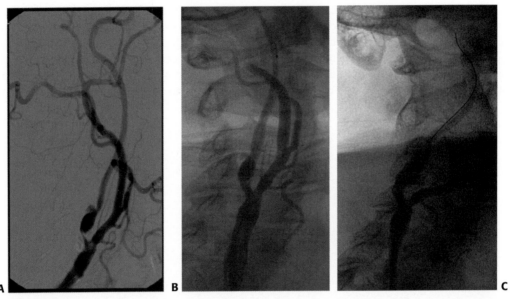

FIGURE 26-5. A 72-year-old patient with symptomatic right internal carotid artery (RICA) lesion. (**A**) An Acunet filter could be delivered only using a buddy wire and the lesion was stented with a 7–10/30 Aculink. (**B**) The filter could not be retrieved despite the use of neck motion, further postdilation, and the use of a JR4 catheter. (**C**) The filter was pulled down and got entangled in the stent, requiring surgical removal. The patient was noted to be blind in the ipsilateral eye postoperatively and remains visually impaired 1 year later.

catheter rather than a straight sheath for access to the CCA is preferred. The guide catheter can be rotated to change the angle of approach to the lesion if either filter delivery or recovery is difficult. Guide rotation may also change the curvature of the vessels to some degree and along with neck rotation often permits device delivery. If these maneuvers do not help, a long 5F JR4 or MP catheter can be used as capture sheaths since the torque control usually permits a change in directionality that helps negotiate the stent edge—this is effective if over-the-wire EPDs are used since the rapid exchange systems are too short (Fig. 26-4). It is helpful to place a long 0.14–in. support wire as a buddy to provide support so that the EPD does not move while the catheter is advanced. Usually these maneuvers are successful in removing the filter, but there are rare cases where surgical removal of the filter has been necessary (Fig. 26-5).

A rare complication that has occurred only once in the authors' experience is total separation of the filter basket from its guidewire (Fig. 26-6). Attempts to snare the filter were unsuccessful and resulted in migration of the filter into the petrous segment of the ICA. The authors chose to deploy bare metal stents in the

CA, trapping the filter between the stent and the vessel wall and restoring normal flow. The patient remained free of symptoms 1 year later.

Other Vascular Complications

Spasm of the ICA due to manipulation of guidewires, catheters, and EPDs has been reported in up to 10% of cases and is more common in smokers (7,8). It is usually transient and responds to vasodilator therapy such as intra-arterial nitroglycerine. Dissection of the common carotid has been rarely reported during sheath or guide placement in the CCA and if detected should be covered with a stent if needed. Perforation of the CA is rare and occurs in far less than 1% of the cases. Most reported cases have used oversized balloons to postdilate a stent placed in calcified arteries. Such lesions have been covered with covered stents or stent grafts (9). Carotid perforation has also been reported in cases of reconstruction of spontaneous dissections. Usually, these have occurred with balloon dilations and have responded to balloon tamponade without the need to use a covered stent. An even rarer complication is the perforation of external CA branches by a Glide wire (Terumo Inc.) placed to advance the sheath or guide (10). The reported cases have involved perforation of the lingual and facial branches with resultant lingual or subglottic hematomas and airway compromise. These patients may complain of dysphagia or a need to swallow as the hematoma develops and may need intuba-

tion or tracheotomy to protect the airway. We avoid wiring the lingual branches, and if the facial branches need to be wired, we preferentially use a nonhydrophilic wire to minimize the risk of perforation. There have been anecdotal cases where the ascending pharyngeal branch has

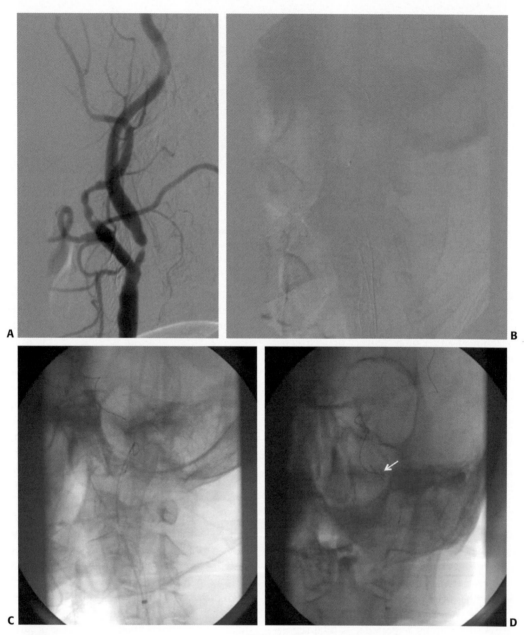

FIGURE 26-6. (**A** and **B**) A 75-year-old man with bilateral symptomatic carotid artery disease presented for intervention on his left carotid artery. The RICA had been stented uneventfully 3 weeks earlier. The lesion was successfully stented with an 8.0/40 Aculink, and the postangiogram revealed normal flow. Attempts to remove the filter revealed free movement of the wire with no motion of the filter. (**C**) Attempts to snare the filter were unsuccessful. (**D**) A decision was made to sandwich the filter between a bare metal stent and the vessel wall (*white arrow*). (*continued*)

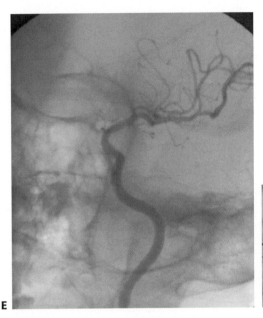

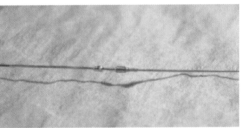

E   F

FIGURE 26-6. (*Continued*) (**E**) The final flow is normal. (**F**) The site where the filter became dislodged from the BHW wire.

been wired erroneously since it can occasionally track along the ICA in its proximal part. Rarely, an EPD has been deployed in this vessel, with resulting retropharyngeal hematoma. The biggest risk again is airway compromise and the treatment involves control of the airway as needed, removal of the EPD, and control of bleeding with deployment of coils to control the bleeding (10). In-depth knowledge of the arterial anatomy with high-quality digital subtraction angiography and the use of roadmapping should prevent such complications.

Cardiovascular Complications

Myocardial infarction occurs in approximately 1% of patients undergoing CAS (Fig. 26-7). Most of these are non-Q wave infarcts with a favorable outcome, and the use of preprocedural statins, antiplatelet therapy, and appropriate antihypertensive therapy is expected to minimize the risk, although there are no randomized data that show efficacy in the setting of CAS.

Hypotension and bradycardia that are symptomatic and require treatment occur in 5% to 10% of CAS procedures but are usually transient. Asymptomatic and clinically insignificant hypotension and bradycardia are much more common and occur in 40% to 50% of cases (11). The mechanism is related to stretching of

afferent carotid sinus baroreceptors and the activation of the medullary vasomotor center. This results in efferent vagal discharge and inhibition of sympathetic outflow, resulting in vasodilatation and bradycardia (Fig. 26-8). Hemodynamic changes are more likely to occur during interventions on calcified lesions involving the carotid bifurcation rather than those proximal or distal to the bulb (11). Conversely, patients with prior carotid endarterectomy appear to be at a lower risk of hemodynamic depression following CAS. The effect is most prominent following postdilation of the stent and can result in profound hypotension and bradycardia and occasional prolonged asystole. The most dramatic response is immediately following postdilation, which starts to improve within seconds of balloon deflation, although some effects can last for up to 24 to 48 hours. Rare cases of prolonged hemodynamic depression have been reported, and in the authors' experience of more than 2,000 cases, the need for a permanent pacemaker is less than 0.1% (unpublished data). While some operators routinely administer prophylactic atropine to all patients, this can result in tachycardia, urinary retention, confusion, and a sense of restlessness, which can be especially problematic in the elderly. The authors reserve the use of atropine to patients who develop

	No. of Patients/No. of Events			
Study	**Carotid Endarterectomy**	**Carotid Artery Stenting**	**Odds Ratio (95% CI)**	**Odds Ratio (95% CI)**
CAVATAS 2001[25]	253/3	251/0		7.03 (0.36–136.76)
SAPPHIRE 2004/8[22,33]	167/12	167/5		2.51 (0.86–7.29)
EVA-3S 2006/8[21,32]	162/2	265/1		2.03 (0.18–22.53)
BACASS 2007[28]	10/0	10/0		
Random effects model	692/17	693/6		2.69 (1.06–6.76)

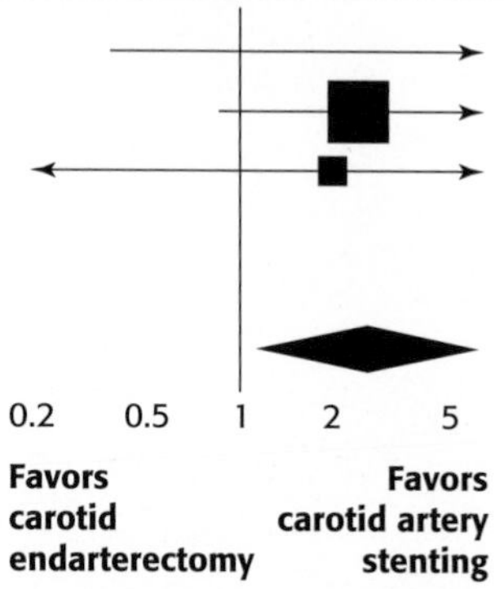

0.2   0.5   1   2   5

Favors carotid endarterectomy   Favors carotid artery stenting

FIGURE 26-7. Forest plot of odds ratios of 30-day risk for myocardial infarction for carotid endarterectomy versus carotid artery stenting. CAVATAS, Carotid and Vertebral Artery Transluminal Angioplasty Study; SAPPHIRE, Stenting and Angioplasty with Protection in Patients at High Risk for Endarterectomy; EVA-3S, Endarterectomy Versus Angioplasty in patients with Symptomatic Severe carotid Stenosis; SPACE, Stent-Supported Percutaneous Angioplasty of the Carotid Artery versus Endarterectomy; BACASS, Basel Carotid Artery Stenting Study. (Reproduced from Meier P, Knapp G, Tamhane U, et al. Short term and intermediate term comparison of endarterectomy versus stenting for carotid artery stenosis: systematic review and meta-analysis of randomised controlled clinical trials. *BMJ.* 2010;340:c467, with permission from BMJ Publishing Group Ltd.)

bradycardia in response to predilation or those with underlying conditions in which even transient bradycardia would be poorly tolerated (e.g., critical aortic stenosis, severe left main coronary artery disease, severe pulmonary hypertension). An alternative strategy in these high-risk patients is to place a temporary pacemaker prior to the procedure, which can be removed once the patient has recovered completely from the hemodynamic depression. There is some evidence that patients who have

prolonged hemodynamic depression have a higher risk of stroke and other major adverse events although this has not been demonstrated in all series (11).

Postprocedural hypotension can be prevented by holding sympatholytic medications prior to the CAS and ensuring adequate hydration. If these measures are not successful, use of oral pseudoephedrine (30–60 mg every 4–6 hours as needed) for asymptomatic hypotension or intravenous dopamine for symptomatic hypotension

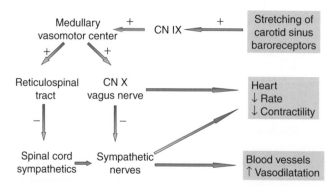

FIGURE 26-8. Mechanisms surrounding the development of periprocedural hypotension and bradycardia. (From Casserly IP, Yadav JS. Carotid Artery Intervention. In: Casserly IP, Sachar R, Yadav JS, eds. *Manual of Peripheral Vascular Interventions.* Philadelphia, PA: Lippincott Williams & Wilkins; 2005.)

is quite effective at ensuring normal blood pressure. Since the underlying mechanism is the inhibition of normal sympathetic outflow, the dose of sympathomimetics required is usually low and the need for high-dose dopamine should prompt search for another cause such as myocardial ischemia or retroperitoneal hemorrhage.

Hypertension after CAS is common and is usually a reflection of the patients' underlying hypertension. Severe hypertension is a major risk factor for cerebral hyperperfusion syndrome (HPS). Cerebral HPS is a rare (1%–2%) but serious complication of carotid revascularization after either carotid endarterectomy or carotid stent placement. Impaired cerebral autoregulation and postrevascularization changes in cerebral hemodynamics are the main mechanisms involved in the development of the syndrome. Predictors of HPS are treatment of a severe ipsilateral stenosis in the presence of a severe contralateral stenosis or occlusion and untreated hypertension (12). HPS presents as a throbbing ipsilateral headache that may be localized to the retroorbital, facial, or temporal area, with accompanying nausea and vomiting. Computed tomography (CT) imaging is usually unremarkable, and there is evidence of increased intracranial flow velocity on transcranial Doppler ultrasound. If untreated, these patients are at high risk of intracerebral hemorrhage (ICH), which is often (80%) fatal. Patients suspected of having post-CAS hyperperfusion need aggressive blood pressure control, using drugs that do not increase cerebral blood flow (e.g., β-blockers, calcium channel blockers). We prefer to use intravenous labetalol while reinstituting patient's oral antihypertensive medications to control blood pressure. It is important to ensure that patient's blood pressure remains under control in the immediate postoperative period, since HPS has been reported to occur up to 14 days after the procedure, although it typically occurs on days 3 to 5 postoperatively. A strategy of aggressive postprocedural blood pressure control with careful outpatient follow-up can drastically reduce the occurrence of this rare but dreaded complication (13).

Neurological Complications

The incidence of stroke and transient ischemic attack (TIA) after CAS varies from 1% to 5% depending on the patient population treated

(symptomatic vs. asymptomatic), the experience of the operators, and the proportion of patients who are treated with an EPD. In experienced centers, the risk of stroke has been very low and less than 3% threshold risk for asymptomatic patients and less than 6% for symptomatic patients. Most strokes occurring after CAS are minor and often resolve by 30 days (14).

The mechanism of stroke is usually embolization of plaque from the site of the intervention and is most common at the time of postdilation of the stent (Fig. 26-9). Embolization can also occur during diagnostic angiography and manipulation of wires and catheters in the aortic arch and the CCA. If a neurological deficit is noticed during the procedure, cerebral angiography should be immediately performed in multiple orthogonal planes with delayed filming that includes the venous phase. If the cerebral angiogram is normal, usually complete recovery can be expected and no further intervention is necessary, although if the patient has a progressive or severe deficit, the presence of an ICH must be considered. If small, an ICH may not have any angiographic manifestations, and only when large and associated with mass effect the classic findings of an intracranial mass are visible on angiography. If the patient has an occlusion of a major intracranial vessel, intracranial rescue intervention should be considered by a

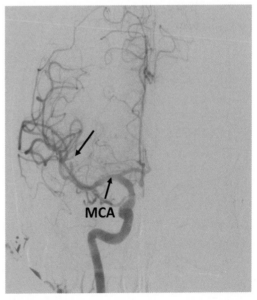

FIGURE 26-9. Distal embolization following carotid artery stenting. MCA, middle cerebral artery.

suitably trained neurointerventionist (see later). If the occlusion involves a small vessel, administration of platelet glycoprotein IIb/IIIa (GPIIb/IIIa) inhibitors can be considered. Also, the activated clotting time (ACT) should immediately be checked, and if it is subtherapeutic, additional heparin should be given.

Strokes and TIAs can also occur later and are usually related to delayed embolization of plaque from the stent or arch or great vessels. When TIA or stroke occurs after the end of the procedure, the final angiogram should be carefully reviewed for the presence of a dissection, particularly in the segment where the EPD was deployed. Patient compliance with the dual antiplatelet regimen should be confirmed and platelet aggregation assays should be performed because of a relatively high incidence of aspirin and clopidogrel resistance (15). In the authors' experience, the only cause of neurological death, other than ICH due to HPS, that they have observed is in patients with acute stent thrombosis due to noncompliance and antiplatelet resistance. These events are fortunately very uncommon, and most TIAs and minor strokes usually resolve spontaneously.

Slow Flow

Slow flow is a phenomenon associated with the use of filter-type EPDs. This is defined as a delay in transit time across the ICA, and it is usually obvious angiographically (Figs. 26-10–26-12). Minor degrees of slow flow manifest as flow in the ICA that is slower than that in the external CA. The likely underlying mechanism is the release of a large amount of plaque debris with occlusion of a large proportion of the filter pores (Fig. 26-13). This phenomenon is mostly noticed after postdilation of the stent, although in some cases, it is evident immediately after stent deployment. Symptomatic lesions; tubular lesions longer than 12 to 15 mm; bulky, soft, and echo lucent carotid plaques; use of large diameter stents and postdilation balloons are major predictors of slow flow (16). Patients with slow flow have suspended debris in the static column of blood, and it is important to aspirate this column by using a manual aspiration catheter prior to filter retrieval. This does not change the flow in the ICA since the filter remains obstructed with plaque debris and immediately after aspirating 40 to 80 ml of

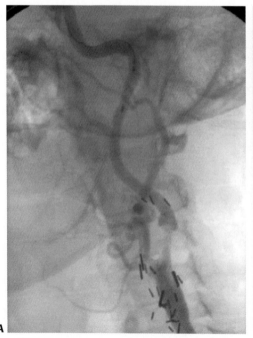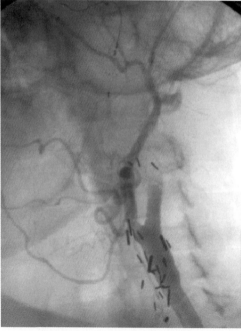

A   **B**

FIGURE 26-10. Slow flow. Angiograms obtained post-PTA (**A**), and poststent placement (**B**). Following stent deployment, there is marked reduction in flow.

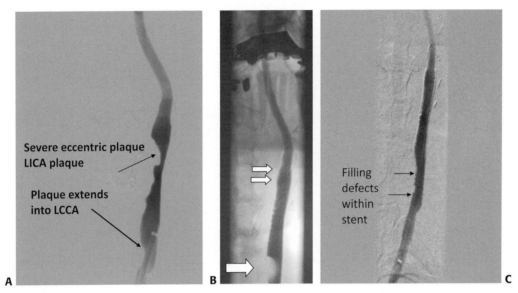

FIGURE 26-11. A 69-year-old patient with occluded RICA and two prior L carotid endarterectomy (CEAs). (**A**) Duplex revealed severe LICA stenosis and evidence of heavy thrombus/plaque burden. Angiography demonstrated severe stenosis involving both the LCCA and LICA. (**B**) Following stenting with a 10 × 40 Precise stent (Cordis Endovascular, Miami Florida), a filling defect was noticed proximally (*large arrow*) along with milder plaque prolapse along the body of the stent (*smaller arrows*). Bivalirudin was administered to ensure adequate anticogulation and in the event of heparin-induced throbocytopenia and another stent was placed proximally. Postdilation with a small-sized balloon resulted in severe slow flow. (**C**) Following aspiration with a thrombecotmy catheter and removal of the filter, the flow was normal. There was, however, evidence of persistent plaque extrusion through the second stent (**C**). The patient was discharged home 2 days later without any neurological deficit.

blood from the ICA, the filter should be removed. Occasionally, severe vasospasm, which is associated with some EPDs more than others (e.g., earlier generations of Emboshield, Abbott

Vascular Inc., Abbott Park Illinois), is the cause of the slow flow. This should be suspected if the markers on the filter basket are not fully separated or if there was excessive movement of the

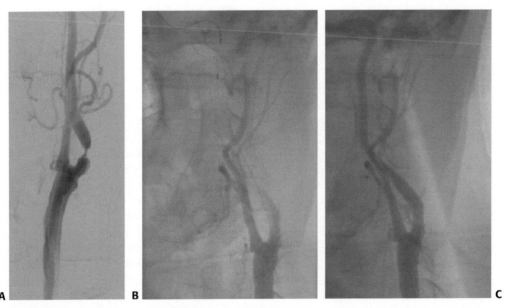

FIGURE 26-12. (**A**) Severe symptomatic LICA stenosis. (**B**) Following postdilation of the stent, there is evidence of severe slow flow. (**C**) Following aspiration and removal of the filter, the flow is normal.

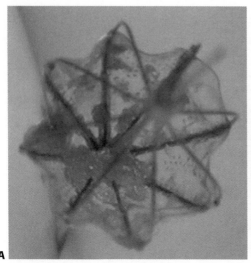
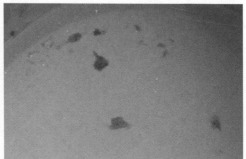

FIGURE 26-13. (A) Debris and emboli on a captured Angioguard™ (Cordis Endovascular, Miami Florida). (B) Slow flow aspirate from the same case in (A).

filter during the procedure. The risk of stroke in patients with slow flow is markedly elevated although most of these strokes are minor.

Plaque Protrusion

A significant degree of plaque prolapse or protrusion through the stent can be observed in rare cases (Fig. 26-11). In the authors' experience, this is most common in patients with long, tubular lesions with bulky plaque or those with aneurismal or ectatic lesions at the site of prior carotid endarterectomy performed using a vein patch. Such lesions should be carefully evaluated prior to the procedure, using CT angiography or carotid Doppler since invasive angiography can underestimate the plaque and thrombus burden, and it may be preferable to consider an alternate strategy such as a covered stent in some cases or endarterectomy. If plaque prolapse is noticed during the procedure, further intervention must be individualized. The first step involves checking an ACT to ensure adequate anticoagulation and consideration of alternate pathology such as procedural thrombosis due to heparin-induced thrombocytopenia or antiplatelet resistance as described earlier. While we are not aware of any such cases in the carotid bed, such events have been noticed in patients undergoing coronary and peripheral interventions. The authors' usual strategy is to switch to a direct thrombin inhibitor in such an event or to add GPIIb/IIIa

antagonists; a drawback to additional anticoagulants or GPIIb/IIIa antagonist use is the increased risk of ICH (see later). The need to cover plaque protrusion with another stent or a stent graft must be individualized and has been our usual approach. The stent used should be the largest diameter available so that when deployed, the stent pore area remains small. Aggressive postdilation must be avoided since it can predispose to embolization.

■ INTRACRANIAL INTERVENTIONS

The most commonly performed intracranial cerebral interventions include acute ischemic stroke (AIS) recanalization, intracranial angioplasty and stenting, and the therapeutic embolization of cerebral aneurysms and arteriovenous malformations. For the most part, the complications associated with these procedures are similar to and are what would be expected with any endovascular procedure on vessels measuring less than 4 mm in diameter. What distinguishes the risk profile of intracranial interventions from interventions on coronary arteries of similar size are the different histological composition of the cerebral vessels and the unforgiving nature of the brain. The intracranial arteries amenable to endovascular therapy and most involved in cerebrovascular disease are the ICAs, the middle cerebral arteries (MCAs), the vertebral arteries (VAs), the basilar artery (BA), and much less commonly the smaller anterior cerebral arteries (ACAs) and the posterior cerebral arteries (PCAs). These vessels differ from muscular arteries in the rest of the body in that they do not have an external elastic lamina or significant adventitia and they have a thin tunica muscularis. They are therefore much more easily injured than the comparably sized coronary arteries. Also, the proximal intracranial ICAs and cervical arteries and VAs often have significant tortuosity that can make device navigation to the brain very difficult if not impossible. These vessels (except for the petrous and cavernous portions of the ICAs) course within the subarachnoid space on the surface of the brain, which is itself enclosed in the noncompliant skull. Perforation or rupture of these vessels can therefore lead to subarachnoid hemorrhage (SAH), elevated intracranial pressure (ICP), and rapid death; this is analogous to cardiac tamponade but is not as easily treated. Also, the MCAs and BA have essential perforating branches that supply the basal ganglia (lenticulostriate branches of the MCA) and the pons, midbrain, and thalami (BA perforators). These branches are typically in the 100- to 200-μm diameter range and therefore may not be visible angiographically, yet their occlusion can result in devastating neurological deficits due to ischemia, and their disruption can result in parenchymal ICH. For the most part, there is no treatment for ICH and SAH and what treatment exists is either ineffective or associated with a high risk of ischemia. The fact that all treatment for cerebral ischemia carries a risk of ICH and all treatment for ICH carries a risk of cerebral ischemia is the single greatest obstacle in the treatment of cerebrovascular disease. Endovascular complications of intracranial interventions thus fall into two broad categories, namely those that cause cerebral ischemia and those that cause ICH.

Risk Factors for Intracranial Complications

The significant tortuosity and fragility of the cerebral vessels described earlier are the major risk factors for complications. The former leads to the need for more aggressive device delivery techniques (e.g., larger, stiffer guide catheters and wires) that combined with the latter greatly increase the risk of vessel injury. As a general rule, stiff wires, highly hydrophilic wires with aggressive tips intended for calcified lesions or to cross chronic total occlusions (CTOs) are contraindicated in the cerebral vessels. Advancing age, uncontrolled hypertension, and more extensive atherosclerosis all increase cerebral vessel tortuosity and fragility. The cerebral vessels may have extensive calcification similar to the coronary arteries. Therefore, stenotic lesion characteristics that would be considered high risk for coronary percutanueous transluminal coronary angioplasty should be considered as high risk if present in the cerebral vessels. CTO of an intracranial vessel should be considered as a contraindication to angioplasty and stenting (17). Advancing age is also a marker for decreasing cerebral neuronal reserve and along with preexisting neurological dysfunction is a marker for increased risk of ischemic injury and reduced potential for recovery. In patients with AIS or those with severely stenotic lesions, hypertension is a major risk factor for ICH (see "Hyperpefusion Syndrome" section earlier). The use of fibrinolytics is associated with higher risks of ICH, and to a lesser degree, anticoagulants and antithrombotics are also risk factors for ICH. In the setting of AIS intra-arterial therapy (IAT), the presence of fibrinolytics should serve as a relative contraindication to the use of any other anticoagulant or antithrombotic including heparin, GPIIb/IIIa antagonists, clopidogrel, and to a lesser degree aspirin (18,19). For IAT procedures, intraoperative heparin may be given but in low doses: typically a 2,000 U bolus is followed by a 500 U/h infusion (20). For non-IAT interventions, therapeutic ACT of 250 to 300 seconds is reasonable, and if stenting is planned, adequate pretreatment with dual antiplatelet agents as in other vascular beds is required. As a general rule, the lowest possible dose of anticoagulant and antithrombotic should be used for intracranial endovascular procedures. Hyperglycemia is a marker for ICH in the setting of AIS, and the size of the baseline hypodensity on CT or the size of the ischemic core on perfusion imaging are also risk factors for ICH and decreased benefit from IAT (21). For elective intracranial revascularization procedures recent (<4 weeks), brain infarction is also a risk factor for ICH but not a contraindication unless the infarct is more than one-third of the territory supplied by the vessel or the patient is disabled by the stroke. In the latter two situations, waiting 4 to 6 weeks if possible may decrease the risk of ICH. Obviously, the presence of ICH on a CT scan or a history of ICH should be considered as contraindications to ischemic endovascular interventions that would require any anticoagulant or antithrombotic.

Inadequate anticoagulation, lack of continuous heparinized flush in catheters and sheaths, aortic arch atherosclerosis, and poor catheter technique can all lead to cerebral embolism and stroke. The risk factors for arterial dissection are self-evident, but in patients with a suspected cervical arterial dissection or history of collagen disorder such as Ehler–Danlos type IV or Marfan syndrome, the risk of iatrogenic dissection is very high. Cerebral angiography and interventions should be avoided in patients with Ehler–Danlos syndrome and performed only when absolutely necessary in others (22). Severe tortuosity or redundant loops in the cervical ICAs and VAs are also risk factors for dissection and vasospasm, and the smallest French devices possible should be used in such cases. Vasospasm occurs in all of the cervical and cranial vessels, especially the VAs.

Ischemic Complications

Embolism and Thrombosis

Embolism and thrombosis are the most likely causes of ischemia during neurointerventional procedures and are not uncommon. For this reason, the authors perform most cerebrovascular interventions in awake patients who are awake and who are assessed neurologically during the procedure particularly at key points of each procedure (e.g., following predilation) (23). If a neurological deficit is found or there has been a change in the status for those with preexisting deficits, an immediate cerebral angiogram of the likely culprit vessel should be performed in multiple orthogonal planes and reviewed closely. If an arterial occlusion is noted, the likely etiology should be determined. If inadequate anticoagulation is found, then more heparin may be considered as long as the occlusion is small and the operator is able to perform neurorescue. If the operator is unable to perform neurorescue, the patient has anything more than a trivial deficit and no other

interventionist is available, then intravenous (IV) Tissue plasminogen activator (tPA) should be considered if a thrombus is suspected and heparin should not be given since it would prevent the use of IV tPA. If a large vessel occlusions is seen (e.g., ICA, MCA trunk, or first-order branch occlusion) or if the patient has a severe neurological deficit, then neurorescue must be rapidly performed.

A full discussion of the techniques of neurovascular recanalization is beyond the scope of this chapter, but the following are generally recommended (19). First, stable access to the culprit vessel is mandatory and a 6F guide catheter should be inserted into the appropriate ICA or VA. Mircrocatheterization of the occluded segment with a 2F to 2.3F microcatheter should be performed if a small thrombus burden is noted and the patient can safely receive fibrinolytics. If the occluded segment is very small (<2 mm), it may be worthwhile to attempt clot disruption with the microcatheter and microwire as it may sometimes be sufficient to completely recanalize the vessel or move the thrombus further downstream to a point that would allow collaterals to supply sufficient flow so as to prevent ischemia. If this not effective or feasible then small aliquots of fibrinolytic (e.g., 1–5 mg tPA, 1 U reteplase), should be given directly into the clot through the microcatheter. If a platelet-rich thrombus is suspected, intra-arterial (or IV) abciximab can be given in low doses (i.e., no more than ¼ to ½ of the usual IV bolus, up to a maximum of ¾ to a full bolus). The dosage should be adjusted on the basis of risk factors for ICH noted earlier, and especially the presence of other anticoagulants or fibrinolytics. Alternatively, particularly if a large thrombus burden is noted, mechanical embolectomy may be performed. The commercially available embolectomy devices (Merci Retriever™, Concentric Medical Inc., Mountain View California and Penumbra™, Penumbra Inc., Alameda California aspiration catheter) have between 50% and 82% recanalization efficacy when combined with pharmacological therapy (24,25). If embolectomy is not successful or if the occlusion is suspected to be in a severely stenotic segment then angioplasty and/or stenting may be successful. For occlusion of the cervical ICA, self-expanding carotid stents are preferred, and for the intracranial vessels, balloon-expandable cobalt–chromium coronary stents are good options as they are far more deliverable (92% delivery success vs. 80% success, A. Abou-Chebl, unpublished data) than any of the stainless steel platforms. If available, the Wingspan (Boston Scientific Inc., Natick Massachusetts) self-expanding cerebral stent may be used, but this device is available only under a humanitarian device exemption for the treatment of refractory intracranial atherosclerosis. Its use for AIS should be discouraged, and if used under that setting, it must be reported to the institutional review board and the manufacturer.

Dissection

Dissection of the cerebral vessels is often asymptomatic if the extracranial ICA or VA are affected, and most heal spontaneously. However, if the dissection is severe and rapidly expands to complete occlusion, ischemia may arise particularly if the dominant VA is affected and the contralateral VA is either occluded or hypoplastic. ICA dissection, even occlusion, may also be asymptomatic as long as the circle of Willis is competent. The authors generally do not treat minor intimal tears that do not spread while being observed over 15 to 30 minutes as long as the patient can tolerate prolonged aspirin or antithrombotic treatment. If the dissection spreads quickly and occlusion is imminent, then treatment should be initiated (Fig. 26-14). Once the lesion is crossed with an appropriate wire, stenting should be performed with a self-expanding stent whenever possible. An exception to the self-expanding stent recommendation is dissection localized to the VA ostium where a balloon-expandable stent is preferred because of the ease of placement and preservation of access to the subclavian artery distal to the VA. In the remainder of the VA, which is highly mobile, self-expanding stents are preferred, and the carotid stents may be used if they can be delivered. The carotid stents are sometimes too big and bulky for the VA, so other smaller devices should be used. There are no commercially available devices designed for the VA, so all stents used would be considered as off-label uses. Stenting of course requires dual antiplatelet therapy.

If the dissection extends intracranially or primarily involves the intracranial vessels, the situation becomes much direr. In the authors' experience, these complications are rarely benign and are often associated with ischemia or SAH. Treatment will have to be individualized since most iatrogenic dissections are secondary to the attempted delivery of devices, which by definition suggests that there is severe tortuosity or severe atherosclerosis and that stenting of the dissected segment will be difficult. For these cases, the self-expanding stents designed for the brain are ideal choices since they are more easily delivered and they do not require balloon inflation, which can make vessel rupture more likely in the presence of an existing intimal tear. Also, the intracranial dissections tend to spread to the next branch and cause occlusion. As in the coronaries, it can be difficult if not impossible to wire the occluded branch without causing a perforation. The best advice is that very rapid action is required when an unsecured dissection is noted to preserve vessel patency. If the dissection is noted poststenting, then it can typically be watched as long as there is no perforation of the vessel.

Intracranial dissections are sometimes associated with delayed complications. Intracranial dissection of the VA in particular is associated with dissecting "pseudoaneurysm" formation, which may lead to delayed and fatal SAH. These expanding intracranial dissecting aneurysms must be treated. Options include vessel sacrifice by embolization, aneurysm coil embolization, and stent-assisted vascular reconstruction (26,27). Surgical clipping is no longer the preferred treatment. Depending on the quality of collateral flow, one approach may be preferred over another. If a dissecting pseudoaneurysm ruptures, neurosurgical consultation is required as these patients may develop the same complications as those with spontaneous SAH due to saccular aneurysm rupture.

Cavernous CA dissection may lead to carotid-cavernous sinus arteriovenous fistula (CC fistula) formation. If symptomatic (i.e., visual loss, ICH), it should be treated. Typically, treatment consists of transvenous embolization of the cavernous sinus, but if a high-flow fistula is present, transarterial embolization from the ICA directly across the fistulous tract into the cavernous sinus can also be performed. Embolization can be performed with coils, glue, or combinations of the two. There have also been reports of stent graft placement to treat CC fistulae (28). If asymptomatic, it can be followed conservatively as long as there is no cortical venous drainage from the fistula, which has a risk of ICH. Temporary internal carotid compression can sometimes be effective at closing the fistula (29).

Vasospasm

Cerebral vasospasm is very common with neurovascular interventions. As with vasospasm elsewhere, it commonly is transient, asymptomatic, and if mild generally does not require treatment. However, severe vasospasm can cause ischemia and more importantly, if not identified, may lead to dissection or vessel perforation. Often aggressive (i.e., distal) positioning of the guide catheter in the cervical ICA or VA

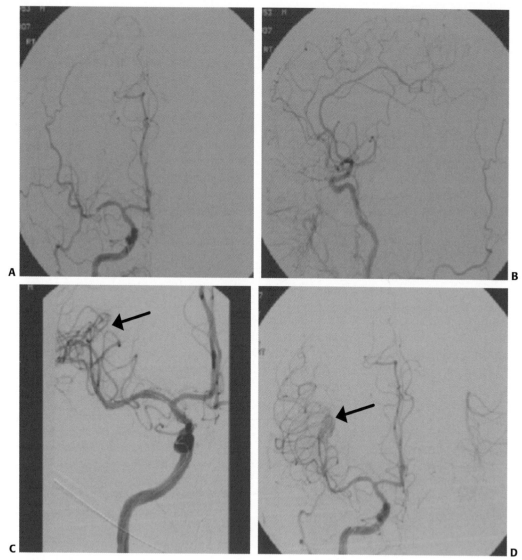

FIGURE 26-14. A 56-year-old Chinese man with a history of HTN presented with recurrent right hemispheric strokes that continued over 72 hours despite induced hypertension, aspirin, clopidogrel, and high-dose statin. Upon standing, his symptoms would worsen. He underwent magnetic resonance imaging under general anesthesia to document the presence of salvageable brain tissue prior to intervention. Intervention was performed under general anesthesia. AP (**A**) and lateral (**B**) angiography revealed a high-grade and flow-limiting distal right middle cerebral artery (MCA) stenosis. (**C**) Intervention was performed with a 0.014-in. system with a soft-tipped wire and cobalt–chromium coronary stent, with excellent immediate angiographic result. Note that the wire tip has no contrast around it on final angiography (*arrow*). (**D**) Upon removal of the wire, tissue was noted on its tip, which prompted immediate angiography revealing active extravasation of contrast into the subarachnoid space (*arrow*). (*continued*)

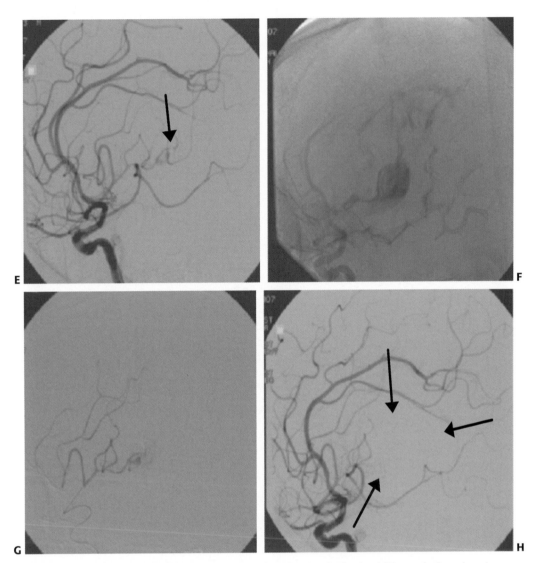

FIGURE 26-14. (*Continued*) (**E**) The point of vessel perforation is clearly visible on the lateral angiogram (*arrow*). The balloon was reintroduced and inflated to 2 atm in the mid-MCA trunk while heparin was reversed and blood pressure was lowered to <100 mmHg. (**F**) After 5 minutes, angiography revealed continued brisk extravasation with development of a large hematoma visible on fluoroscopy. (**G**) A 1.7F neuromicrocatheter was introduced into the MCA branch just proximal to the perforation and the branch was occluded with gelfoam particles. (**H**) Final angiography revealed complete cessation of extravasation but also a moderate area of MCA territory with no arterial flow (*arrows*). The patient awoke from anesthesia with a worsening left hemiparesis and left-sided neglect and had a protracted hospitalization before being discharged to a nursing home.

especially if there are redundant loops proximally in either vessel can cause severe spasm, which can be associated with dissection or cessation of anterograde flow (similar to what can occur in left main coronary artery cannulation with larger guides). For this reason, the authors always monitor the arterial wave form as the guide is being inserted and before any injection of flush or contrast is performed. Even then,

once the guide is placed and the normal arterial wave form is noted, a very gentle puff of contrast is given under fluoroscopy to confirm excellent anterograde flow and normal washout of contrast. If spasm is suspected by the presence of slow flow or if noted on fluoroscopy, depending on the situation, the guide catheter will be withdrawn slightly or completely, vasodilators will be given, and if needed a smaller guide catheter will be used. Nitroglycerin, verapamil, or nicardipine are all effective vasodilators and can be given as boluses or even as continuous infusions when needed. If severe vasospasm is noted while navigating devices intracranially, particularly balloon-expandable stents, vasodilators should be given and the vessel reassessed before delivery is reattempted. Careful attention should be given to wire position and to ensuring that there is flow around the wire. If there is no flow noted in the vessel containing the wire, immediate infusion of vasodilators should be initiated and extreme care should be taken in withdrawing the wire to a larger segment. If spasm is severe or longstanding and the wire is withdrawn too quickly, vessel avulsion and

rupture can occur with catastrophic consequences (Fig. 26-15). Vasospasm occurs frequently in AIS interventions, especially when the mechanical embolectomy devices are used. This can mask recanalization of the vessel and is often associated with SAH if not identified and treated before redeployment of the embolectomy devices. The authors' approach is to give vasodilators liberally after every pass with the Merci Retriever or Penumbra devices. Nitroglycerin in 100 to 200-μg aliquots or calcium channel blockers can all be used. Some operators give continuous infusions of short-acting calcium channel blockers during intracranial interventions to decrease vasospasm. There are no data to support one drug or approach over the other,

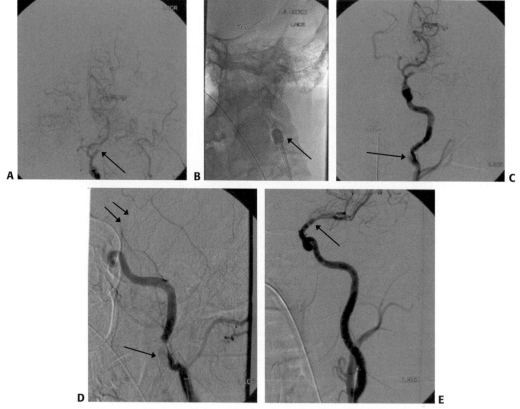

FIGURE 26-15. A 29-year-old woman presented with a dense left middle cerebral artery (MCA) syndrome. (**A**) Angiography revealed internal carotid artery (ICA) terminus occlusion (*arrow*). (**B**) Mechanical embolectomy with the Merci retriever was performed with simultaneous balloon guide occlusion of the ICA (*arrow*). The patient was uncomfortable during retrieval of the Merci device which seemed to "catch on the tip of the guide catheter" as it was withdrawn. (**C**) Immediate angiography revealed that there was an intimal injury with extravasation of contrast within the ICA wall (*arrow*). (**D**) Within minutes, repeat angiography revealed nearly complete occlusion of the ICA, with visible contrast in the false channel (*lower arrow*) with minimal intracranial flow (*upper arrows*). Stenting was performed over a 0.014-in. wire with a self-expanding stent. (**E**) The procedure was then continued with angioplasty of the MCA, which resulted in nearly complete MCA recanalization (*arrow*), and the ICA dissection completely resolved.

except that in the setting of AIS treatment, blood pressures should generally be kept higher to maintain cerebral perfusion until complete recanalization occurs.

Intracerebral Hemorrhage

HPS and Vessel Perforation

Cerebral HPS can occur with any cerebral revascularization procedure although it has been most commonly reported with extracranial ICA revascularization, both surgical and endovascular (see earlier). Nevertheless, it can occur with intracranial revascularization procedures, both elective and emergent (30). The risk factors, clinical manifestations, and treatment are the same as those described earlier for cervical ICA revascularization. When ICH occurs with intracranial interventions, it can be difficult to ascribe an etiology, because the potential causes are many, whereas with extracranial revascularization hyperperfusion is the most likely cause, since devices are most often not introduced intracranially. Intracranial procedures carry the risk of wire perforation, vessel rupture, and dissection, all of which can cause ICH, although typically they are associated with SAH, whereas the majority of HPS-related hemorrhages are parenchymal hematomas (i.e., ICH). When ICH or SAH are related to iatrogenic vessel injury, the clinical manifestations are often immediate rather than delayed for 3 to 5 days as with HPS. Hyperacute ICH has been described with HPS and so only direct angiographic visualization of contrast extravasation can differentiate iatrogenic injury from HPS. Of note in the authors' experience, angiographically visible contrast extravasation into the parenchymal tissue is not common even in the setting of expanding parenchymal hematoma. This is likely related to the fact that for the most part, intraparenchymal hemorrhage occurs from disruption of arterioles and nearly microscopic arteries such as the lenticulostriate or pontine perforators.

If the ICH is detected after the end of the procedure, then the acute treatment is the same regardless of etiology: emergent lowering of blood pressure to low-normal values, reversal of all anticoagulants and antithrombotics (when possible), transfusion of coagulation factors and platelets, close neurological monitoring, and neurosurgical intervention in selected cases. The

former carry the risk of acute stent thrombosis and cerebral embolism, and so the interventionist should be certain of the need for reversal. The latter is of very limited value in the vast majority of ICH complicating endovascular therapy because of the high risk of worsening of ICH associated with craniotomy and ventricular drain (EVD) placement in patients who are anticoagulated or taking dual, potent, antiplatelet agents. Nevertheless, in cases where there is marked elevation of ICP and hydrocephalus, EVD placement may be life-saving. Similarly, in cases of cerebellar hemorrhage, decompressive suboccipital craniotomy may be function and life-saving. Medical measures to control ICP should be strongly considered in all cases, and this may include hyperosmolar therapy and hyperventilation via endotracheal intubation and ventilator support. The latter is often needed as many patients (especially those with SAH) have rapid declines in alertness and may also have cardiopulmonary arrest due to bihemispheric and brain stem compression.

If the ICH or SAH is detected intraoperatively, then along with immediate lowering of blood pressure, temporary cessation of flow to the affected vessel should immediately be performed. As with coronary perforation and tamponade, balloon inflation to achieve occlusion should be performed. For this reason, the authors always perform immediate postangioplasty angiography with the balloon within the lesion rather than withdrawn into the guide. However, unlike the coronary setting, the authors advise caution with balloon inflation directly at the site of vessel rupture since the inflated balloon can worsen the dissection or expand the rupture: the cerebral vessels have essentially no adventitia, no external elastic lamina, and a very thin tunica media. Compliant balloons (Hyperform or Hyperglide, eV3 Inc., Irvine California) are preferred in this setting. However, if a conventional balloon catheter is already in the vessel, it should be used to save time, but at the lowest pressure that achieves occlusion. On the other hand, the often-robust collateral flow from the circle of Willis and/or pial collaterals can retrogradely fill the ruptured segment attenuating the effect of proximal occlusion. If balloon tamponade is not effective or feasible then vessel sacrifice should be strongly considered. As discussed earlier, depending on the location and size of the perforation, the patient may have only minutes before brain death occurs, necessitating that definitive and extreme measures be taken. Vessel sacrifice is often associated with infarction of the relevant territory, but unless the infarct is expected to be fatal (e.g., BA sacrifice or dominant ICA sacrifice in a young individual), it may be the only chance the patient has at survival (Fig. 26-14). Vessel occlusion can be performed with coils or liquid embolic agents (NBCA glue [Codman Inc., Raynham Massachusetts] or Onyx [eV3 Inc., Irvine California]). These devices are often not found in a nonneurointerventional laboratory, and their use requires some prior experience; therefore, other embolic material may be considered as a last resort (e.g., gelfoam, embolic spheres).

In the worst case scenario of massive SAH (unusual without vessel perforation or rupture), patients may have complete cessation of cerebral blood flow when ICP equals MAP and patients may rapidly progress to brain death within 10 to 15 minutes. In such patients, lowering of blood pressure will potentiate cerebral ischemia and the usual emergent treatment of high ICP, i.e. induced hypertension, may cause more bleeding and may further increase ICP. Therefore, in these catastrophic cases, the only treatment option is surgical decompression via EVD or craniotomy, but most patients die before the neurosurgical team can initiate therapy. In the authors' experience, very few patients have survived or benefited from neurosurgical intervention in this setting.

Some patients will have asymptomatic SAH or petechial ICH. Usually this occurs in the setting of acute stroke revascularization and is associated with fibrinolytics and the use of mechanical embolectomy devices. The authors have found that performing acute stroke and elective intracranial interventions in awake patients will decrease the risk of wire perforation and vessel rupture, in contrary to the popular belief that intracranial interventions are not safe in awake patients (31). This is because awake patients will be able to complain of headache with impending rupture or perforation, alerting the interventionist that whatever is being performed at the moment should be stopped. This should be immediately followed by a complete angiographic

evaluation of the vessel being treated as well as a neurological assessment. Common causes of headache include distal wire migration into smaller branches or into tortuous segments, balloon oversizing, device-induced intimal irritation or injury, excessive traction on the vessel from a stiff device, vasospasm, and of course actual ICH or SAH. If the latter are visualized angiographically, the measures described earlier should be immediately initiated. However, if there is no obvious contrast extravasation in multiple angiographic views, the cause of the headache is identified, the headache resolves or quickly improves, and the patient is neurologically intact, then the procedure may be continued if appropriate with more caution and a heightened expectation of impending catastrophe. If there is no obvious extravasation but the headache worsens or there is some neurological deterioration, depending on the setting, immediate CT scan should be performed to assess for ICH and SAH. This is best performed with in-suite CT (e.g., DynaCT [Siemens Medical Systems Inc.] or XperCT [Phillips Medical Inc.]). If such in-suite systems are not available, the interventionist who frequently performs intracranial interventions should strongly consider obtaining these systems because emergent CT outside of the interventional suite is often time consuming and obviates immediate endovascular interventions. Once the CT is completed, if there is no ICH or SAH, the intervention may be resumed if appropriate, although in the authors' experience, except in the direst circumstances (e.g., young person with coma and BA occlusion or partially coiled ruptured aneurysm), it is best not to resume the intervention.

Once the intervention is complete, the patient with ICH or SAH should be monitored closely in a neurological intensive care unit; in addition to the immediate needs of ICP management, such patients are at risk for delayed neurological complications. These include cerebral edema, infarction, cerebral vasospasm, hydrocephalus, seizures, diabetes insipidus, and death. A discussion of the neurological critical care of such patients is beyond the scope of this chapter, and it should be self-evident that these patients should be followed by neurological consultants expert in stroke and neurological critical care. Patients cared for by such experts have improved survival and neurological outcomes.

References

1. Rajagopal V, Yadav JS. Management of carotid artery disease in the high-risk patient with emphasis on the SAPPHIRE study. *Curr Cardiol Rep.* 2007;9:20–24.
2. Roffi M, Yadav JS. Carotid stenting. *Circulation.* 2006;114:e1–e4.
3. Saw J, Gurm HS, Fathi RB, et al. Effect of chronic kidney disease on outcomes after carotid artery stenting. *Am J Cardiol.* 2004;94:1093–1096.
4. Meier P, Ko DT, Tamura A, Tamhane U, Gurm HS. Sodium bicarbonate-based hydration prevents contrast-induced nephropathy: a meta-analysis. *BMC Med.* 2009;7:23.
5. Reed M, Meier P, Tamhane UU, Welch KB, Moscucci M, Gurm HS. The relative renal safety of iodixanol compared with low-osmolar contrast media: a meta-analysis of randomized controlled trials. *JACC Cardiovasc Interv.* 2009;2:645–654.
6. Folmar J, Sachar R, Mann T. Transradial approach for carotid artery stenting: a feasibility study. *Catheter Cardiovasc Interv.* 2007;69:355–361.
7. Cardaioli P, Giordan M, Panfili M, Chioin R. Complication with an embolic protection device during carotid angioplasty. *Catheter Cardiovasc Interv.* 2004;62:234–236.
8. Kwon BJ, Han MH, Kang HS, Jung C. Protection filter-related events in extracranial carotid artery stenting: a single-center experience. *J Endovasc Ther.* 2006;13:711–722.
9. Dieter RS, Ikram S, Satler LF, Babrowicz JC, Reddy B, Laird JR. Perforation complicating carotid artery stenting: the use of a covered stent. *Catheter Cardiovasc Interv.* 2006;67:972–975.
10. Ecker RD, Guidot CA, Hanel RA, et al. Perforation of external carotid artery branch arteries during endoluminal carotid revascularization procedures: consequences and management. *J Invasive Cardiol.* 2005;17:292–295.
11. Gupta R, Abou-Chebl A, Bajzer CT, Schumacher HC, Yadav JS. Rate, predictors, and consequences of hemodynamic depression after carotid artery stenting. *J Am Coll Cardiol.* 2006;47:1538–1543.
12. Abou-Chebl A, Yadav JS, Reginelli JP, Bajzer C, Bhatt D, Krieger DW. Intracranial hemorrhage and hyperperfusion syndrome following carotid artery stenting: risk factors, prevention, and treatment. *J Am Coll Cardiol.* 2004;43:1596–1601.
13. Abou-Chebl A, Reginelli J, Bajzer CT, Yadav JS. Intensive treatment of hypertension decreases the risk of hyperperfusion and intracerebral hemorrhage following carotid artery stenting. *Catheter Cardiovasc Interv.* 2007;69:690–696.
14. Yadav JS, Wholey MH, Kuntz RE, et al. Protected carotid-artery stenting versus endarterectomy in high-risk patients. *N Engl J Med.* 2004;351:1493–1501.
15. Matetzky S, Shenkman B, Guetta V, et al. Clopidogrel resistance is associated with increased risk of recurrent atherothrombotic events in patients with acute myocardial infarction. *Circulation.* 2004;109(25):3171–3175.
16. Casserly IP, Abou-Chebl A, Fathi RB, et al. Slow-flow phenomenon during carotid artery intervention with embolic protection devices: predictors and clinical outcome. *J Am Coll Cardiol.* 2005; 46:1466–1472.
17. Mori T, Mori K, Fukuoka M, Honda S. Percutaneous transluminal angioplasty for total occlusion of middle cerebral arteries. *Neuroradiology.* 1997;39(1):71-74.
18. Tissue plasminogen activator for acute ischemic stroke: the National Institute of Neurological Disorders and Stroke rt-PA Stroke Study Group. *N Engl J Med.* 1995;333(24):1581–1587.
19. Abou-Chebl A, Bajzer CT, Krieger DW, Furlan AJ, Yadav JS: Multimodal therapy for the treatment of severe ischemic stroke combining GPIIb/IIIa antagonists and angioplasty after failure of thrombolysis. *Stroke.* 2005;36:2286–2288.
20. Furlan A, Higashida R, Wechsler L, et al. Intra-arterial prourokinase for acute ischemic stroke: the PROACT II study: a randomized controlled trial. Prolyse in Acute Cerebral Thromboembolism. *JAMA.* 1999;282(21):2003–2011.
21. Adams HP Jr, Brott TG, Furlan AJ, et al. Guidelines for thrombolytic therapy for acute stroke: a supplement to the guidelines for the management of patients with acute ischemic stroke: a statement for healthcare professionals from a Special Writing Group of the Stroke Council, American Heart Association. *Circulation.* 1996;94(5):1167–1174.
22. Freeman RK, Swegle J, Sise MJ. The surgical complications of Ehlers-Danlos syndrome. *Am Surg.* 1996;62(10):869–873.
23. Abou-Chebl A, Krieger D, Bajzer C, Yadav JS. Intracranial angioplasty and stenting in the awake patient. *J Neuroimaging.* 2006;16(3):216–223.
24. Smith WS, Sung G, Saver J, et al. Mechanical thrombectomy for acute ischemic stroke: final

results of the Multi MERCI trial. *Stroke.* 2008; 39(4):1205–1212.

25. The penumbra pivotal stroke trial: safety and effectiveness of a new generation of mechanical devices for clot removal in intracranial large vessel occlusive disease. *Stroke.* 2009;40(8):2761–2768.

26. Higashida RT, Halbach VV, Tsai FY, et al. Interventional neurovascular treatment of traumatic carotid and vertebral artery lesions: results in 234 cases. *AJR Am J Roentgenol.* 1989;153(3):577–582.

27. Cohen JE, Gomori JM, Segal R, et al. Results of endovascular treatment of traumatic intracranial aneurysms. *Neurosurgery.* 2008;63(3):476–485.

28. Wang C, Xie X, You C, et al. Placement of covered stents for the treatment of direct carotid cavernous fistulas. *Am J Neuroradiol.* 2009;30(7): 1342–1346.

29. Higashida RT, Hieshima GB, Halbach VV, et al. Closure of carotid cavernous sinus fistulae by external compression of the carotid artery and jugular vein. *Acta Radiol Suppl.* 1986;369:580–583.

30. Meyers PM, Higashida RT, Phatouros CC, et al. Cerebral hyperperfusion syndrome after percutaneous transluminal stenting of the craniocervical arteries. *Neurosurgery.* 2000;47(2):335–343.

31. Abou-Chebl A, Lin R, Hussain MS, Jovin TG, et al. Conscious sedation versus general anesthesia during endovascular therapy for acute anterior circulation stroke: Preliminary results from a retrospective multi-center study. *Stroke.* In press.

27 Aortic Endovascular Grafting

FRANK C. VANDY, JONATHAN L. ELIASON, JOHN E. RECTENWALD, GUILLERMO A. ESCOBAR, AND GILBERT R. UPCHURCH JR.

Aortic aneurysms are a leading cause of death, with increasing incidence and prevalence. Endovascular aneurysm repair (EVAR) now represents the most common method of aneurysm repair, for both abdominal and descending thoracic aortic aneurysms (TAAs). Ongoing improvements in endovascular stent graft technology have occurred since the first published report of EVAR in 1991. These improvements have led to the approval by the Food and Drug Administration (FDA) of multiple devices, to streamlined operative techniques, and to extended applicability of EVAR. Despite these developments, basic anatomic considerations still eliminate many patients from being offered EVAR. Evolving technology focused on the treatment of the ascending aorta, the aortic arch, and the thoracoabdominal aorta will likely make this treatment paradigm the primary therapy for most aortic aneurysms and other aortic pathology in the near future.

EVAR has many perceived and real advantages over open aneurysm repair. Advantages for EVAR include a less invasive operative exposure, especially true for thoracic EVAR (TEVAR), decreased transfusion requirements, shortened intensive care unit (ICU) and hospital stays, and decreased short-term perioperative mortality (1,2). Utilization of EVAR for ruptured abdominal aortic aneurysms (AAAs) and TAAs appears to be safe and effective, documenting at least clinical equipoise when compared with single-center results with open repair for rupture (1,2). While questions remain regarding the long-term efficacy of EVAR in preventing aneurysm-related death, it is clear that the use of EVAR for

ruptured aneurysms even as a "bridging" technique is life saving (1,3,4).

In the present chapter, we will first provide a brief rationale for treating patients with endovascular therapy, as opposed to open repair. Next, a description of a "standard" endovascular abdominal and TAA repair will follow. Finally, the various modes of endograft failure will be defined, focusing on "endoleaks," to provide illustrative material to help the practitioner avoid and treat the common problems encountered with EVAR.

■ RATIONALE FOR THERAPY

It is important to acknowledge that as many as 80% of aortic aneurysms occur in the abdominal aorta in the infrarenal location. AAAs are conventionally defined as a 50% or greater increase in aortic diameter compared with the normal proximal aorta, and in most patients, this represents a diameter of 3 cm or greater (5). Conventional open surgical repair and EVAR are both viable treatment options. Utilization trends suggest that EVAR has likely become the more common method of repair in the United States (6). TEVAR has also emerged as a viable alternative to open repair for TAAs, with many similarities existing between EVAR and TEVAR.

Prevention of aneurysm rupture is the basis for aneurysm repair, whether by open or endovascular technique. It has been demonstrated in controlled populations that more than half of AAA patients with ruptured aneurysm die at home (7). Large administrative data sets from across the United States revealed that patients with ruptured AAAs who undergo open

TABLE 27-1 **Currently Approved Abdominal Aortic Endografts**

Company Name	Product Name	Fixation Location	Stent Expansion	Stent Material	Graft Material
Cook Medical	Zenith Flex with Z-Trak	Suprarenal	Self-expanding	Stainless steel	Woven Polyester
Endologix, Inc.	Powerlink	Infrarenal, Suprarenal	Self-expanding	Cobalt-Chromium Alloy	High Density ePTFE
Medtronic, Inc.	Talent Advantage	Suprarenal	Self-expanding	Nitinol	Woven Polyester
Medtronic, Inc.	AneuRx AAAdvantage	Infrarenal	Self-expanding	Nitinol	Woven Polyester
W.L. Gore & Associates	Gore Excluder AAA Endoprosthesis	Infrarenal	Self-expanding	Nitinol	ePTFE

(Adapted from *Endovascular Today, 2010 Buyer's Guide*. Vol. 8, No. 12. Wayne, PA: Bryn Mawr Communications; 2009.)

surgical repair have 30-day mortality rates of greater than 40% (8). While in general aneurysm rupture risk increases with aneurysm size, determination of an individuals exact rupture risk is difficult, as variables, such as gender, aneurysm morphology, smoking status, hypertension control, and the presence of chronic obstructive pulmonary disease, must each be considered when calculating individual patient risk. Data suggest that 1-year incidence of AAA rupture exceeds 10% with aneurysm diameters greater than 6.0 cm (9). However, elective open repair of AAA less than 5.5 cm yields no mortality benefit (10–12). With the advent of EVAR, initial in-hospital mortality rates were decreased, while patient outcomes (i.e., fewer transfusions, shorter hospital and ICU stays, lower risk of paraplegia) were improved (1). Based on these observations, multiple trials in the United States and abroad are currently being performed to determine whether lowering the size threshold at which EVAR for AAA should be performed yields any benefit in morbidity or mortality (13).

■ OPEN REPAIR VERSUS EVAR FOR ABDOMINAL AORTIC ANEURYSMS

In 1991, Parodi et al. (14) published the first report of stent graft implantation for AAA in humans. Utilization of this technology had grown at a steady rate, especially in higher-volume hospitals for the treatment of AAA (6). Marketing of five FDA-approved devices is ongoing in the United States, each with slightly different design (Table 27-1). These stent grafts in general utilize radial force from self-expanding stents (passive fixation) or self-expansion in concert with hooks or barbs (active fixation) to prevent endograft migration. Suprarenal support is available from three of the devices as well. With appropriate positioning and adequate fixation, aortic pulsatile flow and shear stress on the wall is prevented from being transmitted to the aneurysm sac, and thus the aneurysm is prevented from rupturing. Evidence to support this intended goal comes from the observation that after EVAR, the majority of aneurysms will either shrink or maintain their size at which they were treated. Multiple studies have suggested there is some variability in this response, believed to be secondary to graft material and structure (15).

At least three randomized controlled clinical trials (RCTs) comparing EVAR with open surgery have been performed. The Dutch Randomized Endovascular Aneurysm Management trial, randomized 351 patients with asymptomatic AAAs greater than 5 cm in diameter with anatomy suitable for EVAR to open or endovascular repair. While this study was underpowered, a strong trend toward a 30-day benefit in mortality favored EVAR in this study (1.2% EVAR vs. 4.6% open surgery; $P = .10$) (16). Two-year follow-up data demonstrated that by 1 year, the trend toward improved survival was lost, with no mortality benefit while using EVAR (17). A second trial, EVAR 1, compared EVAR with open surgical repair in patients with suitable EVAR anatomy and aneurysms 5.5 cm or greater (18). This study contained a large number of patients ($N = 1,082$). Blood product use, length of stay, and perioperative mortality (1.7% EVAR vs. 4.7% open surgery; $P = .009$) all favored EVAR over open repair (19). However, the primary endpoint of all-cause mortality did not show a lasting benefit for EVAR at the 4-year study conclusion. Long-term complication and reintervention rates were also higher in the EVAR group, but a reduction in aneurysm-related death was noted (3.5% EVAR, 6.3% open surgery; $P = .02$) (18). A recent trial from the United States, the OVER trial, performed in Veterans Affairs Hospitals randomized 881 patients to either EVAR or open AAA repair. At a mean follow-up of only 1.8 years, perioperative mortality (30 days or inpatient) was lower for EVAR (0.5% vs. 3.0%; $P = .004$), but by 2 years, there was no significant difference in mortality (7.0% vs. 9.8%, $P = .13$). Similar to the other two trials, patients undergoing EVAR had reduced blood loss and hospital and intensive care unit stay (1 vs. 4 days) but required substantial exposure to fluoroscopy and contrast. There were no differences between the two groups in major morbidity, procedure failure, secondary therapeutic procedures, aneurysm-related hospitalizations, health-related quality of life, or erectile function (20).

Treatment

Patient Selection and Preoperative Planning

Initially, as EVAR was developed, advanced patient age was often a relative indication for EVAR. This was supported by studies that showed an open AAA operative mortality of less than 2% in male patients younger than 65 years of age (21). As trends in the use of EVAR have evolved to the point where it is now the primary therapy for most elective AAA repairs, anatomic criteria are the most important factor in considering when deciding between EVAR and open repair (Table 27-2). Each endograft manufacturer has its own set of instructions for use (IFUs) as mandated by the FDA (Fig. 27-1). It is, however, up to the individual implanting physician to plan an approach that has the highest rate of meeting with success, much of which is predicated on preoperative planning.

Modern imaging techniques are critical to allow the treating physician to model aortic anatomy (Fig. 27-2). Contrast-enhanced, spiral, multislice computed tomography (CT) with three-dimensional reconstructions is the preferred method of evaluation, because it shows the relationship of the lumen to the aneurysmal sac, presence of mural thrombus and calcium that may affect device fixation, and visceral blood supply. Centerline images are often used to better define the anatomy and aid in choosing the appropriate endograft. The most important anatomic reasons patients are not considered EVAR candidates are (1) inadequate proximal or

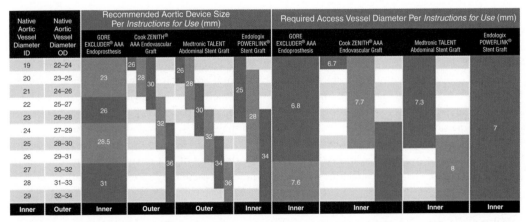

FIGURE 27-1. Current indications for use of four endovascular endografts. (Data from W.L. Gore & Associates, Inc., Cook Medical, Inc., Bloomington, Indiana, Medtronic, Inc., Santa Rosa, California, and Endologix, Inc., Irvine, California.)

TABLE 27-2 **Aortic Endografts and Their Appropriate Size Limitations**

Graft Name (Manufacturer)	Indications for Use
Zenith (Cook Medical, Inc.)	• Adequate iliac/femoral access • Nonaneurysmal proximal infrarenal aortic neck $\geq$ 15 mm in length and between 18 and 32 mm in diameter (outer wall) • Proximal aortic neck angulation $\leq$ 60 degrees relative to the long axis of the aneurysm • Proximal aortic neck angulation $\leq$ 45 degrees relative to the axis of the suprarenal aorta • Iliac artery distal fixation site $\geq$ 10 mm in length and 7.5–20 mm in diameter (outer wall)
Excluder (W.L. Gore & Associates, Inc.)	• Adequate iliac/femoral access • Nonaneurysmal proximal infrarenal aortic neck $\geq$ 15 mm in length and between 19 and 29 mm in diameter (inner wall) • Proximal aortic neck angulation $\leq$ 60 degrees relative to the long axis of the aneurysm • Iliac artery distal fixation site $\geq$ 10 mm in length and 8.5–18.5 mm in diameter (inner wall)
Talent (Medtronic, Inc.)	• Adequate iliac/femoral access • Nonaneurysmal proximal infrarenal aortic neck $\geq$ 10 mm in length and between 18 and 32 mm in diameter (outer wall) • Proximal aortic neck angulation $\leq$ 60 degrees • Distal iliac artery fixation length of $\geq$ 15 mm and 8–22 mm in diameters (outer wall)
Powerlink (Endologix, Inc.)	• Adequate iliac/femoral access $\geq$ 7 mm (large delivery system) • Nonaneurysmal proximal infrarenal aortic neck $\geq$ 15 mm in length and between 18 and 32 mm in diameter (inner wall) • Aortic neck angulation $\leq$ 60 degrees to the body of the aneurysm • Aortic length $\geq$ 1.0 cm longer than the body portion of the chosen bifurcated model • Distal iliac artery fixation length of $\geq$ 15 mm and 10–23 mm in diameters (inner wall) • Iliac artery angulation $\leq$ 90 degrees to the aortic bifurcation • Ability to preserve at least one hypogastric

distal landing zone; (2) inadequate celiac or superior mesenteric artery blood flow to compensate for the loss of the inferior mesenteric artery; (3) excessive calcium, thrombus, or tortuosity of the vessels; and (4) unsuitable iliofemoral arterial access (Table 27-3). Endovascular graft diameter and lengths are individually based on the patient's arterial anatomy and typically should not be oversized by more than 10% to 20% of the diameter at the attachment zone.

Procedure

EVAR can be performed under general, regional, or local anesthesia in an interventional suite or in a hybrid endovascular operating room. While rare, conversion to open repair still occurs and thus personal and staffing should be appropriate. The patient is placed supine on a radiolucent table. Percutaneous access or open exposure of the femoral arteries is performed. Using fluoroscopic guidance, access guidewires and sheaths are introduced. The patient is given intravenous heparin to maintain an activated clotting time (ACT) of 250 seconds. An aortogram is obtained to confirm positioning of the renal arteries, patency of the inferior mesenteric artery and lumbar arteries, and the location of the aortic and iliac bifurcations. This can be performed using carbon dioxide or iodinated contrast (22). In the case of ruptured AAAs, angiography may be the only preoperative imaging available in the hemodynamically unstable patient. In this scenario, an aortic

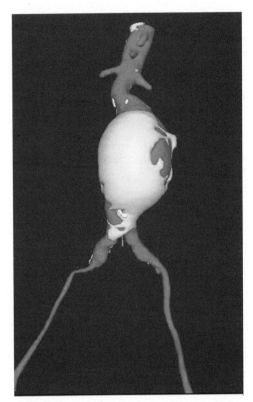

FIGURE 27-2. Aortic three-dimensional reconstruction and modeling allowing for precise anatomical measurements. (See color insert.)

TABLE 27-3 Anatomical Contraindications for Endovascular Aneurysm Repair

Inadequate proximal landing zone
 Aortic neck length too short
 Aortic neck diameter too wide or too narrow,
  ≥32 mm and ≤18 mm, respectively
 Aortic suprarenal neck angulation ≥ 45 degrees
 Aortic infrarenal neck angulation 60 degrees
 Conical aortic neck—Greater than 10% increase
  in diameter
 Irregular calcification, plaque, or thrombus at
  proximal neck

Inadequate distal landing zone
 Nonaneurysmal iliac length ≤ 10 mm

Inadequate visceral blood supply to compensate for
loss of inferior mesenteric artery (IMA)

Excessive tortuosity of the aorta and iliac system

Iliofemoral vessels too small, tortuous, or angulated
to accommodate device

occlusion balloon may be utilized to maintain hemodynamic stability. The endovascular device is oriented and advanced under fluoroscopic guidance over a long, stiff wire, such as an Amplatz super stiff (Boston Scientific Corporation, Natick, Massachusetts) or Lunderquist (Cook Medical Inc., Bloomington, Indiana) wire, until the cephalad portion of the prosthesis is at the proximal landing zone. As most endografts are modular, the main aortic body and the ipsilateral limb of the graft are deployed with an orientation that makes cannulation of the gate area easiest. This typically leaves the contralateral gate area in a lateral or anterior position. A glide wire and catheter, typically a Van Schie or cobra catheter, are advanced via the sheath in the contralateral femoral artery through the contralateral gate. Cannulation of the contralateral limb is confirmed in at least one of three following ways: (1) bilateral oblique "single shots" to document in two projections the glide wire and the sheath in the gate, (2) rotating the catheter inside the aortic graft and watching it move freely inside the endograft, or (3) using a puff of contrast through the catheter inside the aorta to document an aortic graft "shadow." A stiff wire is then placed through the contralateral sheath into the thoracic aorta. Next, the contralateral hypogastric artery is identified, and the contralateral limb is deployed short of the iliac bifurcation. Balloon dilatation is typically done to fully expand the stent grafts and "iron out" folds in the graft material. Postprocedure aortography with runoff is performed to confirm positioning, fixation, and patency of visceral and iliac arteries, as well as to carefully evaluate for endoleaks. All catheters and sheaths are removed and the arteriotomy sites repaired.

■ OPEN REPAIR VERSUS TEVAR FOR THORACIC AORTIC ANEURYSMS

An alternative technique in the treatment of isolated TAAs in the form of stent grafting emerged in the 1990s, with Volodos and colleagues (23) placing the first thoracic aortic endograft. The use of stent graft technology has exploded over the last two decades and has been used to treat a number of thoracic aortic pathologies, including elective and ruptured aneurysms, dissections, and transections. Endovascular TAA repair is associated with less physiologic insult

TABLE 27-4   **Thoracic Aortic Endografts**

Company Name	Product Name	Stent Expansion	Stent Material	Graft Material
Cook Medical	TX2 with Pro-form	Self-expanding	Stainless steel	Woven polyester
Medtronic, Inc.	Talent Thoracic Xcelerant	Self-expanding	Nitinol	Dacron polyester
W.L. Gore & Associates, Inc.	Gore TAG Thoracic Endoprosthesis	Self-expanding	Nitinol	ePTFE

(Adapted from *Endovascular Today, 2010 Buyer's Guide*. Vol. 8, No. 12. Wayne, PA: Bryn Mawr Communications; 2009.)

on the patient, fewer blood transfusions, fewer hospital and ICU stays, and a lower hospital mortality rate compared with open TAA repair (2,24). Similar to endovascular AAA repair, which was originally used to treat elderly patients with significant cardiac, pulmonary, and renal comorbidities, an endovascular approach is now considered by many to be primary therapy for patients with TAAs. This has translated into a relative explosion of TAA repair secondary to the introduction of new technology. Currently, there are three FDA-approved devices on the market available for TEVAR (Table 27-4).

Treatment

Although all of the device-specific trials are prospective, they are not randomized and suffer from primary use of historical controls patients undergoing open TAA repair. In addition, they were not designed to help us determine which patients are best served by stent grafting versus open repair. Three specific trials comparing TEVAR and open TAA repair are worth reviewing. The Gore TAG trial documented 2-year follow-up on the initial multicenter trial involving 140 patients with stent grafts (Gore TAG Thoracic Endograft, Flagstaff, Arizona) versus an open surgical cohort of 94 patients, which included historical and concurrent open controls (25). Perioperative mortality was significantly lower in the endograft (TEVAR) group than in open surgical controls (2.1% for TEVAR vs. 11.7% for open repair, $P > .001$). Perioperative complication rates and intensive care unit and hospital length of stay were also significantly reduced in the TEVAR group. The incidence of endoleaks at 2 years was 9% in the TEVAR group, with three interventions performed in the endograft cohort. At 2 years, Kaplan–Meier analysis revealed no difference in overall mortality. The Cook TX2 trial compared

160 patients undergoing TEVAR with the Zenith TX2 Endovascular Graft (William Cook Europe, ApS, Bjaeverskov, Denmark), with 70 patients undergoing open TAA repair (26). The 30-day survival rate was better for the TEVAR group than for the open group (98.1% vs. 94.3%, $P > .01$). The TEVAR group also had fewer cardiovascular, pulmonary, and vascular adverse events, although neurologic events were not significantly different. No ruptures or conversions occurred in the first year in the TEVAR group. At 12 months, aneurysm growth was identified in 7.1% (8/112) of patients (3.9% endoleak rate). Finally, the Medtronic VALOR Trial (Medtronic Vascular, Santa Rosa, California) for patients with TAAs who were also candidates for open repair documented that patients who underwent TEVAR had a perioperative 2.1% mortality rate (27). Major adverse advents occurred in 41% of the stent graft group, including paraplegia in 1.5%, paraparesis in 7.2%, and stroke in 3.6%. At 12 months, the TEVAR group had an all-cause mortality rate of 16.1% and an aneurysm-related mortality rate of 3.1%.

A recent meta-analysis reviewing open TAA repair and stent grafting included 17 eligible studies totaling 1,109 patients and demonstrated that stenting was associated with a significant reduction in mortality (pooled odds ratio, 0.36; $P > .0001$) and major neurologic injury (pooled odds ratio, 0.39; $P > .0001$), with no difference in the major reintervention rate after elective TAA repair. Importantly, there was no effect on mortality in patients with thoracic aortic trauma or rupture. The authors suggested that TEVAR reduces perioperative mortality and neurologic complications in patients undergoing elective TAA repair (2).

Procedure

Thoracic endovascular aneurysm repair (TEVAR) is performed in a fashion similar to that of EVAR.

Sheath diameters for thoracic aortic endografts are typically larger, and there is a higher incidence of iliofemoral complications. With TEVAR, typically a single iliofemoral exposure is performed, while the contralateral femoral artery is accessed percutaneously for placement of a sheath and marking angiocatheter. The patient is systemically heparinized to an ACT of greater than 250 seconds. A single stiff wire is placed into the ascending aorta, especially in patients with peaked arches. Delivery of the endograft over the wire follows appropriate definition of the anatomy using aortography with specific attention to proximal (left subclavian or common carotid artery) and distal [celiac or superior mesenteric artery (SMA)] landing zones. Serial endografts may need to be deployed depending on the length of thoracic aorta to be treated. Finally, the endografts may subsequently be angioplastied with large diameter balloons to ensure adequate fixation, to make sure the overlap areas are well opposed, and to remove any graft infolding. Completion aortography is performed to ensure exclusion of the aneurysm and to evaluate for endoleaks, especially type 1 and 3. Sheaths and wires are removed and the arteriotomy repaired. Liberal use of spinal drains in patients undergoing TEVAR is routine in our practice.

■ BAILOUT TECHNIQUES
Endoleaks

Type I

Type I endoleaks can be classified into type IA or IB endoleaks. A type IA endoleak is characterized by continued flow around the graft into the aneurysm sac from the proximal seal zone. Seen on angiogram, this is demonstrated by contrast flow around the main body, just below the level of the renal arteries (Fig. 27-3). Type IB

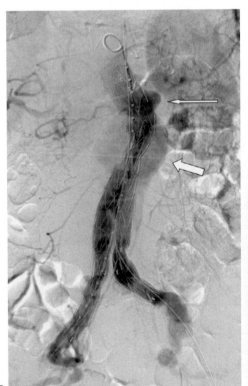
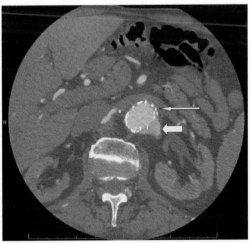

FIGURE 27-3. (**A**) Type IA endoleak after deployment of a Talent endograft (Medtronic, Inc.). The leak is most prominently seen as a small out-pouching on the left posterior aspect of the aorta (*thin arrow*). Note the continued filling of the aneurysm sac (*thick arrow*). (**B**) Type IA endoleak noted on computed tomography. The endoleak shown in this picture corresponds to the leak demonstrated angiographically in **A**. Note the inner metallic stent (*thin arrow*) with persistent contrast filling a misshaped neck (*thick arrow*).

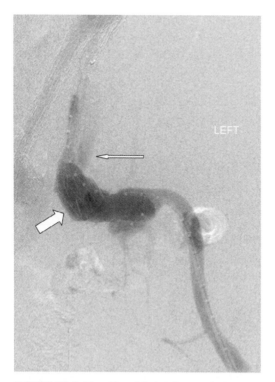

FIGURE 27-4. Type IB endoleak following deployment of a Zenith endograft (Cook Medical, Inc.). Note the contralateral limb resting in a slightly aneurysmal portion of the distal common iliac artery (*thick arrow*). Contrast is seen filling the common iliac artery in a retrograde fashion (*thin arrow*).

endoleak is characterized by persistent back flow into the aneurysm sac from the distal seal zone. On angiography, this can be seen with contrast flowing around either iliac limb into the aneurysm sac (Fig. 27-4). When recognized intraoperatively, this represents a technical failure, and the case should not be terminated until the endoleak is repaired. The simplest option to eliminate this type of endoleak is to reballoon the proximal or distal site with a compliant balloon. Often, success will be achieved with extended inflation times, often 2 to 3 minutes. One must be careful when applying this approach to the proximal seal zone, such that the renal arteries are not being occluded. If this conservative approach is unsuccessful, one must consider the etiology of the endoleak. Does the leak occur because the device was sized incorrectly? Does the leak result from a poor approximation of the graft with the aortic or iliac wall? Often, applying more radial force with an additional large uncovered balloon-expandable stent

can seal the proximal zone (Fig. 27-5). These uncovered balloon mounted stents allow 1 to 2 mm of additional encroachment in the proximal neck that is often not attainable by covered endovascular aortic stents. If a type IA leak continues to persist after the deployment of additional radial force, one must assess the degree of leak. Although not ideal, leaving the operating room with a small, slow endoleak is an option, given that this type of leak has a high likelihood of resolving on its own, especially after reversal of heparinization. Such patients should be followed closely with CT angiography to evaluate aneurysm sac size and resolution of the endoleak. Regardless, after several failed attempts at reballooning and with increased contrast loads, it is wise to terminate the operation unsuccessfully, rehydrate the patient, and formulate an alternative plan. In rare cases, a persistent type IA endoleak needs to be managed with an open operative aneurysm repair. If the patient is unfit for open surgery, in experienced hands, raising the proximal seal zone with a paragraft may be an option (Fig. 27-6).

Type IB endoleaks are often best managed by a distal extension cuff. Iliac cuffs have the option of being flared at the end (up to 28 mm) to achieve an appropriate seal. One might also consider an iliac extension cuff that requires coverage and possible coiling of the ipsilateral hypogastric artery (Fig. 27-7). Unless contraindicated, coil embolization of the ipsilateral hypogastric artery should be performed before covering it with a stent graft to limit the possibility of a type II endoleak (28). This is especially true in large common iliac artery aneurysms. Routine embolization of an ipsilateral hypogastric artery is often performed in the instance of a combined aortoiliac aneurysm necessitating extension of the endograft limb into the external iliac artery. Unilateral embolization of a hypogastric artery may be done in combination with primary repair. If bilateral embolization is necessary, it is recommended this be done in a staged fashion to allow for the development of collateralization to the buttocks and pelvic organs. Alternatively, an external to internal iliac bypass may be performed. More recently, the use of branched endografts into both the internal and external iliac has been demonstrated. It is important to recognize that type I endoleaks may present at

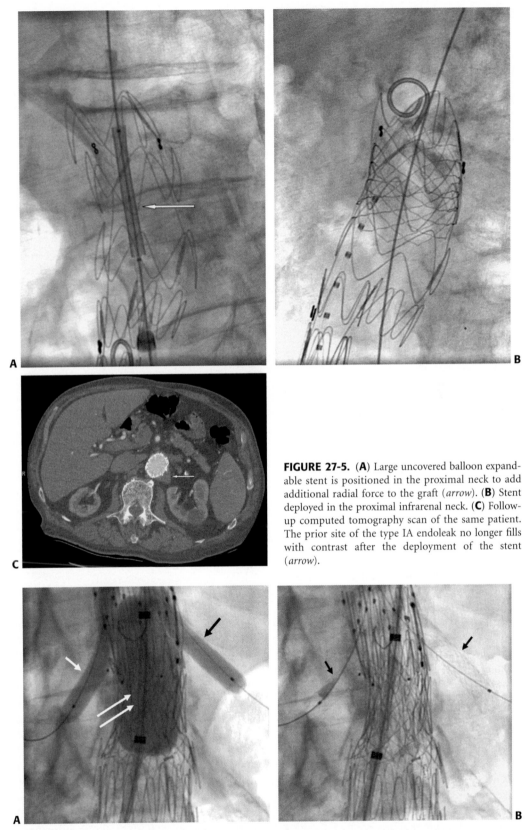

FIGURE 27-5. (**A**) Large uncovered balloon expandable stent is positioned in the proximal neck to add additional radial force to the graft (*arrow*). (**B**) Stent deployed in the proximal infrarenal neck. (**C**) Follow-up computed tomography scan of the same patient. The prior site of the type IA endoleak no longer fills with contrast after the deployment of the stent (*arrow*).

FIGURE 27-6. (**A**) Treatment of a type IA endoleak with a paragraft utilizing simultaneous deployment of bilateral renal stents and a proximal aortic cuff. This technique allows for proximal extension of the endograft with preservation of the renal arteries. *White arrow*, right balloon-expandable renal stent; *black arrow*, left balloon-expandable renal stent; *double arrow*, proximal covered aortic extension cuff. (**B**) Creation of a successful paragraft. *Arrows*, bilateral renal artery stents.

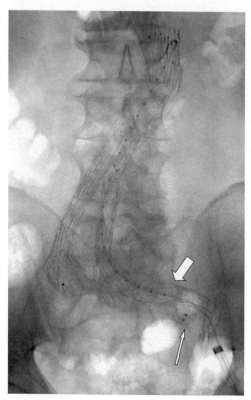

FIGURE 27-7. Unless anatomically inaccessible, the ipsilateral hypogastric artery is routinely occluded (*thin arrow*) before covering it with an iliac extension (*limb thick arrow*). Such a technique limits type II endoleaks from back bleeding of the hypogastric artery. Seen here is occlusion with an Amplatzer vascular plug (AGA Medical Corporation).

any time secondary to graft migration, both proximally and distally (Fig. 27-8). Continued aneurysmal growth of the infrarenal neck leads to the endograft "slipping" down, sometimes even into the sac itself. Conversely, continued iliac aneurysm growth can cause the limb of the graft to "flip" up into the aneurysm sac (Fig. 27-9).

Type II

A type II endoleak is the most common type of endoleak. The hallmark of a type II endoleak is backfilling of the aneurysm sac from a branch artery, such as a lumbar artery or the inferior mesenteric artery. Type II endoleaks are characterized angiographically by late filling of the aneurysm sac. Often, the source of a type II endoleak is difficult to appreciate by CT angiography and duplex. As such, multiple angiographic views may be necessary to identify the

back filling branch artery. Most type II endoleaks resolve by 1 month follow-up. However, even persistent type II endoleaks may be associated with an increased risk of aneurysm rupture (29) (Fig. 27-10). Persistent type II endoleaks often have a combination of an inflow and outflow artery, which contributes to a low likelihood of spontaneous thrombosis. Despite being frequent, most operators do not actively embolize a type II endoleak during the initial EVAR repair due to the high likelihood of spontaneous thrombosis. Accessory renal arteries arising distal to the main renal artery can be a source of a type II endoleak and need to be coiled prior to graft deployment if they originate off the AAA sac. A large, patent, inferior mesenteric artery with minimal aortic laminar thrombus should also likely be embolized before undergoing EVAR, even though specific guidelines have not been published (Fig. 27-11). However, one must be cautioned about the importance of a large patent IMA. In the rare instances of celiac and superior mesenteric artery stenosis, this can lead to severe intestinal ischemia. Embolization of such an artery can be catastrophic and even lethal if not immediately recognized. As a general rule, any branch artery off the aorta has the potential to be a source of a type II endoleak, and this should be considered in the preoperative planning on an individualized basis.

Type III

A type III endoleak is seen as flow in between the modular components of a graft or flow through a tear in the graft. Type III endoleaks are rarely seen following adequate postdeployment balloon dilation. A type III endoleak, similar to a type I endoleak, represents a technical failure and the operation should not be deemed complete until the endoleak is repaired. However, because of the difficulty in appreciating a type III endoleak, the defect can often be mistaken for a type II endoleak. Repairing a type III endoleak due to modular separation can be achieved with additional balloon dilation, with placement of a bare metal stent adding increased radial force, or as a last effort by relining the aorta with a new graft. If graft disruption or tear is suspected, the aorta must be relined with a covered stent. If the leak is never defined, open

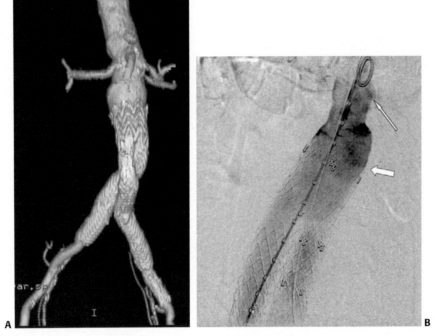

FIGURE 27-8. (**A**) Three-dimensional reconstruction demonstrating distal migration of an Excluder endograft (W.L. Gore & Associates, Inc.). Note the low position in relationship to the renal arteries. Proximal aneurysmal dilation of the aortic neck may be responsible for graft migration. (**B**) Angiography demonstrating distal migration of an AneuRx endograft (Medtronic, Inc.). Note the lower most renal (*thin arrow*) and the top of the graft (*thick arrow*). (See color insert.)

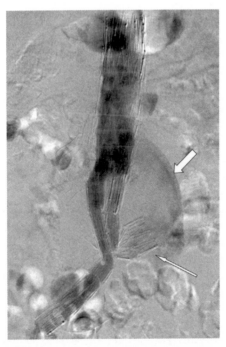

FIGURE 27-9. This late type IB endoleak was discovered incidentally during angiography for unrelated reasons. The left iliac limb migrated proximally and "flipped" up into the aneurysm sac (thin *arrow*). The leak was repaired the following day by endovascular means. Note the persistent filling of the aneurysm sac (*thick arrow*).

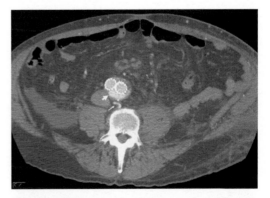

FIGURE 27-10. Type II endoleak noted on follow-up computed tomography scan. *Thin arrow* demonstrates feeding lumbar artery and the *thick arrow* demonstrates contrast filling the aneurysm sac.

469

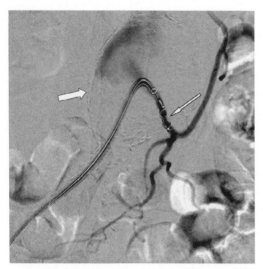

FIGURE 27-11. Large patent IMA noted prior to aortic endograft deployment. IMA embolization may be necessary in the absence of atherosclerosis or laminar thrombus making spontaneous occlusion less likely. Shown here is IMA occlusion with an Amplatzer vascular plug (AGA Medical Corporation) (*thin arrow*). Note the calcified aneurysm sac (*thick arrow*).

repair is reserved for definitive exploration and repair (Fig. 27-12).

Type IV

Type IV endoleak is characterized by flow through the fabric, otherwise known as *graft porosity*. Graft porosity is a bit of a misnomer, as the true etiology of the endoleak is usually small needle holes from the manual fixation of the fabric to the metal stent. Angiographically, a type IV endoleak can be seen as small jets of contrast during the postdeployment run

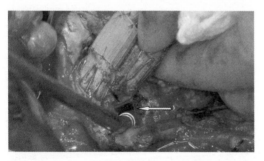

FIGURE 27-12. Type III endoleak noted during open repair. Despite multiple attempts to locate the leak angiographically, it was not until operative exploration that the true origin of the leak was discovered. Note the stream of blood from a small tear in the graft (*arrow*). (See color insert.)

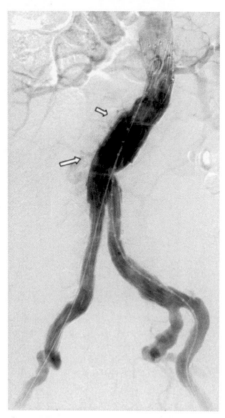

FIGURE 27-13. Type IV endoleak was discovered after graft deployment. Note the individual jets of contrast coming from the graft (*arrows*). The endoleak resolved with reversal of heparin and the follow-up computed tomography scan demonstrated no endoleak.

(Fig. 27-13). Treatment for type IV endoleak is not recommended, as most will resolve with reversal of heparin.

Type V

A type V endoleak is also referred to as *endotension*. In this setting, there are no angiographic findings or CT findings suggestive of continuous flow into the aneurysm sac. Yet, the aneurysm sac will continue to enlarge despite adequate placement of an endograft due to persistent pressurization of the sac. Although the underlying mechanism is unknown, it is proposed that pressure transmission is via thrombus that lines the endograft. In addition, the growth of the aneurysm sac with no discernible endoleak should raise suspicion for graft infection. The treatment for an enlarging aneurysm sac after EVAR with no visible endoleak is operative with explantation of the graft repair of the aneurysm in a conventional fashion (Fig. 27-14).

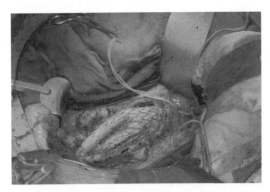

FIGURE 27-14. Despite no evidence of endoleak, this aneurysm sac continued to enlarge, prompting graft explantation and repair of the aneurysm in a conventional fashion. (See color insert.)

Deployment Errors

Covering a Renal Artery

It is important to be familiar with the anatomy of the endograft prior to use. In addition, observation, practice, and repetition of graft deployment is necessary to avoid incorrect graft placement. While some endografts, such as the Excluder, do not allow for small adjustments during deployment; other grafts, such as the Zenith and Talent, are designed for small adjustments during deployment. Using fluoroscopy, the metal component of the endograft may be seen, but the fabric is undetectable. Therefore, it is important to use the radiopaque markers sewn to the graft for accurate placement, not the stent itself. Depending on the presence of aortic calcification and the shape of the aneurysm neck, the graft may "jump" forward proximally a millimeter or two during deployment. This can lead to inaccurate placement and in the worse case scenario, covering branch vessels (Fig. 27-15).

If it is suspected that a renal artery has been partially occluded with the stent graft deployment, the first step is to confirm the suspicion. Deploying the graft with an angiographic catheter at the level of the visceral and renal vessels can give the opportunity to image the vessels before completing the deployment. If the graft in use utilizes a suprarenal fixation stent, and that stent has not been deployed and the graft is still attached to its introducer, the graft should be gently pulled down to the desired level. If the graft is no longer attached to its introducer, suc-

cess can be achieved using a compliant balloon to facilitate pulling the device down. This is done by inflating the device maximally in the graft and then pulling downward. With suprarenal stents and aortic wall "hooks," graft manipulation becomes much more difficult after deployment. One must exercise caution trying to pull a deployed endograft down, for fear of tearing the aortic aneurysm neck. Therefore, if the graft is deployed and a renal artery is covered, the best approach is to stent the renal artery. Often, this entails cannulating the renal artery through a surprarenal stent. If the renal artery is only partially occluded, there is a higher technical success rate than if the renal artery is totally covered. Using a reversed catheter from below or using a brachial approach may offer a higher success rate. If the renal artery is unable to be accessed within a limited amount of time, it is best to convert the procedure to an open repair in the interest of preserved renal

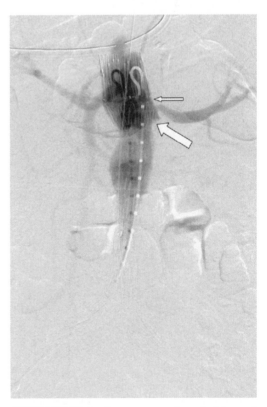

FIGURE 27-15. Inadvertent encroachment of the graft on the left renal artery. Note the end of the metal portion of the graft with extension of the graft fabric (*thin arrow*). Although the renal is almost completely covered, it continues to be perfused by a type IA endoleak (*thick arrow*).

function, especially in the setting of chronic renal insufficiency.

Deployment of Bilateral Limbs in One Iliac Artery

Careful measurements between the lowest renal artery and the aortic bifurcation are necessary when sizing and selecting the main body aortic graft. Successful deployment of the graft should allow the bifurcation of the graft to rest above the bifurcation of the aorta, allowing the contralateral gate to rest over the contralateral iliac artery. Such a configuration will allow for easy access and cannulation of the contralateral limb, facilitating efficient deployment of the ipsilateral limb. Occasionally, the contralateral gate will be positioned in such a manner that cannulation can be extremely difficult (see later). The

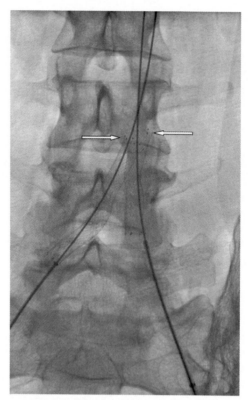

FIGURE 27-17. Caution must be exercised in the setting of bilateral iliac stents. Especially, when, as seen here, the stents were unevenly deployed out of kissing formation. This uneven shelf can cause the contralateral limb to not open properly, or be deployed with in the stent, as noted in Fig. 27-16. *Arrows* demonstrate top of uneven stents.

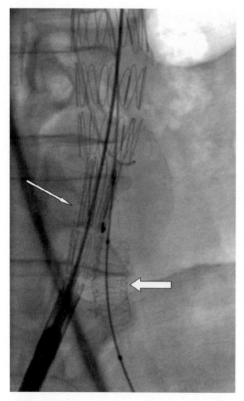

FIGURE 27-16. A Zenith endograft (Cook Medical, Inc.) with two limbs deployed in the ipsilateral iliac (*thin arrow*). This occurred in the setting of bilateral iliac stents for occlusive disease. As shown on the contralateral side, the stents were warped during attempts to pass the main body up both sides of these narrow and diseased iliacs (*thick arrow*). In doing so, the stents were pushed proximally, causing the contralateral limb to be caught in the ipsilateral iliac.

most extreme example of this would be deployment of the both limbs in the ipsilateral iliac artery (Fig. 27-16). This may occur if the graft is sized incorrectly, with deployment of a main body shorter than expected. In addition, if proximal deployment is not done at the level of the lowest renal artery, this may result in the main body extending more proximal than anticipated.

One must be cautious of prior iliac interventions. A history of bilateral iliac occlusive disease with bilateral iliac stenting often results in an artificial rise in the aortic bifurcation. Failing to recognize and incorporate this "new" bifurcation can cause deployment of both limbs into the prior-placed iliac stent (Fig. 27-17). At this juncture, endovascular salvage is determined by one's ability to cross the contralateral gate with a wire. If the contralateral gate has been totally deployed within an iliac artery or stent, it may be technically feasible to raise the main body enough to allow the limb to spring open. This feat may be accomplished by placing a large sheath (9F or greater) into the aortic graft over a stiff wire. By inflating a large compliant molding balloon, such that it is in contact with the graft and resting on top of the sheath, application of gentle forward pressure on the sheath may raise the graft, pushing it proximally. This must be done with caution, as to not cover the visceral or renal arteries. If the limb is partially open and freed from the ipsilateral artery, the task of cannulating the limb will allow for completion of the procedure. Technical tips for cannulation of a difficult limb are discussed later.

If the limb cannot be accessed, consideration must be given to the use of an aorto-uniiliac (AUI) converter. In this instance, a new main body aortic stent graft or AUI converter is deployed within the faulty main body (Fig. 27-18A). The proximal contralateral iliac must be occluded to prevent type IB endoleaks. Occlusion of this limb can be done with a commercial iliac occluder or more recently, an Amplatzer vascular plug (AGA Medical Corporation, Ply-

mouth, MN.) (Fig. 27-18B). Following successful deployment of the AUI converter and occluder device, a surgical femoral artery to femoral artery bypass must be performed to maintain perfusion of the contralateral limb. If one is already employing an open bilateral femoral exposure, the increased morbidity is negligible, with femoro-femoral bypass patency rates improved in the absence of peripheral vascular disease. Completion angiography demonstrates preserved distal perfusion with no detectable endoleak (Fig. 27-18C).

Difficult Contralateral Gate Cannulation

Proper deployment of a main body endograft should allow for easy cannulation of the contralateral gate with nothing more than an angled glide catheter. However, because of anatomical factors and technical error, the contralateral gate can end up in a variety of positions, with misalignment extending as far as an ipsilateral configuration. The first step in successful cannulation begins with proper imaging. The exact position of the gate can be revealed only with

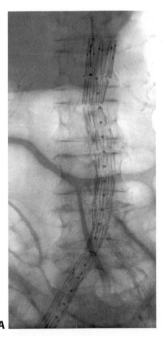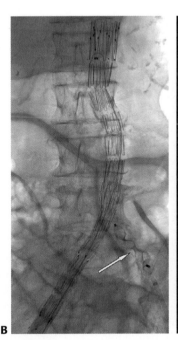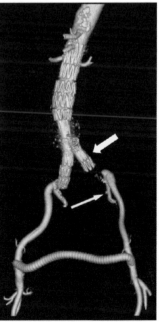

A   **B**   **C**

FIGURE 27-18. (**A**) Deployment of a Renu aorto-uniiliac (Cook Aorto-uniiliac) converter with suprarenal fixation. Note the absence of a contralateral limb. (**B**) Successful deployment of an aorto-uniiliac converter with occlusion of the contralateral iliac using a second generation Amplatzer vascular plug (AGA Medical Corporation) (*arrow*). (**C**) Successful aorto-uniiliac conversion seen on computed tomography angiography at follow-up. Note the contralateral placement of Cook iliac occluder (Cook Medical, Inc.) (*thick arrow*). The femorofemoral bypass is patent and backfills the left external and internal iliac (*thin arrow*). (See color insert.)

the use of multiview fluoroscopy or alternatively, by rotating the image intensifier around the patient. With a wire in the distal aorta, rotating the image intensifier while utilizing fluoroscopy allows visualization of the relationship between the gate, the contralateral iliac, and the main body graft. Catheter and wire manipulation should begin in a projection that allows an understanding of the spatial position of the gate. Often, a double or reversed curve catheter, such as a Beacon Tip Van Schie catheter (Cook Medical, Inc., Bloomington, Indiana) will give excellent results. If multiple attempts are unsuccessful, it may be necessary to confirm the patency and positioning of the contralateral gate with angiography. If the gate is truly unable to be cannulated from the contralateral side, one may attempt to go "up and over" the endograft bifurcation from the ipsilateral side. Unlike a native aortic bifurcation, the bifurcation of an endograft can be rather acute, and appropriate catheter selection for traversing this angle include a Simmons catheter, a SOS Omni flush catheter (Angiodynamics, Inc., Queensbury, NY), a J curve, a right internal mammary catheter, or a shepherd hook. If the gate can be cannulated from the ipsilateral side, the ensuing glide wire needs to be snared in the terminal aorta or contralateral iliac and then pulled extracorporally. At this point, the catheter used should be advanced so that the ends of both the wire and the catheter are extracorporal on opposite sides. The guidewire should then be removed and a stiff wire, such as an Amplatz or Lunderquist wire, should be inserted through the catheter on the contralateral side and advanced over the endograft bifurcation. The catheter can now be removed from the ipsilateral side. The stiff wire can now be gently pulled back until it springs up into the main body of the graft. With wire access established across the contralateral gate, the contralateral limb can be deployed in a standard fashion.

If the endograft bifurcation cannot be traversed by the above-stated technique, a brachial approach may allow successful cannulation. Following brachial access, a guidewire is passed into the main body of the graft. Often, only a straight or an angled glide catheter is needed to cannulate the contralateral gate with this approach. There is little anatomical limitation when this approach is used, as there are only two options

for the guidewire to go: the ipsilateral limb or the contralateral gate. After successful passage of the guidewire into the terminal aorta or contralateral iliac, as described earlier, the guidewire will need to be snared and, along with the catheter, brought extracorporally. The guidewire may be removed and a stiff wire can be used in a retrograde fashion to gain access across the contralateral gate into the main body graft. Not always intuitive, if this approach is used, longer wires and catheters are used as the distance is greatly increased. When using the above-mentioned techniques, it is extremely rare that the contralateral gate cannot be cannulated, requiring conversion to an aorto-uniiliac device with femorofemoral bypass.

Indications for Open Conversion: Short- and Long-Term

With the current, available technology, it is rare that aortic aneurysmal disease thought to be suitable for endovascular repair requires open conversion, either in the acute primary operative setting or after long-term failure of the graft. Even if inadvertent rupture occurs during EVAR, the aneurysm usually can be repaired without open conversion, as studies have shown that infrarenal ruptured AAAs repaired endovascularly have a lower morbidity and mortality than open repair. The use of an intra-aortic balloon occluder can be used as a temporary adjunct to control blood loss. This may be a compliant molding balloon, such as a CODA balloon. If the pressure in the aorta is too great, such that the balloon continuously slips into the distal aorta, allowing continued hemorrhage, success may be achieved by inflating the balloon just outside of a large sheath. The sheath allows for additional support. Alternatively, a brachial approach may be used, permitting the balloon to "hang" in the proximal descending aorta for control. Current indications for acute conversion to open include inadvertent covering of critical renal or visceral main artery branches with demonstrated loss of end organ perfusion.

Perhaps more common than acute conversion of an endovascular repair to an open repair is identifying individual patients in follow-up who will require additional treatment not amenable to catheter-based approaches. Type IA endoleaks seen at follow-up after the primary

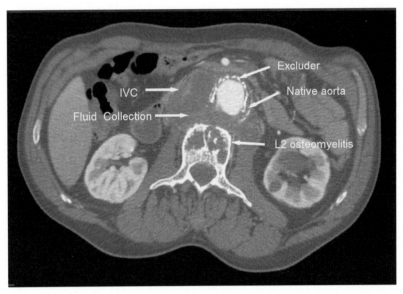

FIGURE 27-19. Continued aneurysm growth in the setting of periaortic infection with concomitant L2 osteomyelitis following aneurysm repair with an Excluder (W.L. Gore & Associates, Inc.). IVC, inferior vena cava.

operation or discovered incidentally need to be repaired in a timely fashion. Older devices appear prone to distal migration (30,31). These endoleaks often can be repaired endovascularly, if an appropriate neck remains to land the new endograft or aortic cuff. In an otherwise healthy patient, with no proximal neck, and an endoleak discovered in follow-up, open aortic reconstruction with graft explantation still remains a viable therapy. However, in those unsuited to undergo such a procedure and in the absence of branched endograft technology readily available, the use of paragrafts may be an option.

Type V endoleaks or endotension are described as a continued growth of the aneurysm sac with no obvious source. This type of endoleak, when identified, is best treated by conventional open repair. Furthermore, rare conditions such as endograft infection, periaortic abscess, and aortitis can all contribute to continued sac growth in the absence of an endoleak (Fig. 27-19). Attempting to repair these aneurysms by endovascular means is unproven and anecdotally results in failure and poor patient outcomes.

Overcoming Anatomical Limitations

The high rate of technical success of EVAR can be attributed to appropriate patient selection and careful preoperative planning. Knowledge

not only of endograft sizing but also of the size of graft delivery systems may influence the decision of which device to use. Angulated or thrombus lined aortic necks may also prohibit accurate placement or a endoleak-free proximal landing zone. Current FDA-approved devices in use are indicated for necks of 1 to 1.5 cm in length. The ongoing PYTHAGORUS trial will hopefully bring to the market the Aorfix graft, capable of managing severely angulated necks (32). In general, a patient should not be taken to the operating room for an endovascular repair if the neck is in question. In the future, branched and fenestrated endografts may widen the patient selection for endovascular repair.

There still remains a subset of patients with aneurysms arising directly distal to the lowest renal artery, with no true neck apparent. While operative treatment remains the mainstay for these patients, it is important to recognize that these patients would incur a high risk of morbidity and mortality, if subject to such a repair. In this particular group, and in the absence of branched endografts, the role for renal artery stenting by snorkel technique and the complex paragraft has evolved (Fig. 27-20). A paragraft overcomes the limitation set forth by the lowest or even both renal arteries by incorporating

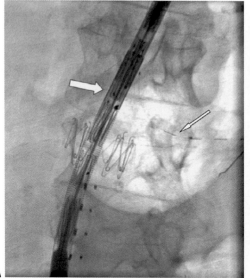

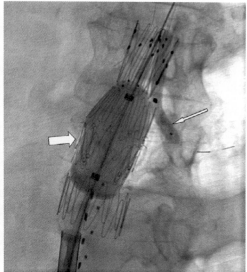

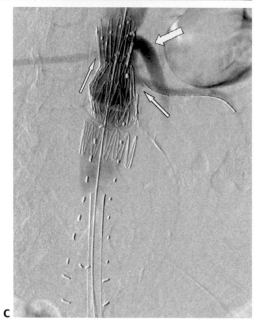

FIGURE 27-20. (**A**) Type IA endoleak occurred secondary to proximal migration of an Ancure endograft (Guidant Corporation). The proximal aortic cuff is brought into place (*thick arrow*). Note cannulation of the left renal artery with an uncovered stent in position for deployment (*thin arrow*). (**B**) The proximal aortic cuff has been deployed. Simultaneous expansion of the cuff with a molding balloon (*thick arrow*) and deployment of the balloon mounted renal stent (*thin arrow*) allows for successful placement of both stents without incurring a crush injury to the device. (**C**) Completion angiogram demonstrates a patent SMA (*thick arrow*) and bilateral renal arteries (*thin arrows*) with proximal extension of the endograft and no endoleak.

them into the proximal landing zone. By simultaneously stenting the renal artery and deploying the proximal main body over the renal arteries, the neck is elongated and a proximal seal can be obtained. As such, the proximal anatomical limiting factor in an aneurysm neck is no longer the renal arteries but rather the superior mesenteric artery. However, successful paragraft performance is complex and requires a carefully orchestrated deployment, which requires many individual operators with a spe-

cific and important role. Femoral access is gained through a cut down as access for the main body endograft. Next, depending on the involvement of one or two renals, unilateral or bilateral brachial access is obtained. If both renal arteries are involved, both renal arteries are selectively cannulated. Long balloon-expandable uncovered stents are positioned in the renal arteries such that there is an extended amount of length proximally in the aorta. The aortic stent graft is brought up and deployed just distal to the SMA, covering the renal arteries. A compliant molding balloon is used to shape the aortic endograft while the renal artery stents are ballooned. The key maneuver is performing the deployment of the renal artery stents and aortic graft molding simultaneous so that neither device is crushed or damaged in any way. The proximal extension of the neck is usually sufficient to obtain a secure proximal landing zone free of type IA endoleaks, while still maintaining adequate renal perfusion.

Another common anatomical area that must be addressed when selecting EVAR candidacy and graft selection is iliac diameter. While most iliac arteries can accommodate the sheath sizes required for EVAR (less so for TEVAR), the iliac must be able to accommodate the delivery system of the aortic graft. Clearly, small arteries with significant atherosclerosis may best be served using low-profile devices. The smallest diameter iliac system should be designated as the contralateral side, while the largest diameter iliac system should be reserved for the main body. True atherosclerotic stenosis can be treated with angioplasty before attempting to deliver the endograft. Alternatively, serial hydrophilic dilators, sizes 16F to 24F, may be passed into the iliac system, progressively dilating the vessel. Severely calcified iliac vessels can rupture with aggressive angioplasty or stenting. Careful attention must be given to vital signs during treatment of severely calcified iliac vessels, especially in the patient undergoing general anesthesia, as a drop in the blood pressure or rise in the heart rate may be the only sign of a ruptured iliac artery.

Occasionally, after progressive dilation or angioplasty and failure to pass the delivery system into the aorta, it may be necessary to intentionally rupture the iliac artery. The iliac is first lined with covered stent grafts (Fig. 27-21). The size of the stent graft, usually 10 mm, should be large enough to accommodate the main body delivery system, but not large enough to cause redundancy. After the iliac, both common and external are lined with stent grafts, an appropriately sized noncompliant balloon is then insufflated until the iliac visibly ruptures (9–10 mm balloon). The rupture is characterized by a brisk but obvious enlargement of the iliac with loss of the angiographic "waist." Wire access should be maintained at all times in case rupture is followed by hemorrhage. Angiography can confirm a successful rupture with no active extravasation. Following rupture, the main body device may be delivered through the covered stent graft with slow and steady but gentle pressure so as to not dislodge the covered stent grafts.

Although rupturing an iliac is an endovascular option, the problem of the small or narrowed iliac artery can also be solved surgically with an iliac conduit (Fig. 27-22). Following iliac exposure with a small retroperitoneal incision, an appropriately sized 10 mm graft is sewn onto the distal common iliac or proximal external iliac. The main body is then delivered into the aorta via the conduit. After the main body is deployed, the conduit can be oversewn or an iliofemoral bypass can be performed and the procedure continued in a standard fashion.

Tortuous iliac anatomy can also make passing the stent grafts difficult. Often, simply using a stiff wire, such as a Lunderquist, and applying slow and steady pressure is enough to allow passage of the main body. If the iliac artery does not straighten out with a stiff wire, it is reasonable to place a second stiff wire to straighten it out enough to accept the delivery system. In addition to tortuous iliacs, a tortuous aorta can make passage of a thoracic endograft difficult. Passage may be eased by creating a stiff monorail system that the graft can be delivered upon. This can be aided through right brachial to femoral access (or flossing). For thoracic grafts in the setting of a tortuous thoracic aortic arch, right arm brachial access is probably more appropriate as it takes the natural curve of the aortic arch. A guidewire and catheter are passed into the terminal aorta from the arm, snared, and brought extracorporally. The guidewire is removed and a stiff Lunderquist wire is left in its place, establishing wire access from the groin to the arm. The wire can then act as a monorail system and the two ends held taught as the endograft is delivered. This should result in enough support to allow the thoracic endograft to be moved into position.

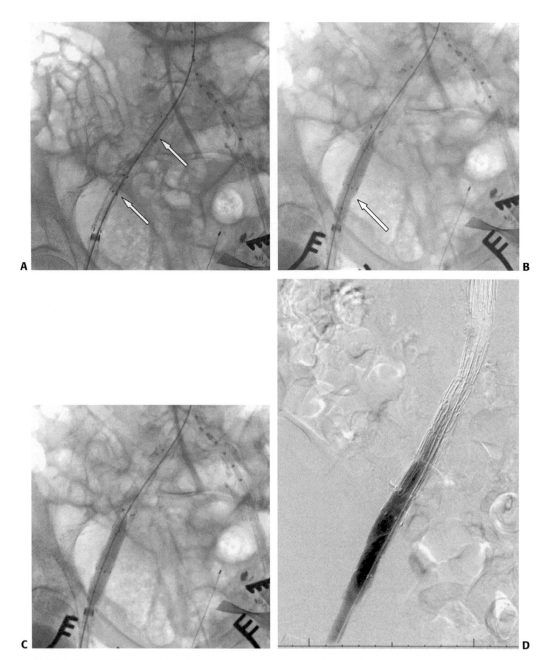

FIGURE 27-21. (A) Narrowed and atherosclerotic right iliac is first lined with covered stent grafts (*arrows*). **(B)** The iliac, now lined with covered stent grafts, is aggressively balloon dilated. Note the distal waist seen in the balloon (*arrow*), corresponding to a tight stenosis. **(C)** During balloon dilation, the stenosis rapidly disappears as the iliac becomes noticeably larger. Of note is the loss of the angiographic waist. The iliac has now been ruptured. **(D)** Following enlargement of the iliac with rupture, the main body is able to pass through the iliac and the ipsilateral limb is brought down in the standard fashion. There is no evidence of active extravasation.

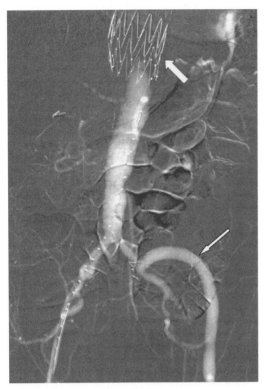

FIGURE 27-22. Aortogram (*thick arrow*) in the setting of bilateral iliac atherosclerotic disease. The conduit (*thin arrow*) serves as a functional iliofemoral bypass.

■ CONCLUSION

Endovascular repair of abdominal and TAAs are now the primary therapy for treatment of these aneurysms. Careful preoperative planning is critical in developing a successful plan for endovascular exclusion of aortic aneurysms. To manage these complex patients with variable arterial anatomy, one must maintain a "tool chest" of techniques to best serve the patient with an aortic aneurysm.

References

1. Lovegrove RE, Javid M, Magee TR, Galland RB. A meta-analysis of 21,178 patients undergoing open or endovascular repair of abdominal aortic aneurysm. *Br J Surg.* 2008;95:677–684.

2. Walsh SR, Tang TY, Sadat U, et al. Endovascular stenting versus open surgery for thoracic aortic disease: systematic review and meta-analysis of perioperative results. *J Vasc Surg.* 2008;47:1094–1098.

3. Karkos CD, Harkin DW, Giannakou A, Gerassimidis TS. Mortality after endovascular repair of ruptured abdominal aortic aneurysms: a systematic review and meta-analysis. *Arch Surg.* 2009;144:770–778.

4. Rayt HS, Sutton AJ, London NJ, Sayers RD, Bown MJ. A systematic review and meta-analysis of endovascular repair (EVAR) for ruptured abdominal aortic aneurysm. *Eur J Vasc Endovasc Surg.* 2008;36:536–544.

5. Johnston KW, Rutherford RB, Tilson MD, et al. Suggested standards for reporting on arterial aneurysms. Subcommittee on Reporting Standards for Arterial Aneurysms, Ad Hoc Committee on Reporting Standards, Society for Vascular Surgery and North American Chapter, International Society for Cardiovascular Surgery. *J Vasc Surg.* 1991;13:452–458.

6. Dimick JB, Upchurch GR Jr. Endovascular technology, hospital volume, and mortality with abdominal aortic aneurysm surgery. *J Vasc Surg.* 2008;47:1150–1154.

7. Mealy K, Salman A. The true incidence of ruptured abdominal aortic aneurysms. *Eur J Vasc Surg.* 1988;2:405–408.

8. Eliason JL, Wainess RM, Dimick JB, et al. The effect of secondary operations on mortality following abdominal aortic aneurysm repair in the United States: 1988–2001. *Vasc Endovascular Surg.* 2005;39:465–472.

9. Lederle FA, Johnson GR, Wilson SE, et al. Rupture rate of large abdominal aortic aneurysms in patients refusing or unfit for elective repair. *JAMA.* 2002;287:2968–2972.

10. Lederle FA, Wilson SE, Johnson GR, et al. Immediate repair compared with surveillance of small abdominal aortic aneurysms. *N Engl J Med.* 2002;346:1437–1444.

11. United Kingdom Small Aneurysm Trial Participants. Long-term outcomes of immediate repair compared with surveillance of small abdominal aortic aneurysms. *N Engl J Med.* 2002;346:1445–1452.

12. Mortality results for randomised controlled trial of early elective surgery or ultrasonographic surveillance for small abdominal aortic aneurysms. The UK Small Aneurysm Trial Participants. *Lancet.* 1998;352:1649–1655.

13. Ouriel K. Randomized clinical trials of endovascular repair versus surveillance for treatment of small abdominal aortic aneurysms. *J Endovasc Ther.* 2009;16(suppl 1):I94–I105.

14. Parodi JC, Palmaz JC, Barone HD. Transfemoral intraluminal graft implantation for abdominal aortic aneurysm. *Ann Vasc Surg.* 1991;5:491–499.

15. Greenberg RK, Deaton D, Sullivan T, et al. Variable sac behavior after endovascular repair of abdominal aortic aneurysm: analysis of core laboratory data. *J Vasc Surg.* 2004;39:95–101.

16. Prinssen M, Verhoeven EL, Buth J, et al. A randomized trial comparing conventional and endovascular repair of abdominal aortic aneurysms. *N Engl J Med.* 2004;351:1607–1618.

17. Blankensteijn JD, de Jong SE, Prinssen M, et al. Two-year outcomes after conventional or endovascular repair of abdominal aortic aneurysms. *N Engl J Med.* 2005;352:2398–2405.

18. Endovascular aneurysm repair versus open repair in patients with abdominal aortic aneurysm (EVAR trial 1): randomised controlled trial. EVAR Trial Participants. *Lancet.* 2005;365: 2179–2186.

19. Greenhalgh RM, Brown LC, Kwong GP, et al. Comparison of endovascular aneurysm repair with open repair in patients with abdominal aortic aneurysm (EVAR trial 1), 30-day operative mortality results: randomised controlled trial. *Lancet.* 2004;364:843–848.

20. Lederle FA, Freischlag JA, Kyriakides TC, et al. Open Versus Endovascular Repair (OVER) Veterans Affairs Cooperative Study Group: outcomes following endovascular vs open repair of abdominal aortic aneurysm: a randomized trial. *JAMA.* 2009;302:1535–1542.

21. Dimick JB, Stanley JC, Axelrod DA, et al. Variation in death rate after abdominal aortic aneurysmectomy in the United States: impact of hospital volume, gender, and age. *Ann Surg.* 2002;235:579–585.

22. Criado E, Kabbani L, Cho K. Catheter-less angiography for endovascular aortic aneurysm repair: a new application of carbon dioxide as a contrast agent. *J Vasc Surg.* 2008;48:527–534.

23. Volodos NL, Karpovich IP, Troyan VI, et al. Clinical experience of the use of self-fixing synthetic prostheses for remote endoprosthetics of the thoracic and the abdominal aorta and iliac arteries through the femoral artery and as intraoperative endoprosthesis for aorta reconstruction. *Vasa Suppl.* 1991;33:93–95.

24. Moainie SL, Neschis DG, Gammie JS, et al. Endovascular stenting for traumatic aortic injury: an emerging new standard of care. *Ann Thorac Surg.* 2008;85:1625–1629.

25. Bavaria JE, Appoo JJ, Makaroun MS, Verter J, Yu ZF, Mitchell RS. Gore TAG Investigators: endovascular stent grafting versus open surgical repair of descending thoracic aortic aneurysms in low-risk patients: a multicenter comparative trial. *J Thorac Cardiovasc Surg.* 2007;133:369–377.

26. Matsumura JS, Cambria RP, Dake MD, et al. TX2 Clinical Trial Investigators: international controlled clinical trial of thoracic endovascular aneurysm repair with the Zenith TX2 endovascular graft: 1-year results. *J Vasc Surg.* 2008;47:247–257.

27. Fairman RM, Criado F, Farber M, et al. VALOR Investigators: pivotal results of the Medtronic Vascular Talent Thoracic Stent Graft System: the VALOR trial. *J Vasc Surg.* 2008;48:546–554.

28. Vandy F, Criado E, Upchurch GR Jr, et al. Transluminal hypogastric artery occlusion with an Amplatzer vascular plug during endovascular aortic aneurysm repair. *J Vasc Surg.* 2008;48:1121–1214.

29. Schlösser FJ, Gusberg RJ, Dardik A, et al. Aneurysm rupture after EVAR: can the ultimate failure be predicted? *Eur J Vasc Endovasc Surg.* 2009;37:15–22.

30. Kelso RL, Lyden SP, Butler B, et al. Late conversions of aortic stent grafts. *J Vasc Surg.* 2009;49:589–595.

31. Zarins CK, Bloch DA, Crabtree T, et al. Aneurysm enlargement following endovascular aneurysm repair: AneuRx clinical trial. *J Vasc Surg.* 2004;39: 109–117.

32. Perdikides T, Georgiadis GS, Avgerinos ED, et al. The Aorfix stent-graft to treat infrarenal abdominal aortic aneurysms with angulated necks and/or tortuous iliac arteries: midterm results. *J Endovasc Ther.* 2009;16:567–576.

Peripheral Vascular Interventions

IMRAN N. AHMAD AND SAMIR R. KAPADIA

T arget vessel complications of peripheral vascular interventions include flow-limiting dissection, spasm and thrombosis, perforation with compartment syndrome, and distal embolization. Depending on the target vessel, area subtended, and adjacent vessels, these complications may have catastrophic consequences. Avoidance through preventative measures and meticulous technique are of the utmost importance. However, at some point one can expect to deal with at least one of these problems. Skill with equipment and experience with bailout techniques can be limb- or lifesaving at these times.

Complications of peripheral vascular interventions can be broadly classified into four categories: local access site, target vessel site, distal vessel, and systemic complications. Local access site and systemic complications have been described in Section 2. The focus of this chapter is on complications and their management as related to upper extremity intervention including subclavian and vertebral artery intervention, renal artery intervention, and lower extremity intervention.

■ INCIDENCE OF COMPLICATIONS

Compared with the percutaneous coronary intervention (PCI) literature, fewer randomized trials exist for peripheral vascular interventions. As a result, case series and cumulative experience are drawn upon heavily when making recommendations regarding complications. It is difficult to draw strong conclusions from case series data because definitions, procedural technique, lesion location, and follow-up vary greatly. Schillinger et al. reported that the overall technical success rates of peripheral interventions tend to be greater than 90% with complication rates of 6% to 10% in the subclavian and vertebral arteries and 4% to 6% in the femoral arteries (1).

Vertebral Artery Interventions

Originating from the first part of the subclavian artery, the vertebral artery can be divided into three extracranial segments (V1 to V3) and one intracranial segment (V4) (Fig. 28-1). The vertebral artery ostium is the most common site of extracranial disease and amenable to percutaneous intervention in the majority of cases with technical success rates of greater than 90%. Because of the tortuous nature and bony encasement, the distal extracranial and intracranial segments can be particularly sensitive to wire or catheter manipulation and carry a higher risk of complication. The most feared complications are posterior circulation CNS ischemic events that occur in approximately 1% of interventions (Table 28-1).

Early experience with percutaneous transluminal angioplasty (PTA) alone for vertebral artery stenosis demonstrated higher rates of success with less restenosis for proximal as compared to distal segment disease. Higashida et al. reported on a case series of PTA in 41 patients who failed medical therapy for symptomatic posterior cerebral ischemia. Of the 34 proximal lesions all were successfully treated with only three transient complications including spasm and TIA. Of the five distal lesions, two major complications occurred including complete vessel occlusion and rupture (2). Terada et al. reported on a case series of PTA in 12 patients with distal vertebral and basilar artery disease. The procedure was successful in eight patients while major complications including two dissections and two distal embolizations occurred in the other four patients (3). In a case series of 16 patients undergoing vertebral artery PTA and stenting, three of the four distal vessel interventions were complicated by dissection with one resulting in a subarachnoid hemorrhage and death (4).

481

TABLE 28-1 Vertebral Artery Interventions Complications

Study	N	Target Vessel	Intervention	Stent Type[a]	Technical Success	Major Complications	Follow-Up (mo)	Residual Stenosis[b]	Restenosis[c]
Coward LJ et al. (30)	8	Vertebral	PTA 75%, Stent 25%	Palmaz-Schatz (1), AVE (1)	100%	25%: 2 TIA	mean 9.6	median 25%	50% (3/6 PTA only arm)
Gupta et al. (9)	49	31 ECVA, 18 ICVA or BA	DES (98%), BMS (2%)	Cypher 26%, Taxus 74%	98%, 1 failed ICVA (success with BMS)	2%: 1 stroke	median 4 ± 2	mean 12% ± 11%	4.9% (2/41 ECVA origin)
Eberhardt et al. (7)	20	9 V0, 2 V3, 5 V4, 4 BA	Stent	Herculine (6), Multilink (1), S670/AVE670 (4), Bx Sonic/Velocity (4), Terumo (1), INX (1)	100%	25%: 2 TIA, 3 stroke (V4 and BA)	median 26	mean V0 3% ± 4%, V3/V4 5% ± 4%, BA 7% ± 3%	23%, (2/4 proximal, 1/9 distal)
Weber et al. (8)	38	Vertebral	Stent	S670, Velocity	100%	7.9%: 2 dissections, 1 TIA	mean 11	13% (5/38), median 10%	38% (10/26), 7.7% (2/26) total occlusion
Janssens et al. (31)	19	Vertebral	PTA	NA	89%	26%: 4 asymptomatic dissections (VA), 1 bilateral iliac dissection	mean 30	47% (9/19), mean 31%	21% (4/19)

[a]Cypher, Palmaz Schatz, and Bx Sonic/Velocity (Cordis), Taxus (Boston Scientific), Herculin and Multilink (Guidant), S670/AVE670 and INX (Medtronic).

[b]Median or mean residual stenosis or percentage with residual stenosis.

[c]Percentage of restenosis in those with angiography or noninvasive imaging at follow-up.

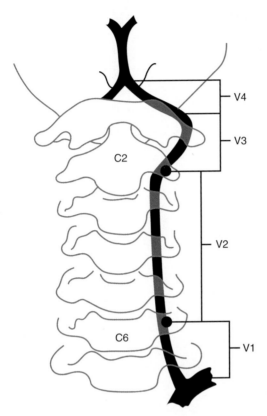

FIGURE 28-1. Schematic of four parts of the vertebral artery. (Adapted from Cloud GC, Markus HS. Diagnosis and management of vertebral artery stenosis. *Q J Med.* 2003;96:27–54.)

Jenkins et al. reported on the safety and efficacy of vertebral artery stenting in 32 patients. Success as defined by less than 20% residual stenosis was achieved in all patients with one TIA (5). Lin et al. reported on 58 patients with 67 ostial vertebral artery lesions who underwent balloon-expandable stent angioplasty. The technical success rate was 100% but complicated by two posterior and one anterior cerebral circulation strokes in the peri-procedural period (6). Eberhardt et al. reported on 20 patients who underwent stenting in the vertebral and basilar arteries. Procedural success was achieved in all patients with minimal residual stenosis. None of the interventions in the proximal vertebral artery resulted in peri-procedural TIA or stroke. Of the five V4 lesions treated, two resulted in peri-procedural stroke and one in recurrent stroke (7). Weber et al. reported on 36 patients with 38 stenoses of the vertebral artery origin who underwent balloon-expandable stent angioplasty. There were only two dissections both successfully treated with further

stenting. However, the angiographic rate of restenosis was 38% in the 26 patients with follow-up. Although the procedure was technically successful in all lesions without recurrent posterior cerebral stroke, the authors concluded that the rate of restenosis was unacceptably high (8).

Because of the relatively high rates of angiographic restenosis with bare metal stents, researchers investigated the use of a drug-eluting stent (DES) in this location. Gupta et al. reported on 59 patients who underwent stenting with a DES to the vertebral or carotid artery. A total of 49 vertebral and basilar artery lesions were treated, 63% of which were proximal vertebral lesions. Successful delivery of a DES was achieved in all proximal lesions. Of the distal lesions, there was one failure of a DES delivery subsequently treated with a BMS and one acute stroke. There was a 7% restenosis rate on follow-up in 27 proximal VA stents and no evidence of restenosis in any of the 14 distal stents with follow-up (9). Typically, the dominant vertebral artery is 4.5 mm to 5.5 mm in diameter. Therefore, the vertebral artery can often times be stented with a 4.0-mm drug-eluting stent and post-dilated to 4.5 mm or even to 5 mm. Intravascular ultrasound (IVUS) examination can determine the reference diameter as well as the extent of disease. The origin of the vertebral artery may be difficult to visualize angiographically because of posterior takeoff and vessel overlap. Ipsilateral shallow angulation with some cranial tilt may help to visualize the origins better.

Subclavian Artery Interventions

Originating from the aortic arch as the third great vessel, the left subclavian artery is the more frequently affected of the two subclavian arteries Table 28-2. Stenosis of the subclavian artery typically occurs proximal to the vertebral artery, while occlusion of the subclavian artery usually extends into the vertebral artery (Fig. 28-2). Total occlusions present a challenge and usually necessitate a brachial approach. During wire manipulation, the tip may enter the subintimal plane causing a dissection that may progress in either a retrograde fashion to involve the aorta or an antegrade fashion to involve the vertebral artery or LIMA. Therefore, proximity of lesions to the vertebral and internal mammary artery should be carefully delineated as patency of these important branch vessels may be jeopardized by an

TABLE 28-2 Subclavian Artery Intervention Complications

Study	N	Target Vessel	Intervention	Stent Type[a]	Technical Success	Major Complications	Follow-Up (mo)	Residual Stenosis[b]	Restenosis[c]
Sixt et al. (15)	108	Subclavian (left 84, both 1) or innominate (24)	PTA 13%, Stent 87%	BES 68%: Palmaz-Schatz (30), Genesis (14), Corinthian (2), Radix (10), PUVA (1), SAXX (1) SES 28%: Dynalink (9), Sinus (3), Wallstent (2), SMART (3)	96% overall, 100% in stenoses (78/78), 87% total occlusions (26/30)	Not specified as treated with provisional stenting	mean 29 ± 20	4 failed total occlusions of left subclavian artery	9% (9/104)
Patel et al. (14)	177	Subclavian (left 142, right 24) or innominate (11)	Stent (214)	BES 71%, SES 29%	98% overall, 99% stenoses (155/156), 91% total occlusions (19/21)	5.8%: 1 embolic stroke, 3 flow-limiting dissections, 1 distal embolization, 1 thrombosis, 1 TIA	mean 35.2 ± 30.8	2 failed total occlusions	16% (22/138)
AbuRhama et al. (13)	121	Subclavian (left 107, right 14)	Stent	BES 100%	98% overall, 100% stenoses (96/96), 92% total occlusions (23/25)	5.8%: 2 distal embolization, 1 brachial artery thrombosis, 1 dissection, 1 CHF, 1 reperfusion edema, 1 pseudoaneurysm	mean 40.8	2 failed total occlusions	5% (6/119)
de Vries et al. (10)	110	Subclavian (left 84, right 26)	PTA	NA	93% overall, 100% stenosis (89/89), 65% total occlusions (13/20)	3.6%: 2 strokes, 2 TIA	mean 34	54% (56/102), 7 failed total occlusions	14% (16/102)
Amor et al. (12)	89	Subclavian (left 74, right 15)	Stent	Palmaz Schatz (55.6%), Corinthian (17.5%)	93% overall, 100% stenosis (76/76), 54% total 1 stroke, occlusions (7/13)	4.5%: 2 distal embolization, 1 TIA	mean 42 ± 24	6 failed total occlusions	17% (15/89)

[a]Balloon Expanadable:Palmaz-Schatz, Genesis, and Corinthian (Cordis), Radix (Sorin Biomedica), PUVA (Devon Medical), SAXX (C.R. Bard) Self-expanding: Dynalink (Guidant), Sinus (Optimed, Wallstent (Boston Scientific), SMART (Cordis).

[b]Median or mean residual stenosis or percentage with residual stenosis.

[c]Percentage of restenosis in those with angiography or noninvasive imaging at follow-up.

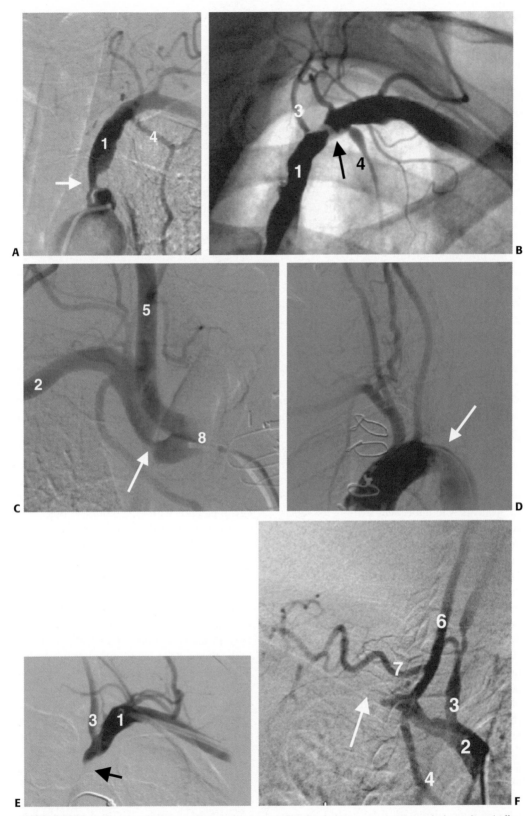

FIGURE 28-2. Spectrum of atherosclerosis in the right and left subclavian arteries. Stenosis (*arrow*) typically occurs in the proximal subclavian artery (**A** and **C**), and rarely distal to the vertebral artery (**B**). Occlusion (*arrow*) of the subclavian artery usually extends from the ostium to the origin of the vertebral artery (**D** and **E**) but occasionally can occur after the vertebral artery (**F**). 1, Left subclavian; 2, Right subclavian; 3, Vertebral; 4, Internal mammary; 5, Right common carotid; 6, Thyrocervical trunk; 7, Suprascapular; 8, Innominate.

unplanned approach. In right subclavian and innominate artery interventions, there is potential for injury to the common carotid artery with embolization to the anterior cerebral circulation.

De Vries et al. reported on 110 patients undergoing PTA of the proximal subclavian artery. Technical success was achieved in 102 lesions. Of the 8 failures, seven were due to an inability to cross a totally occluded proximal lesion with the guidewire and one was due to a major ischemic stroke in the ipsilateral hemisphere of a right subclavian lesion (10). Schillinger et al. reported higher procedural success rates (100% vs. 81%) and one-year patency rates (76% vs. 95%) in patients undergoing stenting versus PTA. Risk factors for failed intervention included complete occlusion and long lesions (11).

Amor et al. reported on 86 patients undergoing stent implantation. Technical success was achieved in all stenoses but in only 54% of total occlusions. The distal embolization rate was 2.2% with one to the arm successfully treated with an aspiration catheter and one to the LIMA requiring stent implantation. One TIA and one major stroke each occurred in the ipsilateral cerebral circulation. Long-term follow-up at 3.51 ± 1.98 years revealed a restenosis rate of 16.8% and reocclusion rate 2.6% (12). AbuRahma et al. reported on 121 patients who underwent stenting for subclavian artery disease, 21% of which were total occlusions. Stenting was successful in all patients except in two cases due to failure to cross total occlusions. The major complication rate was 5.8% and included 4 embolic events treated with lysis and stenting. Long-term patency rates at 3 and 5 years were 78% and 70% (13). Patel et al. reviewed 170 patients who underwent primary stenting of subclavian and innominate artery lesions. The success rate was 99.4% for stenotic lesions and 90.5% for occlusions. Long-term follow up obtained in 151 patients at 35.2 ± 30.8 months demonstrated clinical restenosis rate of 15.9% and target vessel revascularization rate of 14.6% (14).

Sixt et al. reviewed the results of angioplasty alone versus PTA with stenting of the subclavian and innominate artery in 107 patients. All interventions in stenotic lesions were successful and 87% of interventions in total occlusions were successful. Although not statistically significant, there was a trend toward better 1-year patency rates in the stenting versus PTA only group (89% vs. 79% respectively) (15).

In a totally occluded subclavian artery, the antegrade approach via femoral artery access is typically easier, if a "stump" is present for catheter engagement and the aortic arch is not very difficult (Type 1 or 2). The retrograde approach such as through brachial artery access proves easiest in situations where there is a lack of severe subclavian tortuosity. The combined approach using dye injections both proximal and distal to the lesion provides complete anatomical definition and can help minimize complications. Although reentry devices allow the operator to navigate wires through a subintimal plane around a total occlusion, they are only effective from the antegrade approach.

Aorto-Iliac Artery Interventions

Transatlantic Inter-Society Consensus (TASC) Working Group morphologic classification of iliac artery disease stratifies lesions into four types: A through D (Fig. 28-3). Endovascular procedures are favored as the treatment of choice over surgery in patients with type A lesions. In type D lesions, surgery is favored as the treatment of choice. However, controversy exists regarding the optimal management strategy in patients with type B or C lesions.

In a meta-analysis of over 2000 patients from 6 trials of PTA and 8 trials of stenting for aorto-iliac disease, 4-year primary patency rates were higher in patients with stenoses versus total occlusions, claudication versus critical limb ischemia, and stenting versus PTA alone. Complication rates were similar in the two groups (16). In the Dutch Iliac Stent Trial, 279 patients with intermittent claudication from occlusive iliac arterial disease were randomly assigned to direct stenting or primary angioplasty with selective stenting for residual mean gradients greater than 10 mm Hg across the lesion. Selective stenting was performed in 43% of those randomized to angioplasty alone. There was no statistical difference in success rates (81% and 82%) or complication rates (4% and 7%) between direct stenting versus primary angioplasty. Complications included arterial perforation, acute occlusion, embolism, and circulatory collapse. Two patients in the direct angioplasty group required surgical intervention (Table 28-3) (17).

TABLE 28-3 **Aorto-iliac Artery Intervention Complications**

Study	N	Target Vessel	Intervention	Stent Type[a]	Technical Success	Major Complications	Follow-Up (mo)	Residual Stenosis[b]	Restenosis[c]
Murphy et al. (32)	505	88 occlusions, 417 stenosis, 500 iliac, 5 distal aortic	Stent	344 SES, 119 BES, 42 Both, SES: Wallstent, Wallgraft, SMART, BES: Palmaz, Corinthian, AVE-Bridge	98%	7% (24)	mean 33 ± 27	NA	10%
Timaran et al. (19)	178	Iliac, 13 occlusions, 165 stenosis	Stent	BES: Palmaz, AVE Bridge, SES: Wallstent, AVE Bridge SE	96%	11%: 18 dissections, 1 vessel perforation, 1 distal embolization	median 27	40%	15%
Timaran et al. (18)	247	160 CIA, 87 EIA	Stent (42%)/ PTA selective stent (58%)	Palmaz, Wallstent	97%	12 arterial dissections requiring 6 surgical interventions	median 28	43% of selective stent group	NA, no postop surveillance protocol
Tetteroo et al. (17)	365	Common iliac artery (69%), EIA (31%), 29 occlusions	PTA selective stent (53%)/ Stent (47%)	Palmaz					
Bosch & Hunink (16)	2116		1300 PTA/ 816 Stent	Wallstent (46%), Palmaz (34%), Strecker (20%)	96% stent/91% PTA				

[a]Wallstent and Wallgraft (Boston Scientific), SMART, Palmaz, and Corinthian (Cordis), AVE-Bridge (Medtronic).
[b]Median or mean residual stenosis or percentage with residual stenosis.
[c]Percentage of restenosis in those with angiography or noninvasive imaging at follow-up.

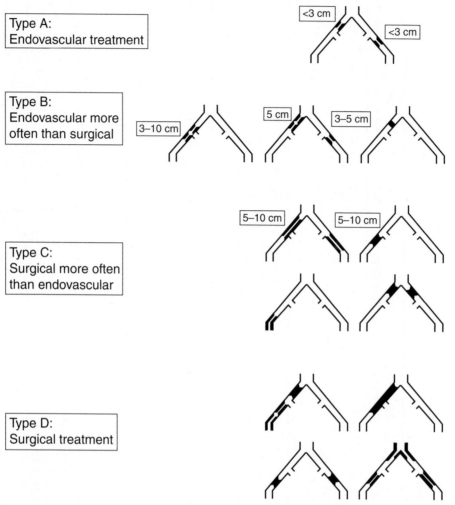

FIGURE 28-3. TASC classifications of aorto-iliac disease. Summary of preferred treatment options for iliac artery lesions by TASC classifications. (Adapted from Dormandy JA, Rutherford RB. Management of peripheral arterial disease (PAD). TASC Working Group. TransAtlantic Inter-Society Consensus (TASC). *J Vasc Surg.* 2000; (31):s1–s296.)

Timaran et al. reviewed the outcomes of 247 iliac angioplasty and stent procedures. Primary stenting was performed in 42% of procedures. Compared to common iliac disease, patients with external iliac artery disease had poorer runoff, smaller vessel size, and more extensive lesions characterized by higher TASC type C lesions. There were 12 arterial dissections, 6 of which required surgical intervention (18). In another series of 178 consecutive iliac angioplasty and stenting procedures in patients with TASC type B and C lesions, there were 18 arterial dissections and 1 vessel perforation (19). In a retrospective analysis of 505 aorto-

iliac stents, the technical success rate was 98% with a major complication rate defined as acute stent thrombosis, distal embolization, arterial rupture, and acute renal failure of 7%. Six patients required surgical intervention. The mortality rate was 0.5% as two patients died within 30 days.

Renal Artery Interventions

As with other vascular beds, renal artery intervention has benefited from the advances in coronary technology, specifically the introduction of guiding sheaths, smaller introducer sheaths, and improved balloon/stent designs.

TABLE 28-4 Renal Artery Intervention Complications

Study	N	Target Vessel	Intervention	Stent Type[a]	Technical Success	Major Complications	Follow-Up (mo)	Residual Stenosis[b]	Restenosis[c]
Patel et al. (34)	203	83% unilateral (169), 17% bilateral (44)	PTA 2.9% (6/203), Stenting 76%: unilateral (154/203), bilateral (44/203)	NA	99% (201/203)	0.5%: 1 death	mean 20.4 ± 18	NA	27% (31/116)
Bax et al. (33)	49	50% unilateral, 50% bilateral	PTA (1), Stent (26)	Palmaz-Corinthian IQ/Palmaz-Genesis	95% (44/46)	10%: 2 perforated renal arteries with death in 30d, 1 infected hematoma with death, 1 dialysis, 2 failures	24	0	20% (1/5)
Rastan et al. (35)	55	90% unilateral (45), 10% bilateral (50)	Stent	Hippocampus	100%	0	12	0	3.50%
Zeller et al. (20)	370	16% bilateral	Stent	Palmaz 104/204 (92), AVE Renal Bridge (35), InFlow Gold (65), Multi-Link Ultra (84), Herculink (23), Corinthian/Genesis (36), NIR/NIRenal (19)	NA	4%: 13 local dissection/perforation, 2 stent displacement	27 ± 15	NA	NA

[a]Palmaz-Genesis/Corinthian IQ (Johnson & Johnson), Hippocampus (Invatec SRL).
[b]Median or mean residual stenosis or percentage with residual stenosis.
[c]Percentage of restenosis in those with angiography or noninvasive imaging at follow-up.

Nonetheless, complications of renal artery intervention occur and include stent misplacement, dissection, rupture, thromboembolic phenomena, and renal infarction (Table 28-4). Prospectively gathered registry data over a 5-year period in 260 patients with renal artery ostial stenosis revealed an overall complication rate of 10% with a nonaccess site complication rate of 6.6%. There were four patients who required permanent hemodialysis, three of which were presumed to be secondary to microembolism and one due to embolism of aortic material in a single functioning kidney. There were 10 ostial dissections after angioplasty treated adequately with stents. One type B dissection occurred after balloon angioplasty from the renal artery origin to the left subclavian artery and was treated medically. Two wire-induced dissections occurred without deterioration of renal function despite a side branch occlusion and an accessory renal artery occlusion. The authors reported reductions in mean sheath diameter, procedural time, and heparin dose over the 5-year period coincident with a reduction in the rate of periprocedural complications (20).

In a trial of 106 patients with atherosclerotic renal artery stenosis randomized to angioplasty or medical therapy, there were two occurrences of acute renal failure and one episode of symptomatic hypotension in the angioplasty group. There were no occlusions, ruptures, or embolic events. Patients with total occlusion of the renal artery, aortic aneurysm requiring surgery, creatinine level greater than 2.3 mg/dL, or stenosis secondary to fibromuscular dysplasia were excluded (21).

Femoropopliteal Artery Interventions

The TASC morphologic classification of SFA disease stratifies lesions into four types: A through D based upon lesion number, length, and presence of stenosis or occlusion (Fig. 28-4). After the origin of the profunda femoral branch, the common femoral artery becomes the superficial femoral artery. The SFA courses through the muscles of the thigh, without any significant branches. It resurfaces at the adductor canal in the adductor magnus muscle. Upon entering the popliteal fossa its name changes to the popliteal artery. The SFA supplies a descending genicular branch to the collateral circulation of the knee, but the majority of the blood it carries is destined for the muscles below the knee. Because the profunda femoral branch is an important supply of collateral circulation in SFA disease, avoiding complications to this vessel is paramount. Compromise of the profunda femoral branch may result in catastrophe in a patient with critical SFA disease.

Femoropopliteal artery interventions in properly selected patients can consistently yield satisfactory results. In a retrospective review of 329 patients who underwent PTA and stenting of the superficial femoral artery, technical success was achieved in 93% of cases. Most failures were secondary to an inability to cross the lesion of interest. Complications such as dissections and perforations occurred in 9% of cases. Embolic events occurred in 3% of patients. One death occurred as a result of an iliac artery rupture (22).

Another retrospective review of 109 patients undergoing stenting of the superficial femoral artery reported rates of perforations and embolism of 5% and 2%, respectively. Early thrombosis defined as stent occlusion less than 30 days from intervention occurred in 9% of cases. Hemodynamic failure defined as an increase in ABI less than 0.15 or failure to heal ischemic ulcers occurred in 4% of patients. There were two infectious complications, an infected stent requiring surgical intervention and a peri-stent abscess requiring percutaneous drainage (23). A meta-analysis of a larger number of patients undergoing balloon angioplasty or angioplasty plus stenting of the femoropopliteal segment reported complication rates of 6% to 11%, respectively (24).

Studies focusing on risk factors for restenosis or reocclusion have yielded variable results. One review of 125 patients including 108 TASC B and 32 TASC C type lesions reported a restenosis or reocclusion rate of 29% at a mean follow-up time of 8.3 months. The technical success rate was 98% and complications were limited to only two pseudoaneurysms and one episode of flash pulmonary edema. Preoperative ABI less than 0.5, increasing lesion length, and hypercholesterolemia were associated with higher rates of restenosis. Angioplasty alone and number of

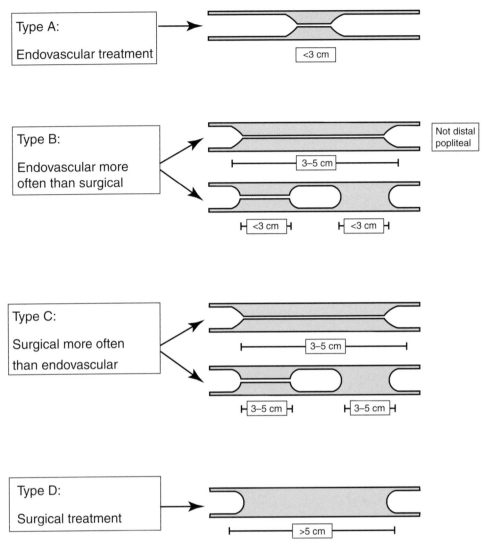

FIGURE 28-4. TASC classifications of femoral disease. Summary of preferred treatment options for femoropopliteal artery lesions by TASC classifications. (Adapted from Dormandy JA, Rutherford RB. Management of peripheral arterial disease (PAD). TASC Working Group. TransAtlantic Inter-Society Consensus (TASC). *J Vasc Surg.* 2000;(31):s1–s296.)

runoff vessels were not associated with higher rates of restenosis or reocclusion (25).

Other studies have focused on risk factors for distal embolization. Continuous Doppler ultrasound monitoring of the popliteal artery for embolic signals was performed in a series of 60 patients undergoing percutaneous treatment of the superficial femoral artery. Embolic signals were identified in all patients during guidewire crossing, balloon angioplasty, stent deployment and/or atherectomy. More signals were noted with plaque excision than other points in the procedure and one patient treated with the excimer laser experienced a single runoff vessel occlusion. Compared to balloon angioplasty, more signals were noted during stenting. Although each step of SFA intervention yielded embolic signals, only one patient experienced an angiographically and clinically significant embolization (26).

Infrapopliteal Artery Interventions

The infrapopliteal arterial tree begins as the popliteal artery branches into the anterior tibial artery and the tibioperoneal trunk just below the level of the knee. The anterior tibial artery courses along the interosseous membrane to supply the muscles of the anterior compartment as well as some of the deep muscles of the posterior compartment. Eventually it becomes the dorsalis pedis artery as it crosses the ankle joint. The tibioperoneal trunk divides into peroneal and posterior tibial artery. The peroneal artery supplies the muscles of the anterior compartment as it courses between the interosseous membrane and the fibula. The posterior tibial artery gives rise to the medial and lateral plantar branches in the foot.

Patients with infrapopliteal artery disease often have multilevel disease including involvement of the more proximal segments. This pattern of diffuse disease often times leads to critical limb ischemia (CLI) defined as chronic ischemic rest pain, ulcerations, or gangrene. CLI is associated with a high risk of major amputation, upwards of 40%, as well as a one-year mortality of 25%. Despite reported one-year primary patency rates of autologous venous conduits greater than 80%, widespread use of bypass surgery has been limited. Issues such as lack of suitable veins in up to 30% of patients undergoing primary revascularization and 50% of patients requiring secondary bypass surgery along with increased risk of wound infections, lack of suitable distal targets, and calcified vessels make an alternate percutaneous approach more attractive. The goal of the infrapopliteal interventions in patients with CLI is to avoid a major amputation by providing complete blood flow to the pedal arch. Angioplasty success rates have ranged from 77% to 100% with lower rates in those with total occlusions (27). Indications for revascularization of the lower extremity include life-style limiting claudication, rest pain, nonhealing ulcerations, and gangrene.

In a meta-analysis of infrapopliteal artery angioplasty for chronic limb ischemia, the reported complication rate was 7.8% in 1743 procedures. The pooled estimate of immediate technical success was 89%. Groin hematomas accounted for 40% of complications. Thromboembolic phenomena, perforation, or dissec-

tion accounted for 50% of complications. Although bypass surgery technical success rates and durability were better than angioplasty, limb salvage rates were similar (28). Other case series have reported the rate of major complications to range between 2% and 6% with higher rates of arterial perforation in the elderly and diabetic patients (29).

■ RISK FACTORS

There are a number of factors recognized through experience that affect the likelihood of an operator encountering a major complication. These factors can be related to the operator, patient, or lesion. Without adequate training and experience, an operator may be ill-equipped to deal with a major untoward event. Clinical presentation and presence of co-morbidities can impact any individual patient's chances of success and risk of complication. Diabetes and chronic renal disease in particular affect outcomes, as these subsets of patients tend to have diffusely diseased distal vessels with substantial calcifications and poor distal run-off. Several lesion-related factors that should always be taken into account prior to an intervention include lesion location, degree of stenosis or occlusion, lesion calcification, vessel tortuosity, and presence of thrombus.

The interventionalist has to make a decision on how to approach the lesion of interest. The approach is a critical factor in determining the difficulty and risk of the procedure and should be based upon not only precise definition of the lesion type and location but also the anatomy of any access and adjacent vessels. For example, in subclavian artery interventions, a totally occluded left subclavian artery that lacks a "stump" on an aortogram would typically necessitate a brachial artery approach. In addition, in iliac artery interventions, an ipsilateral retrograde common femoral artery approach is commonplace. However, for a stenosis located in the distal external iliac artery a contralateral crossover approach from the common femoral artery may be required.

In general, total occlusions tend to be more of a challenge than stenotic lesions. With a total occlusion, the potential to wire into the subintimal plane increases the risk for target vessel dissection. In addition, the risk of distal embolization seems to be higher with total occlusions, especially with long lesions or fresh thrombus. Pre-procedural strategy planning is tantamount and includes defining tortuous or variant anatomy. For example, in patients with acute angulation of the aortic bifurcation or significant iliac artery tortuosity, an ipsilateral antegrade common femoral artery approach to superficial femoral artery interventions tends to give a higher degree of success and a lower risk of complication. Calcified areas of stenosis and tortuosity can add both time and risk to the procedure. In particular, aggressive balloon angioplasty of calcified lesions poses a risk for dissection or rupture.

■ PREVENTION

Appropriate arterial access and catheter selection are the first steps in planning a safe peripheral intervention. Thorough review of all noninvasive imaging studies including CT, MRI/MRA, and ultrasound should be done prior to gaining arterial access. If appropriate definition of the anatomy cannot be gained from noninvasive imaging studies, then diagnostic angiography should be performed in multiple orthogonal views. Pressure monitoring from the injecting catheter is essential, although not uniformly performed in peripheral interventions. Injection of dye should be made only if the pressure waveform from the catheter does not demonstrate pressure dampening. Post-intervention angiograms are done to diagnose any procedural complications such as perforations, thrombus, or dissection. Continuous measurement and display of the patient's vital signs including heart rate, blood pressure, ECG, and pulse oximetry are essential. Because of the risk for adverse CNS events with subclavian or vertebral artery interventions, monitoring of neurological status should be routine. Appropriate procedural anti-coagulation can be assured by routinely checking the activated clotting time (ACT). Also IIb-IIIa inhibitors can be considered in cases with high risk for thromboembolism or inadequate anti-platelet therapy. Dual anti-platelet therapy with aspirin and clopidogrel are typically used. Nitroglycerin, adenosine, and verapamil for intra-arterial administration should be available to manage vasospasm.

Technological advances in the arena of coronary intervention have spilled over into peripheral vascular interventions with a beneficial impact on complication rates. Whenever possible, low-profile rapid-exchange systems should be used. The ostium of the vessels should be engaged carefully with purposeful movements of the guiding catheter or sheath. Proper device sizing relative to the reference vessel diameter can be achieved with the use of intravascular ultrasound. If thrombotic lesions are suspected, proper distal embolic prevention devices should be utilized. Gentle but purposeful manipulation of devices is the key to success.

■ MANAGEMENT AND BAIL-OUT TECHNIQUES

There are several management techniques that are similar for complications seen in different vascular territories. The major complications can be classified into perforations, dissections, and distal embolization. Device embolization is another rare but important complication.

In the event of large-vessel perforation or rupture, the use of a temporary vessel occlusion balloon can be life- or limb-saving. Reversal of anticoagulation and prolonged occlusion can many times stop bleeding. The Coda balloon catheter by Cook Medical comes in 32-mm and 40-mm diameter balloon sizes and can be used to temporarily occlude the aorta in the event of distal aortic or iliac artery rupture. For smaller vessel ruptures, balloon tamponade at the site of perforation is the usual first line of therapy. After stabilization of the situation, a covered stent graft is placed to achieve hemostasis. Covered stent grafts, available as self-expanding or balloon-expandable devices, are composed of metallic scaffolding together with synthetic graft material. The graft material, typically made of polytetrafluoroethylene (PTFE), may be on either side of the stent or in between two layers of stent scaffolding. Some of the available self-expanding stent grafts available include Flair (Baird Peripheral Vascular), aSpire (LeMaitre Vascular, Inc.), Viabahn (Gore), and Wallgraft (Boston-Scientific). There are two balloon-expandable stents currently available in the United States: Jostent and iCast stent. The Jostent is composed of two metal stents with a

PTFE layer in the middle and is limited to diameters of 3 to 5 mm. The Atrium iCast stent is a low-profile microporous PTFE film covered stent available in diameters from 5 to 12 mm. Although FDA-approved for treatment of tracheobronchial strictures, it has been used off-label successfully in the peripheral vascular circulation. In some situations where an active perforation occurs in a vessel without a critical distal bed, such as an ungrafted native left internal mammary artery (LIMA), operators may choose to mechanically occlude the artery through the use of vascular coils.

For dissections, the main treatment goal is to obtain access to the true lumen with the wire to facilitate stenting of the dissection flap. Even though many different wires are available, the 0.014″ diameter wire is primarily used as a first attempt. Adjunctive use of IVUS provides additional aid as a technique to identify the true lumen. Lower and upper limb artery dissections can be wired in a retrograde fashion from a distal artery access site. In certain cases, such as that of long spiral dissections, this is the best option. Once the true lumen is accessed, stent deployment can treat the dissection without much difficulty. For such limb-saving interventions, the preservation of side branches is not usually critical.

Because of a lack of relatively effective treatments, distal embolization is a serious complication that is best prevented. Use of embolic prevention devices is critical for high-risk situations such as when a large visible thrombus is present or the distal vascular territory is in the brain. During proximal subclavian artery interventions, prolonged balloon inflations greater than one minute are performed to prevent distal embolization to the brain. The extended periods of balloon inflation induce a flow reversal in the vertebral artery system. Use of distal protection devices have been attempted in renal artery interventions, but because of early bifurcation, adequate protection with conventional devices is not feasible. It is also not clear that distal embolic prevention with current devices lead to any difference in outcome. Furthermore, the larger amounts of contrast associated with embolic protection devices make it less attractive when many patients with renal stenosis have renal insufficiency. During ostial carotid or innominate artery interventions, the use of an embolic protection device is sometimes difficult because a 0.014-inch wire may not allow enough support for the accurate placement of the stent in the ostium. Employing a double wire technique by placing a stent on two wires can lead to success in these situations. In the lower extremity when dealing with highly thrombogenic situations, the use of a filter wire is recommended. If there is distal embolization, then mechanical thrombectomy, aspiration thrombectomy, or spray lytics with mechanical thrombectomy can be considered. Pharmacologic approaches include anti-coagulants, IIb-IIIa inhibitors, and lytics. Use of these agents has to be individualized based on patient and lesion characteristics while balancing risks and potential benefits.

Various retrieval devices should be available to recover fragments of debris, thrombus, catheters, sheaths, stents, balloons, and wires. The Amplatz Goose Neck snare and Microsnare kit are composed of a nitinol cable with a gold plated pre-formed tungsten loop. The snare loop forms a 90-degree angle with the shaft remaining coaxial with the vessel lumen. The Micro Elite snare by Vascular Solutions is a helical loop retrieval device with a 0.014-inch profile permitting delivery through microcatheters and balloon catheters. Jaw snares, used in urological interventions, work particularly well when significant force is required to retrieve larger devices such as an IVC filter.

In the following paragraphs interesting cases are shown with specific methods used for management of complications in different vascular territories. Some of the cases described highlight what should be done to prevent such complications.

Vertebral Artery Intervention

A patient with a totally occluded left carotid artery presented with acute dizziness and syncope. Noninvasive imaging diagnosed bilateral vertebral artery disease. Diagnostic angiography (Fig. 28-5) confirmed 90% stenosis of the right vertebral artery and 70% stenosis of the left vertebral artery. After proper anticoagulation, the right vertebral artery was wired using a "non-touch" technique. For this, a Wholey wire is advanced into the right subclavian and a JR-4 guide catheter is advanced in close proximity to the ostium of the right vertebral artery without engagement. Using a hydrophilic wire, the lesion

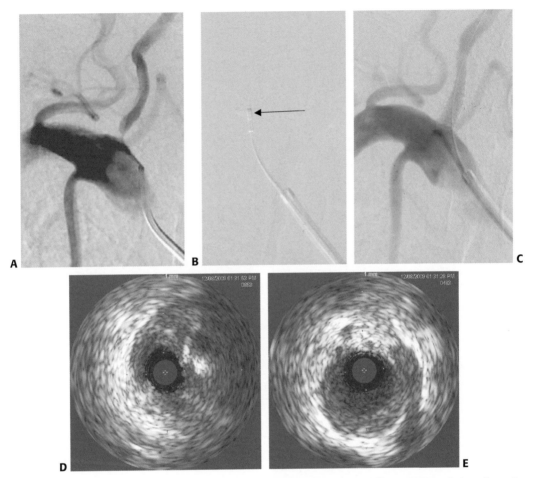

FIGURE 28-5. Severe symptomatic ostial stenosis of the right vertebral artery (**A**). An IVUS study is performed (**B**) to examine the ostium and reference diameter. IVUS identifies the ostial disease (**D**) and reveals a long lesion with diffuse disease (**E**). Given a reference diameter of aproximately 4 mm, the lesion was stented with a 4.0/12 mm coronary stent with good angiographic result (**C**).

was crossed and gently pre-dilated followed by IVUS interrogation. IVUS is helpful in three main ways: (i) assessment of reference diameter which is critical for stent selection, (ii) defining the nature of disease as diffuse or focal, and (iii) locating the ostium because sometimes angiographically it may be difficult to "see." In this patient, a 4-mm reference diameter allowed a 4.0-mm stent to be successfully placed. Longer inflation of the balloon with slow deflation may induce flow reversal in the vertebral artery and minimize stroke risk. A distal protection device was not used in this case because of concerns of diffuse disease and a tortuous artery.

In another case (Fig. 28-6), as the stent was being advanced to cover the lesion in sub-clavian artery after stenting the vertebral artery, it was noted that the stent length was not accurate. During attempts at stent with-drawal, the stent caught the leading edge of the guiding catheter, dislodging it from the balloon but remaining on the wire. A small balloon was used to bring it back to the iliac artery. The gooseneck snare was then used to remove the stent from the sheath. Careful withdrawal of stents is necessary especially when working in angulated arteries like the vertebral origin.

Subclavian Artery Intervention

In a patient with severe innominate stenosis, placement of an embolic protection device in

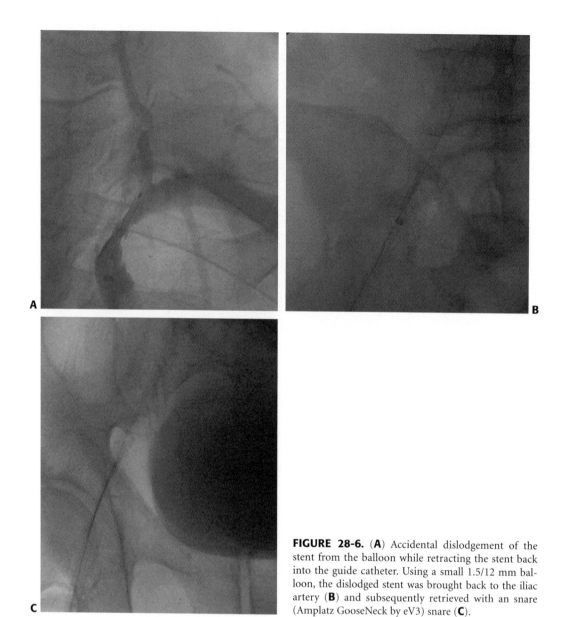

FIGURE 28-6. (**A**) Accidental dislodgement of the stent from the balloon while retracting the stent back into the guide catheter. Using a small 1.5/12 mm balloon, the dislodged stent was brought back to the iliac artery (**B**) and subsequently retrieved with an snare (Amplatz GooseNeck by eV3) snare (**C**).

the internal carotid may mitigate the risk for adverse CNS events (Fig. 28-7). However, at times the 0.014-inch system does not provide enough support for accurate placement of the stent in the ostium. A buddy wire in the subclavian is an option but this is at times not very stable. Use of another 0.014-inch stiff wire in the right carotid artery provides adequate support for stent delivery. A 0.035-inch stent is placed on both wires, making the system ideal for accurate stent placement. This unique method of stenting

for ostial arch vessels has good safety and adequate support.

As with coronary angiography, orthogonal views of the region of interest allow the peripheral interventionalist to accurately define anatomy. Failure to do so may result in a case of "mistaken identity". Figure 28-8 shows a series of images from an intervention on a totally occluded left subclavian artery that is complicated by a misplaced stent in the left internal mammary artery. An aortogram

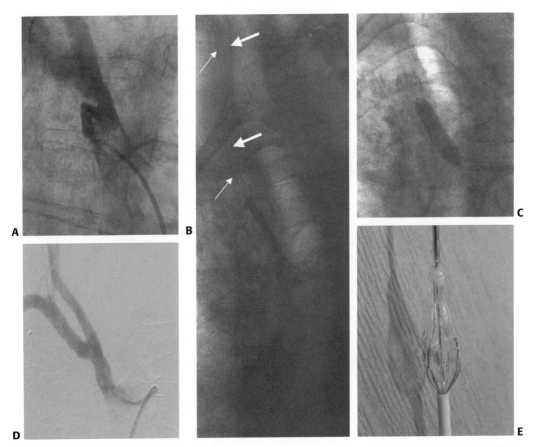

FIGURE 28-7. Use of an embolic protection device during intervention on a severe innominate stenosis (**A**). A 0.014-inch wire is placed into the external carotid artery (*thick arrows*) while a distal embolic protection device (Guidant ACCUNET filter) is placed into the internal carotid artery (*thin arrows*) (**B**). The stent mounted on a 0.035-inch balloon is deployed over both wires (**C**) with a good angiographic result (**D**). After embolic protection device removal, debris is identified in the filter (**E**).

reveals total occlusion of the left subclavian artery with late filling via collateral vessels from the external carotid artery taken in the LAO projection. Left brachial artery access is obtained and a wire is passed in the LAO projection appearing to be have crossed the lesion with the distal end resting in the ascending aorta. Repeat angiogram and aortogram in the LAO projection appear to confirm the position of the wire. Angioplasty and stent placement is then performed with evidence of acute vessel closure. Repeat angiography after RAO movement of the image intensifier finally reveals misplacement of the stent in the LIMA. Angiography after further advancement of the catheter into the stent demonstrates arterial

rupture at the distal aspect of the stent. The distal LIMA and stent are treated with vascular coils with resolution of the rupture. This is a type of complication that should not happen in experienced hands.

Aorto-Iliac Artery Intervention

Complications in the peripheral circulation can stem from almost any percutaneous vascular intervention. The availability of a skilled peripheral interventionalist can prove worthwhile in these circumstances. Figure 28-9 shows a series of images from an aortic balloon valvuloplasty complicated by balloon rupture and inability to remove the balloon from the iliac artery. A segment of balloon

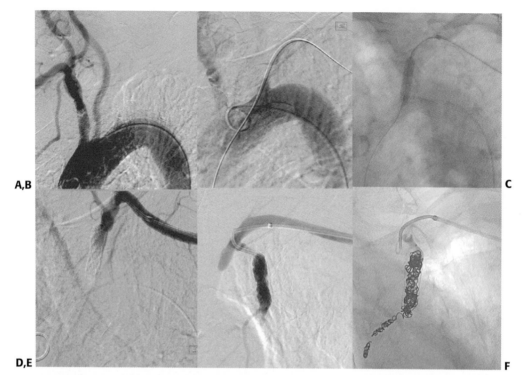

FIGURE 28-8. A patient undergoing intervention on a totally occluded left subclavian artery (**A**). (**B**) Wire advancement in the LAO projection from a left brachial artery approach appears successful. (**C** and **D**) Subsequent balloon-expandable stent deployment. Patient complained of severe chest pain and it is clear on RAO projection (**E**) that the wire never crossed the total occlusion and in fact was in the left internal mammary artery complicated by arterial perforation. (**F**) This was treated with multiple coils. This underscores the importance of imaging in multiple planes while performing interventions.

was lost in the iliac artery and could not be retrieved despite the use of a gooseneck snare from the contralateral groin. Typically snaring the wire from the contralateral groin and then pulling the balloon piece out is possible (lower panel in Fig. 28-9) but was not feasible in this patient because of severe tortuosity. A few hours after the procedure, the patient experienced acute vessel closure of the right iliac artery. An SOS catheter was chosen to guide a stiff-angled Glidewire into the right internal iliac artery. Following wire exchange for an Amplatz SuperStiff wire, the SOS catheter was removed. Next a 7-F Balkan 40-cm sheath was advanced into the distal common iliac artery. Telescoping through a 4-F angled Glide catheter, the occlusion in the external iliac artery was wired successfully

with an angled Glidewire. Despite multiple balloon angioplasty attempts, there was no reconstitution of flow. At this point, an 8-mm × 100-mm S.M.A.R.T Control stent (Cordis) was deployed from the proximal superficial femoral artery to the right external iliac artery with successful restoration of blood flow. In order to exclude the balloon fragments from the bloodstream and prevent thrombosis, an 8 mm × 60 mm Atrium iCast covered stent was overlapped with the previously placed stent. At 3-years of follow ups patient had continued patency of the right femoral system.

Figure 28-10 shows a patient who had rupture of the left iliac artery after a large sheath removal.

The patient rapidly became hemodynamically unstable. Volume resuscitation was instituted and contralateral access allowed an 8.0/20 mm balloon to occlude the ruptured iliac artery.

Another possible approach in this situation is to occlude the distal aorta to control the hemorrhage. However, definitive treatment requires successful wiring of the iliac artery. In this case, a covered balloon-expandable stent was deployed with immediate restoration of hemodynamic stability and antegrade blood flow to the left lower extremity.

Femoropopliteal Artery Intervention

A patient with total occlusion of the left superficial femoral artery presented to the catheterization laboratory for a peripheral

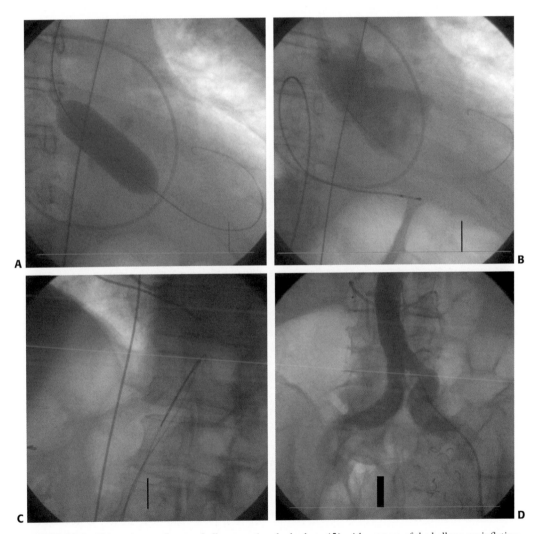

FIGURE 28-9. This patient underwent balloon aortic valvuloplasty (**A**) with rupture of the balloon on inflation (**B**). Balloon could not be retrieved from the groin and distal piece was left in the iliac artery. Snaring from the left groin could not get the balloon to go across the distal aortic bifurcation (**C**). Surgical removal was not possible because of the general condition of the patient. The right iliac artery was open at the end of the procedure (**D**) but closed in a few hours (**E**). Patient had to be brought to the catheterization laboratory and the balloon was stented to the side of the vessel from contralateral groin (**F to H**). On 3-year follow up patient had patent iliac and common femoral arteries. (**I**) Piece of balloon recovered from snaring from the opposite groin in a different patient. In this patient it was not possible to retrieve the balloon by snaring from opposite groin. (*continued*)

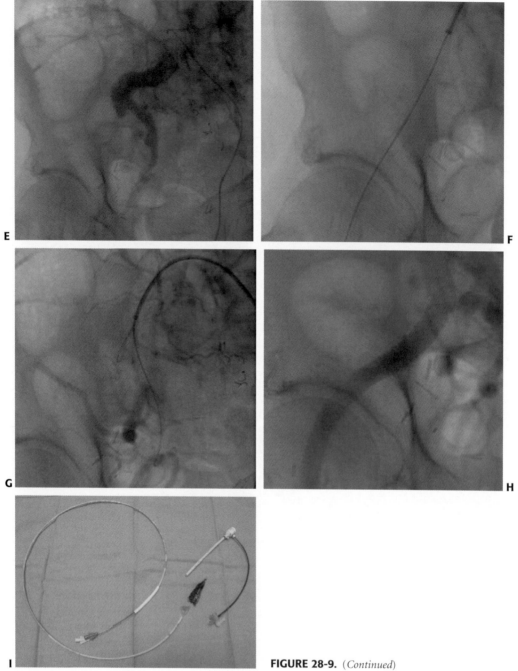

FIGURE 28-9. (*Continued*)

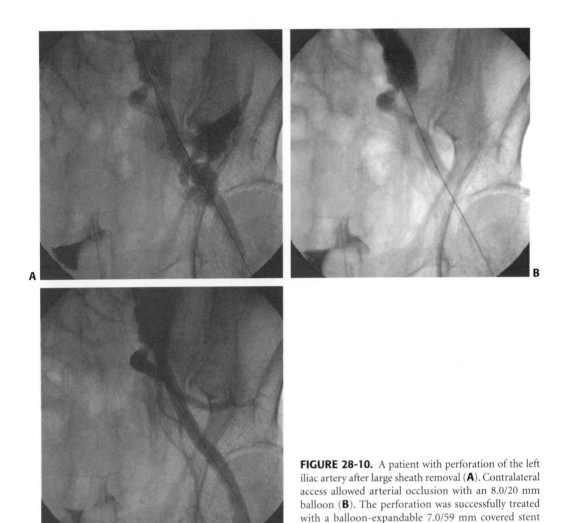

FIGURE 28-10. A patient with perforation of the left iliac artery after large sheath removal (**A**). Contralateral access allowed arterial occlusion with an 8.0/20 mm balloon (**B**). The perforation was successfully treated with a balloon-expandable 7.0/59 mm covered stent (Atrium iCast).

intervention (Fig. 28-11). Using an angled Glide catheter and a 0.035-inch stiff angled glidewire, the lesion was recanalized and subsequently stented. A few days later the patient returned to the catheterization lab with acute vessel closure. It was clear that a distal edge dissection and a severe lesion in the stent outflow (popliteal artery) were missed contributing to the stent closure. Proper angiography is critical to prevent such complications. The patient underwent successful intervention with placement of another stent distal to the lesion as well as rotational atherectomy (Diamondback by Cardiovascular Systems) of the popliteal lesion.

In another case of total occlusion of the right SFA (Fig. 28-12), wiring was complicated by a dissection with extravasation of blood into the lower extremity compartment. Two re-entry catheters, Outback (Cordis) and Stingray (Bridgepoint Medical), were unable to be advanced beyond the occlusion due to preferential entry into a large side branch. Using IVUS in the false lumen, a Glide catheter with a stiff 0.035-inch glidewire was directed and advanced into the true lumen. This case demonstrates that perforation as long as it is not free-flowing combined with thoughtful perseverance can lead to a successful intervention.

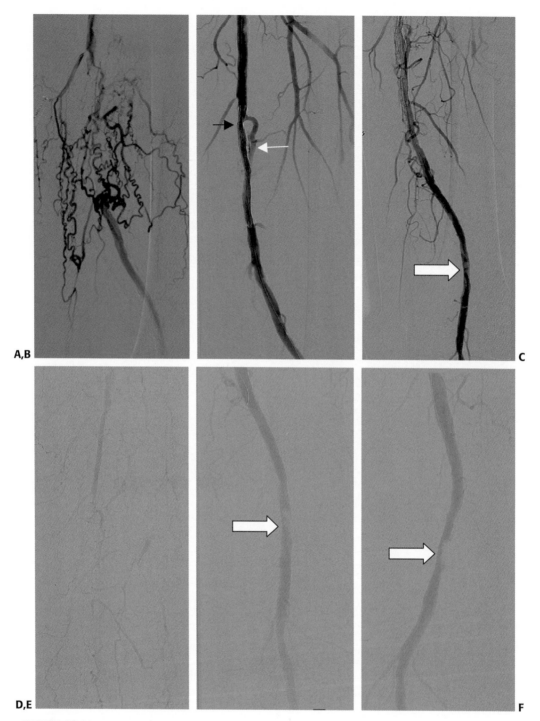

FIGURE 28-11. Intervention on a total occlusion of the left superficial femoral artery (**A**). The first intervention (**B** to **C**) is notable for residual inflow stenosis (*black arrow*), proximal stent dissection (*thin white arrow*), and distal segment haziness (*thick white arrow*). After returning to the catheterization laboratory with acute stent closure (**D**), restoration of flow reveals the distal haziness to be a severe lesion in more steep angulation (**E** and **F**). (*continued*)

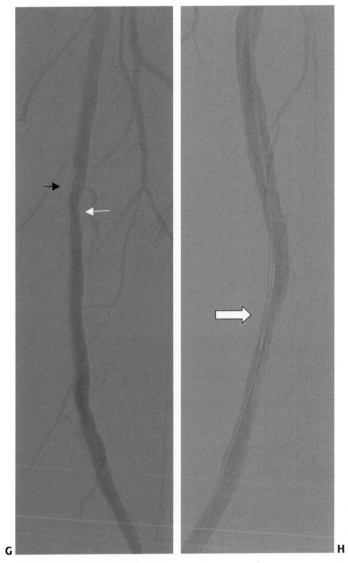

FIGURE 28-11. (*Continued*) (**G** and **H**) Final result with good inflow and outflow.

Renal Artery Interventions

When performing renal artery interventions, it is important to note the angle from which it arises from the aorta. For example, in an inferiorly oriented renal artery brachial access may be optimal. This is because excessive force during stent positioning and deployment from groin access may result in perforation or dissection of the renal artery. Figure 28-13 shows a proximal renal artery perforation due to the use of a 0.035-inch

stiff wire distorting the artery in combination with an oversized stent. This was managed with reversal of anti-coagulation and prolonged balloon inflations. Although the prior cases highlights a complication related to the use of 0.035-inch stiff wire in the renal artery, wire related dissections may also occur with the use of a 0.014-inch wire. A patient with an ostial stenosis of the right renal artery in Figure 28-14 developed a small non-flow limiting distal vessel dissection which should have been managed

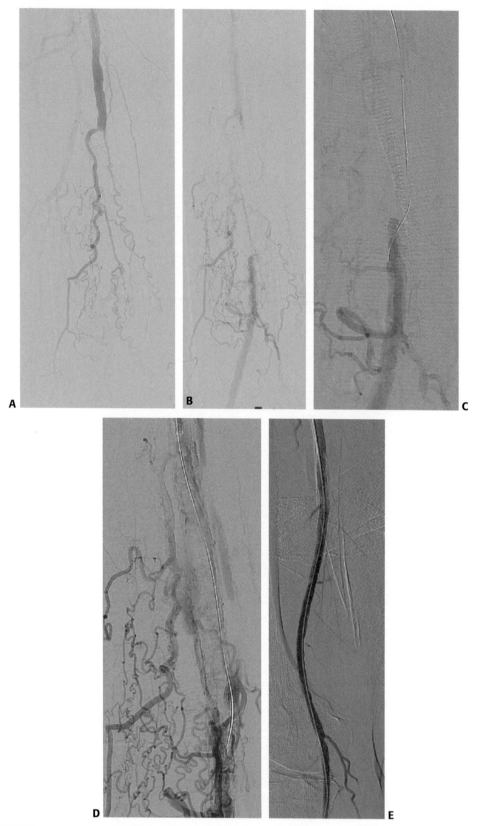

FIGURE 28-12. Intervention on a totally occluded SFA with reconstitution distally by collaterals (**A** and **B**). Wiring results in a subintimal course with perforation and extravasation of dye (**C** and **D**). With IVUS imaging in the false lumen, access was gained to the distal vessel and the lesion treated with a self-expanding stent giving an excellent angiographic result (**E**).

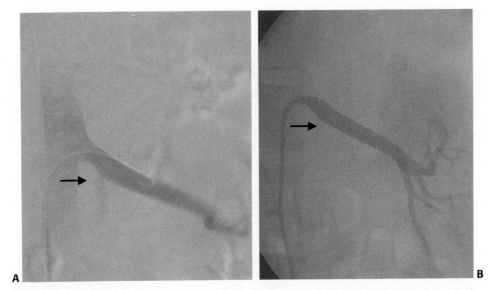

FIGURE 28-13. Perforation of the proximal renal artery with use of a stiff 0.035-inch wire and oversized stent (**A**). Reversal of anti-coagulation and prolonged balloon inflation gave a good angiographic result (**B**).

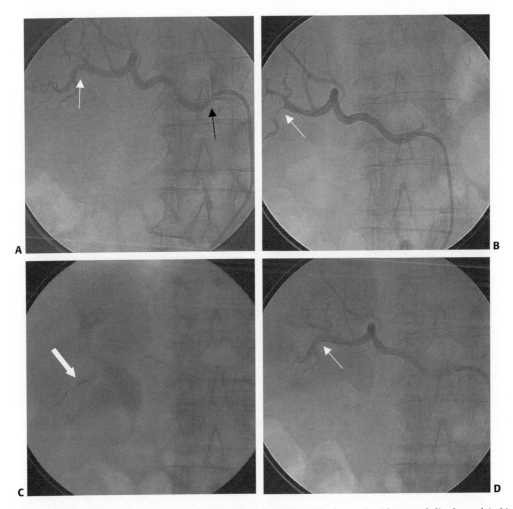

FIGURE 28-14. (**A**) Severe ostial stenosis of the right renal artery (*black arrow*) with normal distal vessel (*white arrow*). (**B**) Wire dissection of the distal vessel (*white arrow*). Attempts at balloon angioplasty (**C**) resulted in propagation of the dissection proximally (**D, E**) requiring stenting that resulted in a suboptimal result, side branch compromise (*double arrows*), and excessive use of contrast (**F**). (*continued*)

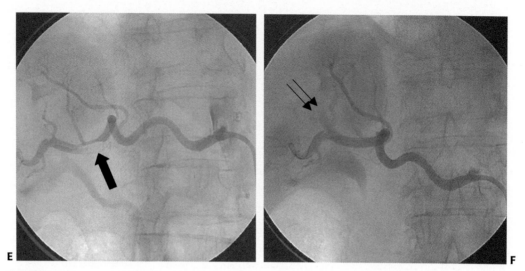

FIGURE 28-14. (*Continued*)

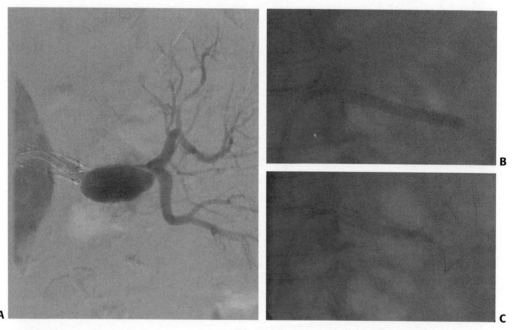

FIGURE 28-15. Patient with a left renal artery aneurysm with plans to place a proximal covered stent followed by "V" stenting into the bifurcation (**A**). The first stent was deployed in the proximal segment (**B**) followed by kissing balloon angioplasty into the bifurcation (**C**). (*continued*)

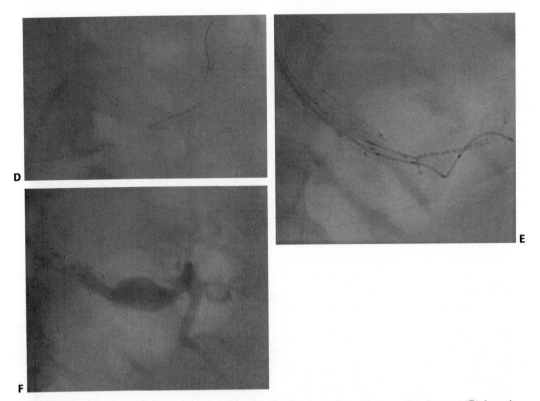

FIGURE 28-15. (*Continued*) Attempts at passing stents distally is complicated by stent dislodgement (**D**) from the balloon. The EN Snare device was used to retrieve the stent (**E**) and final angiography did not reveal any evidence of dissection or perforation (**F**).

conservatively. However, repeated attempts to treat the dissection with angioplasty enlarges the spiral dissection to included the mid renal artery segment. Despite distal and mid vessel stenting, a residual dissection flap remains with a compromised side branch. Sometimes nonflow limiting dissections can be treated conservatively.

Figure 28-15 shows a patient with an aneursym of the left renal artery. The initial plan was to exclude the proximal aneurysm with a proximal covered stent followed by "V" stenting into the bifurcation to exclude the distal aneurysm. However, after placement of the covered stent, attempts to advance into the bifurcation resulted in stent dislodgement and embolization. In our experience and others, covered stents seem more prone to slip off their balloon then non-covered stents. In addition, little wire purchase, poor stent trackability, and lack of support all pointed to this as an unusually optimistic plan. Stent retrieval was successful using arm access and a snare device (EN Snare by Merit Medical Systems).

References

1. Schillinger M, Minar E. Complications in Peripheral Vascular Interventions. London, UK: Informa Healthcare, 2007.
2. Higashida RT, Tsai FY, Halbach VV, et al. Transluminal angioplasty for atherosclerotic disease of the vertebral and basilar arteries. J Neurosurg. 1993;78(2):192–198.
3. Terada T, Higashida RT, Halbach VV, et al. Transluminal angioplasty for arteriosclerotic disease of the distal vertebral and basilar arteries. *J Neurol Neurosurg Psychiatry.* 1996;60(4):377–381.
4. Hauth EA, Gissler HM, Drescher R, et al. Angioplasty or stenting of extra- and intracranial vertebral artery stenoses. *Cardiovasc Intervent Radiol.* 2004;27(1):51–57.
5. Jenkins JS, White CJ, Ramee SR, et al. Vertebral artery stenting. *Cathete Cardiovasc Interv* 2001;54 (1):1–5.
6. Lin YH, Juang JM, Jeng JS, et al. Symptomatic ostial vertebral artery stenosis treated with tubular coronary stents: Clinical results and restenosis analysis. *J Endovas Ther.* 2004;11(6):719–726.

7. Eberhardt O, Naegele T, Raygrotzki S, et al. Stenting of vertebrobasilar arteries in symptomatic atherosclerotic disease and acute occlusion: Case series and review of the literature. *J Vasc Surg.* 2006;43(6):1145–1154.

8. Weber W, Mayer TE, Henkes H, et al. Efficacy of stent angioplasty for symptomatic stenoses of the proximal vertebral artery. *Eur J Radiol.* 2005; 56(2):240–247.

9. Gupta R, Al-Ali F, Thomas AJ, et al. Safety, feasibility, and short-term follow-up of drug-eluting stent placement in the intracranial and extracranial circulation. *Stroke.* 2006;37(10):2562–2566.

10. de Vries J, Jager L, van den Berg J, et al. Durability of percutaneous transluminal angioplasty for obstructive lesions of proximal subclavian artery: Long-term results. *J Vasc Surg.* 2005;41(1):19–23.

11. Schillinger M, Haumer M, Schillinger S, et al. Risk stratification for subclavian artery angioplasty: Is there an increased rate of restenosis after stent implantation? *J Endovasc Ther.* 2001; 8(6):550–557.

12. Amor M, Eid-Lidt G, Chati Z, et al. Endovascular treatment of the subclavian artery: Stent implantation with or without predilatation. *Catheter Cardiovasc Interv.* 2004;63(3):364–370.

13. AbuRahma AF, Bates MC, Stone PA, et al. Angioplasty and stenting versus carotid-subclavian bypass for the treatment of isolated subclavian artery disease. *J Endovasc Ther.* 2007;14(5): 698–704.

14. Patel S, White C, Collins T, et al. Catheter-based treatment of the subclavian and innominate arteries. *Catheter Cardiovasc Interv.* 2008;71(7): 963–968.

15. Sixt S, Rastan A, Schwarzwälder U, et al. Results after balloon angioplasty or stenting of atherosclerotic subclavian artery obstruction. *Catheter Cardiovasc Interv.* 2009;73(3):395–403.

16. Bosch JL, Hunink MG. Meta-analysis of the results of percutaneous transluminal angioplasty and stent placement for aortoiliac occlusive disease. *Radiology.* 1997;204(1):87–96.

17. Tetteroo, Graaf Y, Bosch JL, et al. Randomised comparison of primary stent placement versus primary angioplasty followed by selective stent placement in patients with iliac-artery occlusive disease. *The Lancet.* 1998;351(9110):1153–1159.

18. Timaran CH, Stevens SL, Freeman MB, et al. External iliac and common iliac artery angioplasty and stenting in men and women. *J Vasc Surg.* 2001;34:440–446.

19. Timaran CH, Prault TL, Stevens SL, et al. Iliac artery stenting versus surgical reconstruction for TASC (TransAtlantic Inter-Society Consensus) type B and type C iliac lesions. *J Vasc Surg.* 2003;38:272–278.

20. Zeller T, Frank U, Müller C, et al. Technological advances in the design of catheters and devices used in renal artery interventions: impact on complications. *J Endovas Ther.* 2003;10(5):1006–1014.

21. van Jaarsveld BC, Krijnen P, Pieterman H, et al. The effect of balloon angioplasty on hypertension in atherosclerotic renal-artery stenosis. Dutch Renal Artery Stenosis Intervention Cooperative Study Group. *N Engl J Med.* 2000;342(14): 1007–1014.

22. Surowiec SM, Davies MG, Eberly SW, et al. Percutaneous angioplasty and stenting of the superficial femoral artery. *J Vasc Surg.* 2005;41(2): 269–278.

23. Ihnat D, Duong S, Taylor Z, et al. Contemporary outcomes after superficial femoral artery angioplasty and stenting: The influence of TASC classification and runoff score. *J Vasc Surg.* 2008;47(5): 967–974.

24. Mwipatayi B, Hockings A, Hofmann M, et al. Balloon angioplasty compared with stenting for treatment of femoropopliteal occlusive disease: A meta-analysis. *J Vasc Surg.* 2008;47(2):461–469.

25. Baril D, Marone L, Kim J, et al. Outcomes of endovascular interventions for TASC II B and C femoropopliteal lesions. *J Vasc Surg.* 2008;48(3): 627–633.

26. Lam R, Shah S, Faries P, et al. Incidence and clinical significance of distal embolization during percutaneous interventions involving the superficial femoral artery. *J Vasc Surg.* 2007;46(6):1155–1159.

27. Nair V, Chaisson G, Abben R. Strategies in Infrapopliteal Intervention: Improving Outcomes in Challenging Patients. *J Interv Cardiol.* 2009;22:27–36.

28. Romiti M, Albers M, Brochado-Neto FC, et al. Meta-analysis of infrapopliteal angioplasty for chronic critical limb ischemia. *J Vasc Surg.* 2008;47:975–981.

29. Tsetis D, Belli AM. The role of infrapopliteal angioplasty. *Br J Radiol.* 2004;77:1007–1015.

30. Coward LJ, McCabe DJ, Ederle J, et al. Long-term outcome after angioplasty and stenting for symptomatic vertebral artery stenosis compared with medical treatment in the Carotid And Vertebral Artery Transluminal Angioplasty Study (CAVATAS): A randomized trial. *Stroke.* 2007;38:1526–30.

31. Janssens E, Leclerc X, Gautier C, et al. Percutaneous transluminal angioplasty of proximal vertebral artery stenosis: Long-term clinical follow-up of 16 consecutive patients. *Neuroradiology.* 2004;46:81–84.

32. Murphy TP, Ariaratnam NS, Carney WI Jr, et al. Aortoiliac insufficiency: Long-term experience with stent placement for treatment. *Radiology.* 2004;231:243–249.

33. Bax L, Woittiez AJ, Kouwenberg HJ, et al. Stent placement in patients with atherosclerotic renal artery stenosis and impaired renal function: A randomized trial. *Ann Intern Med.* 2009;150:840–848.

34. Patel VI, Conrad MF, Kwolek CJ, et al. Renal artery revascularization: Outcomes stratified by indication for intervention. *J Vasc Surg.* 2009; 49(6):1480–1489.

35. Rastan A, Krankenberg H, Müller-Hülsbeck S, et al. Improved renal function and blood pressure control following renal artery angioplasty: The renal artery angioplasty in patients with renal insufficiency and hypertension using a dedicated renal stent device study (PRECISION). *EuroIntervention.* 2008;4(2):208–213.

29 Inferior Vena Cava Filters

KYUNG J. CHO AND JAMES J. SHIELDS

enous thromboembolic disease (VTE) including deep vein thrombosis (DVT) and pulmonary embolism (PE) is a common venous disease that mainly affects hospitalized patients. Anticoagulation therapy with intravenous heparin and oral warfarin remains the mainstay treatment of VTE. Vena cava filters are used for the prevention of PE if anticoagulation is contraindicated or cannot be continued in patients with VTE. Compared with anticoagulation alone, placement of an inferior vena cava (IVC) filter reduces the incidence of PE but appears to increase the likelihood of recurrent DVT. Although the evidence for this latter effect is limited, this is the main reason contributing to the increased demand for retrievable filters.

The Mobin–Uddin umbrella, introduced in 1967, was the first IVC filter utilized to prevent PE. Its manufacture was discontinued in 1986 (1). The filter was associated with many adverse events, including migration, caval thrombosis, and caval perforation. Although the filter has not been implanted for more than 20 years, patients who received this filter may still seek medical attention because of lower extremity swelling associated with caval/filter occlusion (Fig. 29-1). Led by the introduction of the Greenfield filter (2) (Boston Scientific, Natick, Massachusetts) in 1972 (Fig. 29-2), the search continues for an ideal filter. At least 10 additional filters are now available on the U.S. market. Criteria that have been considered for the ideal filter include the capability of trapping life-threatening emboli with facilitation of lysis of the captured clots and maintenance of caval patency. It must remain fixed securely within the vena cava and be structurally strong for the prevention of fracture. All filters currently approved by the U.S. Food and Drug Administration (FDA) are relatively safe and effective but all have been associated with some adverse events occurring at filter placement or noticed at follow-up.

This chapter reviews indications for vena caval filters and describes the currently available vena cava filters with respect to the filter design, characteristics, and placement techniques. We also discuss risk factors, and the prevention and management of adverse events with filter placement.

■ INDICATIONS FOR VENA CAVA FILTER PLACEMENT

The indications can be grouped into the generally accepted indications and special indications for selected patients (3). The generally accepted indications include contraindication to anticoagulation in patients with VTE, VTE with hemorrhage secondary to anticoagulation, worsening DVT or recurrent PE despite anticoagulation, inability to achieve adequate anticoagulation, massive PE in patients at risk for further PE, free-floating iliofemoral or IVC thrombosis, severe cardiopulmonary disease and VTE, and poor compliance with anticoagulant medications. The special indications include patients with severe trauma (closed head injury, spinal cord injury, and multiple long bone or pelvic fractures) and high-risk patients (immobilized, intensive care patients, prophylactic preoperative placement and in patients with multiple risk factors for VTE).

Occasionally, IVC filters are placed above the level of the renal veins. The indications for suprarenal filter placement include

511

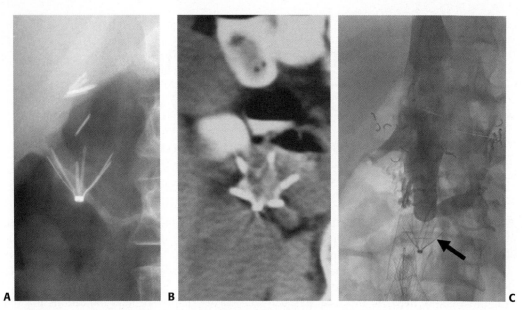

FIGURE 29-1. The Mobin–Uddin umbrella (Edwards Laboratories, Santa Ana, California). The Mobin–Uddin filter had an umbrella-shaped silicone membrane with six radiating stainless steel alloy spokes. The apex of the filter is pointed caudally and the silicone membrane of the filter had 18 fenestrations. (**A**) Radiograph showing a Mobin–Uddin filter placement in the inferior vena cava. (**B**) Computed tomography scan at the level of the filter showing low-density within the filter representing clot. (**C**) Inferior vena cavogram in a 45-year-old man, showing vena caval occlusion at the level of the filter (*arrow*). The patient had undergone successful caval recanalization with placement of Wallstents.

contraindication to anticoagulation in patients with PE and renal vein thrombosis, IVC thrombosis extending above the renal veins, DVT during pregnancy or in women of child-bearing age, thrombus extending above previously placed infrarenal filter, contraindication to anticoagulation in patients with PE and gonadal vein thrombosis, and the presence of certain venous anatomic variants: duplicated IVC and low insertion of retroaortic left renal vein. The indications for vena cava filter placement are summarized in Table 29-1. There are no known absolute contraindications to vena cava filter placement. Sepsis is not a contraindication to filter placement.

■ TECHNIQUE

Selection of the proper catheterization equipment and development of a facile percutaneous technique are essential in performing safe filter placement. Prior to filter placement, the procedure should be explained in detail to the patient. Patients should be informed about the potential benefits of the filter, the relative merits of permanent and retrievable filters, and the complications that can occur. Potential complications include access site hematoma, contrast allergy and nephrotoxicity, filter misplacement and filter migration. Patients should also be informed of the unusual but severe complications, such as filter migration to the chest, fracture/embolization, and caval penetration by the filter limbs. A mild sedative and an analgesic are given just before percutaneous venous puncture. If carbon dioxide (CO_2) is used as a contrast agent, sedation is limited as the signs and symptoms of excessive sedation may mimic the cardiovascular or ventilatory effects of air contamination, a known potential complication of CO_2 angiography (4).

The Seldinger technique for percutaneous vascular access is used. The veins that have been used for access for filter placement are the femoral, jugular, subclavian, and antecubital veins. Of these, the femoral approach is preferred by most operators. Prior to filter insertion, vena cavography should be performed to demonstrate caval

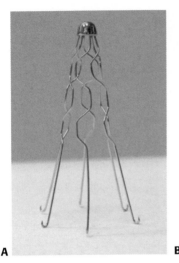
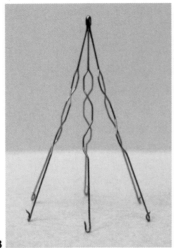
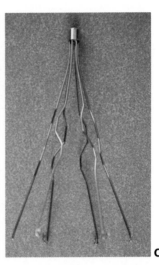

A   B   C

FIGURE 29-2. Greenfield filters. (**A**) Original stainless steel Greenfield filter has a conical design with six legs and an aperture for passage of a guidewire. Each strut has a hook for fixation on the wall of the cava. The filter is 46 mm in height and 30 mm in width. (**B**) Titanium Greenfield filter also has a conical design but without an aperture for passage of a guidewire. The filter is 50 mm in height and 38 mm in width. (**C**) Percutaneous stainless steel Greenfield filter also has a conical shape with the central aperture for passage of a guidewire. The filter is 52 mm in height and 32 mm in width. (See color insert.)

patency, the level of renal veins, any venous anomaly, and to measure caval diameter. Caval diameter should be measured at the intended level of filter placement after correction for magnification.

As the filter is placed commonly below the lowest renal vein, knowledge of the caval

| TABLE 29-1 | Indications for Vena Cava Filter Placement |

- Contraindication to anticoagulation in patients with venous thrombosis or pulmonary embolism PE
- Recurrent embolism despite adequate anticoagulation
- Development of complications during anticoagulation in patients with venous thromboembolic disease
- Patients at high risk with a free-floating thrombus
- Chronic, recurrent PE associated with pulmonary hypertension and cor pulmonale
- Massive PE requiring vasopressors
- Recurrent embolism after filter placement
- Patients at high risk with severe trauma but without venous thrombosis or PE
- Patients at high risk for PE (e.g., immobilized, intensive care patients, prophylactic preoperative placement in patients with multiple risk factors for venous thrombosis or PE)

anatomy and anomalies is important. The preaortic left renal vein (80%–93%) is found at the level of first or second lumbar vertebra. The retroaortic left renal vein (3.7%) usually courses inferomedially and passes behind the aorta before joining the IVC. If the segment of the IVC caudal to the retroaortic left renal vein is too short for filter placement, the filter should be placed above the renal veins. In the presence of circumaortic left renal vein, the filter should be placed suprarenally if the IVC caudal to the caval entry of the retroaortic segment is too short for filter placement. Duplicated IVC represents persistence of the right and left supracardinal veins and occurs at the rate of 0.2% to 3.0%. Crossover in such duplications usually occurs at the level of the iliac and renal veins. In the absence of crossover at the level of the iliac veins, the left-sided IVC can be hidden if venography is performed from the right femoral approach. The findings that suggest the presence of a left-sided IVC on the right femoral vena cavogram include a small infrarenal caval size with the absence of flow from the left iliac vein and a large flow defect from unopacified blood from the left renal vein (Fig. 29-3) (5). The left-sided IVC can be confirmed by advancing a hydrophilic coated guidewire through the left

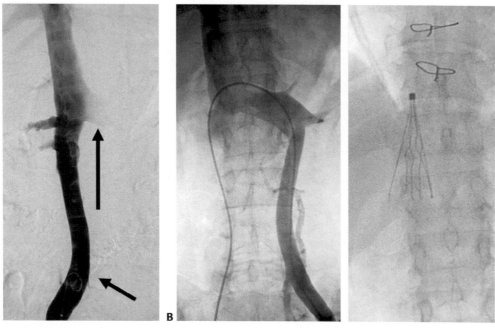

FIGURE 29-3. Duplicated inferior vena cava (IVC) and suprarenal Greenfield filter placement in a 66-year-old woman with deep vein thrombosis and pulmonary embolism and a contraindication to anticoagulation. (**A**) Inferior vena cavogram with the injection of contrast medium into the right iliac vein. The infrarenal portion of the IVC is small in diameter with the lack of flow defect from the left common iliac vein (*shorter arrow*) and a large flow defect from the left renal vein (*longer arrow*). (**B**) The left-sided IVC was catheterized through the left renal vein. (**C**) Anteroposterior radiograph after suprarenal placement of a stainless steel Greenfield filter, showing proper placement of the Filter.

renal vein into the left-sided IVC. In the presence of duplicated inferior vena cava, a filter is placed above the renal veins or, alternatively, two filters may be placed (one in the right-sided and one in the left-sided IVC). When the IVC diameter is greater than 28 mm, either bi-iliac filter placement or a Bird's Nest filter with strut diameter of 60 mm is recommended (6).

When the use of iodinated contrast medium is contraindicated because of renal failure or contrast allergy, alternative imaging methods may be used, including CO_2 angiography or intravascular ultrasonography. CO_2 is the only proven safe contrast agent in renal failure or contrast allergy. After percutaneous catheterization of the right femoral vein, a 5F Cobra catheter is introduced into the left common iliac vein, CO_2 digital subtraction venography is performed with the injection of 40 to 50 cc of CO_2. If the left femoral vein has been accessed, CO_2 is injected into the left external iliac vein (Fig. 29-4). Because of the low viscosity of the gas, an end-hole catheter is used for CO_2 delivery, permitting

catheterization of the contralateral iliac vein and left renal vein if needed (6). The plastic bag delivery system is the safest method and should be used for CO_2 delivery.

Intravascular ultrasound (IVUS) can be used to guide filter placement (7). It is particularly useful in extremely obese patients, traumatized patients, or pregnant women for whom fluoroscopy is contraindicated. This technique involves standard percutaneous femoral vein access and the introduction of the filter delivery sheath over the guidewire. The IVUS catheter is then introduced, identifying the contralateral iliac vein, the aorta, the renal veins, and the right atrium. The IVUS catheter is then retracted to just below the renal vein, and the filter delivery sheath is advanced to the tip of the IVUS catheter, and the filter is deployed. Procedure-related complications with the IVUS-guided filter placement include insertion site hematoma and misplacement of the filter into the iliac vein. The latter can be prevented by careful identification of the reference vessels including the supra-

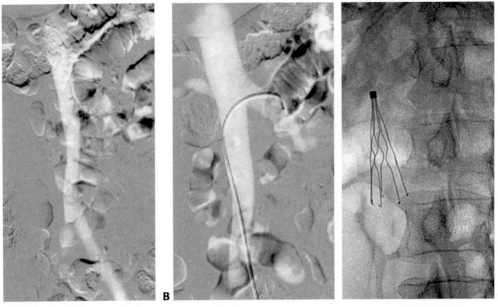

A   **B**   **C**

FIGURE 29-4. CO_2-guided vena cava filter placement in a patient with deep vein thrombosis and a contraindication to anticoagulation. (**A**) CO_2 vena cavogram from left femoral vein approach. No left-sided inferior vena cava is seen. (**B**) Because of no filling of left renal vein, the 5F Cobra catheter used for the vena cavogram was advanced into the left renal vein, and a CO_2 renal venogram was obtained to identify its location. (**C**) Postplacement radiograph showing the stainless steel Greenfield filter in a good position.

and infrarenal IVC, renal veins, and iliocaval junction.

Suprarenal Filter Placement

The technique of suprarenal filter placement is the same as the infrarenal filter placement regarding venous access sites, selection of the filter, and deployment techniques (8). Inferior vena cavography is performed, which depicts the entire IVC from the common iliac vein to the cavoatrial junction. If the suprarenal IVC is too short to place a filter due to suprarenal thrombus, an original Greenfield filter should be used as it allows capturing the thrombus and advancing it toward the renal veins for placement of the filter (Fig. 29-5). When a captured clot propagates cephalically, a second filter is placed suprarenally (Fig. 29-6). The apex of the filter should be placed just caudal to the cardiophrenic angle, thereby ensuring filter placement below the right atrium and above the renal veins (Fig. 29-7). Placing the filter too near the renal veins may lead to migration of the filter or slippage of its limbs into the renal vein since the IVC is widest at the level of renal veins.

Greenfield et al. (9) reported 73 suprarenal Greenfield filter placements and concluded that such placement was safe and efficacious with a minimal risk of caval occlusion or renal failure. The rate of recurrent PE in patients with suprarenal Greenfield filter placement has been reported to be 8% and the caval occlusion rate to be 2.7%.

Superior Vena Cava Filter Placement

The incidence of upper extremity DVT has increased with the increased use of central venous catheters. Vena cava filters are placed in the superior vena cava (SVC) when PE originates from the axillosubclavian or internal jugular vein and there is a contraindication to anticoagulant therapy. SVC filters can be placed from the jugular or femoral approach. If the femoral approach is used, a superior vena cavogram is performed with the injection of contrast medium into the left brachiocephalic vein, which can help identify the junction of the brachiocephalic vein and the SVC. If a filter is to be placed from the internal jugular approach, contrast medium is injected into the

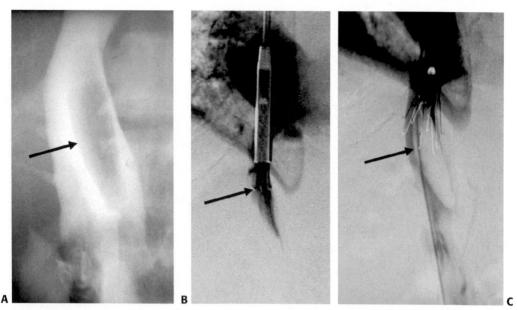

FIGURE 29-5. Free-floating thrombus in the suprarenal portion of the inferior vena cava (IVC). (**A**) Suprarenal inferior vena cavogram. A large free-floating thrombus is seen in the suprarenal segment of the IVC (*arrow*). (**B**) Because the length of the IVC above the level of the thrombus was too short for a filter, an original Greenfield filter was used to capture the thrombus (*arrow*) and was advanced caudally to place the filter below the cavoatrial junction. (**C**) Inferior vena cavogram showing proper placement of the Filter capturing the thrombus (*arrow*). (Courtesy of Dr. David Williams, University of Michigan.)

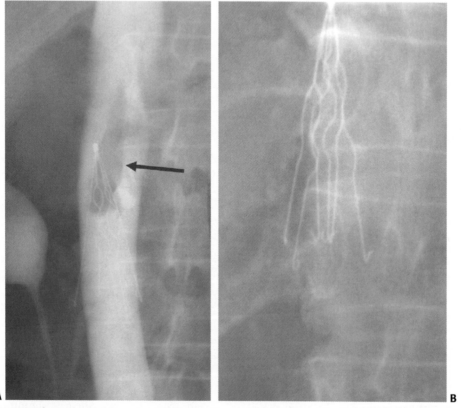

FIGURE 29-6. Recurrent pulmonary embolism (PE) after the placement of a titanium Greenfield filter in a 75-year-old woman with breast cancer. (**A**) Inferior vena cavogram obtained 1 year after filter placement shows cephalic propagation of the captured clot (*arrow*). (**B**) A second titanium Greenfield filter was placed in the suprarenal inferior vena cava. She has not had recurrent PE for 6 years after placement of a second filter.

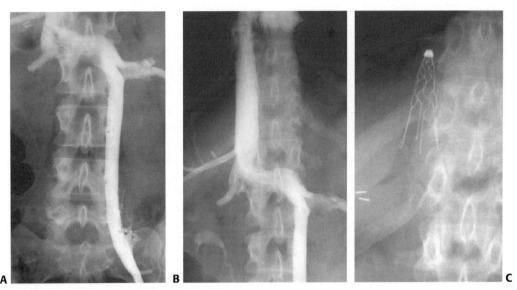

FIGURE 29-7. Duplicated inferior vena cava (IVC) and suprarenal filter placement. (**A**) Left-sided vena cavogram with the injection of contrast medium into the left iliac vein. The left IVC joins the left renal vein, which continues a normal course to the IVC. (**B**) Suprarenal vena cavogram showing patent suprarenal IVC. (**C**) Anteroposterior radiograph after placement of an original Greenfield filter showing proper placement of the filter.

right or left brachiocephalic vein. The filter introducer is then advanced over a guidewire to the intended level of filter placement. The hooks of the filter are placed just caudal to the junction of the SVC with the left brachiocephalic vein (Fig. 29-8).

When placing a filter with a conical shape in the SVC, selection of the filter is essential for proper filter orientation, as these filters are designed for unidirectional use. When either the Greenfield filter or the Günther Tulip filter (Cook, Inc., Bloomington, Indianna) is to be

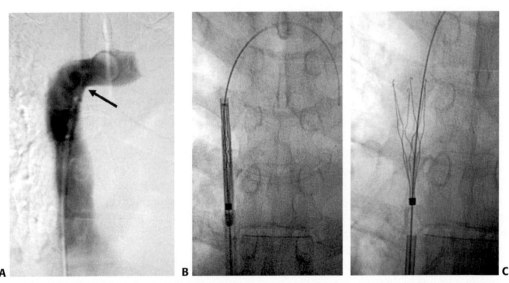

FIGURE 29-8. Superior vena cava (SVC) filter placement in a patient with upper extremity deep vein thrombosis and a contraindication to anticoagulation. (**A**) Superior vena cavagram. The beginning of the SVC can be better identified due to the injection of contrast medium into the left brachiocephalic vein (*arrow*). (**B**) The carrier of the stainless steel Greenfield filter is positioned in the SVC just caudal to the junction of the brachiocephalic vein and SVC. The Amplatz superstiff guidewire is positioned in the left brachiocephalic vein. (**C**) The filter was placed in the SVC.

placed from the femoral approach, the jugular filter set should be used, whereas the femoral filter set should be used from the jugular approach. Greenfield filters have been the most commonly used filter for SVC placement. Other filters that have been used for SVC placement are Vena Tech filter (VTF, B. Braun Vena Tech, Evanston, Illinois), Simon Nitinol filter (SNF, BARD Peripheral Vascular, Tempe, Arizona), TrapEase filter (Miani, Florida), Günther Tulip filter (Cook, Inc., Bloomington, Indiana), OptEase filter (Cordis, Miami, Florida), Recovery filter (BARD Peripheral Vascular, Tempe Arizona), and the Bird's Nest filter (Cook, Inc. Bloomington, Indiana).

SVC filters have been shown to be safe and effective in preventing PE. (10) Reported procedure-related complications included pneumothorax, hemorrhage, and filter misplacement. Long-term complications included migration, caval occlusion, SVC perforation with pericardial tamponade, and caval perforation with erosion into the ascending aorta (11,12).

Postplacement Imaging Follow-Up

Clinical and imaging follow-up after placement of permanent and retrievable filters is important. Although uncommon, all available and previously available filters have demonstrated occasional complications at long-term follow-up. Post placement follow-up may include clinical examination, radiography, and Duplex ultrasound at 1, 6, and 12 months. Beyond 1 year after placement, routine follow-up will not be necessary unless the patient develops clinical symptoms that might be related to the filter.

Migration of a vena cava filter within the IVC can be difficult to quantify as it involves the comparison of a moving vessels to a fixed skeletal structure. The magnitude of a filter's movement within the IVC is not the most significant consideration; rather it is the effect of migration that is important. The acceptable amount of movement within the IVC for an IVC filter is 10 mm. Apparent penetration up to 5 mm beyond the caval wall on computed tomography (CT) is often due to tenting of the caval wall with incorporation of the hooks into the wall of the vena cava.

Changes in the diameter of the filter on follow-up radiography may indicate caval penetration. It is important to recognize the respiratory variation of the caval diameter. When compared with previous radiographs, both inspiratory and

expiratory radiographs should be examined when assessing filter diameter and intracaval movement.

■ CURRENTLY MARKETED VENA CAVA FILTERS

The vena cava filters can be grouped as permanent filters and retrievable filters. All retrievable filters are approved by the FDA for permanent placement and are sometimes referred to as *optional filters*. No filters currently available in the United States are made for "temporary use only." The permanent (not designed for retrieval) vena cava filters are Greenfield filters, VTF, Vena Tech LP filter (VTF-LP, B. Braun), Simon Nitinol filter (Bard Peripheral Vascular), Bird's Nest filter (Cook, Inc.), and TrapEase filter (Cordis Endovascular). The retrievable filters include Günther Tulip filter, Celect (Cook, Inc.), G2 Express Filter (Bard Peripheral Vascular), and Option filter (Angiotech) (Fig. 29-9). All filters except for TrapEase, OptEase, and Bird's Nest have a conical design. The cone of the filter can capture a large volume of clot without interfering significantly with the caval flow. Studies have demonstrated that clot filling 70% of the filter depth results in blockage of only 40% of the cross-sectional area.

Original Greenfield Filter

The stainless steel Greenfield filter has six corrugated legs arranged in a conical shape, extending from the apex with an aperture. The base of each strut has a fine hook for fixation on the wall of the cava. It is 46 mm tall and 30 mm wide (Fig. 29-2). It is designed to capture large emboli within the cone, permitting continued flow and lysis of emboli. The rate of recurrent PE has been reported to be 2% to 4% and the caval patency rate is reported to be 95% to 98% (13). Minor filter movement of no clinical significance has been reported in 8% of cases. The Greenfield filters have been placed in the IVC below and above the renal veins and in the SVC (Figs. 29-5 and 29-7). This filter was designed originally to be inserted through a surgical cutdown of the jugular or femoral vein, using an operator-loaded delivery system. For percutaneous insertion, a 24-Fr sheath is required for the introduction of the filter carrier. The introductions of the lower profile titanium Greenfield filter and percutaneous stainless steel Greenfield filter have caused marked reduction in the use of this filter.

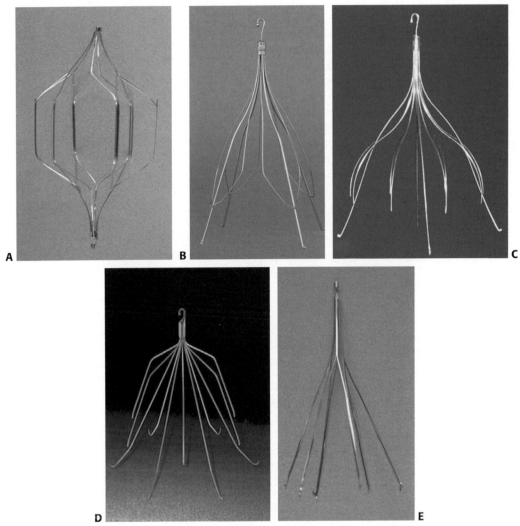

FIGURE 29-9. Retrievable filters. (**A**) OptEase filter (Cordis Endovascular, Warren, New Jersey). (**B**) Günther Tulip filter (Cook Medical, Bloomington, Indiana). (**C**) Celect (Cook Medical, Bloomington, Indiana). (**D**) G2 Express (Bard Peripheral Vascular, Tempe, Arizona). (**E**) Option filter (Angiotech Interventional, Gainesville, Florida). The dimensions of each filter do not reflect the actual height and width of the filter. (See color insert.)

Complications have occurred at placement and have been found in follow-up. The most serious complication at surgical placement was intracardiac misplacement resulting in inadvertent ejection of the filter into the right atrium. Attempts at removal have been hazardous. Surgical or percutaneous methods have been used to remove misplaced filters with some successes and failures (14,15). An attempt at percutaneous removal caused migration of the filter into the pulmonary artery where it was described as clinically asymptomatic. Atrial misplacement of the filter has been largely prevented with the proper use of a guidewire and fluoroscopy. Other known complications have involved penetration of adjacent organs, cardiac arrhythmias, limb fractures, filter migration caudally with filter deformation, and cephalic migration to the right atrium, right ventricle, and pulmonary artery, as well as intra-aortic misplacement (16–19). "Quad cough" chest physical therapy that is used for the treatment of pulmonary secretions in quadriplegics has been shown to cause migration of the filter that may be associated with deformation of the filter and caval penetration (20). Most often, caval penetration is asymptomatic, and leg fracture and intracaval filter migration do not require intervention.

Titanium Greenfield Filter

A titanium version of the Greenfield system (TGF) was developed to facilitate percutaneous insertion. The TGF retains the conical shape of the original Greenfield filter and is inserted through a 15F sheath. The original TGF has undergone hook modification, and this has improved caval fixation (Fig. 29-2). Because the filter is advanced through the sheath without a guidewire, sheath kinking with difficulty of insertion has occurred when inserting from the left femoral approach. Insertion of the filter is technically easier when the right femoral or jugular approach is used. The TGF is longer than the original Greenfield filter with a length of 4.7 cm as compared with the 4.4 cm length of the stainless steel Greenfield filter (SGF). The TGF is broader at the base (38 mm) than the SGF (30 mm).

The results of the multicenter clinical trial of the TGF with modified hooks (TGF-MH) revealed recurrent PE in 3%, caval patency in 98%, insertion site thrombosis in 8.7%, incomplete opening in 2%, leg asymmetry in 5.4%, insertion site hematoma in l%, and apical penetration of the cava during insertion in 1% (21). The reported complications have involved migration, penetration, filter deformity, incomplete opening, and leg asymmetry. The serious complications reported include filter migration into the pulmonary artery and intra-aortic misplacement. Successful attempts have been made at retrieving the migrated TGF from the left pulmonary artery (22,23) and from intra-aortic misplacement of the filter (24).

Asymmetry of the TGF has been discussed extensively but no statistical correlation between asymmetric positioning and recurrent PE was found. The factors contributing to leg asymmetry may include the absence of a guidewire at discharge of the filter, caval geometry, and caval thrombosis. Asymmetric leg distribution can often be corrected by transvenous manipulation using a Cobra catheter and a guidewire. The filter is durable, allowing its placement in children. Limb fracture is extremely uncommon and likely insignificant.

Percutaneous SGF

The continued quest for the ideal filter led to the development of the percutaneous stainless steel Greenfield filter (PSGF). It is similar to the TGF in design and clinical outcome (Fig. 29-2). The use of a guidewire (Amplatz superstiff wire) for insertion of the filter has improved centering and the ease of placement (25,26). This filter has alternating hooks and was evaluated in a prospective clinical trial with placement of the filter in 75 patients and follow-up with radiographs and ultrasound scans at 30 days after placement. There were four cases of limb asymmetry (5.5%) without clinical sequelae and one incidence of failure to completely span the vena cava. There was no recurrent PE. Caval penetration occurred in 1.7%, and caval occlusion was confirmed in 5%. Serious complications related to the placement of PSGF have rarely occurred.

No mortality has been attributed to this filter. Subsequent mortality is usually from underlying malignancy and cardiac disease. Clinical outcomes regarding recurrent PE and caval patency appear to be comparable with the TGF. Because of the use of an Amplatz superstiff guidewire, asymmetry of the leg distribution encountered with the TGF has significantly improved. Inadvertent guidewire entrapment remains a problem with subsequent "blind" central venous catheterization as with other filters. The PSGF can be introduced from the jugular and femoral veins and is also effective for suprarenal and SVC placement.

Bird's Nest IVC Filter

The Bird's Nest filter was introduced for clinical trial in 1982 and approved by the FDA in 1989. It is made of a 100 cm length of stainless steel wire attached to the two sets of rigid struts, which form a mesh when deployed in the IVC. The maximum width of the struts is 60 mm, but the filter is recommended for mega cava with a diameter only up to 40 mm (Fig. 29-10). It is delivered through the 11F introducer. The insertion technique involves the deployment of the initial V-shaped struts at the level of the renal veins, followed by the formation of a wire mesh. Before deploying a second V-shaped strut, the delivery system is advanced to over the apex of the initial struts. During deployment of the wire mesh, the delivery sheath is rotated counterclockwise for 360 degrees twice to form a tight mesh, thereby preventing wire prolapse. Wire prolapse is commonly seen on abdominal radi-

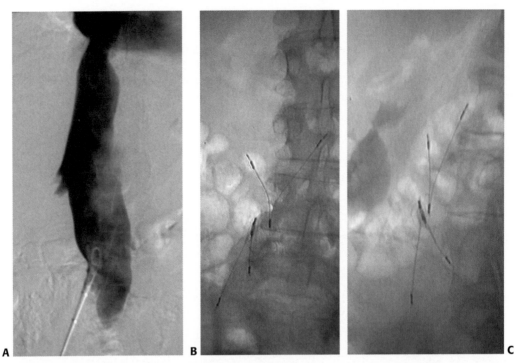

FIGURE 29-10. Bird's Nest filter placement in a 65-year-old woman with a mega cava who had pulmonary embolism and retroperitoneal bleeding while on anticoagulation. (**A**) Inferior vena cavogram showing a mega vena cava measuring 32 mm in transverse diameter. (**B** and **C**) Postplacement radiographs of the filter in the anteroposterior and lateral views showing proper placement of the filter.

ographs, but it does not increase risk for PE. Recurrent PE has been reported in up to 2.7% and IVC occlusion in 4.7%. Asymptomatic perforation of the caval wall by the struts is commonly seen on CT.

Limited data have been published since the introduction of this device. Vesely et al. (27) summarized problems that may be encountered during placement of this filter. Some considerations have been described: although both V-shaped struts are visible, the wire mesh is difficult to see under fluoroscopy; the length of the IVC should be at least 7 cm for successful placement of the filter; the filter has been implanted in both the suprarenal IVC and SVC, but if it is deployed incorrectly, the filter will likely occupy the longer length of the vena cava. Training and experience are necessary for correct placement. Reported complications include caval obstruction, caval penetration and fracture of a strut of the filter requiring surgical removal because of the associated abdominal pain, caval penetration with symptomatic hydronephrosis, and migration to the right atrium. Rogoff et al. (28) reported two cases of

cephalic migration of the filter, which was related to a massive thromboembolism after the filter placement. Percutaneous retrieval of the migrated filter was successful in one patient. A patient who developed pericardial tamponade required emergency open heart surgery for removal of the filter. The presence of a Bird's Nest filter in the IVC does not preclude the passage of a guidewire or a catheter through the filter. This filter has been used in a pediatric patient; however, the most commonly used filters in pediatric patients are Greenfield filters and TGFs.

Simon Nitinol Filter

The SNF is made of nitinol alloy that has the thermal shape–memory properties. It has a conical design with two-level filtering capability and traps thrombi as small as 3 mm. The femoral or jugular vein is normally used for placement of this filter. If neither approach is possible, the antecubital approach can be used because of the low profile delivery system.

The antecubital SNF is delivered through the 7F, 100-cm long introducer catheter following access to the basilic vein in the arm, using ultrasound guidance. A 5F pigtail catheter is advanced into the left common iliac vein, and a vena cavogram is obtained. Over the guidewire, the filter introducer catheter is loaded and is advanced until the tip of the introducer reaches the IVC approximately 5 cm below the lowest renal vein. The guidewire and dilator are removed, and the filter is advanced until it reaches the end of the introducer. Inadvertent discharge may occur because

the system is not very radiopaque and because the more radiopaque junction between the upper and lower level filter components can be mistaken for the hooks of the filter. If one fails to recognize the base of the filter and the filter is discharged, it will be deployed lower than the intended level. Upon discharge from the sheath, the dome of the filter shortens caudally (Fig. 29-11). In a very small vena cava, the filter may form a spindle shape if there is not enough room for its dome to form. Advancing

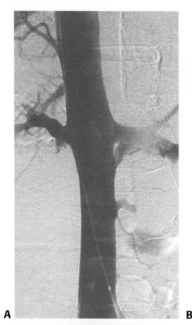

A

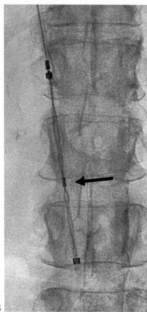

B

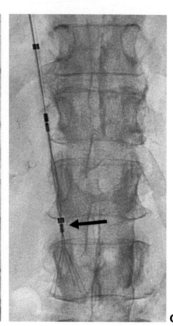

C

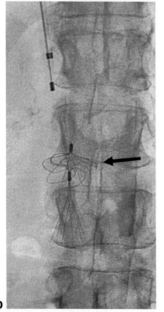

D

FIGURE 29-11. Antecubital Simon nitinol filter placement in a 76-year-old woman with end-stage renal disease, congestive heart failure, peripheral arterial occlusive disease, and deep vein thrombosis. She is to undergo below-knee amputation. (**A**) Inferior vena cavogram from left arm vein approach. Both renal veins were filled with contrast medium because of the end-stage renal disease. (**B**) The filter introducer with a Simon nitinol filter is positioned at the intended level of the IVC. The junction between the lower and upper level filtration (*arrow*) is positioned immediately below the renal veins, which should not be mistaken for the hooks of the filter. (**C**) The lower level of the filter was opened (*arrow*). (**D**) The filter was fully discharged. The upper level of the filter has dropped while forming its umbrella shape (*arrow*).

the sheath caudally during or after discharge of the filter will help the formation of the filter dome. In some cases, formation of the dome may be delayed but still may occur naturally.

Although this filter has been safe and effective, long-term results are lacking, particularly regarding caval patency. Simon et al. (29) reported 4.5% recurrent PE and 9% symptomatic vena cava occlusion in 44 patients. Grassi et al. (30) reported a 28% rate of caval occlusion. This high caval occlusion rate was attributed to reduced venous inflow in patients with prior nephrectomy or pelvic neoplasms, pelvic venous compression by tumor mass, and hypercoagulable states. In vitro hemodynamic evaluation of the filter suggested that the extended region of stagnant flow near the midsection of the umbrella region might lead to organization of thrombus and fibrin mesh network development with resultant caval occlusion (31).

Reported complications have involved the difficulty of discharging the filter from the introducer, misplacement into an ascending lumbar vein, incomplete formation of the filter in a narrow IVC, caval occlusion, migration of the filter to the chest, caval penetration, eccentric filter position, partial filter disruption, kinking of the filter, and retraction with inversion following transvenous intervention (32–34). Of these, vena caval occlusion seems to be a significant complication that may be likely related to the filter design. Acute and chronic vena caval occlusion associated with the filter can be recanalized using an endovascular method. The technique involves balloon dilatation through the occluded filter from the femoral approach and placement of two parallel metallic stents through the filter. In vitro study the umbrella part of the filter can be dilated up to 18 mm in diameter. In a patient with an occluded filter, two parallel balloons and stents are usually required to dilate the IVC sufficiently to maintain caval blood flow.

Vena Tech Filter

The VTF is made from a biocompatible nonferromagnetic alloy, Phynox wire. It has a six-legged conical design with six stabilizer bars that are intended to improve centering within the vena cava. This filter is introduced through a 10F introducer catheter. Ricco et al. (35) reported a 2% rate of recurrent PE and an 8% rate of caval

occlusion in 90 patients. In a Canadian study of 64 patients, recurrent PE occurred in 3% of cases. IVC thrombosis occurred in 22% and this was symptomatic in 9% (36). Reported complications include proximal propagation of thrombus, insertion site thrombosis, migration, tilting, fracture, and incomplete opening.

A related filter, VTF-LP, is a permanent, low-profile wire filter with a conical design with stabilizing bars and hooks. This filter is also made from Phynox, placed through a 7F introducer. A European multicenter prospective study of VenaTech LP in 106 patients revealed a frequency of 3.9% for filter tilting but revealed no signs of recurrent PE or undesired device-related events. A 3-month mortality rate was reported to be 21% (37). The basilic or brachial vein can be used for placement of this filter.

TrapEase Filter

The TrapEase filter differs from the standard conical design. It consists of two short, conical trapping surfaces joined by six fixation struts of broad flat wire bounded by 12 hooks. It is a double-basket symmetric filter that is laser-cut from nickel-titanium (nitinol) tubing. The filter was approved by the FDA in 2000. The cephalic and caudal baskets of the filter consist of baskets in a six-diamond or trapezoidal shape configuration. The baskets are then connected by six straight struts that provide proximal and distal hooks for fixation within the IVC. The filter is placed through a 6F sheath and can be inserted through the femoral, jugular, or antecubital venous approach. The unexpanded length of the filter is 64 mm; the expanded filter length depends upon the IVC diameter.

The filter demonstrates excellent clot capturing ability and resistance to migration but greater pressure response to clot volume loading in the filter. It has been postulated that the double tier trapping surface of the filter disturbs caval flow and reduces lysis, subsequently leading to caval/filter occlusion (38). This has been demonstrated in an ovine model where clots were captured at the lower trapping level in contact with the caval wall. A large amount chronic clot with extensive fibrin webbing covered the filter lumen at 60 days (Fig. 29-12).

The result of a multicenter prospective study with 65 patients showed no cases of filter migration or other filter-related complications (39).

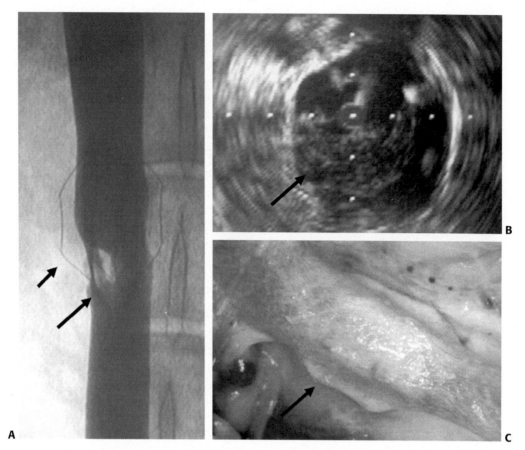

FIGURE 29-12. TrapEase in sheep at 60 days postplacement. Clot was injected into the inferior vena cava (IVC) after filter placement. (**A**) Inferior vena cavogram showing a large amount of clot within the inferior basket (*arrow*). The filter struts extended outside the contrast filled IVC lumen (*shorter arrow*). (**B**) Intravascular ultrasound image at the level of residual clot showing a large intraluminal echogenic thrombus (*arrow*). The images obtained at the fixation struts demonstrated distortion of the cava wall and penetration. (**C**) Gross photograph of the vena cava showing pericaval penetration of the fixation struts. Thick fibrous tissue is seen around the penetrated filter (*arrow*). (See color insert.)

Kalva et al. (40) reported the result of TrapEase filter placement in 751 patients: groin hematoma (0.4%), symptoms of PE (7.5%), fracture of filter components (3%), thrombus within the filter (25.2%), caval occlusion (0.7%), and no migration.

Life-threatening filter migration to the chest has been reported. Porcellini et al. (41) reported a case of delayed intracardiac migration of a TrapEase filter within 1 week after placement. Sudden venous hypertension and caval dilation resulting from filter occlusion by large captured emboli was blamed for migration of the filter. Sudden increase in right atrial pressure associated with the migrated filter caused paradoxical embolism in the presence of a patent foramen ovale. Hadda-

dian et al. (42) reported a case of sudden cardiac death caused by the migration of a TrapEase vena cava filter. Six days after filter placement for massive PE, the patient had cardiopulmonary arrest, and autopsy of the heart showed the IVC filter entrapped within the tricuspid valve.

OptEase Retrievable Vena Cava Filter

The OptEase filter is of a similar design and is constructed from nitinol. It has a double-basket design, identical to TrapEase, and is introduced through a 6F sheath. The filter has a central caudal hook for snaring and retrieval. It has six superior barbs to prevent central migration (Fig. 29-9). The side struts help self-centering and reduce filter tilting. The clot trapping pattern

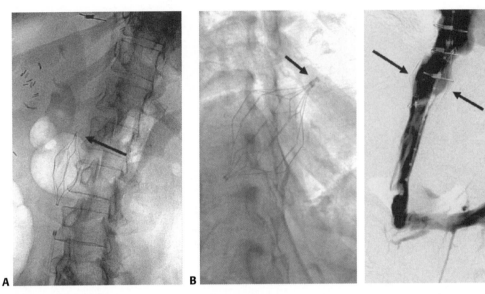

FIGURE 29-13. Incorrect orientation of OptEase filter. (**A**) OptEase filter was placed in the inferior vena cava (IVC) in an incorrect orientation in a 63-year-old woman with ovarian cancer and deep vein thrombosis. The postplacement image shows the hook of the filter in incorrect orientation (*arrow*). (**B**) The image taken 50 days after placement showing cephalic migration of the filter. (**C**) Inferior vena cavagram. The filter wire extends outside the caval lumen (*arrows*) and partial thrombosis of the suprarenal IVC. The infrarenal IVC was thrombosed, which was treated with balloon angioplasty and stent placement. Retrieval of the filter was unsuccessful because of the incorporation of the filter into the wall of the vena cava.

and caval hemodynamic alteration associated with the OptEase filter is similar to that of TrapEase filter. The filter is retrieved from the femoral vein approach, and the recommended dwell time is up to 12 days. After 2 months of placement, retrieval of the filter has been shown to be difficult due to strut protrusion through the caval wall. Like all other filters, this filter may be implanted permanently. The filter is constrained in a plastic tube indicating the correct orientation for femoral or jugular approach. Failure to identify the appropriate orientation of the filter storage tube at deployment can lead to incorrect placement with the risk for central migration (Fig. 29-13). The hook of the filter is visible through the clear plastic tube, allowing confirmation of correct orientation.

A multicenter prospective trial (43) demonstrated that OptEase can be safely used as both a permanent and a temporary filter. This study reported filter migration and filter-associated DVT in 0.9% and 0.8%, respectively, at 1 month. When followed up to 6 months, there were no new cases of filter migration or filter-related DVT. Filter fracture was reported in two patients (1.8%) without clinical sequelae.

The OptEase filter can be easily retrieved by using a Goose Neck snare from the femoral vein or popliteal vein within 2 weeks and potentially can be retrieved up to 4 to 8 weeks after placement, but late retrieval may be difficult because of incorporation of the filter into the wall of the cava. Because of the broad area of stasis along the caval wall and near the apex of the filter, lysis of the trapped emboli and thrombi may be slowed or new thrombus may be formed there. A study reported by Mahrer et al. (44) reported failure of retrieval in 22% of patients because of large intrafilter thrombi.

Günther Tulip Vena Cava Filter

The Günther Tulip vena cava filter is made of nonferromagnetic conichrome wire. It has a conical shape with four primary legs with fixation hooks and eight secondary legs. The filter is 30 mm in base diameter and 50 mm in height (Fig. 29-9). The filter should not be placed when the cava diameter is greater than 30 mm. Multiple clinical studies have documented that the filter is safe and effective with a 94% probability of successful retrieval at 12 weeks after placement (45).

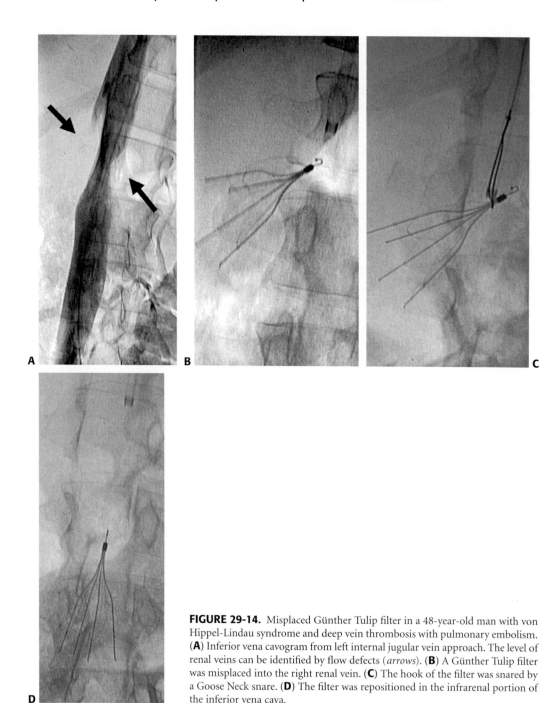

FIGURE 29-14. Misplaced Günther Tulip filter in a 48-year-old man with von Hippel-Lindau syndrome and deep vein thrombosis with pulmonary embolism. (**A**) Inferior vena cavogram from left internal jugular vein approach. The level of renal veins can be identified by flow defects (*arrows*). (**B**) A Günther Tulip filter was misplaced into the right renal vein. (**C**) The hook of the filter was snared by a Goose Neck snare. (**D**) The filter was repositioned in the infrarenal portion of the inferior vena cava.

Known complications associated with Günther Tulip vena cava filter at placement include misplacement and migration. A misplaced filter should be snared and removed or repositioned (Fig. 29-14). If the filter is incorporated into the wall of the vena cava, retrieval may be difficult or unsuccessful (Fig. 29-15). Reported complications are migration of the filter to the heart and caval penetration. Galhotra et al. (46) reported two cases of migration of Günther Tulip vena cava filters. In the first case, the filter migrated to the main pulmonary artery during filter placement. In the second case, a Günther Tulip vena cava filter was found to have migrated to the tricuspid valve after the patient sustained cardiopulmonary arrest and

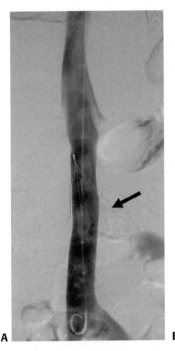
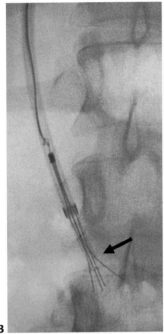
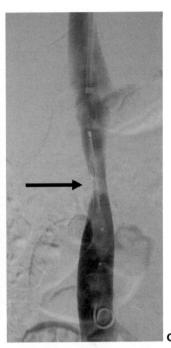

A   B   C

FIGURE 29-15. Failure to retrieve Günther Tulip filter in a 24-year-old man with Wegner granulomatosis, pulmonary embolism, and pulmonary hemorrhage. (**A**) Inferior vena cavogram obtained 3½ months after filter placement shows caval penetraton of the struts (*arrow*). (**B**) Despite considerable force used to disengage the lower limbs and hooks from the caval wall, retrieval was unsuccessful (*arrow*). (**C**) Inferior vena cavogram obtained immediately after release of the legs showing moderate retraction of the filter with narrowing of the inferior vena cava (*arrow*). There were no clinical sequelae from the attempted retrieval. Computed tomography scan and radiographs obtained 1 month later showed reexpansion of the filter to the preretrieval shape.

subsequent resuscitation. Both filters were removed by open surgery. Bochenek et al. (47) reported a case of filter migration to the right atrium immediately after placement from the right subclavian approach. The filter was successfully removed by using the EnSnare device (Merit Medical Systems, Inc. South Jordan, Utah). A delayed complication of symptomatic caval penetration into the vertebra, aorta, and duodenum was reported by Parkin et al. (48). In that case, surgical intervention was required to remove the filter.

Percutaneous removal of the Günther Tulip vena cava filter is generally safe and usually technically easy. Difficult or unsuccessful retrievals may be secondary to excessive tissue ingrowth at filter legs, the hook being oriented toward the caval wall, incorporation of the hook into the wall of the cava, and excessive entrapped clot in the filter (49). Additional reported complications from filter retrieval have included mild caval stenosis, filter fracture and embolization to the lung, and PE.

Cook Celect Filter Vena Cava Filter

The Cook Celect Vena Cava filter is made of a nonferromagnetic conichrome wire. It has a conical shape with four primary legs with fixation hooks and eight secondary legs. It is 30 mm in diameter and 48 mm in height (Fig. 29-9). Unlike Günther Tulip vena cava filter, the secondary legs are not connected to the primary legs. It has a retrievable hook at the apex of the filter. This filter is introduced from the femoral or jugular vein. For the jugular vein approach, the filter must be manually loaded into the peel-away sheath. The NavAlign delivery is available on Günther Tulip and Celect filters. It includes a hemostatic valve and push-button filter deployment.

The filter should not be placed when the IVC diameter is greater than 30 mm or less than 15 mm. The filter is retrieved from the jugular vein using the Cook retrieval set or an Amplatz Goose Neck snare. Prior to filter retrieval, inferior vena cavography should be performed in the anteroposterior and lateral views. The filter should

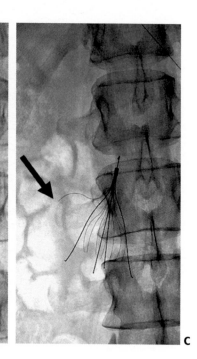

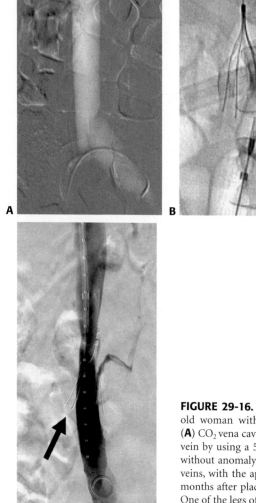

FIGURE 29-16. Migration and penetration of a Celect filter in a 46-year-old woman with pulmonary embolism and subarachnoid hemorrhage. (**A**) CO_2 vena cavagram with the injection of CO_2 into the left common iliac vein by using a 5F Cobra catheter. The inferior vena cava (IVC) is patent without anomaly. (**B**) A Celect filter was placed in the IVC below the renal veins, with the apex of the filter at the level of L1–2 interspace. (**C**) Seven months after placement, the filter has migrated caudally and tilted (*arrow*). One of the legs of the filter has penetrated into the duodenum on computed tomography scan (*not shown*). (**D**) Inferior vena cavogram with contrast medium prior to filter retrieval shows limb penetration (*arrow*) and mild caval stenosis. Filter retrieval was successful.

not be retrieved when the filter cone is filled with clot in greater than 25% of the depth of the cone.

A multicenter registry study with 95 patients showed a probability of successful filter retrieval rate of 100% at 50 weeks and 74% at 55 weeks after placement. No adverse events from the retrieval procedures were reported (50). Other studies reported significant rates of caudal or

cephalic migration and caval penetration (22% and 14%, respectively), and frequent tilting.

Sadaf et al. (51) reported a young woman with PE and a large left lower extremity arteriovenous malformation that developed back pain 9 days after placement of a Celect filter. CT and inferior vena cavogram demonstrated caudal migration associated with caval penetration into the adjacent organs. Figure 29-16 demonstrates a similar case of caudal migration and IVC penetration. Caval stenosis, penetration, contrast extravasations, retroperitoneal hematoma, and infection have been seen after retrieval.

Bard Recovery Filter, G2 and G2 Express Filters

The Bard Recovery filter provides two levels of filtration with six upper arms and six elastic hooks. The Recovery filter was approved by the FDA in 2002. This filter was modified to a second-generation filter to prevent migration and fracture. The modified filter, called *G2*, was introduced in 2005 and has a wider leg span and thick fixation hooks. G2 Express is the G2 filter with the addition of the hook at the apex of the filter to allow snaring for retrieval (Fig. 29-9). It has 12 nitinol wires emanating from a central nitinol sleeve with a retrieval hook at the apex of the filter and is delivered through a 7F introducer sheath.

G2 Express is retrieved by using either a Goose Neck snare or the Bard recovery cone device. Unlike other retrievable filters, G2 filter is retrieved by withdrawing the filter into the sheath rather than advancing the sheath over the filter. Retrieval can be very difficult if the filter apex is tilted and embedded in the caval wall. Various techniques have been described, including the use of the loopsnare, endobronchial forceps, and balloon-assisted manipulations. No serious complication has been reported after retrieval of the filters.

The reported complications after insertion include filter migration, fracture, caval penetration, and caval thrombosis (Fig. 29-17). Hull et al. (52) evaluated 14 filters with unenhanced CT scans at various intervals and found arm caval perforation in 56% and leg perforation in 11%. Images obtained after a mean of 899 days demonstrated filter arm perforation in all 14 patients followed and leg perforations in 35%. There were four fractures with migration in 21% of patients. It was concluded that Recovery filter limb caval perforation increases over time with a 21% incidence of fracture and migration. Early retrieval and follow-up imaging after placement were recommended. Nazzal et al. (53) also reported two cases of filter arm penetrations of the caval wall associated with filter deformity. In one of the patients, one arm was fractured and migrated into the peripheral pulmonary artery during retrieval. Hull et al. (54) reported a case of

filter arm perforation, subsequent fracture, and migration to the right ventricle that caused chest pain and ventricular tachycardia. The filter fragment was successfully retrieved percutaneouly using an EnSnare device.

Saeed et al. (55) reported a rare case of right ventricular migration of a fractured arm of the filter that resulted in pericardial tamponade. Open heart surgery was required to remove the fractured filter fragment. Bui et al. (56) reported asymptomatic right ventricular migration of a G2 filter that was discovered 3 months after placement. Vergara et al. (57) reported spontaneous migration of a Recovery filter into the right atrium, causing tricuspid regurgitation and perforation of right atrium and cardiac tamponade. Gupta et al. (58) reported symptomatic caval penetration of a G2 filter in which the arm penetrated into the aortic lumen. Ganguli et al. (59) reported fracture and migration of a suprarenal Recovery filter 67 days after placement in a pregnant woman. This reported central migration of the filter seems to relate to inadequate fixation of the filter to the wall of the cava.

Option Retrievable Vena Cava Filter System

The Option filter (Angiotech Interventional, Gainesville, Florida) is laser cut from nitinol tubing into a conical shape with a retrievable hook at the apex of the filter. The filter was approved by the FDA in June 2009 (Fig. 29-9). The filter is indicated for use in both permanent and retrievable placement in caval diameters up to 30 mm. Filter placement is done with the use of an over-the-wire curved pusher system. It is delivered using a 5F introducer. The same cartridge is used for insertion by the femoral or jugular vein. Filter retrieval is recommended within 175 days following placement. The IVC filter is retrieved from the jugular vein by using 8F sheath and EnSnare or Goose Neck snare. The SVC filter is retrieved from the femoral vein.

The results of a prospective multicenter study enrolled with 100 patients showed no filter embolization, fracture, or caval penetration (60). Retrieval was successful in 92% (mean implantation time, 67 days). The reported complications from this study included 4% of filter tilt (>15 degrees), 5% of suspected PE, and 2% of symptomatic caval occlusion.

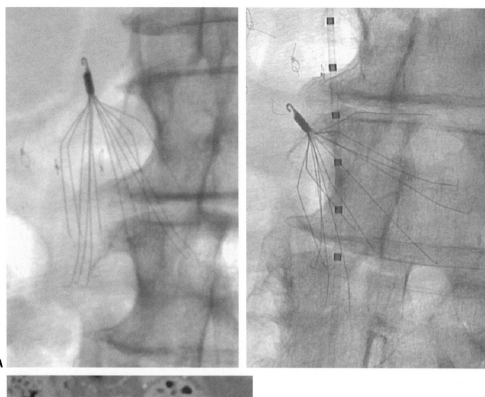

A   B

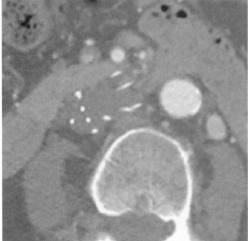

C

FIGURE 29-17. Migration, penetration, and fracture of a G2 Express filter in a 74-year-old woman with pulmonary embolism and traumatic subarachnoid hemorrhage. (**A**) G2 Express filter was placed below renal veins. The filter is slightly tilted. (**B**) Thirty-four days after the placement, the filter migrated with caval wall penetration. (**C**) Computed tomography scan at the level of the filter, showing caval wall penetration by three limbs into the retroperitoneal structures. The filter was removed successfully.

■ COMPLICATION IN VENA CAVA FILTER PLACEMENT

Complications associated with vena cava filter placement are grouped as complications related to contrast medium used for vena cavography, insertion site complications, complications at placement, complications after placement, complications of retrieval, and entrapment of wires and catheters by the filter.

Contrast Reactions and Contrast-Induced Nephropathy

Although the amount of contrast medium used for vena cavography is usually less than 50 mL in volume, iodinated contrast medium should be avoided in patients with a history of contrast allergy and renal failure. Steroid preparation or CO_2 should be used for patients with contrast allergy. CO_2 is the only known safe contrast agent in patients with renal failure. The plastic bag system is used for CO_2 delivery. CO_2 digital subtraction venography can provide the necessary vascular roadmap for safe filter placement.

Insertion Site Complications

The use of smaller sheath for filter placement has decreased the risk for insertion site complications. Complications of venous catheterization include puncture site venous thrombosis, arterial injury, and arteriovenous fistula. Facile catheterization technique with the venous puncture using a 21-gauge needle under ultrasound guidance has decreased the risk of puncture site complications.

Complications at Placement

Vena cava filters have been misplaced in various locations, including the iliac, subclavian, renal, hepatic, and gonadal veins and the right atrium and aorta (61–63). The use of preplacement vena cavography and fluoroscopy combined with the facile technique has decreased the incidence of misplacement. When a filter is misplaced or migrates to the chest, it must be retrieved immediately. If a permanent filter has been misplaced in a tributary vein, it may be left there since retrieval may result in vessel injury and bleeding. If a temporary filter has been misplaced, it should be retrieved using the standard retrieval snare. If the filter introducer with a dilator is pushed inadvertently without a guidewire, it can penetrate the caval wall with errant placement of the filter. If the apex of the filter has penetrated through the wall of the cava, it should be retrieved. If the repositioned filter has been deformed, a second filter should be placed above the first filter. If a filter has failed to expand fully upon discharge, a second filter should be placed above the first filter from the jugular approach. Manipulation of the incompletely opened filter by a guidewire or catheter may result in central migration of the filter. Tilting and asymmetric leg distribution should be left without intervention as they have not been associated with recurrent PE.

Complications After Filter Implantation

After placement of a filter, complications may develop, including migration, penetration, fracture/embolization, iliocaval thrombosis, retroperitoneal hematoma, and recurrent PE. Generally, there have been no clinical sequelae from minor migration and caval penetration, and this argues against unnecessary interventions. If a retrievable filter shows migration, fracture, caval penetration, or deformity, it should be removed when anticoagulation can be resumed or the risk period for PE has passed. If not, a second filter should be placed. If a filter or filter fragment has migrated into the right ventricle with or without pericardial tamponade, it should be removed by using a percutaneous method or surgically. Migration of a filter into the pulmonary artery is extremely rare, and removal of the filter may be difficult. If a retrievable filter has migrated into the pulmonary artery, it should be removed using a snare. Removal is not recommended for asymptomatic PE of filter fragments.

The incidence of vena cava occlusion has increased with the increased use of filters. This may be asymptomatic or may cause bilateral lower extremity swelling. Most symptomatic vena cava occlusions have involved infrarenal placement. Very few incidences of caval occlusion have been associated with suprarenal or SVC placement. Symptomatic occlusion of the vena cava harboring a filter requires endovascular intervention with catheter-directed thrombolysis or mechanical thrombectomy, balloon dilation, and stent placement through the filter. When the filter is incorporated within the occluded IVC, retrieval is usually difficult; and therefore, stents should be placed through the filter to achieve caval patency. If acute vena cava thrombosis is associated with bilateral DVT, thrombolysis of both femoral and iliac veins and IVC is performed before mechanical recanalization of the occluded IVC followed by stent placement of the IVC and both iliac veins. Recanalization can be achieved even for the chronically occluded IVC that harbors a filter.

Complications Associated with Filter Retrieval

Retrieval of vena cava filters is usually straightforward and safe when retrieval is attempted within the recommended dwell time. The OptEase filter is retrieved from the femoral approach and has the shortest dwell time of 2 weeks. If the filter has been placed for more

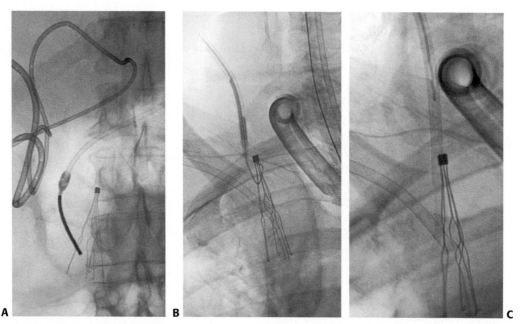

FIGURE 29-18. Guidewire dislodgment of a Greenfield filter. (**A**) Percutaneous stainless steel Greenfield filter was placed in the inferior vena cava (IVC) below the renal veins because of pulmonary embolism and a contraindication to anticoagulant therapy. (**B**) One week later, a J-tipped guidewire was entrapped by the filter, and the filter was pulled to the right brachiocephalic vein during a central venous catheter placement. (**C**) The guidewire was disengaged by advancing a catheter toward the hooks of the filter. The filter was left in the vein.

than 1 month, retrieval may be difficult. Recovery and G2 Express filters have much longer recommended dwell times, and retrieval may be possible after a year of placement. Prolonged dwell time and increasing patient age influence retrievability of these filters. Potential adverse events associated with retrieval include caval injury, caval stenosis, PE, DVT, filter fracture, migration, retrieval site bleeding, and contrast extravasation.

Guidewire Dislodgment of Vena Cava Filters

Dislodgement of IVC filters as a result of guidewire entrapment is a potential complication of the subsequent insertion of a central venous catheter (Fig. 29-18) (64). This complication can be avoided by limiting the distance that a guidewire is advanced during the insertion of a central venous catheter or by inserting the straight end of the guidewire. If the guidewire is caught in the filter, it should be disengaged by advancing a catheter or a guiding catheter caudally under fluoroscopy. If a filter is present in the SVC, fluoroscopy should be used when carefully inserting a central venous catheter. Fluoroscopy should also be used when a Swan–Ganz catheter is inserted from the femoral approach in the presence of a filter in the IVC.

■ DISCUSSION

The filter performance with respect to clot resolution and mechanical stability appears to be linked to the characteristics of the filter design (65). It appears that the simple conical design with separate filter limbs provides effective clot capturing and stability (Fig. 29-19). The hooks of each separate limb are found to be well incorporated into the wall of the cava covered by fibrous tissue. Because of its tenting effect on the thin caval wall, the filter hooks may appear to penetrate the caval wall (Fig. 29-20) (66). It has been documented that the original conical design of the Greenfield filter can trap significant amount of thrombus while maintaining normal caval blood flow, thus preventing caval occlusion. Other important factors that should be taken into consideration in the selection of filter may include the age of the patient, caval diameter, mechanical and structural stability,

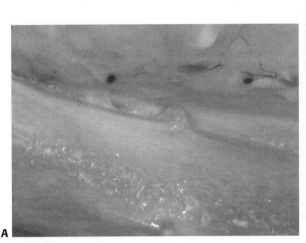
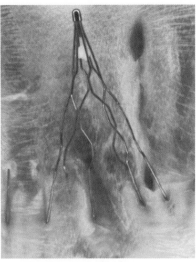

FIGURE 29-19. Titanium Greenfield filter in an ovine model. (**A**) Gross photograph of the inferior vena cava (IVC) at 60 days after filter placement. The hooks are well incorporated into the wall of the cava, and the extruded hook points are covered with a fibrous nodule. (**B**) Opened cava. The distal limbs and hooks are well incorporated, whereas the cone part of the filter is free of adhesion to the caval wall. (See color insert.)

magnetic resonance imaging compatibility, retrievability, patient life expectancy, and thrombogenicity.

Despite many efforts to produce an "ideal" filter for more than three decades, the currently marketed filters have shown adverse events that may occur during or after placement. Known adverse events may include death, misplacement, migration, penetration, fracture, and caval/filter occlusion. The most serious complications are cephalic migration of the filter or filter fragments to the heart and caudal migration associated with leg penetration into the pericaval structures. Both the percutaneous and surgical interventions have been used to remove filters from the right atrium and ventricle. Symptomatic caval penetration of permanent filters usually requires surgical intervention for

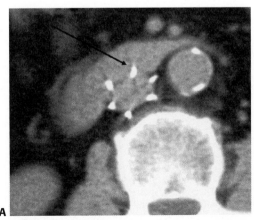
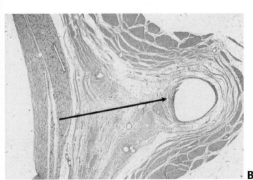

FIGURE 29-20. Pseudocaval penetration. (**A**) A computed tomography scan of a Greenfield filter shows the hooks projecting outside the caval wall, suggesting caval penetration. (**B**) Studies on animal have shown that the hooks that appear to have penetrated caval wall were in fact well incorporated with pericaval tissue (*arrow*).

removal whereas most retrievable filters with caval penetration have been removed using snaring devices.

The concept of a retrievable filter was introduced in 1986. There are two types of retrievable filters: the tethered temporary filter and the option filter. The tethered temporary device must be removed as it is tethered or attached to a catheter. It has been used in conjunction with catheter-directed thrombolysis or mechanical thrombectomy. There is no FDA-approved tethered temporary filter currently available for

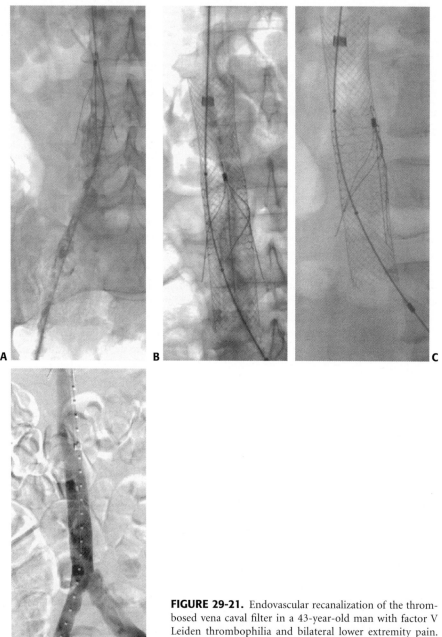

FIGURE 29-21. Endovascular recanalization of the thrombosed vena caval filter in a 43-year-old man with factor V Leiden thrombophilia and bilateral lower extremity pain. (**A**) Iliac and vena cavogram showing thrombosed inferior vena cava (IVC) and filter. (**B**) Placement of Wallstent through the IVC filter with additional Palmaz stent at the level of the filter showing compression of the caval filter. (**C**) Poststenting cavogram showing patent IVC.

standard use. The option filter is used increasingly as a nontethered temporary filter or a permanent filter. It may be removed when the risk of PE is over or anticoagulation can be resumed. Despite the general acceptance of option filters, the advantages for their use instead of using a permanent filter remains unproven.

In general, vena cava filters are 95% to 97% effective in preventing recurrent symptomatic PE, but symptomatic recurrent DVT appears to be higher at 35.7% with filter placement as compared with anticoagulant therapy alone at 27.5% (67). For this reason, IVC filters are often requested for removal when anticoagulation can be resumed in patients with venous thrombosis or PE. However, symptomatic PE is lower at 6.2% with filter placement as compared with anticoagulation at 15.1% (67). There are potential problems with retrievable vena cava filters. The current option filters approved by the FDA are approved for permanent placement, allowing the filters to remain permanently. No long-term data on the performance of retrievable filters are available. In current practice, less than 50% of retrievable filters are removed. Retrievability decreases with the increasing dwell time, particularly with the OptEase and Günther Tulip filters. As the retrievable filters are designed for removal, filter wires and fixation hooks seem to be soft, with resultant risk of fracture, penetration, and migration. Retrieval of the option filter is not without risks. Caval stenosis at the site of filter placement has occurred, which may lead to caval occlusion. Once the filter has been removed, there is risk for recurrent PE. It is unknown whether risk of retrieval is less than the risk of keeping a filter permanently. Retrieving the filter increases the cost. This additional cost of retrieval should be justified. The preferred indication for retrievable filters is the known time for risk for anticoagulation or DVT/PE. The advent of retrievable (option) filters has led to the increased use of the filter for prophylaxis as in trauma patients.

Filter retrieval is usually safe and easy in uncomplicated cases. If retrieval is performed within the recommended dwell time, retrieval success rates are 90% to 100%. Retrieval can be difficult when the filter is adhered with incorporation of the apex of the filter into the wall of the cava, forcing the interventionists to use various adjunctive techniques. Acute or chronic IVC occlusion after filter placement is not uncommon and requires advanced endoluminal techniques to reestablish caval blood flow (Fig. 29-21).

The current vena cava filters, both permanent and option filters, provide safe and effective protection against PE. Complications associated with filter placement may occur at placement or at follow-up. The use of vena cavography and thorough understanding of placement techniques can eliminate most adverse events at filter placement, but complications after placement appear to be related to the characteristics of the filter. Efforts to determine the characteristics of an "ideal" filter, defining appropriate indications and understanding the benefits of retrievable filters are ongoing. Accumulated data from careful clinical and imaging follow-up after filter placement will provide the basis for future development of an ideal filter and understanding of its appropriate clinical applications.

References

1. Senties AC, Carrera NF, Gordillo OG. Inferior vena cava ligation versus the Mobin-Uddin filter for prevention of recurrent pulmonary embolism. *Int Surg.* 1977;62:420.

2. Greenfield L, McCurdy J, Brown P, et al. A new intracaval filter permitting continued flow and resolution of emboli. *Surg.* 1973;73:599.

3. Grassi CJ, Swan TL, Cardella JF, et al. Quality improvement guidelines for percutaneous permanent inferior vena cava filter placement for the prevention of pulmonary embolism. *J Vasc Interv Radiol.* 2003;14:S271.

4. Cho KJ, Hawkins IF. *Carbon Dioxide Angiography: Principles, Techniques, and Practices.* London, England: Informa Healthcare; 2007.

5. Trigaux JP, Vandroogenbroek S, De Wispelaere J-F, et al. Congenital anomalies of the inferior vena cava and left renal vein: evaluation with spiral CT. *J Vasc Interv Radiol.* 1998;9:339.

6. Reed RA, Teitelbaum GP, Taylor FC, et al. Use of the bird's nest filter in oversized inferior venae cavae. *J Vasc Intervent Radiol.* 1991;2:447.

7. Bonn J, Liu JB, Eschelman DJ, et al. Intravascular ultrasound as an alternative to positive-contrast vena cavography prior to filter placement. *J Vasc Interv Radiol.* 1999;10:843.

8. Kalva SP, Chlapoutaki C, Wicky S, et al. Suprarenal inferior vena cava filters: a 20-year single-center experience. *J Vasc Intervent Radiol.* 2008;19:1041.

9. Greenfield L, Cho KJ, Proctor M, et al. Late results of suprarenal Greenfield vena cava filter placement. *Arch Surg.* 1992;127:969.

10. Usoh F, Hingorani A, Ascher E, et al. Long-term follow-up for superior vena cava filter placement. *Ann Vasc Surg.* 2009;23:350.

11. Hussain SM, McLafferty RB, Schmittling ZC, et al. Superior vena cava perforation and cardiac tamponade after filter placement in the superior vena cava—a case report. *Vasc Endovascular Surg.* 2005;39:367.

12. Cousins GR, DeAnda A Jr. Superior vena cava filter erosion into the ascending aorta. *Ann Thorac Surg.* 2006;81:1907.

13. Greenfield LJ, Proctor MC. Twenty-year clinical experience with the Greenfield filter. *Cardiovasc Surg.* 1995;3:199.

14. Patterson R, Fowl RJ, Lubbers DJ, et al. Repositioning of partially dislodged Greenfield filters from the right atrium by use of a tip deflection wire. *J Vasc Surg.* 1990;12:70–72.

15. Braun MA, Collins MB, Sarrafizadeh M, et al. Percutaneous retrieval of tandem right atrial Greenfield filters. *AJR Am J Roentgenol.* 1991;157: 199.

16. Carabasi R, Moritz M, Jarrell B. Complications encountered with the use of the Greenfield filter. *Am J Surg* 1987;154:163.

17. Appleberg M, Crozier JA. Duodenal penetration by a Greenfield caval filter. *Aust N Z J Surg.* 1991; 61:957.

18. Messmer JM, Greenfield LJ. Greenfield caval filters: long-term radiographic follow-up study. *Radiology.* 1985;156:613.

19. Taheri S, Kulaylat M, Johnson E, Hoover E. A complication of the Greenfield filter: fracture and distal migration of two struts—a case report. *J Vasc Surg.* 1992;16:96.

20. Balshi JD, Cantelmo NL, Menzoian JO. Complications of caval interruption by Greenfield filter in quadriplegics. *J Vasc Surg.* 1989;9:558.

21. Greenfield LJ, Cho KJ, Proctor M, et al. Results of a multicenter study of the modified hook titanium Greenfield filter. *J Vasc Surg.* 1991;14: 253.

22. Mitchell WB, Bonn J. Percutaneous retrieval of a Greenfield filter after migration to the left pulmonary artery. *J Vasc Interv Radiol.* 2005;16:1013.

23. Friedell ML, Goldenkranz RJ, Parsonnet V, et al. Migration of a Greenfield filter to the pulmonary artery: a case report. *J Vasc Surg.* 1986;3:929.

24. Xenos ES, Minion DJ, Sorial EE, et al. Endovascular retrieval of an intraaortic Greenfield vena cava filter. *Vasc Endovascular Surg.* 1986;3:929.

25. Cho KJ, Greenfield LJ, Proctor MC, et al. Evaluation of a percutaneous stainless steel Greenfield filter. *J Vasc Interv Radiol.* 1997;8:181.

26. Greenfield LJ, Proctor MC. The percutaneous Greenfield filter: outcomes and practice patterns. *J Vasc Surg.* 2000;32:888.

27. Vesely T, Darcy M, Picus D, Hicks M. Technical problems associated with placement of the Bird's Nest inferior vena cava filter. *AJR Am J Roentgenol.* 1992;158:875.

28. Rogoff PA, Hilgenberg AD, Miller SL, et al. Cephalic migration of the Bird's nest inferior vena cava filter: report of two cases. *Radiology.* 1992;184:819.

29. Simon M, Athanasoulis C, Kim D, et al. Simon nitinol inferior vena cava filter: initial clinical experience. *Radiology.* 1989;172:99.

30. Grassi CJ, Matsumoto A, Teitelbaum G. Vena caval occlusion after Simon Nitinol filter placement: identification with MR imaging in patients with malignancy. *J Vasc Interv Radiol.* 1992;3:535.

31. Leask RL, Johnston KW, Ojha M. In vitro hemodynamic evaluation of a Simon nitinol vena cava filter: possible explanation of IVC occlusion. *J Vasc Interv Radiol.* 2001;12:613.

32. McCowan T, Ferris EJ, Carver DK, Molpus M. Complications of the Nitinol vena caval filter. *J Vasc Interv Radiol.* 1992;3:401.

33. LaPlante JS, Contractor FM, Kiproff PM, et al. Migration of the Simon nitinol vena cava filter to the chest. *AJR Am J Roentgenol.* 1993;160: 385.

34. Poletti PA, Becker CD, Prina L, et al. Long-term results of the Simon nitinol inferior vena cava filter. *Eur Radiol.* 1998;8:289.

35. Ricco JB, Crochet D, Sebilotte P, et al. Percutaneous transvenous caval interruption with "LGM" filter. *Ann Vasc Surg.* 1988;2:242.

36. Millward SF, Marsh JI, Peterson RA, et al. LGM (Vena Tech) vena cava filter: clinical experience in 64 patients. *J Vasc Interv Radiol.* 1991;2:429.

37. Le Blanche AF, Benazzouz A, Reynaud P, et al. The VenaTech LP permanent caval filter: effectiveness and safety in the prevention of pulmonary embolism—a European multicenter study. *J Vasc Interv Radiol.* 2008;19:509.

38. Harlal A, Ojha M, Jonston KW. Vena cava filter performance based on hemodynamics and reported thrombosis and pulmonary embolism patterns. *J Vasc Interv Radiol.* 2007;18:103.

39. Rousseau H, Perreault P, Otal P, et al. The 6-F nitinol TrapEase inferior vena cava filter: results of a prospective multicenter trial. *J Vasc Interv Radiol.* 2001;12:299.

40. Kalva SP, Wicky S, Waltman AC, et al. TrapEase vena cava filter: experience in 751 patients. *J Endovasc Ther.* 2006;13:365.

41. Porcellini M, Stassano P, Musumeci A, et al. Intracardiac migration of nitinol TrapEase vena cava filter and paradoxical embolism. *Eur J Cardiothorac Surg.* 2002;22:460.

42. Haddadian B, Shaikh F, Djelmami-Hani M, et al. Sudden cardiac death caused by migration of a TrapEase inferior vena cava filter: case report and review of the literature. *Clin Cardiol.* 2008;31:84.

43. Ziegler JW, Dietrich GJ, Cohen SA, et al. PROOF trial: protection from pulmonary embolism with the OptEase filter. *J Vasc Interv Radiol.* 2008; 19:1165.

44. Mahrer A, Zippel D, Garniek A, et al. Retrievable vena cava filters in major trauma patients: prevalence of thrombus within the filter. *Cardiovasc Intervent Radiol.* 2008;31:785.

45. Hoppe H, Nutting CW, Smouse HR, et al. Günther tulip filter retrievability multicenter study including CT follow-up: final report. *J Vasc Interv Radiol.* 2006;17:1017.

46. Galhotra S, Amesur NB, Zajko AB, et al. Migration of the Günther Tulip inferior vena cava filter to the chest. *J Vasc Interv.* 2007;18:158.

47. Bochenek KM, Aruny JE, Tal MG. Right atrial migration and percutaneous retrieval of a Günther Tulip inferior vena cava filter. *J Vasc Interv Radiol.* 2003;14:207.

48. Parkin E, Serracino-Inglott F, Chalmers N, et al. Symptomatic perforation of a retrievable inferior vena cava filter after a dwell time of 5 years. *J Vasc Surg.* 2009;50:417.

49. Marquess JS, Burke CT, Beecham AH, et al. Factors associated with failed retrieval of the Günther Tulip inferior vena cava filter. *J Vasc Interv Radiol.* 2008;19:1321.

50. Lyon SM, Riojas GE, Uberoi R, et al. Short- and long-term retrievability of the Celect Vena Cava filter: results from a multi-institutional registry. *J Vasc Interv.* 2009;20:1441.

51. Sadaf A, Rasuli P, Olivier A, et al. Significant caval penetration by the Celect inferior vena cava filter: attributable to filter design? *J Vasc Interv Radiol.* 2007;18:1447.

52. Hull JE, Robertson SW. Bard recovery filter: evaluation and management of vena cava limb perforation, fracture, and migration. *J Vasc Interv Radiol.* 2009;20:52.

53. Nazzal M, Abbas J, Shattu J, et al. Complications secondary to the Bard retrievable filter: a case report. *Ann Vasc Surg.* 2008;22:684.

54. Hull JE, Han J, Giessel GM. Retrieval of the recovery filter after arm perforation, fracture, and migration to the right ventricle. *J Vasc Interv Radiol.* 2008;19:1107.

55. Saeed I, Garcia M, McNicholas K. Right ventricular migration of a recovery IVC filter's fractured wire with subsequent pericardial tamponade. *Cardiovasc Intervent Radiol.* 2006;29:685.

56. Bui JT, West DL, Pinto C, et al. Right ventricular migration and endovascular removal of an inferior vena cava filter. *J Vasc Interv Radiol.* 2008;19:141.

57. Vergara GR, Wallace WF, Bennett KR. Spontaneous migration of an inferior vena cava filter resulting in cardiac tamponade and percutaneous filter retrieval. *Catheter Cardiovasc Interv.* 2007;69:300.

58. Gupta P, Lopez JA, Ghole V, et al. Aortic and vertebral penetration by a G2 inferior vena cava filter: report of a case. *J Vasc Interv Radiol.* 2009;20:829.

59. Ganguli S, Tham JC, Komlos F, et al. Fracture and migration of a suprarenal inferior vena cava filter in a pregnant patient. *J Vasc Interv Radiol.* 2006; 17:1707.

60. Johnson MS. The safety and effectiveness of the Retrievable Option™ Inferior Vena Cava Filter: a prospective, multicenter U.S. clinical study in patients at permanent or temporary risk for pulmonary embolism. *J Vasc Interv Radiol.* 2009; 20(suppl):S13.

61. Schneider RC. A misplaced caval filter: its removal from the heart without cardiopulmonary bypass. *Arch Surg.* 1980;115:1133.

62. Lahey SJ, Meyer LP, Karchmer AW, et al. Misplaced caval filter and subsequent pericardial tamponade. *Ann Thorac Surg.* 1991;51:299.

63. Kaufman JL, Berman JA. Accidental intraaortic placement of a Greenfield filter. *Ann Vasc Surg.* 1999;13:541.

64. Liddell RP, Spinosa DJ, Matsumoto AH, et al. Guidewire entrapment in a Greenfield IVC Filter: "rail and reins technique." *Clin Radiol.* 2000;55:878.

65. Proctor MC, Cho KJ, Greenfield LJ. In vivo evaluation of vena cava filters: can function be linked to design characteristics? *Cardiovasc Intervent Radiol.* 2000;23:460.

66. Proctor MC, Greenfield LJ, Cho KJ, Moursi MM, James EA. Assessment of apparent vena caval penetration by the Greenfield filter. *J Endovascul Surg.* 1998;5:251.

67. The PREPIC Study Group. Eight-year follow-up of patients with permanent vena cava filters in the prevention of pulmonary embolism: the PREPIC (Prevention du Risque d'Embolie Pulmonaire par Interruption Cave) randomized study. *Circulation.* 2005;112:416.

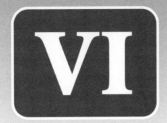
Specific Complications of Pediatric Interventions

CHAPTER

30

Cardiac Catheterization in Children

THOMAS R. LLOYD

Cardiac catheterization of children presents substantial challenges. Pediatric cardiologists must obtain accurate diagnostic information and perform effective interventions on patients with an astonishing array of cardiovascular malformations, many of whom have undergone any of a dizzying number of surgical interventions. Although only 2 decades of age separate the newborn from the young adult, the body size range of this patient population spans more than two orders of magnitude.

Newborns exemplify these challenges, beginning with the problem of gaining access to their small central vessels. Catheter diameters of 4 to 5 French are usually required for adequate angiocardiographic flow rates and diagnostic fidelity of intracardiac pressure recording. Typical diagnostic catheters occupy a very large proportion of the diameter of a neonate's femoral artery or vein, which predisposes to access site complications. Right heart catheterization is particularly important in congenital heart disease, and the anatomy is often complex. Even when the intracardiac anatomy is not particularly challenging, the small heart requires catheter courses with turns of very short radius, yet the sort of high-torque, preformed catheter that would seem ideal for these purposes presents a substantial risk of perforation in these thin-walled, highly compliant hearts. Because of their small size, newborns are very sensitive to blood loss, so blood waste is unacceptable, but essentially all newborns have intracardiac shunts, so reinfusion of withdrawn blood risks systemic embolization of any air or thrombus present. In addition, many newborns who require catheterization have lesions with hemodynamics which are fundamentally incompatible with extrauterine life.

Catheterization through the full spectrum of the pediatric age range requires familiarity not only with patients of widely different sizes and hemodynamics (both normal and pathologic), but also with the full range of human intellectual and emotional development. This has substantial impact on patient cooperation and response to sedation, and is complicated by well-known associations of congenital heart disease and developmental disabilities in certain syndromes. Although those of us who also care for adults with congenital heart disease (who comprise one-fifth of the catheterization procedures performed at the University of Michigan C.S. Mott Children's Hospital) are well aware of the different challenges in these patients, those involved in the emerging field of fetal interventional cardiology have an entirely different set of challenges which are well beyond the scope of this chapter.

Although the complications of catheterization in children have been a matter of clinical interest and study since the beginning of the practice, contemporary data is relatively sparse in the literature. Patient numbers are small overall (very few institutions perform as many as 1000 in a year), and the wide variety of diagnoses and patient sizes hinder collection of homogeneous populations of sufficient size for statistically valid clinical studies. Published reports tend to be highly focused on particular procedures, on individual complications, and to involve small numbers of patients. More comprehensive reviews are further hampered by the lack of consensus on best practices in identifying and collecting complications, which events to consider as complications, and how best to classify and analyze the events collected.

The University of Michigan Congenital Heart Center's quality assurance program requires identification of complications observed during each procedure in the cardiac catheterization laboratories at C.S. Mott Children's Hospital, with complications entered into a database common to all the laboratories. Complications can be entered by the recording technician, the circulating nurse, or the attending physician, and entry of complications or an affirmative statement of no complications is required to end each procedure.

For the roughly one-third of our patients who are hospital inpatients, a catheterization laboratory nurse collects information on complications arising during the 24 hours following the procedure from the patient's inpatient nurse. For patients discharged on the day of catheterization, complications noted in the post-catheterization recovery area are entered by the recovery nurses. In addition, a pediatric cardiology nurse practitioner contacts the family after 24 hours to identify any complications occurring after discharge. Complications noted within 24 hours of catheterization in both inpatients and outpatients are then added to the database. All complications are evaluated, tabulated, and summarized by the medical director of the catheterization laboratories, and then reviewed and discussed at pediatric cardiology quality assurance meetings.

Complications are classified as major or minor. Major complications are those which are considered life-threatening, which threaten or result in permanent sequelae, or which require additional invasive procedures or prolong hospital stay. All other complications are considered minor. Thus, an instance of transient complete heart block treated with atropine is considered a minor complication, but a similar instance in which chest compressions are initiated will be considered a major complication. Similarly, a case in which an occlusion device embolizes and is retrieved during the index catheterization is counted as a minor complication, but it is a major complication if the device is retrieved at a subsequent catheterization or at surgery.

For analysis purposes, cases with major complications are assigned to one of a series of hierarchical categories, the first of which is death. Any death occurring within 30 days of catheterization is included in the database, with two exceptions: 1) deaths following and reasonably related to a subsequent procedure, for example, surgery, except when the subsequent procedure was necessitated by complications of the index catheterization, and 2) deaths resulting from withdrawal of support when the decision to withdraw support was based on the findings of cardiac catheterization rather than its complications (1). The second category includes patients requiring resuscitation who survived, and the third category is patients who suffered central nervous system events. The fourth category is patients who required unplanned endotracheal intubation, and the fifth includes those treated for hypotension. The remaining categories include patients with myocardial perforation, complications related to device embolization or placement, and complications not otherwise categorized.

■ COMPLICATIONS OF CATHETERIZATION

Table 30-1 summarizes complication rates from several contemporary series (2–6) of pediatric cardiac catheterization procedures, as well as 10 years' data from the University of Michigan Congenital Heart Center. Those series denoted as *comprehensive* include all procedures (diagnostic, interventional, and electrophysiologic) and all identified complications. Those series denoted as *limited* were restricted to certain interventional procedures and focused on intraprocedural complications. Complications were identified by anesthesiologists in the series from Birmingham (4) and by cardiologists in the series from Toronto, Paris, and Cincinnati (2,3,5,6). Despite the diverse methodology employed, the rates of minor complications, major complications, and death were remarkably consistent in these 6 reports from 5 institutions in 4 nations on 2 continents.

The most common minor complication reported at C.S. Mott Children's Hospital was emesis, which occurred in 295, or 35% of the 847 cases with minor complications. Emesis is not considered a complication of catheterization in any other reported series, but we have considered it beneficial to our patients to reduce the occurrence of emesis after catheterization, and have therefore monitored it as a complication. Arrhythmias were reported in 157 patients (18.5% of minor complications, 1.9% of the population). These are fairly equally divided

TABLE 30-1 **Complications of Catheterization in Children**

Institution, Years	Procedures	Minor (%)	Major (%)	Deaths (%)
Comprehensive series[a]				
HSC, 1987–1993 (2)	4952	458 (9.25)	102 (2.06)	7 (0.14)
HSC, 1993–2006 (3)	11,073	663 (5.99)	195 (1.76)	25 (0.23)
BCH, 1993–2001 (4)	4454	323 (7.25)	91 (2.04)	4 (0.09)
UMCHC, 1997–2006	8409	847 (10.07)	99 (1.18)	10 (0.12)
Limited series[a]				
GHNEM, 1997–2004 (5)	1282		23 (1.79)	4 (0.31)
CHMC, 1996–20006[b]	578		11 (1.90)	1 (0.17)

[a]*Comprehensive series* report major and minor complications from all catheterization laboratory procedures performed; *limited series* include only interventional procedures, and the report of major complications and deaths.
[b]Schroeder et al. (6) is limited to complications requiring emergent surgical procedures.
BCH, Birmingham Children's Hospital, Birmingham, UK; CHMC, Children's Hospital Medical Center, Cincinnati, Ohio; GHNEM, Groupe Hospitalier Necker Enfants Malades, Paris, France; HSC, Hospital for Sick Children, University of Toronto School of Medicine, Toronto, Ontario, Canada; UMCHC, University of Michigan Congenital Heart Center, C.S. Mott Children's Hospital, Ann Arbor, Michigan.

between heart block and supraventricular tachycardia, with 3 cases of ventricular tachycardia and 1 case of persistent right bundle branch block. Catheter entry site complications were reported in 147 patients (17.4% of minor complications, 1.7% of procedures), of which 67 (46%) had hematomas, 48 (33%) had bleeding requiring pressure, and 32 (22%) were noted to have diminished pulse.

Vascular complications were the most common events in the Toronto reports (2,3), and ultrasound studies have reported iliofemoral thrombus in up to 10% of children 24 hours after catheterization (7). Depending on the condition of the limb, patients with diminished distal pulse can be managed expectantly or treated with systemic heparin or thrombolytics (8). Minor respiratory depression (requiring stimulation, repositioning, or supplemental oxygen) was reported in 113 of our patients (13.3% of minor complications, 1.3% of procedures). This complication is limited to procedures done under sedation, and the series of Mehta et al. (3) and Bennett (4) et al. employed general anesthesia in all cases; general anesthesia is used in 30% of procedures done at our institution. Embolization of an occlusion device, coil, stent, guidewire, or catheter fragment occurred in 29 cases (3.4% of minor complications, 0.3% of procedures), similar to the 4.8% of minor complications reported by Mehta et al. (3) and the 3.9% of minor complications reported by Vitiello et al. (2) Minor perforations

of the myocardium, often incidental to transseptal puncture, were noted in 13 cases (1.5% of minor complications, 0.2% of procedures), again similar to the rates of 1.7% and 1.4% of minor complications reported in the Toronto series.

The 99 major complications observed in the Michigan series consisted of 10 deaths, 20 instances of successful resuscitation, 8 central nervous system events, 21 unplanned intubations, 11 patients treated for hypotension, 11 myocardial perforations, 12 device embolizations or unsatisfactory placements, and 6 otherwise unclassified events. Newborns and infants under 6 months of age accounted for 43 of the major complications, including 8 of the 10 deaths (newborns make up less than 10% of our catheterization volume). Interventional procedures were involved in 46 of the cases with major complications, including 7 of the 10 deaths. In 17 of these cases, the interventional procedure was valvuloplasty, angioplasty, or stenting, whereas occlusion procedures were involved in 14 cases. The remaining 15 cases involved atrial septal puncture, septostomy, or radiofrequency ablation.

■ RISK FACTORS

The study of Vitiello et al. (2) identified patients under the age of 2 years and those having interventional procedures as being at higher risk of any complication, with inconsistent but statistically significant effects of the year in which catheterization was performed. Major complications were more frequent in patients under the age of 6 months, those having interventional procedures, and those who were hospital inpatients at the time of catheterization. Of the 7 patients who died, 5 were newborns or young infants, and cardiac or aortic perforation occurred in 4. Mehta et al. (3) reported as independent risk factors for complications younger age, male sex, and inpatient status, with patient age being the only consistent risk factor for major complications. Bennett et al. (4) noted higher complication rates in patients less than 1 year of age and modest risk of complications for occlusion of patent ductus arteriosus or atrial septal defect compared to other interventions or to diagnostic catheterization; further analysis of these data is complicated by the authors' inability to identify the nature of the complication in 161 of their cases (for purposes of Table 30-1 these have been assumed to be minor complications). Agnoletti et al. (5) studied interventional procedures only, excluding atrial septostomies, and reported significant association of major procedural complications with technical challenge of the procedure, critical clinical condition of the patient prior to catheterization, in-training status of the primary operator, and equipment failure during the procedure. They also noted a significant contribution of operator error to the risk of complications.

Schroeder et al. (6) studied surgical emergencies which occurred during interventional catheterizations, adding endomyocardial biopsy, transhepatic vascular access, and transseptal puncture to the usual suite of interventional procedures. No procedures were identified as being particularly prone to eventuation of surgical emergency. Carmosino et al. (9) reported a series of 141 cardiac catheterizations on children with pulmonary artery hypertension with major complications in 5% and death in 1.4%. Risk was especially high in patients with suprasystemic pulmonary artery pressure. Pulmonary artery hypertensive crisis was considered responsible for 3 of our 11 patients with hypotension and 2 of the 20 patients who survived resuscitation.

As mentioned in the preceding text, and in contradistinction to the other reports discussed, most catheterization procedures at C. S. Mott Children's Hospital do not involve general anesthesia, and therefore unplanned endotracheal intubation is a more prominent major complication in our series. Of the 21 instances of this complication, 5 occurred late enough after catheterization to raise substantial doubt as to a direct relationship to the procedure. In an additional 4 cases, patients sent from intensive care units with endotracheal tubes in place were inadvertently extubated in the catheterization laboratory, requiring reintubation. The remaining 12 cases are instructive: Four patients were neonates receiving prostaglandin infusion, a well-known risk factor for apnea. Sedative medications were thought to be responsible for respiratory failure in four cases, with one patient receiving multiple doses of sedation for a prolonged procedure and the other three responding in an apparently idiosyncratic fashion. Upper airway obstruction contributed to failure of sedation in the remaining four cases, with two cases of vocal cord paralysis and two cases of obstructive sleep apnea.

Central nervous system events are rightly feared by all practitioners of cardiac catheterization. Although intracardiac thrombus is uncommon in pediatric patients and atherosclerotic plaque disruption is exceedingly rare, most pediatric patients will have intracardiac shunts which permit paradoxical embolization of venous thrombi to the systemic circulation. Of the 8 patients in our series who had central nervous system events (0.09%), 6 had thromboembolic strokes. Of this number, five had cyanotic heart disease, three had prolonged procedures, and in three cases heparin administration was not documented. The sole thromboembolic stroke patient without cyanosis was an adolescent with ectopic atrial tachycardia who underwent a 5-hour ablation procedure. One patient suffered apparent air embolism from aortography and recovered completely with the aid of hyperbaric oxygen therapy. The final patient, an adolescent with a history of prior ablation of atrioventricular nodal tachycardia and a seizure disorder, developed intractable seizures during an electrophysiologic study and was transferred to the pediatric intensive care unit, where video-EEG studies demonstrated pseudoseizures. Liu et al. (10) studied neurologic complications of catheterization at the Children's Cardiac Centre of the University of Hong Kong, identifying 14 cases in 12 years (0.38%). Half of these were embolic in nature, with three cases of hypoxic-ischemic encephalopathy from cerebral underperfusion, two cases of subdural hemorrhage (one from therapy for femoral artery thrombosis), and single cases of hypoglycemic brain injury and brachial plexus injury from positioning under general anesthesia. Agnoletti et al. (5) reported stroke in 0.10% of their patients, and stroke rates were 0.10% and 0.13% in the Toronto series (2,3). Compression neuropathies, including brachial plexus, cranial nerve, and femoral nerve injuries, were reported in 0.06% (3) and 0.10% (5).

■ MANAGEMENT AND BAILOUT TECHNIQUES

Complications specific to valvuloplasty, pulmonary artery or coarctation angioplasty or stenting, and occlusion of septal defects or the ductus arteriosus will be discussed in subsequent chapters. Balloon atrial septostomy, the first catheter intervention to find widespread clinical acceptance (11), is performed less frequently now that neonatal repair of transposition of the great arteries is routine, but complications are still observed.

In two of our cases, hypotension was successfully treated with volume and pressors, but a third patient who developed an occlusive dissection of the ductus arteriosus required resuscitation with ECMO. Two patients who required blade septostomies suffered major complications, one requiring surgical repair of left atrial perforation and the other, who was moribund on arrival, expiring despite ECMO support. In all, myocardial perforation contributed to major complications in 18 cases, including 4 deaths and 3 survivors of resuscitation. Surgical repair was required in 4 of the 14 survivors and was also performed in 2 of the fatal cases. Transseptal puncture was responsible for one case requiring surgical repair in an infant, and two cases that were treated with percutaneous drainage. Both these patients were adolescents who had ablation procedures for accessory connections. Another patient who developed acute hemopericardium requiring drainage had radiofrequency ablation in the right atrium only, without transseptal puncture. Surgical repair was required in one of the two newborns with

significant perforations of the right ventricular infundibulum by guidewires and in one of the four newborns with guidewire perforations of the left ventricle. This baby, who died, had critical aortic stenosis, as did the two neonates who survived resuscitation.

Newborns with hypoplastic left heart syndrome complicated by intact atrial septum or highly restrictive atrial septal defect cannot survive with medical therapy alone and are poor candidates for surgical palliation (12). Blade septostomy, static balloon septostomy, or atrial septal stenting is usually performed to improve survival, but these patients are very high risk because they possess multiple risk factors: all are neonates, all have pulmonary artery hypertension (due to pulmonary venous hypertension), all have hemodynamics incompatible with postnatal survival, and most have a very thick atrial septum with a tiny left atrial cavity, with the septum typically in a very abnormal position. Four of our patients with major complications suffered from this condition; one required surgical repair of perforation, one required resuscitation with ECMO, and two expired (one after surgical repair of perforation). A high index of suspicion for myocardial perforation must be maintained when performing catheterization in children, and operators should be skilled in percutaneous drainage of the pericardium. Tamponade is the likeliest cause of pulseless electrical activity arrest in the pediatric catheterization laboratory, and pericardiocentesis should be initiated without delay for echocardiographic confirmation. If confirmation of the diagnosis is needed, a small amount of radiographic contrast can be injected through the pericardiocentesis needle prior to advancing the guidewire. Autotransfusion of blood withdrawn from the pericardial space is useful in supporting patients acutely, and if drainage continues to be brisk, emergency surgical repair is indicated.

Hypotension was the major complication in 11 of our patients and was responsible for cardiac arrest in 9 of the 20 patients, who survived resuscitation, as well as 2 deaths. In addition to the 3 previously mentioned balloon atrial septostomy patients and the 5 patients with pulmonary hypertensive crises, 6 of these events were attributed to the effects of general anesthesia. Two were managed without further complication, and were thought to be idiosyncratic, but four cases, all of whom had myocardial disease, required resuscitation. Blood loss was considered responsible for hypotension in two neonates, both of whom responded well to transfusion. However, one of these patients developed necrotizing enterocolitis and died. Four of our patients had a specifically catheter-related cause of hypotension. In one patient, a 2-month-old who required ECMO support after cardiac surgery, refractory hypotension occurred during a catheterization requested to document the status of the coronary circulation. The pigtail catheter in the aortic root was found to be stenting the aortic valve open, and the hypotension resolved with withdrawal of the catheter. In three other cases, hypotension was caused by interventional sheaths across the tricuspid valve in patients with elevated right ventricular pressure. Resuscitation was required in two of these cases, one in a young infant needing pulmonary artery stenting and one in an infant with multiple ventricular septal defects having transcatheter occlusion of a large muscular defect. In both cases, substitution of a less stiff guidewire in the interventional sheath allowed the procedure to be finished safely. In the other case, again an infant with multiple ventricular septal defects, hypotension occurred each time the occluder device was advanced into the heart, and the procedure was terminated.

Otherwise unclassified major complications included single instances of hypercyanotic spell and lobar pneumonia in young infants with tetralogy of Fallot and a case of pulmonary hemorrhage complicating diagnostic catheterization performed under general anesthesia. The remaining cases had vascular access site complications. A retroperitoneal hematoma occurred in a child who had transcatheter occlusion of an atrial septal defect, but did not require surgical intervention. Superficial femoral artery thrombosis was treated surgically in a middle aged obese man who had his aortic coarctation stented. An 8-month-old child with persistent postoperative cyanosis due to previously unrecognized persistent left superior vena cava returning to the left atrium developed hemothorax requiring percutaneous drainage after transcatheter occlusion of the anomalous vessel from the left subclavian vein approach. The subclavian artery had been entered inadvertently prior to achieving subclavian vein access, and it was unclear whether the bleeding was due to arterial puncture, the venous access site, or injury to the left superior vena cava from the occlusion procedure.

Bailout from an unusual access site complication is shown in Figure 30-1. Shortly after placement of a 6-French sheath in the right femoral artery, moderate hemorrhage was noted from a small perforation in the proximal portion of the sheath. Rather than replacing the dilator and guidewire, which would have controlled the bleeding and permitted replacement of the sheath in a simple fashion, pressure was applied to the sheath, resulting in complete fracture of the sheath and migration of the fractured end under the skin, where it formed an arteriocutaneous fistula, resulting in brisk hemorrhage. Had any portion of the sheath remained external, it might have been removed with an instrument or by passing a balloon catheter into the lumen for hemostasis and to remove the sheath remnant. Instead, pressure was applied to the entry site to control bleeding and the left femoral artery was entered, passing a 4-French Judkins left 2.5 catheter into the right iliac artery retrogradely. A 10-mm Amplatz Goose Neck snare was passed through the coronary catheter and used to snare the sheath remnant. This was then pulled back to the iliac bifurcation, whereupon the sheath remnant buckled at the snare site, allowing it to be withdrawn to the tip of the left femoral sheath. A 0.018-inch Cope wire was passed into the 6-French left femoral artery sheath alongside the 4-French left coronary catheter, and the sheath fragment, snare and coronary catheter, and femoral sheath were removed en bloc, leaving the Cope wire in place to maintain access for the procedure. Angiography of the iliac arteries at the conclusion of the catheterization showed no adverse consequences of this adventure. Figure 30-2 illustrates how bailout procedures can have their own complications. In this patient, an occlusion coil embolized to the right iliac artery and could not be retrieved with a snare. Retrieval forceps were used to extract the coil, resulting in the dissection seen in Figure 30-2. The dissection progressed to complete occlusion, requiring stenting as illustrated. Although lower extremity blood flow

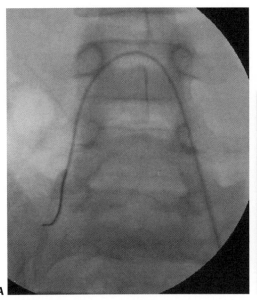
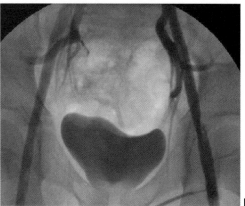

FIGURE 30-1. (**A**) A 10-mm Amplatz Goose Neck Snare (ev3 Endovascular) is grasping the fragment of a 6-French sheath in the right femoral artery which is functioning as an arteriocutaneous fistula (see text for details). The snare has been passed through a 4-French Judkins left coronary artery catheter inserted through a left femoral artery sheath which has been placed for the purpose of retrieving the fractured right femoral sheath. (**B**) After completion of the catheterization through the left femoral artery, injection at the iliac bifurcation demonstrates patency of both iliac and femoral arteries.

was well preserved, this patient suffered lumbar plexus nerve injury which eventually resolved.

Some complications of cardiac catheterization may not become apparent until long after the procedure. Occlusion of the femoral or iliac veins or the infrarenal inferior vena cava may only be noted when future attempts to cannulate the vessels are frustrated. Although alternative

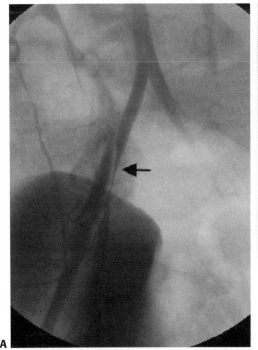
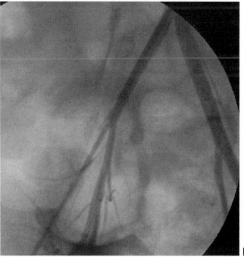

FIGURE 30-2. (**A**) Injection through the arterial sheath after retrieval of an embolized coil shows dissection of the right common iliac artery (*arrow*). (**B**) After completing the planned procedure, a second injection through the sheath shows iliac artery occlusion. (*continued*)

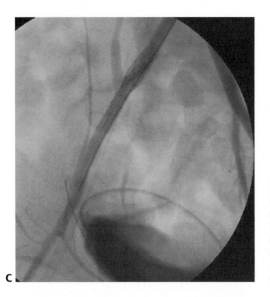

FIGURE 30-2. (*Continued*) (**C**) After placement of P154 stents (Johnson & Johnson Interventional) in the common and external iliac arteries, injection shows patency of these arteries as well as the right femoral artery. The right internal iliac artery remains occluded and is jailed by the external iliac artery stent. This infant suffered a lumbosacral plexus nerve injury, which required months to resolve.

routes of access, such as transhepatic puncture (13) have been developed, the femoral veins have many advantages. It is therefore exciting that methods of restoring patency to iliofemoral veins and inferior venae cavae are being devel-

oped (14). Another catheterization complication which, in our experience, has only been recognized in follow up is femoral arteriovenous fistula. We reported a technique for transcatheter occlusion of these fistulae which we

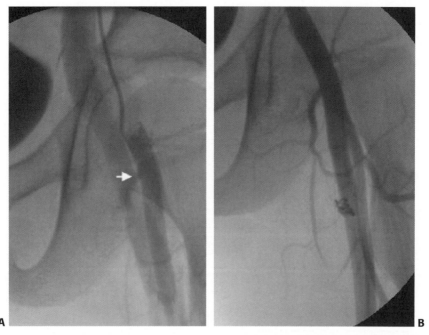

FIGURE 30-3. (**A**) Injection of the left femoral artery demonstrates a femoral arteriovenous fistula (*arrow*). This patient was 7 years old, and had previously been catheterized through both femoral veins for placement of stents at the bifurcation of his right ventricle to pulmonary artery conduit, which was part of his repair of truncus arteriosus. A thrill in the groin had been noted on a follow-up examination. (**B**) Angiography after coil embolization of the arteriovenous fistula shows patency of the left femoral artery with complete occlusion of the fistula.

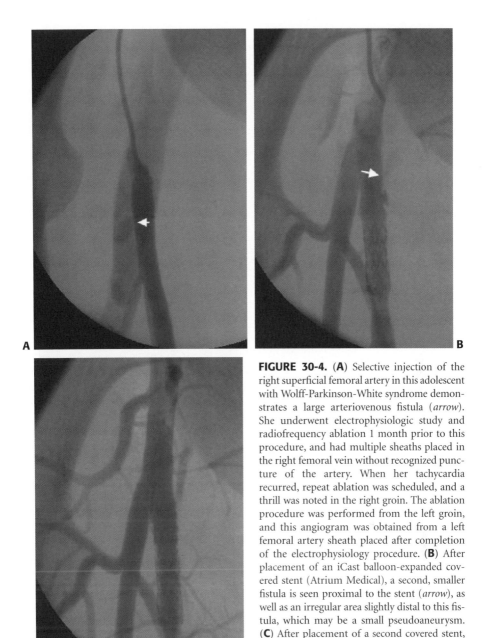

FIGURE 30-4. (**A**) Selective injection of the right superficial femoral artery in this adolescent with Wolff-Parkinson-White syndrome demonstrates a large arteriovenous fistula (*arrow*). She underwent electrophysiologic study and radiofrequency ablation 1 month prior to this procedure, and had multiple sheaths placed in the right femoral vein without recognized puncture of the artery. When her tachycardia recurred, repeat ablation was scheduled, and a thrill was noted in the right groin. The ablation procedure was performed from the left groin, and this angiogram was obtained from a left femoral artery sheath placed after completion of the electrophysiology procedure. (**B**) After placement of an iCast balloon-expanded covered stent (Atrium Medical), a second, smaller fistula is seen proximal to the stent (*arrow*), as well as an irregular area slightly distal to this fistula, which may be a small pseudoaneurysm. (**C**) After placement of a second covered stent, there are no further arteriovenous fistulae and the possible small pseudoaneurysm has been excluded from the circulation.

applied to a toddler with a functional single ventricle (15). We have subsequently confirmed the usefulness of this technique in a 7-year-old with truncus arteriosus and have had success with new balloon-expanded covered stents in an adolescent with Wolff-Parkinson-White syndrome (Figs. 30-3 and 30-4).

■ SUMMARY

Cardiac catheterization in children presents particular risks related to patient size, the nature of lesions encountered, delicacy of tissues, typical lack of patient cooperation, and the nature of the interventions frequently performed in this population. Minor complications are observed in 6% to 10% of procedures, with major complications in 2% and death in 0.1% to 0.3%. Neonates and young infants are particularly at risk, as are patients having interventional procedures. Airway status, cardiac perforation, thromboembolic stroke, and catheter-site complications require particular attention.

References

1. desJardins SD, Crowley DC, Beekman RH, et al. Utility of cardiac catheterization in pediatric cardiac patients on ECMO. *Catheter Cardiovasc Interv.* 1999;46:62–67.
2. Vitiello R, McCrindle BW, Nykanen D, et al. Complications associated with pediatric cardiac catheterization. *J Am Coll Cardiol.* 1998;32:1433–1440.
3. Mehta R, Lee K, Chaturvedi R, et al. Complications of pediatric cardiac catheterization: A review in the current era. *Catheter Cardiovasc Interv.* 2008;72:278–285.
4. Bennett D, Marcus R, Stokes M. Incidents and complications during pediatric cardiac catheterization. *Paediatr Anaesth.* 2005;15:1083–1088.
5. Agnoletti G, Bonnet C, Boudjemline Y, et al. Complications of paediatric interventional catheterization: An analysis of risk factors. *Cardiol Young.* 2005;15:402–408.
6. Schroeder VA, Shim D, Spicer RL, et al. Surgical emergencies during pediatric interventional catheterization. *J Pediatr.* 2002;140:570–575.
7. Kulkarni S, Naidu R. Vascular ultrasound imaging to study immediate postcatheterization vascular complications in children. *Catheter Cardiovasc Interv.* 2006;68:450–455.
8. Balaguru D, Dilawar M, Ruff P, et al. Early and late results of thrombolytic therapy using tissue-type plasminogen activator to restore arterial pulse after cardiac catheterization in infants and small children. *Am J Cardiol.* 2003;91:908–910.
9. Carmosino MJ, Friesen RH, Doran A, et al. Perioperative complications in children with pulmonary hypertension undergoing noncardiac surgery or cardiac catheterization. *Anesth Analg.* 2007;104:521–527.
10. Liu X, Wong V, Leung M. Neurologic complications due to catheterization. *Pediatr Neurol.* 2001; 24:270–275.
11. Rashkind WJ, Miller WW. Creation of an atrial septal defect without thoracotomy. A palliative approach to complete transposition of the great arteries. *JAMA.* 1966;196(11):991–992.
12. Lloyd TR. Prognosis of the hypoplastic left heart syndrome. *Prog Pediatr Cardiol.* 1996;5:57–64.
13. Shim D, Lloyd TR, Beekman RH. Transhepatic therapeutic cardiac catheterization: A new option for the pediatric interventionalist. *Catheter Cardiovasc Interv.* 1999;47:41–45.
14. Frazer JR, Ing FF. Stenting of stenotic or occluded iliofemoral veins, superior and inferior vena cavae in children with congenital heart disease: Acute results and intermediate follow up. *Catheter Cardiovasc Interv.* 2009;73:181–188.
15. Maher KO, Lloyd TR. Coil occlusion of a femoral arteriovenous fistula. *Catheter Cardiovasc Interv.* 2000;51:308–311.

31

Valvuloplasty, Angioplasty, and Stent Placement in Children

AIMEE K. ARMSTRONG

■ PULMONARY VALVULOPLASTY

The first report of percutaneous balloon valvuloplasty was in a patient with valvar pulmonary stenosis in 1982 (1). Balloon pulmonary valvuloplasty is now the standard-of-care treatment for moderate and severe valvar pulmonary stenosis with an intact ventricular septum. The balloon tears either the valve leaflets along the fused commissures or the leaflet tissue itself.

Complications from this procedure are more common in infants than in adults, and infants younger than 1 month are at particularly high risk (2). These complications include pulmonary insufficiency, tricuspid valve injury, arrhythmias (heart block, ventricular tachycardia, and ventricular fibrillation), hemodynamic compromise, disruption of the pulmonary valve or annulus, pulmonary artery dissection, perforation of distal pulmonary vessels, and perforation of the right ventricular outflow tract. Stanger et al. (2) reported the complications from the Valvuloplasty and Angioplasty of Congenital Anomalies (VACA) Registry, in which there were 822 balloon pulmonary valvuloplasty procedures performed at 26 institutions from 1981 through 1986 (Table 31-1) (2). Only five patients (0.6%) had major complications, including two patients (0.2%) who died. The first death was in a 12-month-old infant who had an annular disruption, despite using a balloon that was only 100% of the annulus diameter, which is significantly less than the recommended balloon size of 120% to 140% of the annulus. The second death was in a 5-day-old infant, in whom a double balloon technique was used, which resulted in the inability to withdraw the catheters from the body and subsequent laceration of the inferior vena cava. One newborn had perforation of the right ventricular outflow tract with tamponade. Two patients developed significant tricuspid regurgitation. The first was a 4-year-old patient, who suffered avulsion of the anterior papillary muscle following the use of a 6-cm long balloon. The second patient of unknown age developed tricuspid regurgitation as a result of the balloon being too proximal during inflation. Minor complications occurred in 11 patients (1.3%) and included two arrhythmias requiring treatment, both of which occurred during balloon inflation. One patient had a possible avulsion of the anterior pulmonary valve leaflet, and the others had femoral vessel complications and respiratory depression from morphine (2).

The development of some degree of pulmonary insufficiency is common but occurs to a lesser degree when compared with surgical pulmonary valvotomy. Moderate pulmonary valve insufficiency occurs in 44% of patients after surgery, compared with 11% after balloon valvuloplasty (3). Long-term follow-up over an average of 8.7 years of 533 patients after an initial balloon pulmonary valvuloplasty revealed moderate pulmonary insufficiency in 7% of patients and no one with severe insufficiency (4). Balloon movement during inflation increases the risk of pulmonary insufficiency, and this can be minimized with the use of a stiff wire that is secured in a distal pulmonary artery branch. The slack should be eliminated from the wire, and a slight forward push should be maintained on the wire to minimize movement of the balloon (5).

TABLE 31-1   **Complications of Balloon Pulmonary Valvuloplasty (822 Procedures)**

Complications	Age	%
Major complications: death		0.24
1 annular tear	12 mo	
1 vein tear	5 d	
Major complications: other		0.35
1 perforation and tamponade	8 d	
2 tricuspid regurgitations	?, 4 y	
Minor complications		1.34
5 vein thrombosis	5 d, 8 d, 11 mo, 11 mo, 6 y	
2 vein tears	6 d, 2 mo	
1 respiratory arrest	4 d	
1 leaflet avulsion	3 mo	
2 arrhythmias	6 y, 7 y	
Incidents		2.55
6 arrhythmias	1 mo, 2 mo, 5 mo, 12 mo, 12 mo, 16 y	
3 hypoxia	4 mo, 22 mo, 23 mo	
1 perforation	17 mo	
1 hypotension	4 mo	
7 bleeding from catheterization site	1 mo, 1 mo, 5 mo, 10 mo, 2 y, 2 y, 10 y	
2 arterial thrombosis	7 mo, 8 mo	
1 hemoptysis	21 y	

(From Stanger P, Cassidy C, Girod DA, et al. Balloon pulmonary valvuloplasty: results of the Valvuloplasty and Angioplasty of Congenital Anomalies (VACA) registry. *Am J Cardiol.* 1990;65:775–783.)

The development of moderate tricuspid regurgitation is reported to occur in 1% to 4% of patients, and it is severe in 0% to 1% (2,3,6). To avoid damage to the tricuspid valve, the balloon of the wedge catheter should be fully inflated while still in the right atrium, before crossing the tricuspid valve. If the balloon enters the tricuspid valve fully inflated and stays inflated at least until it is just beneath the pulmonary valve, the catheter will be less likely to pass between chordae or between chordae and the septum. This wedge catheter is then exchanged over a stiff wire for the angioplasty balloon. If the wedge catheter has passed through chordae during the initial placement, then the angioplasty balloon could be in a location that could rupture chordae during inflation or removal of the balloon. Care should be taken also to use the shortest balloon available, which is a 2 cm balloon for infants and young children, and to avoid displacing the balloon too proximally during inflation. Use of a stiff

wire helps to stabilize the balloon during inflation, and a forward push on the balloon catheter during inflation helps to keep the balloon out of the tricuspid valve.

Transient complete heart block can occur from the stiff wire impinging on the conduction system. The subclavian and internal jugular approaches, in particular, cause the catheter to lie on the atrioventricular node, and transient complete heart block is more common (2.2%) (7). A vagal response can also occur from balloon inflation. Prophylactic atropine can be given, particularly in patients with systemic or suprasystemic right ventricular pressure or who are hemodynamically unstable (8). Ventricular arrhythmias can also occur as a result of the stiff wire passing through the right ventricle, and access to a defibrillator should be readily available.

Hemodynamic compromise can occur as a result of the angioplasty balloon obstructing all of the cardiac output while it is inflated. If an atrial septal defect or patent foramen ovale is present, patients will develop hypoxemia during inflation but may have preserved cardiac output. These defects are a source for paradoxical embolism, and attention needs to be paid to proper anticoagulation and flushing of catheters. In older children and adults, hemodynamic instability can be minimized by using a double balloon technique to allow more flow through the valve both during and at full inflation (5).

Disruption of the pulmonary valve annulus and transmural tears in the right ventricular outflow tract have been reported (9). This is usually due to balloon oversizing, which can be avoided with accurate measurement of the annulus using a reliable calibration system and by keeping the balloon 140% or less of the annulus diameter. While this major complication is usually fatal, immediate drainage of the pericardial and/or pleural spaces with autotransfusion and transfer to the operating room for surgical repair should be attempted (5).

Pulmonary artery dissection and tears have also been reported but are usually asymptomatic. They can be diagnosed by postvalvuloplasty right ventricular angiography showing an irregular bulge or linear radiolucency in the anterior wall of the pulmonary artery. Perforation of distal pulmonary vessels can occur due to the stiff wire tips. These wires must be well controlled and consideration given to using a stiff wire with a J-tip.

The development of dynamic subpulmonary obstruction is considered more of a result than a complication of pulmonary balloon valvuloplasty. Because of the relief of the high pressure just proximal to the pulmonary valve, the dynamic subpulmonary obstruction can occur immediately after the balloon dilation, particularly in older children who have developed significant right ventricular hypertrophy. If the right ventricular pressure remains elevated after valvuloplasty, the level of obstruction can be delineated by a precise end-hole catheter pullback or by the response to a fluid bolus. If the right ventricular pressure decreases with a fluid bolus, then the obstruction is likely at the subvalvar area. This can be treated acutely with propranolol and fluid and usually improves with time.

The risk of right ventricular outflow tract perforation is highest in the neonate and can be decreased by using a 4F wedge catheter with a 0.018-in. angled glidewire to cross the pulmonary valve. Care should be taken to keep the catheter tip pointing posteriorly, while attempting to cross the valve, and not anteriorly and superiorly at the right ventricular outflow tract. Having an echocardiography machine in the catheterization laboratory and turned on, prior to the start of the procedure, facilitates immediate evaluation for pericardial effusion, if hemodynamic compromise occurs or if there is a suspicion of perforation. It also allows for prompt ultrasound guidance for pericardiocentesis. In addition, having supplies to perform an emergency pericardiocentesis available on the catheterization table decreases the time to drainage of effusions. Many of the complications of pulmonary balloon valvuloplasty can be avoided with planning and attention to detail.

◼ AORTIC VALVULOPLASTY

Still considered an experimental treatment throughout the 1980s, percutaneous aortic valvuloplasty lagged behind pulmonary valvuloplasty as the standard of care for valvar aortic stenosis. The risk of complications is greater with aortic valvuloplasty than with pulmonary valvuloplasty, with major and minor complications occurring in 9.3% to 15.4% and 20.8% to 26.4%, respectively (10,11). Balloon aortic valvuloplasty had the highest percentage of complications (42%) of 17 types of interventions in a review of 1,412 catheterizations (11). Similar to pulmonary valvuloplasty, neonates remain the highest risk group.

The early mortality rate for balloon valvuloplasty in neonatal critical aortic stenosis is 9% to 10% (12,13). When neonates are excluded, the mortality rate is 0.7% and major complications occur in less than 3% (14). Complications pertaining to balloon aortic valvuloplasty for the neonate through the young adult include severe aortic insufficiency (1.6%), avulsion of the aortic valve (0.2%), stroke (0.2%), dissection or aortic injury (0.5%), perforation of the left ventricle (1.1%), mitral valve damage, arrhythmia (ventricular arrhythmias, left bundle branch block, and complete heart block), and femoral artery injury or thrombosis (2.1%) (12).

The most common complication is the development of aortic insufficiency. Excluding the neonatal population, the degree of aortic insufficiency increases in 10% to 58% of patients and is grade three or four in 12.8% (14,15). Risk factors for increased aortic insufficiency are young age (1–5 years), history of valvotomy, and a higher grade of aortic insufficiency prior to valvotomy (14). Aortic insufficiency can be caused by avulsion, prolapse, or perforation of a leaflet. The risk of aortic insufficiency has been shown to increase with increasing balloon size in some studies (Fig. 31-1) (12,15). but not in all (14). Balloon instability or excessive movement during inflation increases the risk of damage to the valve and of incompetence. Balloon stabilization is created by use of a double balloon technique, long balloons (2 cm for neonates, 3 cm for 1–3 years, 4 cm for 4–12 years, 5–6 cm for >12 years), stiff wires, adenosine to stop contractions temporarily, or rapid ventricular pacing in the right ventricle at approximately 200 paces per minute to decrease the blood pressure by half of the normal value. If rapid ventricular pacing is used, defibrillation

pads should be applied before pacing, in case defibrillation is needed. Perforation of a leaflet can occur from the tip of a stiff wire during retrograde crossing of the aortic valve. This can be avoided by the anterograde approach, which has its own risks, however. Leaflet perforation can also be avoided by very gently and rapidly bouncing off the leaflet with a soft-tipped angled glidewire or catheter. Once the wire has passed into the left ventricle, the catheter should be advanced very carefully across the valve. If any resistance is met when advancing the catheter, the wire may have perforated a leaflet, and the catheter should not be advanced.

Avulsion of the aortic valve is rare and can be avoided by not oversizing the balloon and by using valid calibration for annulus measurements. The initial balloon should be 90% to 100% of the valve annulus, and the balloon size can be increased by up to 10% for repeat dilation, if the initial balloon does not produce significant aortic insufficiency or improvement in gradient (5).

Central nervous system complications occur from embolization of a clot or air while catheter manipulations are performed in the left atrium, left ventricle, and/or aortic arch. This can be prevented by meticulous flushing of catheters, by keeping the activated clotting time (ACT) at more than 200 to 250 seconds, and by keeping all catheters and wires in the descending aorta when they are not in use.

Perforation of the left ventricle is caused by the tip of a straight wire passing through the myocardium as it is passed through the aortic valve. In addition, if the balloon milks into the ventricle during inflation, the stiff portion or transition zone of the wire, which is curled in the apex of the ventricle, can be pushed against the myocardium, causing perforation (5). The operator should take care not to advance the straight wire too far into the ventricle, after the wire has passed through the aortic valve. Balloon catheters should be used over J-tipped wires with curves manually placed on the end to allow the wires to conform to the shape of the ventricular apex, and stiff wires should be avoided in the neonate. Easy access to an echocardiography machine can facilitate rapid diagnosis and treatment of this complication.

Injury to the mitral valve is more common with the anterograde technique than with the retrograde approach, but perforation or tear of

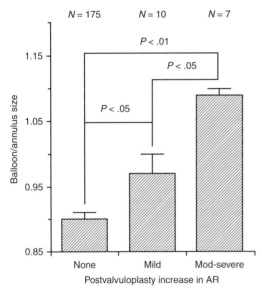

FIGURE 31-1. The relationship between the ratio of valvuloplasty balloon size to aortic annulus size and development of aortic regurgitation (AR) after balloon valvuloplasty in the VACA Registry. All values are mean ± standard error of the mean. Mod-severe, moderate to severe. (Reprinted from Rocchini AR, Beekman RH, Shachar GB, et al. Balloon aortic valvuloplasty: results of the valvuloplasty and angioplasty of congenital anomalies registry. *Am J Cardiol.* 1990;65:784–789, with permission from Elsevier.)

the mitral leaflets can occur with either method. Disruption of the mitral chordae can occur with the retrograde approach, if the balloon is entrapped in the chordae. When this entrapment occurs, the balloon appears to have a more posterior position in the left ventricle and does not move freely (5).

Femoral arterial thrombosis, damage, or permanent pulse loss occurred in 31.6% of children younger than 1 year undergoing this procedure prior to 1990, but these complications are much less common in the current era of low-profile balloons (5,15).

Hemodynamic compromise is not uncommon in the neonate with critical aortic stenosis undergoing aortic valvuloplasty, and these patients usually need inotropic and pressor support before, during, and after the procedure. The hemodynamic, acid–base, and respiratory status should be as optimized as much as possible before the valvuloplasty. Ventricular arrhythmias can occur when the wire and/or catheter enter the left ventricle. In critical aortic stenosis, it can be impossible to defibrillate successfully, until the valvuloplasty is performed. If fibrillation occurs, a rapid valvuloplasty is advised, followed by defibrillation. In these neonates, left ventricular angiograms are not recommended, prior to valvuloplasty, because of the risk of severe ventricular arrhythmias prior to the intervention. Defibrillation patches and a defibrillator should be readily available during these cases.

■ PULMONARY ARTERY ANGIOPLASTY

As branch pulmonary artery stenoses can be inaccessible surgically, pulmonary balloon angioplasty is used to treat stenotic pulmonary arteries by causing intimal interruption, as well as medial tears, which usually extend to the adventitia (16). Vascular remodeling and healing occur at a larger diameter (17). The major complication rate, including major vessel rupture and death, is 3.2% to 3.8%, and this has not changed over the last three decades (10,18). Complications include perforation or rupture of the pulmonary artery, bleeding requiring transfusion, acute pulmonary artery aneurysm formation, hemodynamic compromise, pulmonary edema from reperfusion injury, arrhythmia, and death (Table 31-2) (5,8,18).

TABLE 31-2 **Complications of Balloon Angioplasty of Branch Pulmonary Arteries: Occurrence in 182 Procedures in 156 Patients with Possible Risk Factors**

Complications	Age ≤ 2 y	Balloon Diameter > 3 × Stenosis Diameter	Balloon Rupture	Total #
Tear or perforation of pulmonary artery	1	2	1	9
Death	2	1	0	5
Technical failure	1	· · ·	· · ·	4
Bleeding requiring transfusion	1	0	0	3
Arrhythmia	1	0	0	2
Acute aneurysm formation	1	0	0	2
Interstitial lung edema	0	0	0	1
Paradoxical embolus	1	1	0	1
Cerebral accident	1	1	0	1
Loss of arterial pulse	0	0	1	1

(Reprinted from Kan JS, Marvin WJ, Bass JL, Muster AJ, Murphy J. Balloon angioplasty-branch pulmonary artery stenosis: results from the Valvuloplasty and Angioplasty of Congenital Anomalies registry. *Am J Cardiol.* 1990;65:798–801, with permission from Elsevier.)

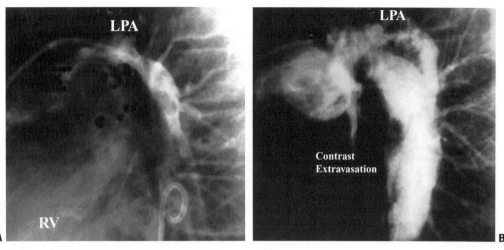

FIGURE 31-2. Pre–balloon dilation left pulmonary artery angiogram (**A**, lateral view) from a patient with left pulmonary artery stenosis demonstrates discrete area of stenosis in the proximal artery. Post–balloon dilation left pulmonary artery angiogram RV, right ventricle; LPA, left pulmonary artery. (**B**, lateral view) reveals extravasation of contrast as a result of a small arterial tear caused by dilation procedure. (Reprinted from Schroeder VA, Shim D, Spicer RL, et al. Surgical emergencies during pediatric interventional catheterization. *J Pediatr.* 2002;140:573, with permission from Elsevier.)

Pulmonary artery rupture is the most common cause of morbidity and mortality in this procedure and occurs in 5.8% of cases (18). It is caused by overdilation of stenotic lesions and, more commonly, of the adjacent vessel distal to the narrowing and by balloon rupture (Fig. 31-2) (9). Rupture of the pulmonary artery is increased in native stenoses with no surgical scar tissue around the lesion, which is resistant to tearing and dissection. Therefore, more aggressive dilation can be performed in old (>6 months) postsurgical lesions (5). Balloon diameter greater than three times the dimension of the stenosis is usually needed for success. For old postoperative lesions, the balloon diameter should be limited to no greater than 50% to 75% of the diameter of the adjacent normal vessel or 3 to 4 times the diameter of the stenosis, whichever is smaller. For native stenoses, the diameter of the balloon should be limited to 10% to 15% larger than the adjacent normal vessel and no more than three times the diameter of the stenosis (5). Pulmonary artery rupture can also be caused by placing the guidewire in a small distal branch. Poststenotic arteries tend to be thin-walled, and when the stenosis is dilated, the distal small branch may also be dilated, leading to rupture in this area. Care should be taken to keep the distal guidewire in the largest distal branch and to avoid the use of compliant

angioplasty balloons. Compliant balloons will expand to larger than the advertised diameter in areas of less vessel resistance, leading to injury of the normal vessel (5). Another cause of pulmonary artery injury is balloon rupture. Balloon rupture usually occurs longitudinally and can cause a very sudden, high-pressure jet of fluid to be released into the pulmonary artery. This can be avoided by paying careful attention to the rated burst pressure of the balloon and by using a pressure-controlled inflation device for all inflations. The odds of pulmonary artery trauma increase with increasing main pulmonary artery pressure, and ruptures exposed to high pressure are more likely to lead to significant hemorrhage (19). Finally, pulmonary artery rupture can occur at areas of recent surgical anastomoses or augmentation. Healing of vessels occurs in the initial 6 to 8 weeks postoperatively, but significant scarring does not occur for 6 to 12 months.

The operator should maintain wire access across the pulmonary artery that is being dilated until it has been proven by angiography that a rupture or tear did not occur. Angiography should be performed by hand through a long sheath, additional venous catheter, or via a monorail catheter. If extravasation of contrast is noted on angiography, a cardiac surgeon should be alerted. Next, a dilation balloon should be gently inflated with low pressure in the area of

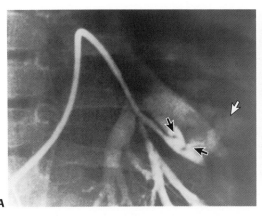 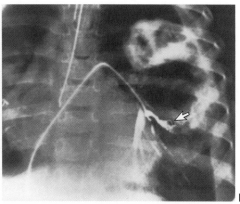

FIGURE 31-3. Unconfined tear. (**A**) An anterior–posterior frame from an angiogram demonstrating a large tear (*black arrows*) in the left pulmonary artery after balloon dilation. Free flow of contrast into the pleural space can be seen (*white arrow*). (**B**) The same pulmonary artery after coil occlusion (*white arrow*) of the tear, demonstrating no further extravasation of contrast. (Reprinted from Baker CM, McGowan FX Jr, Keane JF, Lock JE. Pulmonary artery trauma due to balloon dilation: recognition, avoidance and management. *J Am Coll Cardiol.* 2000;36:1687, with permission from Elsevier.)

the rupture to tamponade the bleeding, and the patient should be supported hemodynamically. Hemoptysis can occur, and the anesthesiologists should be alerted to watch for this complication. Once the patient has been stable for approximately 30 minutes (60 minutes for a large vessel under high pressure), another angiogram should be performed with the balloon deflated. If two attempts at tamponade are not successful, a covered stent, if available, can be placed to cover the area of rupture or a vascular occlusion device, such as an Amplatzer Vascular Plug II (AGA Medical Corporation, Plymouth, Minnesota), or embolization coils can be used to occlude the vessel proximal to the rupture (Fig. 31-3) (19). Surgical therapy should also be considered, as it may be preferable to occluding a large pulmonary vessel permanently.

If the wire position has been lost, a balloon-tipped catheter can be passed to the branch pulmonary artery, proximal to the rupture to occlude it. A balloon wedge catheter can be used in small children and a Medi-tech occlusion balloon (Boston Scientific, Natick, Massachusetts) in older patients. After 30 to 60 minutes of hemodynamic stability, the balloon should be slowly deflated, and hand angiography should be performed to observe for extravasation, as described earlier (5).

Perforation of the pulmonary arteries can also be caused by perforation of the distal vessels by the stiff tip of the wire used for the procedures. This is detected by hemoptysis, coughing, an increasing density around the wire tip on flu-

oroscopy, or by extravasation of contrast on angiography. If this occurs, the wire should be withdrawn very slightly but not removed from the vessel. An angioplasty or balloon-tipped, end-hole catheter should be used to temporarily occlude blood flow to that area of the distal pulmonary artery. After 30 minutes, the balloon can be deflated slowly, and a hand injection of contrast should be performed looking for continued extravasation. If bleeding continues, that area of the distal pulmonary artery can be occluded with embolization coils (5). Mortality can be reduced by routinely coil occluding vessels with unconfined hemorrhage (8). Urgent resuscitative management, including intubation with positive pressure ventilation, evacuation of hemothoraces, and transfusion with blood products, may be required.

Pulmonary artery aneurysm formation occurs in 3% to 5% of vessels undergoing angioplasty, and this occurs mostly in the small branches distal to the stenoses that are inadvertently dilated during the angioplasty of the stenotic regions (Fig. 31-4) (17,20). Aneurysm formation does not seem to be related to larger balloon:artery ratios or to inflation pressures (17). Patients with William syndrome may be more prone to this complication, and this has been reported to lead to late rupture 2 weeks after dilation in one patient with significant main pulmonary artery hypertension (21).

Cutting balloons are used to treat pulmonary artery stenoses that are resistant to standard

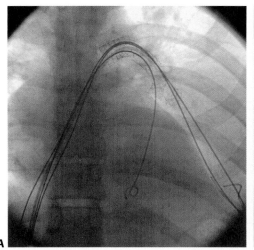
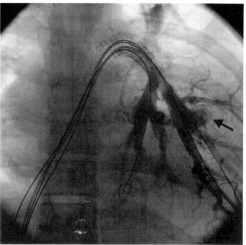

FIGURE 31-4. Multiple stents in congenital branch pulmonary artery stenosis (**A**) before redilatation and (**B**) after redilatation, demonstrating pseudoaneurysm formation (*arrow*) secondary to distal vessel damage. (Reproduced from Duke C, Rosenthal E, Qureshi SA.. The efficacy and safety of stent redilatation in congenital heart disease. *Heart.* 2003;89:910, with permission of BMJ Publishing Group Ltd.)

angioplasty, and the cutting balloon size is generally 1 mm larger than the waist of the standard angioplasty balloon. A long sheath should be placed just proximal to the site of cutting balloon angioplasty to avoid withdrawing the deflated cutting balloon across valves. The blades of the cutting balloon can be avulsed from the balloon with any rough handling, and a long sheath can cover a damaged balloon during withdrawal (5). During withdrawal of the cutting balloon into the long sheath, the distal portion of the sheath should be parallel to the balloon. If there is an angle between the cutting balloon and the tip of the sheath, the blades of the deflated balloon can slice the sheath longitudinally. Filling defects, caused by intimal flaps or an irregular lumen, are common after cutting balloon angioplasty (22).

Patients with main pulmonary artery hypertension, particularly suprasystemic pressures, are not only at increased risk of hemorrhage from rupture but are also at increased risk of hemodynamic compromise during angioplasty. Their cardiac output is significantly compromised during occlusion of one pulmonary artery, and a prophylactic atrial septostomy should be considered if the main pulmonary artery pressure is more than 10 mmHg higher than the systemic pressure (5,8). This will allow temporary right-to-left shunting at the atrial level and help to preserve cardiac output at the expense of oxygenation, and these small atrial

septal defects created with static balloon dilation typically close spontaneously.

Transient pulmonary edema occurs in 3% of cases from reperfusion injury in areas of the lung that were previously poorly perfused. Edema is seen on chest radiograph in segmental areas of the lung where angioplasty was performed, and the patients may develop hemoptysis. Treatment is with positive pressure ventilation with increased positive end-expiratory pressure, diuretics, and supportive care (8).

Preparation for the potential occurrence of pulmonary artery rupture includes general anesthesia with endotracheal intubation, at least two large bore peripheral intravenous lines, rapid accessibility to a cardiac surgeon and cardiac operating room, consideration given to two points of central venous access (one for tamponade of the vessel and one for angiography) or a long sheath in the pulmonary artery, and rapid access to packed red blood cells for emergency transfusion. The operator should be vigilant to observe for the development of hemoptysis, systemic hypotension, and opacification on fluoroscopy of the lung segment in the area of dilation. Recrossing a recently dilated vessel with a wire or catheter should be avoided as to prevent further injury to the recently disrupted intima and media.

Extra caution should be taken in patients with isolated peripheral pulmonary stenosis, particularly those with Williams syndrome, and in patients with elevated main pulmonary artery pressures, as these patients are at the highest risk for pulmonary artery rupture and hemorrhage (19). In fact, patients with Williams syndrome, can have cardiovascular collapse with passage of an uninflated balloon into the branch pulmonary arteries and with inflation of the balloon (17,18).

■ PULMONARY ARTERY STENTING

Complications from pulmonary artery stenting include all of those noted earlier in the section on "Pulmonary Artery Angioplasty," but pulmonary artery rupture is much less common, because balloons do not need to be larger than the adjacent vessel on either side of the stenosis. Stenting, however, has the added complication risk of stent embolization and an increased risk of balloon rupture on the stent. This can lead to surgical emergencies with need for stent/balloon removal in 2.5% of cases (9). The risk of distal pulmonary vessel perforation is more so with stenting than with angioplasty because the wires used for stenting are stiffer, and the treatment is outlined in the previous section.

Stent embolization can range from displacement of the stent on the unexpanded balloon to the stent embolizing proximally or distally after inflation. If the unexpanded stent displaces on the balloon while the stent is still within the long sheath, the stent, balloon, and long sheath should be removed over the wire. A new long sheath is placed over the wire, and the procedure is begun again. If the unexpanded stent slips distally on the balloon while the stent is outside of the sheath, the operator should not attempt to withdraw the stent back into the sheath, since this will usually cause the stent to slip further distally on the balloon. Advancement of the original deflated balloon further through the stent will also likely continue to push it distally. It is preferable to replace the deflated balloon with a smaller, lower-profile balloon to catch the stent and then pull the partially inflated balloon and stent back into position. Similarly, if an unexpanded stent slips distally completely off the balloon, a smaller, lower profile balloon is advanced through the stent. Either serial inflations are performed in a safe location in the

distal pulmonary artery until the stent is fixed, or the smaller balloon is used to pull the stent back into position where it can be inflated serially. If the stent displaces proximally and cannot be inflated there, an attempt can be made to relocate it to the contralateral branch pulmonary artery. An end-hole catheter from a second venous access site is passed through the stent and to the contralateral pulmonary artery. A stiff wire is placed through the end-hole catheter, and the original balloon and the wire are removed. A new balloon is placed over the wire that is in the contralateral pulmonary artery and is inflated gently. Once the stent is fixed onto the balloon, the unit can be advanced carefully into the contralateral pulmonary artery and advanced as distally as possible for inflation (5). The main pulmonary artery is usually too large for stent implantation, and stents in this area can compress coronary arteries. It is generally not advised to attempt to withdraw a stent into the right ventricle and right atrium from the pulmonary arteries, when it is outside of a sheath, to avoid damaging the pulmonary and tricuspid valves. The operator should consult with a cardiac surgeon before attempting this maneuver.

During inflation of a stent, the inflation should be stopped immediately if the stent starts to slip on the balloon. If it has slipped proximally, the operator should advance the long sheath to the proximal end of the stent to stabilize it while the balloon is repositioned, which requires a slight deflation of the balloon (8). If a partially inflated stent slips distally, advancement of the original deflated balloon through the stent will likely continue to push it distally. It is preferable to replace the balloon with a smaller, lower-profile balloon to catch the stent and then pull the balloon and stent back into position (8). If a partially inflated stent milks off the balloon completely and is distal to the stenosis, the balloon should be replaced with a low-profile balloon that is slightly larger than the current diameter of the stent. This balloon can be passed distal to the stent and expanded until it is the same size as the stent. With the stent on the catheter shaft, an attempt can be made to withdraw the entire catheter—stent–balloon unit backward over the wire, until the stent is at the original area of stenosis. The stent can be inflated initially with the small balloon, which can then be replaced with a larger balloon (5). If this is not possible, the embolized stent can be inflated to an appropriate size in a distal vessel.

Once a stent is expanded, it can be displaced during the removal of the balloon from the stent. This can be prevented by advancing the sheath into the stent over the deflated balloon, prior to removal of the balloon. If this is not possible and the balloon is stuck within the stent, a second catheter from an additional venous access site can be used to buttress the stent while the balloon is jiggled free from the stent (5).

While balloon rupture in pulmonary artery angioplasty usually occurs because of inflation at pressures higher than the rated burst pressure, rupture during stenting usually occurs because of balloon rupture on the sharp points on the distal ends of the stent. This tends to occur even at relatively low inflation pressures but usually is less damaging to the vessel. It does, however, cause incomplete inflation of the stent, which increases the risk of stent embolization. The operator should choose a balloon that is only a few millimeters longer than the stent on either end to avoid an excessive dumbbell shape of the inflating balloon, which causes the sharp ends of the stent to cut into the balloon. Using stents with rounded ends also helps to avoid this complication.

If a balloon ruptures inside of a stent and the stent is expanded fully, the operator should attempt to advance the long sheath over the balloon. If the balloon does not come into the sheath but comes out of the stent, the wire can be left in place, as the balloon and sheath are removed together from the patient. A new long sheath can then be placed over the wire. If the stent is only partially expanded and the balloon will not come out of the stent, a second wire can be passed from an additional sheath in another venous access site through the stent, and a second, smaller angioplasty balloon can be placed over this wire to inflate the stent further. Once the stent is fixed in place, the ruptured balloon can usually be removed. If the stent is only partially expanded but the sheath can be advanced over the balloon inside of the stent, a second catheter from another access site can be used to apply pressure to the proximal stent to prevent it from slipping proximally. The ruptured balloon can be withdrawn into the sheath and replaced with a larger balloon to dilate the stent (5).

In addition to stent displacement, stent embolization, and balloon rupture, other complications of pulmonary artery stenting are crushed stents, stent erosion, and restenosis. If bilateral proximal branch pulmonary artery stents are placed, they should be placed simultaneously to prevent the balloon in one stent from crushing the contralateral stent. If they are placed sequentially, then a balloon should be inflated in the first stent while the contralateral stent is being placed. Stent erosion is very rare but can occur when a pulmonary artery stent is compressed by a markedly dilated aorta and when there has been previous surgery on one of the vessels (5). Restenosis is also rare, especially when the stents are not overdilated at implantation, but can occur at areas between two stents in a series where the stents do not overlap. Intimal build-up occurs between the stents. Therefore, overlapping stents should overlap by at least 5 to 6 mm to allow for longitudinal growth of the vessel (5).

Prevention of pulmonary artery stent complications requires meticulous attention to stent preparation, when mounting the stent onto the balloon. The operator should dilate the stent slightly on a sheath dilator that is one French size smaller than the sheath used for delivery. This opens the stent slightly to prevent injury to the balloon when the stent is advanced onto it. The stent should be carefully crimped onto the center of a balloon that is only a few millimeters longer than the stent, avoiding friction between the stent and the balloon during the crimping process. A stent that is crimped off center on the balloon has a higher risk of displacement and embolization. In addition, the operator should avoid using balloons with a hydrophilic coating, which can cause the stent to slip on the balloon. The stent and balloon should be dipped into contrast to help affix the stent to the balloon. A cover can be cut from a short sheath that is one French size smaller than the size of the delivery sheath to assist in advancing the balloon and stent through the bleed-back device of the long delivery sheath. This cover should be just longer than the balloon and should be removed from the bleed back device, once the balloon and stent have entered the delivery sheath. The balloon catheter should be advanced carefully through the long sheath, and the operator should make sure that the stent is still centered on the balloon, before the balloon is advanced outside of the sheath tip. A stiff wire should be used to stabilize the stent and balloon from movement during inflation, and the transition point of the wire should be well past the area of stenosis. The operator should pay close attention to the tip of the straight wire in the distal pulmonary artery to prevent perforation of distal vessels.

■ COARCTATION ANGIOPLASTY

Balloon angioplasty is used to treat both native coarctation, particularly in children outside of infancy, and recoarctation after surgical repair at any age. Major complications occur in 2.8% of angioplasty for native coarctations and in 3.9% of procedures for recoarctation (10). Total complications are similar for both groups, with 15% experiencing complications in the native group and 13% in the recoarctation group (23). Complications include aortic tear, rupture, disruption, and aneurysm; femoral artery thrombosis and injury; central nervous system injury; paraplegia; and death. In the early era of angioplasty for coarctation, prior to 1990, the mortality was 0.7% for native coarctations and 2.5% for recoarctation (24,25). More recent examination showed the mortality for both native and recoarctations to be 0.7% (23) and to be related to the condition of the patient prior to the procedure. The only significant differences in complications between the two groups were an increased risk of intimal tear or flap in the native coarctation group (5.2% vs. 1.6%) and an increased need for blood product transfusion in the recurrent coarctation group (15% vs. 4.1%) (23).

Aortic tear, rupture, and dissection are caused by using a balloon too large for the aorta to accommodate. The coarctation segment should not be dilated to more than three times the diameter of the stenosis, and the dilation balloon should not be larger than the diameter of the adjacent narrowest aorta (5). Aortic rupture is very rare and is primarily related to balloons with very tight waists (8). In a large cohort of patients undergoing balloon angioplasties, there were no transmural aortic tears in the native coarctation group and only 0.7% in the recoarctation group (23). If there is progressive extravasation of contrast from the aorta, a cardiac surgeon should be notified immediately. The balloon should be reinflated at a low pres-

sure in the area of the extravasation, and the patient should be taken to the operating room for repair. Alternatively, a covered stent can be used, if available, to cover the region of the rupture. Intimal dissection with the creation of an intimal flap occurs in 1% to 1.5% of angioplasty for recoarctation (25,26). Rigid dilation balloons can injure the aorta proximal to the stenosis, if the balloon is too long and straightens in the aortic arch. Furthermore, the aorta can be damaged by readvancing catheters or wire across a freshly dilated area.

Aneurysms occur in 2% to 7% of patients undergoing angioplasty for native coarctation and in 1% of those with recoarctation (8,24,26,27,28). They usually occur in the area of dilation and can occur early or late. Early, discrete aneurysms can be covered by a large covered stent, if one is available at the time of catheterization, but early aneurysms can remodel and decrease in size with time. Progression of the aneurysms is rare. In a group of 53 patients who underwent balloon angioplasty of discrete, native coarctations, four patients developed aneurysms, all of which were small and did not change in size at a mean follow-up of 11.8 years (4–18 years) (27). Aneurysms should be followed serially with imaging every 1 to 2 years.

Femoral arterial thrombosis and injury are less common in the current era of lower-profile balloons. The area of the femoral sheath should be infiltrated with local anesthesia prior to removal, since pain causes vasospasm, which increases the risk of thrombosis (5). Pulse loss is treated with heparin until the pulse returns, and a vascular surgeon should evaluate the patient if a popliteal pulse cannot be obtained by Doppler interrogation.

Neurologic events occur in 1.5% to 2.2% of angioplasty cases for recoarctation (25,28). Central nervous system complications occur from embolization of a clot or air while catheter manipulations are performed in the aortic arch. This can be prevented by meticulous flushing of catheters, by keeping the ACT at more than 200 to 250 seconds, and by keeping all catheters and wires in the descending aorta when they are not in use. The operator should also avoid placing the distal end of a wire in the carotid or vertebral arteries. Paraplegia has been reported only once, in a 2-month-old patient with complex congenital heart disease who underwent balloon angioplasty of a recoarctation, and the cause remains unknown (29).

■ COARCTATION STENTING

Stent implantation is an accepted treatment for native and recurrent coarctation in older children and adults. If an aortic stent is implanted in a child, it should be a stent large enough to be dilated ultimately to the size of the adult aorta. This typically limits the procedure to children who weigh more than 30 to 35 kg. Complications of coarctation stenting include all of those described earlier for coarctation angioplasty with the added technical complications of stent migration and balloon rupture. A multi-institutional report of 565 aortic stent procedures in children and adults revealed complications in 14.3% of procedures, although complications were less frequent after 2002, occurring in 9% (30). Complications were most frequent in the group of patients who were older than 40 years (30).

Forbes et al. (30) reported that aortic wall complications occur in 3.9% of aortic stent procedures (1.4% with intimal tears, 1.6% with aortic dissection), and these were more common after present balloon angioplasty, with abdominal aortic coarctation, and in adults older than 40 years. Of nine aortic dissections, three were managed with emergency surgery, with two of these patients dying as a result of severe neurologic injuries, and three were managed with covered stent placement. The other three patients were managed medically with antihypertensive agents (30). Aortic dissection should be treated emergently with a covered stent (Fig. 31-5) (31) or repaired in the operating room. Present high-pressure angioplasty should not be performed, since this may increase the risk of aortic wall complications. The physician should carefully weigh the risk and benefits of aortic stent placement in adults of advanced age, in patients with vasculitis, and in patient with conditions associated with a vasculopathy, such as Turner syndrome, since stenting can lead to serious complications and death in these patients (32,33).

Aortic aneurysm is present at intermediate follow-up in 9% of cases, and the risk is not

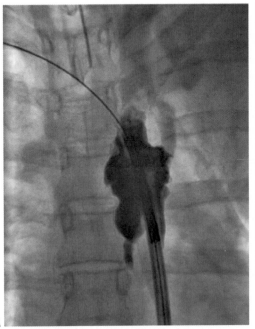
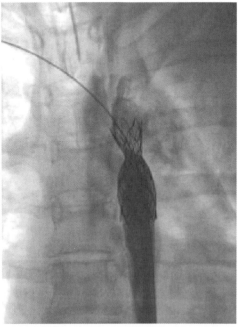

FIGURE 31-5. (**A**) Anteroposterior angiogram of descending aorta through the long sheath with stent across the coarctation site and extravasation of contrast from the aorta. (**B**) Following deployment of the covered stent, repeat angiography demonstrates containment of contrast within the stented aorta. (From Kenny D, Margey R, Turner MS, et al. Self-expanding and balloon expandable covered stents in the treatment of aortic coarctation with or without aneurysm formation. *Catheter Cardiovasc Interv.* 2008;72:69. Copyright 2008. Reprinted with permission of John Wiley & Sons, Inc.)

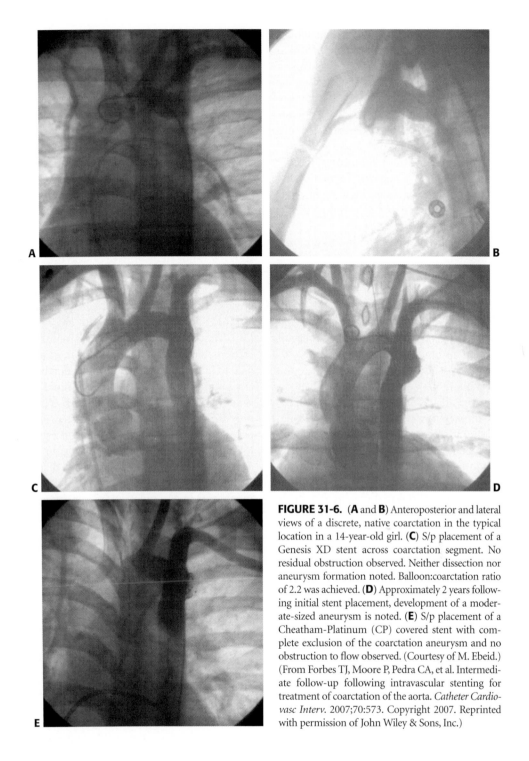

FIGURE 31-6. (**A** and **B**) Anteroposterior and lateral views of a discrete, native coarctation in the typical location in a 14-year-old girl. (**C**) S/p placement of a Genesis XD stent across coarctation segment. No residual obstruction observed. Neither dissection nor aneurysm formation noted. Balloon:coarctation ratio of 2.2 was achieved. (**D**) Approximately 2 years following initial stent placement, development of a moderate-sized aneurysm is noted. (**E**) S/p placement of a Cheatham-Platinum (CP) covered stent with complete exclusion of the coarctation aneurysm and no obstruction to flow observed. (Courtesy of M. Ebeid.) (From Forbes TJ, Moore P, Pedra CA, et al. Intermediate follow-up following intravascular stenting for treatment of coarctation of the aorta. *Catheter Cardiovasc Interv.* 2007;70:573. Copyright 2007. Reprinted with permission of John Wiley & Sons, Inc.)

different between native and recoarctation groups (34). The aneurysms usually occur at the area of the narrowest coarctation segment, but they can also occur proximal to the stent (Fig. 31-6) (34). The majority of these aneurysms are small, and intervention is needed in only about 30% of cases (34). Exceeding a balloon:coarctation ratio of 3.5 at the initial procedure increases the occurrence of aortic wall injury, including aneurysm, as does present angioplasty (34). The diameter of the balloon should be determined by the smallest normal vessel diameter adjacent to the coarctation. The balloon should be no larger than 1 to 2 mm than the proximal unaffected aorta. Balloons should not be sized to the aorta just distal to the coarctation, as there is often significant poststenotic dilatation. Decreased aortic compliance may be a contributing factor to aneurysm formation, and compliant balloon testing has been advocated (32,34). Patients should be monitored for the development of late aneurysm formation by follow-up magnetic resonance imaging or computed tomography, starting at 6 months after stent placement (32).

Technical complications unique to the procedure are stent migrations, which occur in 0% to 6% of these procedures, and balloon rupture, which occurs in 0% to 4% (30). Causes of stent migration are delivery of the stent on a balloon that is more than 2 mm larger than the aorta proximal to the coarctation site and delivery of the stent on an undersized balloon. Delivery of the stent in a pseudocoarctation, which is a fold in the aorta and not a true stenosis, and balloon rupture are other causes (30). Distal displacement of the stent can be prevented by decreasing stroke volume, blood pressure, and pulse pressure during implantation (32). This can be done by the administration of adenosine or by rapid ventricular pacing in the right ventricle. If the stent is displaced distally, the stent is repositioned in the distal aorta and implanted so that is does not cover any vital side branches.

Balloon rupture is more common with the use of P8 series Palmaz stents than with the P10 series Palmaz, LD, eV3, Genesis, Cheatham-Platinum, or other covered stents (30). This complication has been implicated in stent migration, cerebrovascular accidents, and need for surgical removal of balloon fragments. Balloon rupture can be avoided in part by maintaining a straight wire and catheter course. A straight catheter course decreases the chance that the sharp ends of the stent will puncture the balloon upon inflation. This may require parking the tip of the wire in the right or left subclavian artery, as opposed to in the ascending aorta or left ventricle. The carotid arteries should not be used for wire placement. Balloon rupture also can be caused by the use of a single large-diameter balloon that expands at the ends first, causing the ends of the stent to evert and protrude radially from the center, potentially causing balloon rupture and/or aortic wall injury. The NuMed Balloon-in-Balloon (BIB) catheter has a smaller inner balloon and a larger outer balloon. Initial inflation of the inner balloon allows the stent to open uniformly along the length (32). Use of the BIB catheter also allows manipulation of stent position after inflation of the inner balloon for precise placement and may decrease the risk of stent migration. Single balloon catheters are lower profile, however, and may be needed in children to decrease the risk of femoral arterial injury.

Other complications include cerebrovascular accidents, femoral arterial injury, in-stent stenosis, and stent fracture. Cerebrovascular accidents are reported in 0.7% of these procedures, and the incidence increases when there are technical complications, such as stent migration or balloon rupture, and with older patients (30). The ACT should be kept at more than 250 seconds, and meticulous attention should be paid to limiting the time that wires and balloons are in the aortic arch. Significant femoral arterial injury has been reported to occur in 2.3%, with only 0.5% requiring therapy. In-stent stenosis occurs in 11% of aortic stents at intermediate follow-up and is associated with a younger age at implantation, smaller poststent diameters, and higher poststent gradients (34). Stent fracture occurs in 4% and primarily in native coarctations. Most require repeat stent placement or redilation due to reobstruction (34).

References

1. Kan JS, White RI, Mitchell SE, Gardner TJ. Percutaneous balloon valvuloplasty: a new method for treating congenital pulmonary valve stenosis. *N Engl J Med.* 1982;307:540–542.

2. Stanger P, Cassidy C, Girod DA, et al. Balloon pulmonary valvuloplasty: results of the Valvuloplasty and Angioplasty of Congenital Anomalies (VACA) registry. *Am J Cardiol.* 1990;65:775–783.

3. Peterson C, Schilthuis JJ, Dodge-Khatami A, et al. Comparative long-term results of surgery versus balloon valvuloplasty for pulmonary valve stenosis in infants and children. *Ann Thorac Surg.* 2003;76:1078–1082.

4. McCrindle BW. Congenital heart disease: independent predictors of long-term results after balloon pulmonary valvuloplasty. *Circulation.* 1994; 89:1751–1759.

5. Mullins CE. *Cardiac Catheterization in Congenital Heart Disease: Pediatric and Adult.* Malden, MA: Blackwell Futura; 2006.

6. Witsenburg M, Talsma M, Rohmer J, Hess J. Balloon valvuloplasty for valvular pulmonary stenosis in children over 6 months of age: initial results and long-term follow-up. *Eur Heart J.* 1993;14:1657–1660.

7. Zeevi B, Berant M, Fogelman R, et al. Acute complications in the current era of therapeutic cardiac catheterization for congenital heart disease. *Cardiol Young.* 1999;9:266–272.

8. Lock JE, Keane JF, Perry SB, eds. *Diagnostic and Interventional Catheterization in Congenital Heart Disease.* 2nd ed. Norwell, MA: Kluwer Academic; 2000.

9. Schroeder VA, Shim D, Spicer RL, et al. Surgical emergencies during pediatric interventional catheterization. *J Pediatr.* 2002;140:570–575.

10. Mehta R, Lee KJ, Chaturvedi R, Benson L. Complications of pediatric cardiac catheterization: a review in the current era. *Catheter Cardiovasc Interv.* 2008;72:278–285.

11. Vitiello R, McCrindle BW, Nykanen D, et al. Complications associated with pediatric cardiac catheterization. *J Am Coll Cardiol.* 1998;32:1433–1440.

12. McCrindle BW for the VACA Registry Investigators. Independent predictors of immediate results of percutaneous balloon aortic valvotomy in childhood. *Am J Cardiol.* 1996;77:286–293.

13. Egito ES, Moore P, O'Sullivan J, et al. Transvascular balloon dilation for neonatal critical aortic stenosis: early and midterm results. *J Am Coll Cardiol.* 1997;29:442–447.

14. Moore P, Egito E, Mowrey H, et al. Midterm results of balloon dilation of congenital aortic stenosis: predictors of success. *J Am Coll Cardiol.* 1996;27:1257–1263.

15. Rocchini AR, Beekman RH, Shachar GB, et al. Balloon aortic valvuloplasty: results of the valvuloplasty and angioplasty of congenital anomalies registry. *Am J Cardiol.* 1990;65:784–789.

16. Edwards BS, Lucas RV, Lock JE, Edwards JE. Morphologic changes in the pulmonary arteries after percutaneous balloon angioplasty for pulmonary arterial stenosis. *Circulation.* 1985;71:195–201.

17. Rothman A, Perry SB, Keane JF, Lock JE. Early results and follow-up of balloon angioplasty for branch pulmonary artery stenoses. *J Am Coll Cardiol.* 1990;15:1109–1117.

18. Kan JS, Marvin WJ, Bass JL, et al. Balloon angioplasty-branch pulmonary artery stenosis: results from the Valvuloplasty and Angioplasty of Congenital Anomalies registry. *Am J Cardiol.* 1990;65:798–801.

19. Baker CM, McGowan FX, Keane JF, Lock JE. Pulmonary artery trauma due to balloon dilation: recognition, avoidance, and management. *J Am Coll Cardiol.* 2000;36:1684–1690.

20. Duke C, Rosenthal E, Qureshi SA. The efficacy and safety of stent redilation in congenital heart disease. *Heart.* 2003;89:905–912.

21. Zeevi B, Berant M, Blieden LC. Late death from aneurysm rupture following balloon angioplasty for branch pulmonary artery stenosis. *Cathet Cardiovasc Diagn.* 1996;39:284–286.

22. Bergersen L, Jenkins KJ, Gauvreau K, Lock JE. Follow-up results of cutting balloon angioplasty used to relieve stenoses in small pulmonary arteries. *Cardiol Young.* 2005;15:605–610.

23. McCrindle BW, Jones TK, Morrow WR, et al., for the VACA Registry Investigators. Acute results of balloon angioplasty of native coarctation versus recurrent aortic obstruction are equivalent. *J Am Coll Cardiol.* 1996;28:1810–1817.

24. Tynan MT, Finley JP, Fontes V, et al. Balloon angioplasty for the treatment of native coarctation: results of VACA registry. *Am J Cardiol.* 1990;65:790–792.

25. Hellenbrand WE, Allen HD, Golinko RJ, et al. Balloon angioplasty for aortic recoarctation: results of VACA registry. *Am J Cardiol.* 1990;65:793–797.

26. Reich O, Tax P, Bartakova H, et al. Long-term (up to 20 years) results of percutaneous balloon angioplasty of recurrent aortic coarctation without use of stents. *Eur Heart J.* 2008;29:2042–2048.

27. Hassan W, Awad M, Fawzy ME, et al. Long-term effects of balloon angioplasty on left ventricular hypertrophy in adolescent and adult patients with native coarctation of the aorta: up to 18 years follow-up results. *Catheter Cardiovasc Interv.* 2007;70:881–886.

28. Yetman AT, Nykanen D, McCrindle BW, et al. Balloon angioplasty of recurrent coarctation: a 12-year review. *J Am Coll Cardiol.* 1997;30:811–816.

29. Ussia GP, Marasini M, Pongiglione G. Paraplegia following percutaneous balloon angioplasty of aortic coarctation: a case report. *Catheter Cardiovasc Interv.* 2001;54:510–513.

30. Forbes TJ, Garekar S, Amin Z, et al., for the Congenital Cardiovascular Interventional Study Consortium. Procedural results and acute complications in stenting native and recurrent coarctation of the aorta in patients over 4 years of age: a multi-institutional study. *Catheter Cardiovasc Interv.* 2007;70:276–285.

31. Kenny D, Margey R, Turner MS, et al. Self-expanding and balloon expandable covered stents in the treatment of aortic coarctation with or without aneurysm formation. *Catheter Cardiovasc Interv.* 2008;72:65–71.

32. Golden AB, Hellenbrand WE. Coarctation of the aorta: stenting in children and adults. *Catheter Cardiovasc Interv.* 2007;69:289–299.

33. Fejzic Z, van Oort A. Fatal dissection of the descending aorta after implantation of a stent in a 19-year-old female with Turner's syndrome. *Cardiol Young.* 2005;15:529–531.

34. Forbes TJ, Moore P, Pedra CAC, et al. Intermediate follow-up following intravascular stenting for treatment of coarctation of the aorta. *Catheter Cardiovasc Interv.* 2007;70:569–577.

32

Ventricular Septal Defect, Patent Ductus Arteriosus, Fontan Fenestration, and Arteriovenous Fistula

RANJIT AIYAGARI

■ VENTRICULAR SEPTAL DEFECT

Percutaneous closure of ventricular septal defects (VSDs) was initially reported by Lock and colleagues (1) by using a Rashkind double umbrella device in 1988. The basic technique which was developed includes creating an arteriovenous (AV) rail by passing a catheter and wire from the arterial system retrograde through the aortic valve, into the left ventricle, and across the defect. This is followed by snaring the wire from the venous system, exteriorizing the wire, using this wire position to place a long venous sheath with its tip in the left ventricle, and finally by delivering a device across the septum. Various adaptations of this technique, including a venovenous rail with transseptal access to the left atrium and ventricle, continue to be used today. Over the last 5 to 10 years, new devices have made transcatheter VSD occlusion more feasible, with significantly lower complication rates than previously reported (Table 32-1). Still, this is a long and technically demanding procedure, typically performed under general anesthesia with echocardiographic guidance.

The complex geometry of the ventricular septum makes a "one device fits all" approach unsuitable for VSD closure. Therefore, selection of device and delivery approach must be tailored to the patient and defect location and size. In general, the delivery sheath is placed in the IJ

venous route for mid-to-apical muscular VSDs, and in the femoral venous route for more anterior muscular VSDs. Usually, this decision regarding access can be made on the basis of the preprocedure echocardiogram, but in some cases, it rests on the intraprocedure angiograms.

The most commonly used devices at this time for VSD closure are the Amplatzer occluders (AGA Medical, Plymouth, Minnesota). Within the Amplatzer "family" of occluders, the perimembranous and the muscular occluders (Fig. 32-1) are the two devices most commonly used for VSD closure. Other devices that are currently in use for VSD closure include the CardioSEAL and STARFlex (Nitinol Medical Technologies, Boston, MA).

Congenital VSDs Versus Posttraumatic and Post–Myocardial Infarction VSDs

Literature on traumatic and postinfarction VSDs is fairly limited (2). Various devices have been reported as successful, including the Amplatzer atrial septal occluder (ASO), Amplatzer patent ductus arteriosus (PDA) occluder, Amplatzer muscular VSD occluder, and a specialized Amplatzer postinfarction VSD device. These are particularly challenging cases because of the bizarre shape and course of these defects. In addition, there is the potential for

TABLE 32-1 Summary of Large Published Series of Amplatzer Devices (More Than 20 Patients) for Closure of Ventricular Septal Defects

Study	VSD Device Type	No. of Patients	Median Age/Median Weight	Procedural Success	Significant Adverse Events or Procedural Complications	High-Grade AV Block	Procedure-Related Death	Median Follow-up
Perimembranous, single institution (Zhou, 2008) (13)	pmVSD	210	6.7 y/28 kg	206 (98%)	8 (3.8%)	6 (2.9%)	0	0.9 y
Adults, single institution (Chessa, 2009) (64)	mVSD and pmVSD	40	38 y/67 kg	40 (100%)	4 (10%)	1 (2.5%)	0	3.0 y
European registry, 23 centers (Carminati, 2008) (65)	mVSD and pmVSD	430	8 y/28 kg	410 (95%)	24 (5.6%)	16 (3.7%)	1 (0.2%)	2.0 y
Infants, single institution (Diab, 2007) (67)	mVSD	20	0.4 y/4.6 kg	19 (95%)	4 (20%)	0	0	3.8 y
Perimembranous, single institution (Butera, 2007) (14)	pmVSD and mVSD	104	14 y/26.5 kg	100 (96%)	15 (14%)	9 (8.7%)	0	3.2 y
Perimembranous International Registry (Holzer, 2006) (11)	pmVSD	100	9 y/27.5 kg	93 (93%)	15 (15%)	3 (3%)	0	0.5 y

Study	Type	N	Age/Weight	Success				Follow-up
Perimembranous U.S. Phase I Trial (Fu, 2006) (67)	pmVSD	35	7.7 y/25 kg	32 (91%)	7 (20%)	2 (5.6%)	0	0.5 y
Italy, single center (Carminati, 2005) (9)	mVSD and pmVSD	122	15 y/35 kg	119 (98%)	8 (6.6%)	5 (4.1%)	0	1.7 y
Muscular, U.S. Registry (Holzer, 2004) (19)	mVSD	75 (83 total procedures)	1.5 y/?	72 (87%)	34 (45%)	6 (8%)	2 (2.7%)	0.6 y
Multicenter initial pmVSD experience (Bass, 2003) (68)	pmVSD	27	13.8 y/42.6 kg	25 (93%)	0	0	0	0.1 y
Single center mVSD (Thanopoulos, 2005) (69)	mVSD	30	5.8 y/22 kg	28 (93%)	1 (3.3%)	1 (3.3%)	0	2.2 y
Single center mVSD (Arora, 2004) (70)	mVSD	48	3–28 yr/?	48 (100%)	0	0	0	0.3–8 yr
Multicenter pmVSD (Masura, 2005) (71)	pmVSD	186	15.9 y/43.5 kg	186 (100%)	2 (1.1%)	2 (1.1%)	0	1 y

pmVSD, perimembranous ventricular septal defect; mVSD, muscular ventricular septal defect; AV, arteriovenous.

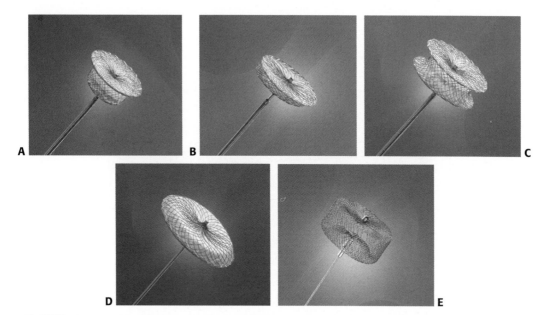

FIGURE 32-1. Amplatzer devices commonly in use. (**A**) Amplatzer septal occluder. (**B**) Amplatzer membranous VSD occluder (not for sale in the United States). (**C**) Amplatzer muscular occluder. (**D**) Amplatzer duct occluder. (**E**) Amplatzer vascular plug. (Courtesy of AGA Medical Corporation, Plymouth, Minnesota.)

enlargement of the VSD necrosis at the margin in post–myocardial infarction (MI) cases. Transesophageal echocardiography is especially useful in these cases to assess defect size and shape and to look for residual shunt. The overall likelihood of some residual shunt is much higher in these cases.

There is a paucity of literature on closure of these types of defects, given their rarity and heterogeneity. The initial series published by Landzberg and Lock (3), using older, pre-Amplatzer devices, reported a procedural success for percutaneous closure in 17 of 18 patients (94%), but the overall survival was only 10 of 18 (55%) at a median of 54 months (3). The multicenter U.S. registry, which employed the Amplatzer postinfarction VSD device, contained 18 adult post-MI patients. There was a procedural success of 89% with two patients requiring a second procedure to close a residual VSD, an overall complication rate of 22% (blood loss, bradycardia, and LV dysfunction), no procedure-related death, a 30-day mortality of 28%, and an overall mortality of 41%. This was noted to compare favorably with surgery in this setting (2). In a recent series of 10 adult patients with postinfarction and traumatic VSDs from the Mayo clinic, Martinez et al. (4) reported 100% success

with no major complications and one death due to renal and central nervous system disease.

Complications of Percutaneous VSD Closure and Bailout Techniques

Hemodynamic Instability during Catheter and Wire Manipulation

This is observed in a significant percentage of cases and is particularly a problem because of the extensive left heart manipulation involved in this procedure, including multiple exchanges using long wires and long sheaths. Constant invasive blood pressure monitoring is therefore critical, as is effective communication between the cardiologist and the anesthesiologist.

Entrainment of Air into the Left Side of the Heart

As is the case with percutaneous atrial septal defect (ASD) closure, introduction of air or clot must be avoided. It is important to be methodical and careful during all exchanges. Heparin 100 units/kg is administered at the outset of the procedure, and additional doses at intervals thereafter, with a goal of keeping the activated clotting time between 275 and 350 seconds.

Wire Rail Establishment

Arrhythmias, getting wires caught in the tricuspid valve apparatus, damage to valves, or impingement upon valves by holding them open, leading to sudden, free valve regurgitation and cardiovascular collapse have all been observed. In addition, the so-called sawing effect of a tensioned superstiff wire on tissue must be avoided (5). It is helpful to minimize the time spent with a "naked" wire within the heart, attempting to keep a catheter over the wire as a protective covering. In addition, it is imperative not to tighten loops of a "naked" wire within the heart. Finally, during the initial crossing of the defect from the arterial side, a balloon catheter is preferable to cross the true VSD. However, if this fails, a precurved catheter such as a Judkins Right can be helpful. Once the defect is crossed, if it is difficulty snaring the wire from the pulmonary artery, it can be helpful to use an EnSnare (MD Tech, Gainesville, Florida), which has three loops.

Cardiac Perforation

With the multitude of wires, catheters, and long stiff delivery sheaths used in this procedure, perforation is a significant risk. Transesophageal or intracardiac echocardiographic monitoring should be employed to identify the problem quickly. Obviously, the use of soft-tipped wires and balloon catheters to cross valves and defects is warranted when feasible.

Snagging of Cardiac Valves or Chordae

Any device has the potential of snagging on valvular structures or chords, especially those related to the tricuspid valve. This may be a greater problem with CardioSEAL or StarFLEX devices because of their design (5). The likelihood of this complication is greater if a wire was used to cross the defect (as opposed to a catheter). In general, this complication is less likely if the tricuspid valve is crossed with a balloon catheter as well, making sure everything passes through the largest orifice rather than within or between chords. Be careful if there is any resistance during any step of the procedure. Intraprocedural echocardiography is usually diagnostic, and the device should be removed and redelivered (Fig. 32-2).

Embolization

Correct sizing of the defect and a thorough assessment of the geometry of the VSD are both critical. In sizing, the use of multiple redundant methods including echocardiography and angiography is helpful. Balloon sizing is usually not necessary and may complicate the procedure, but some have routinely accomplished it. The ventricular septum is less deformable than the atrial septum, making the echocardiographic measurement more reliable. If a VSD device embolizes, it can travel to either side of the heart or into a great vessel. Most embolized devices can be retrieved percutaneously with the application of the general techniques for retrieval of Amplatzer devices that were developed for ASOs.

General Technique for Retrieval of Amplatzer Devices (6,7)

The design factors common to each Amplatzer device result in similar retrieval techniques for all devices, although those with external screw mechanisms are easier (Fig. 32-3). The goal is to remove the device doing as little harm to intracardiac structures (such as AV valves) as possible. If percutaneous retrieval is not possible, the goal becomes to stabilize the device so that no additional harm will take place while getting the patient to surgery for definitive retrieval.

1. Stabilize the device in a location where it will not acutely harm the patient, using a snare, bioptome, or wire (or combination of these).
2. For devices with exposed microscrews (e.g., ASO, patent foramen ovale (PFO) occluder, perimembranous VSD [pmVSD] device), grab the microscrew with a 10 mm snare advanced either through the implantation sheath or through a separate access site. For devices with unexposed microscrews (e.g., Amplatzer duct occluder [ADO], muscular VSD device; Fig. 32-4), it may not be possible to snare the microscrew, and an alternative approach is to snare the waist of the device.
3. Remove the bioptome or wire, and pull the device either taut against the sheath or preferably into the sheath. Drag the device out of the heart.
4. Place a stiff wire through the device to limit its ability to migrate back (Fig. 32-5), then remove the snare.
5. Change out the implantation sheath for a long, stiff sheath (at least 2F larger if the

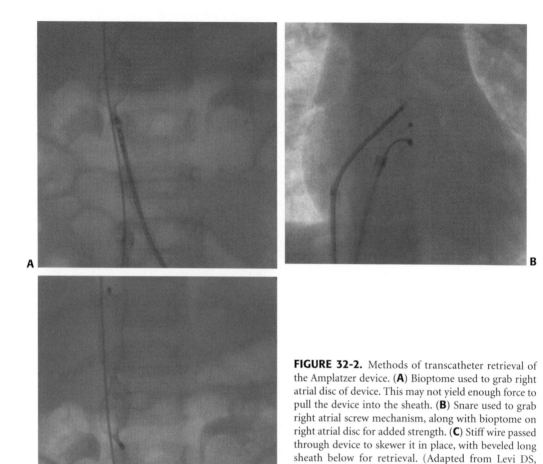

A

B

C

FIGURE 32-2. Methods of transcatheter retrieval of the Amplatzer device. (**A**) Bioptome used to grab right atrial disc of device. This may not yield enough force to pull the device into the sheath. (**B**) Snare used to grab right atrial screw mechanism, along with bioptome on right atrial disc for added strength. (**C**) Stiff wire passed through device to skewer it in place, with beveled long sheath below for retrieval. (Adapted from Levi DS, Moore JW. Embolization and retrieval of the Amplatzer septal occluder. *Catheter Cardiovasc Interv.* 2004;61: 543–547. Reprinted with permission of Wiley-Liss, Inc., a subsidiary of John Wiley & Sons, Inc.)

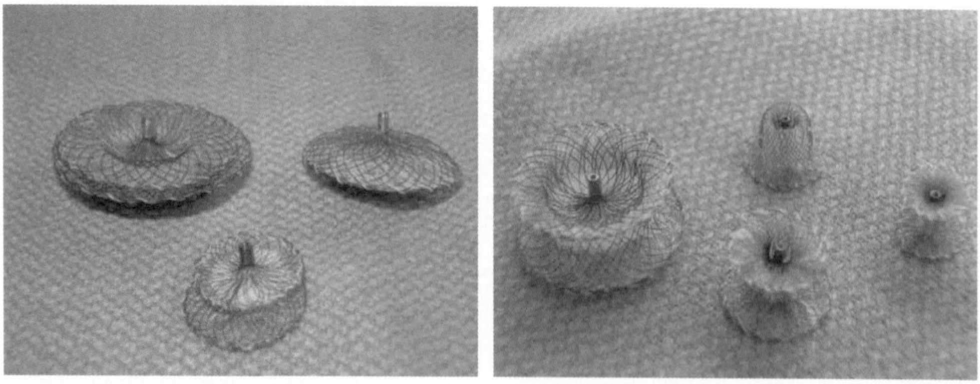

A

B

FIGURE 32-3. The ability to snare the screw mechanism on the Amplatzer device depends on whether it is exposed. (**A**) Devices with exposed screw mechanisms are easily snared: atrial septal occluder device (**left**), per-imembranous ventricular septal defect (VSD) device (**center**), and PFO device (**right**). (**B**) Devices with recessed screw mechanisms are much more difficult to snare: duct occluder device (**back center**) and multiple muscular VSD devices (**left, right, and front center**). (Adapted from Tan CA, Levi DS, Moore JW. Embolization and transcatheter retrieval of coils and devices. *Pediatr Cardiol.* 2005;26:267–274, with kind permission from Springer Science and Business Media.)

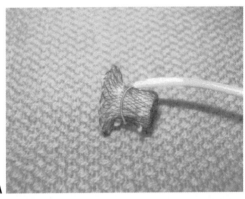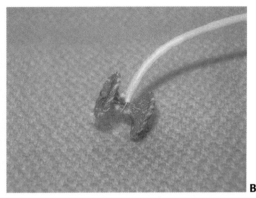

FIGURE 32-4. Snaring an Amplatzer device without an exposed screw mechanism. (**A**) The waist of the duct occluder device is snared. (**B**) The waist of the muscular ventricular septal defect device is snared. (Adapted from Tan CA, Levi DS, Moore JW. Embolization and transcatheter retrieval of coils and devices. *Pediatr Cardiol.* 2005;26:267–274, with kind permission from Springer Science and Business Media.)

microscrew was snared, or at least 4 F larger if the device waist was snared). This is more likely to be able to recapture the device. It may also be helpful to cut a bevel in the tip of this sheath (Fig. 32-6). Both the Cordis Brite Tip (Cordis Corp., Miami Lakes, Florida) and Cook Flexor sheaths (Cook Inc., Bloomington, Indiana) are useful for this purpose.

6. Reinsert the snare and resnare the device at the microscrew. Remove the stiff wire, and collapse the device into the larger sheath. If

the device still does not collapse, the other end of the device can be pulled through a separate access site (such as the IJ, if the device is in the inferior vena cava (IVC)) to collapse it further.

A similar approach can be performed for embolized CardioSEAL or STARFlex devices. In this case, the snare is used to grab one of the device legs. Pulling the device into the sheath is considerably harder for these devices and usually requires a long, stiff sheath that is at least 3F larger than the delivery sheath.

Hemolysis with Incomplete Closure

As is the case with incomplete closure of a PDA, if a VSD device is placed and results in incomplete closure with anything more than a small residual "smoke-like" shunt on postdevice angiography,

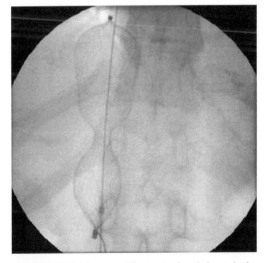

FIGURE 32-5. A superstiff wire is placed through the large Amplatzer device while in the inferior vena cava, limiting its ability to migrate back into the heart. (Adapted from Tan CA, Levi DS, Moore JW. Embolization and transcatheter retrieval of coils and devices. *Pediatr Cardiol.* 2005;26:267–274, with kind permission from Springer Science and Business Media.)

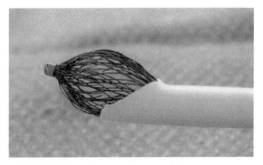

FIGURE 32-6. Beveling of a long, stiff sheath allows for easier retrieval of the Amplatzer device. (Adapted from Tan CA, Levi DS, Moore JW. Embolization and transcatheter retrieval of coils and devices. *Pediatr Cardiol.* 2005;26:267–274, with kind permission from Springer Science and Business Media.)

the high-velocity jet can result in hemolysis. In some cases, this has necessitated device removal. An alternative approach is to try putting in an additional device first to see whether the shunt can be eliminated. Intravascular hemolysis related to device placement can be intractable and sequelae including renal failure have been reported (8).

Loss of Sheath Position or Damage to the Sheath

It is unfortunately easy to have the long delivery sheath with its tip in the left ventricle slip out. This can negate all wire rail establishment efforts and prolong the procedure significantly. Therefore, it is helpful to maintain a catheter and wire from the opposite end of the rail into the long sheath at all times until one is truly ready to deliver the device. In addition, severe kinks can develop in the long sheath, especially if any attempt is made to advance it without the dilator in place. Strategies that have been proposed to counteract this include placing an 0.018-in. wire alongside the device within the delivery sheath, loading the delivery sheath through an Arrow-Flex sheath (Arrow International, Reading, Massachusetts) that is 2F larger, or substituting a Cook Flexor sheath for the Amplatzer delivery sheath (9).

Endocarditis or Vegetation

This seems to be a fairly rare complication, reported chiefly in case reports (10). Subacute bacterial endocarditis prophylaxis is recommended for at least 6 months after device placement, and potentially longer if there is a residual shunt at the margin of the device or if inadequate endothelialization is suspected.

Vascular Complications

As with any procedure involving large sheaths, local vascular complications such as hematomas and arteriovenous fistulae (AVFs) may arise. The general techniques to prevent this, such as using as small an arterial sheath as possible, apply. Some have proposed a venovenous wire loop, in which transseptal access to the left atrium is used, obviating the need for an arterial sheath. It is not clear whether this lowers the complication rate.

Device-Specific Issues

Amplatzer Perimembranous VSD Device

In an international registry of 100 patients undergoing pmVSD closure with the Amplatzer pmVSD device, risk factors for lack of proce-

dural success included weight less than 10 kg, inlet extension of the pmVSD, and aortic cusp prolapse into the VSD (11).

Aortic Valve Injury, Entrapment, or Significant Aortic Insufficiency

Careful assessment of the aortic rim before attempting device placement is of critical importance. Even though the Amplatzer perimembranous device is eccentric with a 1 mm superior rim, a superior rim of approximately 3 mm seems to be the minimal safe distance. Some worsening of aortic insufficiency occurs in approximately 10% of patients, but most cases are mild and have not required treatment. It is critical to assess for aortic insufficiency carefully by echocardiography once the device is in place but not yet released, so that the device can be removed if necessary. One common mechanism leading to the development of aortic insufficiency is for the device to pinch the right coronary cusp of the aortic valve (12).

Tricuspid Valve Injury or Regurgitation

This is usually mild and less likely to require treatment than device-related aortic insufficiency. Again, the mechanism should be carefully assessed by echocardiography before releasing the device, and a judgment must be made whether the device should be removed.

Heart Block or Other Conduction Abnormalities

This is perhaps the Achilles' heel of the Amplatzer pmVSD device. Conduction abnormalities may be immediate but can also be late (even months after the procedure). The incidence varies in published series (see Table 32-1) but seems to average approximately 3% to 8% (13). If any left bundle branch block or complete heart block is encountered during device placement, the device should be removed or repositioned. If these continue to recur, the device should be removed and the procedure abandoned. If the procedure is abandoned and no device is placed, the majority of patients will recover sinus rhythm within 24 hours. Some have advocated treatment of a presumed local inflammatory reaction with steroids. This seems to be a more frequent complication in younger patients; in one series of pediatric patients, all patients who developed complete heart block (CHB) were younger than 6 years (14). Not all patients require pacemaker insertion, but it is still not clear who will (i.e., even transient heart block with recovery places one at risk for late heart block) (15).

Zhu et al. (16) retrospectively analyzed the risk factors for early arrhythmias after transcatheter closure of pmVSDs in a large series of patients ($N = 358$) and found larger device size, nonsymmetrical device used (such as the Amplatzer pmVSD device), short distance from the defect to the tricuspid valve, and the presence of a ventricular septal aneurysm all to be risk factors (16).

Amplatzer Muscular VSD Device

Incomplete Closure

As many muscular VSDs (mVSDs) are really multifenestrated areas of the septum, the operator relies on the overhang of the device to occlude nearby minor defects. It is helpful to cross the VSD from the left ventricular side with a balloon catheter with the balloon partially inflated to ensure that the central, largest orifice is crossed rather than these minor defects. If it is difficult to cross the defect in this manner, a "tip deflector"–type wire such as the 0.035-in. Amplatz controllable deflector wire (Cook Inc., Bloomington, Indiana) can redirect the balloon catheter toward VSD.

Hybrid Approach

Delivery of the mVSD device in a "perventricular" fashion through the right ventricular wall has received a fair amount of attention recently and is commonly employed especially in small infants weighing less than 5 kg or in patients undergoing an open heart procedure for another reason. In this approach, the chest is opened, the right ventricle (RV) is entered with a needle, a short sheath is placed into the ventricle, the defect is crossed with a wire or catheter under transesophageal echocardiographic guidance, the sheath is advanced into the left ventricle (LV), and the device is delivered. This approach carries the attractiveness of utilizing short sheaths, with no need for a wire loop, so the procedural time is considerably shorter. A brief period of cardiopulmonary bypass is necessary in a minority of cases, which may negate some of the advantages compared with surgery. There is obviously a lower risk of vascular complication, but there is some risk of mediastinitis (17). Various adaptations of this technique have

been reported, including suturing the device to the septum to prevent migration (18), but these have not been adopted as standard approaches.

In an international registry of 75 patients (including many very young patients) undergoing device closure of mVSDs through percutaneous and perventricular approaches, the main risk factor for complications was low weight. Interestingly, the number of VSDs and the size of VSD were not risk factors in this series (19).

CardioSEAL Device

There is limited published literature on the use of this device in VSD closure. It is a non–self-centering device with a larger (10F–11F) delivery system and limited retrievability. Because the device is intended to be oversized (ideally twice the minimum diameter of the VSD), its arms can interfere with the AV valves. Late arm fracture has been reported for some generations of this device. There is a significant risk of kinking the long delivery sheath during placement (5).

■ PATENT DUCTUS ARTERIOSUS

Transcatheter closure of the PDA has been in fairly routine clinical use since the early 1990s. In the current era, surgical closure of a PDA is extremely rare outside the neonatal period. Catheter-based PDA occlusion was initially reported using such cumbersome devices such as the Rashkind PDA occluder (20) and the Porstmann plug (21), followed shortly thereafter by an alternative double-umbrella device (22) and a buttoned device (23). Placement of both free and detachable coils became the standard technique for occlusion of many PDAs by the mid-1990s. The introduction of the Amplatzer PDA occluder in the late 1990s greatly expanded the types and sizes of PDAs that were amenable to transcatheter closure.

New devices are in development to tackle the large neonatal PDA, which has heretofore remained a largely surgical lesion in most centers due to the small size of the patient and the relatively large size of the ductus. Following the availability of the ADO, there have been considerable advances in the ability to close large PDAs in fairly small infants. A recent series of 28 patients weighing less than 6 kg with large PDAs (>4 mm) showed a 93% procedural success with 85% of patients having ADOs implanted and 15% having bioptome-aided large coils placed.

Weight less than 6 kg is currently listed as a contraindication for ADO placement on the ADO instructions for use. Newer modified "angled" ADOs, designed to achieve closure of the large ductus in the young infant without impingement on the aorta or embolization, are on the horizon.

Closure of the ductus arteriosus can be accomplished from both arterial and venous routes, depending on the device chosen.

PDA Types

A simplified version of Krichenko classification (25), eliminating numerical subtypes, results in five major types of PDA, lettered "A" to "E" (Fig. 32-7). In general, types A, D, and E can potentially be occluded by coils, while types B and C, in general, require devices. The very short type B ducts may be better approached with a septal occluder device than with an ADO (26), and some tubular type C ducts may be more easily occluded with the Gianturco–Grifka vascular occlusion device, or more simply, with a slightly oversized Amplatzer vascular plug (AVP). At this time, the Gianturco coil can be used for many small- to medium-sized PDAs with favorable anatomy, whereas the ADO can be used for the vast majority of medium- to large-sized PDAs.

Complications of Percutaneous PDA Closure and Bailout Techniques

Coils

Coil Embolization

This can occur with either free release or detachable coils, without appreciable difference in incidence (7) (approximately 4%). Because the direction of flow in most PDAs is from aorta to pulmonary artery, any object that is placed properly but undersized or not firmly anchored

within the ductus will generally embolize to the pulmonary arteries. However, a coil that is improperly placed can embolize in either direction. The probability of embolization depends in large part on the following factors:

1. Sizing accuracy—Accurate biplane angiography, with the anteroposterior camera slightly right anterior oblique (RAO) and the lateral camera directly lateral, usually profiles the PDA best. The anatomic type, length, and the narrowest dimension of the PDA should be determined. A coil that is greater than twice the minimum diameter of the PDA and that is long enough (at least three loops, ideally four) should be used (27). In general, PDA up to 1.7 mm can be closed with 3-mm diameter coils, and up to 2.2 mm with 5-mm diameter coils. For PDA 2.3 mm and more, a device should be considered as initial therapy.

2. Adequacy of the ampulla—The majority of the coil loops (usually 2–3 loops) are placed in the aortic ampulla, which is what makes Gianturco coils less attractive options for type B and otherwise very short PDAs.

3. Catheter used to deliver coil—Several end-hole catheters have been used for coil delivery. The most commonly employed are the Judkins right coronary (e.g., JR 3.5) and the Bentson (e.g., JB1) catheters. The JR coronary catheter tends to have more friction and pull back the coil more easily; therefore, it is the job of the operator to make sure not to pull the entire coil into the aorta. Conversely, the JB1 glide catheter tends to be more slippery and squirt the coil forward; with

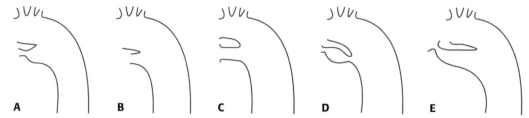

FIGURE 32-7. Schematic of the major anatomic subtypes of the ductus arteriosus, A through E. (**A**) Medium-length with narrowing at pulmonary artery end. (**B**) Short, window-like, with narrowing near aorta. (**C**) Tubular with no discrete narrowing. (**D**) Complex with multiple narrowings. (**E**) Long with narrowing at PA end.

this catheter, the operator needs to make sure not to put too much loop in the pulmonary artery or the coil will embolize there.

4. Use of bioptome-aided technique—This has generally been employed with larger (0.052-in.) coils and may now be only of historical interest, as the need for large coils has been largely superseded by the availability and ease of use of the ADO.

5. Technique and expertise of the operator.

Retrieving Embolized Coils

To Aorta

In this case, the key is to maintain the coil stuck to the catheter if at all possible. In general, while most of these coils are delivered through 4F sheaths, a short 6F sheath is necessary for retrieval. This can be placed in the other femoral artery if necessary. A 10 mm snare and end-hole catheter are advanced to the coil and any portion of the coil is snared. The coil should be able to fold over on itself within the 6F sheath and thereby be removed from the body. A bioptome can be used in rare cases where this snare technique fails.

To Pulmonary Arteries

If a small coil (0.035-in. or less) is used, these will generally embolize very distally. In such cases, the coil may not need to be retrieved and, in fact, may not be possible to retrieve. Coils of size 0.038 in. and larger generally can be retrieved via a long, at least 6F, sheath. The use of a long sheath avoids dragging the coil through right-sided cardiac structures (7). As with aortic retrieval, a 10 mm snare and an end-hole catheter are employed, with a bioptome used if the snare technique fails.

It is helpful (and perhaps superstitious) to get access in both the femoral artery and vein at the start of case prior to heparinization, even in the case of a tiny PDA where no right heart catheterization is performed, in case the retrieval is needed.

It remains to be seen whether newly available detachable, expanding "hydrocoils" will have any utility in PDA closure. In theory, the properties of these coils should decrease the likelihood of embolization (Fig. 32-8).

Inadequate Closure and Hemolysis

One must completely eliminate the shunt to avoid this problem, which arises when there is a residual small high-velocity jet through or around the coil or device. Therefore, postprocedure angiography is critical, and incomplete closure should not be tolerated by the operator. Additional coils or devices should be placed until the entire shunt is eliminated. There is one case report of hemolysis after the Dacron was

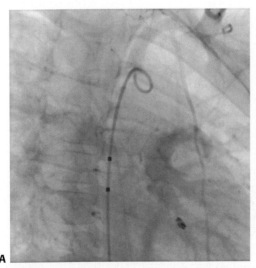 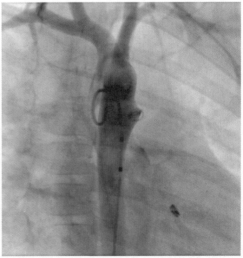

FIGURE 32-8. (**A**) Accidental embolization of a coil from the ductus arteriosus to the left pulmonary artery. (**B**) The embolized coil is left alone, and a new coil is placed successfully within the ductus.

stripped off a Gianturco coil by the bioptome in a bioptome-assisted coil deployment (28).

Endocarditis

As is the case with hemolysis, there is a higher risk with an open PDA or with residual shunt after device placement. Subacute bacterial endocarditis prophylaxis is recommended for 6 months after device placement, and potentially longer if there is any residual shunt.

Amplatzer Duct Occluder

This device is recapturable and has a recessed Amplatzer screw mechanism. It is fairly versatile although probably a bit more cumbersome than a coil for small straightforward PDAs. The ADO is generally placed through a 6F to 8F sheath from the venous side. One challenge during ADO placement is actually crossing the PDA from the venous side, which can be more difficult than from the arterial side due to the multiple turns required and the direction of blood flow. If this is particularly difficult, a catheter can be passed from the arterial side, with a snare placed through it, and a wire can be dragged across the PDA into the descending aorta. There does not seem to be a particular PDA morphology that is not amenable to ADO placement.

ADO Impingement on Aorta or Left Pulmonary Artery

It is worthwhile to obtain angiograms, including a lateral view aortogram and a left pulmonary artery (LPA) angiogram, via hand injection through the side port of the delivery sheath, before releasing the ADO. The ADO does have a fairly large aortic retention skirt, which raises the

concern of iatrogenic coarctation, especially within small aortas. In addition, it is recommended that the ADO be removed if greater than 3 mm juts into the LPA or more than half of the LPA lumen is occupied by the device. However, the incidence of clinically significant coarctation of the aorta or LPA stenosis from an ADO is extremely low. In the U.S. Amplatzer PDA occlusion device trial, in which 435 patients had ADO devices placed, although 101 (23%) had a gradient from ascending to descending aorta, the median gradient was only 4 mmHg and only 1 patient had a gradient greater than 15 mmHg. Similarly, with respect to the LPA, although 227 (54%) had a gradient between the main pulmonary artery (MPA) and LPA, the median gradient was only 3 mmHg, and only 8 patients had gradients of greater than 10 mmHg (29).

Device Embolization

If too short a device is used for the length of the PDA, the ADO can embolize into the pulmonary arteries (Fig. 32-9) (30). In patients with elevated pulmonary vascular resistance, the "stopper" shape of the device does not prevent embolization from pulmonary artery into aorta (Fig. 32-10). In patients with suspected elevated pulmonary vascular resistance, one must proceed with care. It is useful to check the pulmonary vascular reactivity to oxygen and nitric oxide, reconsider whether PDA closure is clinically indicated, and if so, to consider other devices. However, this approach should be regarded with caution. Retrieving an embolized ADO is performed in a similar fashion to retrieval of an embolized ASD or VSD device;

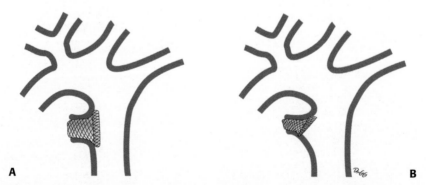

FIGURE 32-9. (**A**) Correct positioning of Amplatzer duct occluder within the PDA. (**B**) An Amplatzer duct occluder device that is too short for the ductus arteriosus. In this case, the retention disc is angled and pulled too far into the ductus. The device is at risk of embolization to the pulmonary arteries.

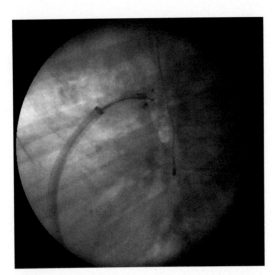

FIGURE 32-10. Embolization of an Amplatzer duct occluder device into the aorta in the setting of elevated pulmonary vascular resistance. The device is snared around its waist in preparation for retrieval. (Courtesy of Daniel S. Levi, MD.)

however, it can be challenging since the screw mechanism is quite well hidden and difficult to snare (7) (see Figs. 32-3B and 32-4A).

Inadequate Closure and Hemolysis

In general, clinically significant hemolysis in the setting of an ADO is quite rare. Because the device changes configuration once released, some apparent residual shunts will be eliminated. Residual shunting seems less likely with the ADO than with a coil (11% the day after procedure, decreased to less than 2% at 1-year follow-up) (29) and decreases significantly at follow-up, likely due to polyester fabric within the device promoting thrombosis. An initial "smoke-like" shunt through the center of the device is common and does not appear to be a risk factor for hemolysis or persistent patency of the ductus (29).

Improper Sizing

The pulmonary artery disc ("B" dimension or smaller number in ADO nomenclature) should be 2 mm larger than the narrowest dimension of the PDA. Some have reported success in very small infants by using a device with a pulmonary artery disc up to 1 mm larger than the smallest PDA dimension, provided that the aortic disc is not larger than the diameter of the descending aorta. (24) The length of the device

and the PDA are also worthy of note. Except for the smallest (5–4) ADO, these devices are all 7 to 8 mm long. Especially in very small children or those with short PDAs, it is important to look carefully at the length and make sure there is room to place the device without impinging on the aorta or LPA.

The overall complication rate with the ADO is quite low. A large multicenter U.S. trial showed a 99% procedural success rate, with a 2.3% major complication rate (29) (Table 32-2). Long-term outcome data are limited but appear to be very good for the ADO, with 100% complete closure rate and no deaths or late major complications in a series of 64 patients followed for a median of 58 months. Approximately 3% of these patients had mildly elevated descending aortic peak flow velocity, which persisted at 4 to 5 years, suggesting that such patients need to be followed serially. One patient had an elevated LPA flow velocity that resolved with time (31).

Other Devices

A new "ADO II" device was recently released. This device is symmetric, it has a somewhat lower profile than the ADO, and it is delivered through 4F and 5F catheters. There is limited published experience with this device. Another device that has been used successfully to close small to moderate PDAs is the DuctOcclud coil (pfm AG, Cologne, Germany) with a few small series published showing good results. The AVP has been used in some PDA, although there is a report of one device placed in a large type C PDA embolizing (32).

■ PDA STENTING

This is a newer procedure that essentially provides an alternative to a surgical systemic pulmonary artery shunt. Its main indications are to provide a source of pulmonary blood flow in right heart lesions such as pulmonary atresia variants and some forms of Ebstein anomaly and to provide a source of systemic blood flow as part of transcatheter palliation for hypoplastic left heart variants. There is one report of PDA stenting as a means for retraining the LV in D-transposition of the great arteries with intact ventricular septum (D-TGA/IVS) (33). Even a recently closed PDA has been successfully recanalized by manipulation of

TABLE 32-2 Summary of Large Published Series of Amplatzer Duct Occluder Devices (More Than 50 Patients) for Closure of the Patent Ductus Arteriosus

Study	No. of Patients	Median Age/ Median Weight	Procedural Success	Complete Closure Verified	Significant Adverse Events or Procedural Complications	Procedure-Related Death	Median Follow-up
ADO single institution (Wang, 2007) (72)	68	3.3 y/15.3 kg	66 (97%)	66 (97%)	1 (1.5%)[a]	0	0.5 y
ADO single institution (Masura, 2006) (31)	64	3.4 y/15 kg	64 (100%)	64 (100%)	0	0	4.8 y
Multicenter U.S. trial (Pass, 2004) (29)	439	1.8 y/11 kg	435 (99%)	428 (97%)	10 (2.3%)[b]	1 (0.2%)	1.0 y
Early experience multicenter (Ebeid, 2001) (73)	106	7.1 y/21.4 kg	105 (99%)	105 (99%)	0	0	0.1 y
Early experience single center (Bilkis, 2001) (30)	209	1.9 y/8.4 kg	205 (98%)	204 (98%)	5 (2.4%)[c]	0	0.7 y
Early multicenter international trial (Faella, 2000) (74)	316	2.1 y/10.7 kg	313 (99%)	? (95%–100%)	9 (2.8%)[d]	1 (0.3%)	0.3 y

ADO, Amplatzer duct occluder.

[a] 1 device embolization.

[b] 1 death, 2 device embolizations, 5 groin complications, 2 partial left pulmonary artery (LPA) obstruction.

[c] 3 device embolizations, 2 major blood loss.

[d] 1 death, 2 device embolizations, 2 major blood loss, 2 catheter fracture, 1 asystole, 1 partial LPA obstruction, 1 coarctation.

a hydrophilic, high-support coronary guidewire, resulting in the ability to place an open cell stent in a patient with ductus-dependent Ebstein anomaly (34).

In this procedure, either a venous or arterial approach can be used. For the venous approach, the PDA is crossed with a small (0.014 in.) coronary guidewire, a 5F coronary guiding sheath is placed across the duct, and a small premounted coronary stent (usually 3.5–4 mm diameter, length 1–2 mm longer than the PDA) is placed. For the arterial approach, the PDA is crossed with a small coronary guidewire and coronary stents (usually 3.5–4 mm diameter) are directly implanted without placing a sheath across the duct (35). Self-expanding stents may be used but size choices are limited, and control over delivery location is reduced with this approach.

The most important aspect of this procedure is to cover the entire length of the PDA with the stent but without impinging significantly on the pulmonary artery or descending aorta (Fig. 32-11) (35). If the length of the duct is not completely covered by the stent, placement of an additional stent is indicated. In general, the procedure can be accomplished via the arterial approach through a 3F to 4F arterial sheath. In some cases, an axillary artery approach allows for more direct access and improves the ability to cross the PDA with a coronary guidewire (J.P. Cheatham, personal communication).

Most operators will stop prostaglandin infusion anywhere between 4 to 6 hours before the procedure and the start of the procedure to promote mild ductal constriction to "grip" the stent within the duct.

Stent Selection

Flexible stents are probably better for longer, more tortuous ducts, and less flexible, stronger stents are probably better for short, straight ducts, but there is no good evidence to back this.

There are few published series on PDA stenting, nearly all of which focus on duct-dependent pulmonary blood flow. Initial reports from the late 1990s showed high rates of procedural failure, thrombosis, restenosis, and death (36). As technology and techniques have evolved, these figures continue to improve. Part of the reason for this is the recognition of the importance of covering the complete length of the ductus.

In a series of 21 infants who underwent placement of 28 ductal stents to maintain pulmonary blood flow, stents were expanded to 4 to 5 mm, and there were two procedural failures, but there were two early deaths due to right heart failure. The restenosis rate was high (43%); still, overall survival was 86% at 6 years (37). In a more recent series of 10 neonates with duct-dependent pulmonary blood flow and short, straight ducts, procedural success was achieved in all 10 patients (13 stents) without procedure-related complications. This resulted in relief of cyanosis over a median follow-up period of 5 months (35).

Complications of PDA Stenting

Restenosis

The most frequent complication is restenosis, either due to incomplete stenting with ductal constriction at the margins of the stent or due to

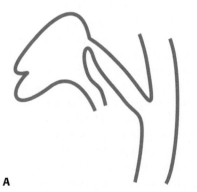 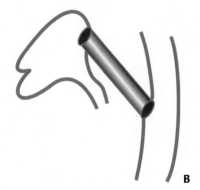

A   **B**

FIGURE 32-11. Schematic of ideal stent placement within the ductus arteriosus. (**A**) Patent ductus arteriosus. (**B**) Stent should cover the entire length of ductus with minimal encroachment into pulmonary artery and no encroachment into aorta.

neointimal formation. Nearly all of these stents will develop neointimal proliferation and in-stent stenosis over a period of months. They are generally responsive to redilation and placement of an additional stent if necessary. Both of these frequent complications increase with the time the stent is left in place.

Embolization

As is the case with a PDA closure device, a PDA stent can embolize to either the aortic or pulmonary arterial circulation. Once expanded, these stents are not retrievable by percutaneous means. Therefore, they are best left and further expanded in a benign location if possible; otherwise, they should be removed surgically.

Pulmonary Overcirculation

Depending on PDA diameter and distal pulmonary artery size and anatomy, the stented PDA can be physiologically similar to an aortopulmonary shunt that is too large. In the case of hypoplastic left heart syndrome (HLHS), this is the expected course, and PDA stenting is performed in conjunction with bilateral pulmonary artery bands (or implantation of flow restrictors).

Stent Thrombosis

Anticoagulation is controversial in this setting. Antiplatelet therapy is generally agreed to be indicated to prevent the formation of thrombi that could either occlude the PDA or embolize.

Iatrogenic Coarctation or Left Pulmonary Artery Stenosis

As is the case with the ADO, a stent that is too long can impede flow within the aorta or LPA. Given the choice, it is better to overhang a little bit of the stent into the pulmonary artery than into the aorta, especially in these fairly small patients.

As with any stent, fracture can occur and result in decreased radial strength. Furthermore, as with any interventional procedure, vascular complications, particularly arterial injury, can arise. If the patients require eventual surgical palliation, these stents can be coil-occluded in the catheterization laboratory in the majority of cases, and crushed by the surgeon in a minority of cases.

Risk Factors for Complications

In the case of PDA stenting for ductal-dependent pulmonary blood flow, a long, tortuous PDA, lower weight and lower aortic diameter,

and the use of hand-crimped stents (due to a much higher risk of the stent slipping off the balloon) have been identified as risk factors for PDA stent complications (37).

In a series of 40 patients with HLHS, 39 (97%) underwent successful PDA stenting, although with a 25% rate of significant technical or procedural complications. There was a 5% late complication rate, mostly coarctation at the aortic end of the stent, and one death. In HLHS, the PDA is much larger (mean diameter 6.6 mm); and therefore, larger stent diameters are needed (range of 7–12 mm). The authors categorized patients by ductal angulation, concluding that the most favorable anatomy was a leftward angulation in the vertical plane and that mesoversion or rightward angulation were risk factors for technical difficulty (38).

■ **FONTAN FENESTRATION**

Fontan fenestration evolved as a technique to protect cardiac output in the early postoperative period after the Fontan operation at the expense of mild hypoxemia. For a lateral tunnel Fontan, this simply involves using a punch to create a small (approximately 3 mm), perfectly circular hole in the piece of Gore-Tex used to create the Fontan baffle. On the other hand, for an extracardiac conduit Fontan, "fenestration" is considerably more complex and generally involves placing a Gore-Tex tube (essentially a shunt) from the Fontan to the systemic atrium. Interventions on Fontan fenestrations can come in many flavors.

Fenestration Closure

Most commonly, Fontan fenestrations within a lateral tunnel Fontan are closed in a subset of patients who either are hypoxemic at baseline or develop hypoxemia with exertion. The majority of these defects can be closed satisfactorily with the Amplatzer ASO device. Assuming the size of the fenestration is already known, balloon sizing is not necessary. However, many operators will perform balloon test-occlusion for a variable duration (typically approximately 10 minutes) to assess the impact of fenestration occlusion on pulmonary artery pressure and systemic oxygen saturations. Typically, since these fenestrations are less than 4 mm in diameter, the 4-mm ASO device will suffice. Oversizing is not necessary since there are no floppy rims, just rigid Gore-Tex, surrounding the fenestration. This can be accomplished safely in the vast majority of patients, with an acceptably low complication rate (39). A variety of other devices have been reported to be successful for this purpose.

Complications of Fenestration Closure

Device Misplacement or Embolization

As with ASD or VSD closure, a device implanted across the Fontan baffle that is either undersized or misplaced can embolize either into the pulmonary arteries or into the "left" side of the circulation. Standard techniques for recapturing Amplatzer devices apply (see earlier section on VSD closure for detailed steps). Surgery is a last resort if other efforts fail.

Device Not Lining Up Properly with Septum

Because the angle between the IVC-RA junction and the typical Fontan fenestration is nearly 90 degrees, it can be difficult to get an Amplatzer device to align correctly. The easiest way around this is to deliver the *entire* device on the systemic side, then pull it back taut against the baffle wall, recapture the "right atrial" disc, and deliver on it within the Fontan. Alternate approaches around this problem include beveling the delivery sheath to change the angle, or using a different, straighter access route such as transhepatic.

Residual Shunt

This is extremely rare with the Amplatzer device and is usually of no real consequence, as the resulting jet is of low velocity.

Changes in Protein-Losing Enteropathy

There are several anecdotal reports of worsened protein-losing enteropathy (PLE) following fenestration closure, which may or may not be reversible once the fenestration is reopened. There is no reliable hemodynamic predictor for this complication.

General Anesthesia

If the procedure is performed under general anesthesia, it is important to remember that, within the context of Fontan physiology, positive pressure ventilation itself can lead to a marginal-low cardiac output state.

"Fenestrations" within extracardiac conduit Fontans, as well as baffle leaks (vascular channels) from intracardiac Fontans, can be closed with a variety of devices, depending on the size and configuration of the communication. These are highly variable and require specific angiographic evaluation and on-the-fly planning in the catheterization laboratory. Devices reported in the literature for these purposes include covered stents such as the Cheatham-Platinum stent, detachable coils, Amplatzer ASOs and ADOs, and Helex devices.

Fenestration Creation

Fenestration creation, either in a nonfenestrated Fontan circulation or in the setting of a previously closed fenestration generally involves perforating from the Fontan pathway into the systemic atrium and using either a balloon or a stent to enlarge the resulting communication. This is a challenging procedure and is best achieved with a combination of fluoroscopic and echocardiographic guidance (either transesophageal or intracardiac). In the setting of a tough Gore-Tex membrane, perforation with transseptal needles is extremely difficult and requires a fair amount of force, often enough to distort the entire plane of the "septum" being perforated into a perpendicular plane. A transhepatic approach may be beneficial in that it creates a straighter path (40). Cutting balloons are particularly useful for creating a reasonably sized hole. Stents have been used but are likely to "dogbone" and may not be entirely stable in the setting of a thin membrane with no length. If a device is already present in the septum, device removal could be attempted (unlikely to work unless device has not been in longer than a few weeks) or creation of a side channel within an Amplatzer by placing a small stent. There are no large published series on this procedure.

Note that although fenestration creation is often performed in the setting of PLE with the idea that decompressing the Fontan will lower portal venous pressure and reverse the process, published results show that resolution of PLE after this procedure is unlikely and even more unlikely to be long-lasting (41).

Fenestration creation has been reported in extracardiac conduit Fontans by placing a longer covered stent to bridge from the Fontan to the systemic atrium (42). This would be anticipated to require a high degree of technical ability and have a significant risk of bleeding, and investigators continue to attempt alternative methods of achieving the goal of fenestration creation in the extracardiac conduit Fontan.

Complications of Fenestration Creation

Cardiac Perforation with Resulting Tamponade

As with any transseptal procedure, perforation is a potential complication of fenestration creation. The typical rules of transseptal catheterization apply: if a small wire or transseptal needle perforates, bleeding will usually be controlled if the wire or needle is removed. If a dilator, sheath, or catheter perforates, there is likely to be a hole large enough to require surgical closure, and the object should be left in place to reduce the risk of tamponade in the interim.

Embolization of Air or Balloon Material

Air embolism can be either systemic or pulmonary and underscores the importance of carefully eliminating all air from sheaths, catheters, and balloons. CO_2 preparation of balloons can be helpful before filling them with diluted contrast.

Creation of Too Large a Fenestration with Resulting Severe Cyanosis

It is expected to see an oxygen saturation drop, typically from the 90s into the 80s, after this procedure. If saturations fall to critical levels, this could reflect either pulmonary embolism or too large a fenestration resulting in lack of pulmonary blood flow. To temporize in this situation, while maintaining wire access across the fenestration, a balloon catheter can be advanced back across it and inflated. A more precise diagnosis can then be made and intervention planned.

General Anesthesia

As is the case with fenestration closure, if the procedure is performed under general anesthesia, it is important to remember that, within the context of Fontan physiology, positive pressure ventilation itself can lead to a marginal-low cardiac output state.

■ ARTERIOVENOUS FISTULAE

AVFs can occur anywhere within the circulation. Those typically approached by the interventional cardiologist include aortopulmonary collaterals, pulmonary AVF, and coronary AVF, while cerebral and hepatic AVF are typically managed by interventional radiologists, but there is considerable overlap and room for collaboration.

The original AVP has been shown to be reasonably safe and effective for collaterals, pulmonary AVF, coronary AVF, transhepatic tracts, and central shunts, with an average complete occlusion rate of 94% within 10 minutes and a very low rate of procedure-related complications (32) (Fig. 32-12). The AVP and more recently released AVP II have a fairly low profile and are becoming the default choice for many AV fistulas.

Peripheral AVFs and Complications

These are often high-flow lesions such as hepatic AVF and cerebral AVF. Collaboration with interventional radiology may be useful. Both the AVP and coils can be useful. There is a high risk of embolization due to high flow. There are numerous reports of catastrophic embolization with cyanoacrylate and related glues, even in experienced hands; these make the use of cyanoacrylate and related glues a less attractive option. New expanding "hydrocoils" offer the potential of some promise in this regard.

Coil or Device Embolization

This can occur distally into the venous system and right heart, or proximally into the arterial system. Retrieval techniques depend on the type of device used but follow the standard routine of

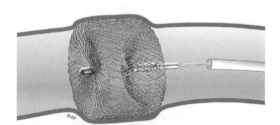

FIGURE 32-12. Schematic of an Amplatzer vascular plug (AVP) situated within a blood vessel. In general, the AVP is sized 30% to 50% greater than the vessel diameter by angiography.

getting to the device, using a snare or bioptome to grasp it, using sheath at least 2F larger than that used to deliver the device, collapsing or at least folding the device into the sheath, and removing the device while trying to minimize dragging a sharp device through intracardiac structures.

Pulmonary AVFs and Complications

Most data on occlusion of these fistulae are in the setting of hereditary hemorrhagic telangiectasia, where pulmonary AVF are quite common (43). Again, collaboration with interventional radiology may be warranted. The standard techniques for small to moderate pulmonary AVFs involve selective catheterization of the feeding artery with a guiding catheter, insertion of a coaxial hydrophilic catheter through the catheter, and delivery of platinum coils or detachable balloons through the catheter. Larger pulmonary AVFs can be treated with standard devices such as the AVP, using a device size between 130% and 150% of the vessel diameter (44).

Coil or Device Embolization

Embolization can occur and is best avoided by (1) anchoring the coil in side branches; (2) using larger, higher radial force coils and then packing behind them with smaller, lower radial force coil; or (3) perhaps most definitively, balloon occluding the feeding artery to allow for safe delivery of coils in the setting of high-flow lesions (43).

Pleural effusion, pleural pain, and air embolism are other potential complications of occlusion for pulmonary AVF.

Coronary AVFs and Complications

Catheter-based occlusion of coronary AVF represents one of the most daunting interventional procedures, with perhaps the least uniformity of techniques. The first transcatheter closure of a coronary AVF was reported using detachable balloons in 1983 (45), with multiple cases being reported starting in the early 1990s. Coronary AVF are often detected in asymptomatic children as continuous murmurs. Presence of ischemia and dilation of the proximal coronary artery are both indications for closure, but this is controversial, and many advocate intervention in the absence of symptoms.

Coronary AVFs have a highly variable source, destination, course, and size, necessitating a diverse armamentarium of devices. In 1997, Mavroudis et al. (46) concluded that coil embolization was possible in "only a very small, select group of patients" (35%–40% of coronary fistulas), restricting them to those which should be cannulated safely, without important large branch vessels that might be occluded, without multiple fistulous communications, and those with a single, restrictive drainage site into the cardiac chamber. Today, although by no means are all coronary AVFs amenable to transcatheter closure, the advent of new devices has increased this number significantly.

A retrograde approach is typically used to access the fistula and perform angiography. Devices used in the past have included gelfoam, polyvinyl alcohol foam, detachable balloons, coils, and various devices (47). If there is a stable position, a coil or a device such as an AVP can be delivered via this approach (48). Free-release coils are useful for small fistulas but have an unacceptably high embolization rate in larger fistulas; controlled-release coils can lower this rate somewhat (49). A coaxial technique can provide improved stability with precise coil delivery into the distal portion of a fistula (50). Often, with very large or complex fistulas, an AV wire loop is desired for more security and for delivery from the venous side. This is also helpful if higher profile devices need to be inserted, as they limit arterial sheath size.

Other devices may be more appropriate depending on anatomy. A small series of patients with short, nontortuous fistulas with a proximal origin underwent fistula closure with the ADOs (six ADOs in six patients, five complete closures, one small residual shunt). There were no embolizations, device misplacements or deaths (51). The ADO has even been used in neonates with large coronary fistulas (52) and has been delivered retrogradely in adults, obviating the need for an AV wire loop (53). In one report, a 2.4-kg neonate underwent sequential placement of a 12-mm Amplatzer mVSD device, seven Flipper coils, a 10/8 ADO, and a 9-mm Gianturco–Grifka vascular occlusion device within a giant coronary AVF (54). As evidenced by this report, the tremendous anatomic variability of coronary AVF necessitates adaptability and a wide armamentarium of devices.

Another approach is using "stent grafts" (covered stents) to obstruct the wall of the fistula. The advantage of this approach is that there is obviously less risk of clot propagation back into the coronary, but there is a potential risk of neointimal growth within the stent. This approach has been applied in a small number of adult patients with some success (55).

In one series of transcatheter closures of coronary fistulas in 45 patients, there was a 91% complete closure rate, with 93% of patients symptom-free and complication-free. Procedural mortality was similar for coils and surgery at 1.4% to 2.2% (56). A more recent series from France included 25 patients undergoing 30 procedures, with a wide range in ages from children to adults. Various devices (17 coils, 9 detachable balloons, 5 microparticles, 2 Amplatzer devices) were used, with an overall success rate of 92% and an acceptable 4% complication rate with no deaths (57).

Embolization

The major complication of device and coil placement within a coronary AVF is embolization. Retrieval is accomplished via the usual techniques depending on the location of embolization. With coils, the use of detachable rather than free-release coils can be helpful. To avoid distal migration or embolization, it is helpful to start with a larger coil and to use a

"backstop" technique of packing smaller coils behind it. To avoid proximal migration, the coil should be delivered as distally as possible. When placing coils into very distal, tiny vessels, it may be helpful to use 0.018-in. microcoils, which can be delivered through tiny coaxial 3F microcatheters (58). When using an AVP to occlude a coronary AVF, sizing greater than 150% of vessel size is useful.

Ischemia

This obviously arises from occlusion of the flow in the coronary artery from which the fistula arises; ST and T wave changes must be looked for carefully, recognized immediately, and dealt with expediently to avoid precipitating infarction. Test occlusion with a balloon tipped catheter may be useful, especially in infants, to predict effect of closure and the best location for closure (52). Following creatine kinase-MB and troponin levels may be helpful. Both early and late infarction have been reported, with one report of an apparent clot propagating back from the fistula into the left circumflex and resulting in complete occlusion (59). Fatal occlusion of a larger coronary artery can occur with coils that work their way back during deployment. It is important to deliver coils distally (Fig. 32-13), being careful not to use a longer coil than necessary (47). It is quite dangerous to try to snare, retrieve, and drag coils within

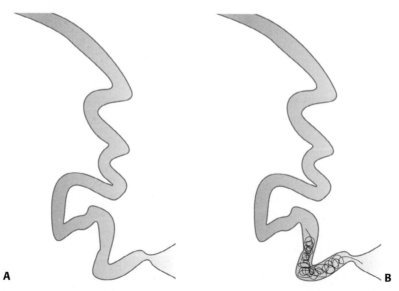

FIGURE 32-13. Ideal site of coronary fistula occlusion with coils. (**A**) Long, tortuous feeding artery leading toward fistula. (**B**) Multiple coils placed distally within feeding artery, occluding fistula.

epicardial coronaries as they can easily be dissected (60). In this case, the ADO and AVP are both more easily repositioned.

Arrhythmias

Right bundle branch block and transient junctional tachycardia have both been reported (61).

Guidewire Entrapment

This has been reported especially with small 0.014-in. coronary guidewires. These are generally retrievable with a snare to prevent fracture (62).

Residual Shunt

This is quite common immediately postintervention but does decrease with time. If the residual shunt is not audible and seen only by echocardiography, it is not clear whether the patient is at elevated risk for endocarditis, but prophylaxis seems reasonable in this setting (47).

Persistent Coronary Artery Dilation

Many patients with coronary AVF have continued coronary dilation even after closure. Despite the absence of good data, antiplatelet agents are generally used with more aggressive anticoagulation reserved for aneurysms and severe dilation (63).

Unfortunately, there is a general paucity of large series on transcatheter closure of coronary AVF. Pediatric data are sparse, with many case reports and a few case series, and current efforts are ongoing to collect multicenter registry data on these challenging cases.

■ ACKNOWLEDGMENTS

The author thanks Dr. Daniel Levi for generously providing several images, Dr. Albert Rocchini for carefully reviewing the manuscript, and Donna Wilkin for expertly preparing all of the figures used in this chapter.

References

1. Lock JE, et al. Transcatheter closure of ventricular septal defects. *Circulation.* 1988;78(2):361–368.
2. Holzer R, et al. Transcatheter closure of postinfarction ventricular septal defects using the new Amplatzer muscular VSD occluder: results of a U.S. Registry. *Catheter Cardiovasc Interv.* 2004;61(2): 196–201.
3. Landzberg MJ, Lock JE. Transcatheter management of ventricular septal rupture after myocar-

dial infarction. *Semin Thorac Cardiovasc Surg.* 1998;10(2):128–132.
4. Martinez MW, et al. Transcatheter closure of ischemic and post-traumatic ventricular septal ruptures. *Catheter Cardiovasc Interv.* 2007;69(3): 403–407.
5. Mullins CE. *Cardiac Catheterization in Congenital Heart Disease.* Malden, MA: Blackwell Futura; 2006.
6. Levi DS, Moore JW. Embolization and retrieval of the Amplatzer septal occluder. *Catheter Cardiovasc Interv.* 2004;61(4):543–547.
7. Tan CA, Levi DS, Moore JW. Embolization and transcatheter retrieval of coils and devices. *Pediatr Cardiol.* 2005;26(3):267–274.
8. Spence MS, et al. Transient renal failure due to hemolysis following transcatheter closure of a muscular VSD using an Amplatzer muscular VSD occluder. *Catheter Cardiovasc Interv.* 2006;67(5): 663–667.
9. Carminati M, et al. Transcatheter closure of congenital ventricular septal defect with Amplatzer septal occluders. *Am J Cardiol.* 2005;96(12A): 52L–58L.
10. Scheuerman O, et al. Endocarditis after closure of ventricular septal defect by transcatheter device. *Pediatrics.* 2006;117(6):8.
11. Holzer R, et al. Transcatheter closure of perimembranous ventricular septal defects using the amplatzer membranous VSD occluder: immediate and midterm results of an international registry. *Catheter Cardiovasc Interv.* 2006;68(4): 620–628.
12. Kenny D, Tometzki A, Martin R. Significant aortic regurgitation associated with transcatheter closure of perimembranous ventricular septal defects with a deficient aortic rim. *Catheter Cardiovasc Interv.* 2007;70(3):445–449.
13. Zhou T, et al. Complications associated with transcatheter closure of perimembranous ventricular septal defects. *Catheter Cardiovasc Interv.* 2008;71(4):559-563.
14. Butera G, et al. Transcatheter closure of perimembranous ventricular septal defects: early and long-term results. *J Am Coll Cardiol.* 2007;50(12): 1189–1195.
15. Yip WC, Zimmerman F, Hijazi ZM. Heart block and empirical therapy after transcatheter closure of perimembranous ventricular septal defect. *Catheter Cardiovasc Interv.* 2005;66(3):436–441.
16. Zhu XY, et al. Risk factors for early arrhythmias post transcatheter closure of perimembranous

ventricular septal defects. *Zhong Hua Xin Xue Guan Bing Za Zhi.* 2007;35(7):633–636.

17. Bacha EA, et al. Multicenter experience with perventricular device closure of muscular ventricular septal defects. *Pediatr Cardiol.* 2005;26(2): 169–175.

18. García-Valentín A, et al. Device migration in hybrid technique for apical muscular ventricular septal defects closure. *Interact Cardiovasc Thorac Surg.* 2007;6(6):780–782.

19. Holzer R, et al. Device closure of muscular ventricular septal defects using the amplatzer muscular ventricular septal defect occluder: immediate and mid-term results of a U.S. registry. *J Am Coll Cardiol.* 2004;43(7):1257–1263.

20. Lock JE, et al. Transcatheter closure of patent ductus arteriosus in piglets. *Am J Cardiol.* 1985; 55(6):826–829.

21. Bussmann WD, Sievert H, Kaltenbach M. Transfemoral occlusion of persistent ductus arteriosus. *Dtsch Med Wochenschr.* 1984;109(35):1322–1326.

22. Babic UU, et al. Double-umbrella device for transvenous closure of patent ductus arteriosus and atrial septal defect: first experience. *J Interv Cardiol.* 1991;4(4):283–294.

23. Rao PS, et al. Transcatheter closure of patent ductus arteriosus with buttoned device: first successful clinical application in a child. *Am Heart J.* 1991;121(6, pt 1):1799–1802.

24. Sivakumar K, Francis E, Krishnan P. Safety and feasibility of transcatheter closure of large patent ductus arteriosus measuring ≥4 mm in patients weighing ≤6 kg. *J Interv Cardiol.* 2008;21(2): 196–203.

25. Krichenko A, et al. Angiographic classification of the isolated, persistently patent ductus arteriosus and implications for percutaneous catheter occlusion. *Am J Cardiol.* 1989;63(12):877–880.

26. Rao PS. Percutaneous closure of patent ductus arteriosus: state of the art. *J Invasive Cardiol.* 2007; 19(7):299–302.

27. Lloyd TR, et al. Transcatheter occlusion of patent ductus arteriosus with Gianturco coils. *Circulation.* 1993;88(4, pt 1):1412–1420.

28. Gupta K, Rao PS. Severe intravascular hemolysis after transcatheter coil occlusion of patent ductus arteriosus. *J Invasive Cardiol.* 2005;17(10):7.

29. Pass RH, et al. Multicenter USA Amplatzer patent ductus arteriosus occlusion device trial: initial and one-year results. *J Am Coll Cardiol.* 2004; 44(3):513–519.

30. Bilkis AA, et al. The Amplatzer duct occluder: experience in 209 patients. *J Am Coll Cardiol.* 2001;37(1):258–261.

31. Masura J, et al. Long-term outcome of transcatheter patent ductus arteriosus closure using Amplatzer duct occluders. *Am Heart J.* 2006; 151(3):755.e7–755.e10.

32. Hill SL, et al. Evaluation of the AMPLATZER vascular plug for embolization of peripheral vascular malformations associated with congenital heart disease. *Catheter Cardiovasc Interv.* 2006;67(1): 113–119.

33. Sivakumar K, et al. Ductal stenting retrains the left ventricle in transposition of great arteries with intact ventricular septum. *J Thorac Cardiovasc Surg.* 2006;132(5):1081–1086.

34. Santoro G, et al. Neonatal patent ductus arteriosus recanalization and stenting in critical Ebstein's anomaly. *Pediatr Cardiol.* 2008;29(1):176–179.

35. Gewillig M, et al. Stenting the neonatal arterial duct in duct-dependent pulmonary circulation: new techniques, better results. *J Am Coll Cardiol.* 2004;43(1):107–112.

36. Gibbs JL, et al. Fate of the stented arterial duct. *Circulation.* 1999;99(20):2621–2625.

37. Michel-Behnke I, et al. Stent implantation in the ductus arteriosus for pulmonary blood supply in congenital heart disease. *Catheter Cardiovasc Interv.* 2004;61(2):242–252.

38. Boucek MM, et al. Ductal anatomy: a determinant of successful stenting in hypoplastic left heart syndrome. *Pediatr Cardiol.* 2005;26(2):200–205.

39. Cowley CG, et al. Transcatheter closure of fontan fenestrations using the amplatzer septal occluder: initial experience and follow-up. *Catheter Cardiovasc Interv.* 2000;51(3):301–304.

40. Recto MR, Sobczyk WL, Austin EH. Transcatheter fenestration of autologous pericardial extracardiac fontan via the transhepatic approach. *J Invasive Cardiol.* 2005;17(11):628–630.

41. Vyas H, et al. Results of transcatheter fontan fenestration to treat protein losing enteropathy. *Catheter Cardiovasc Interv.* 2007;69(4):584–589.

42. Michel-Behnke I, et al. Fenestration in extracardiac conduits in children after modified fontan operation by implantation of stent grafts. *Pediatr Cardiol.* 2005;26(1):93–96.

43. De Cillis E, et al. Endovascular treatment of pulmonary and cerebral arteriovenous malformations in patients affected by hereditary haemorrhagic teleangiectasia. *Curr Pharm Des.* 2006;12(10):1243–1248.

44. Farra H, Balzer DT. Transcatheter occlusion of a large pulmonary arteriovenous malformation using the amplatzer vascular plug. *Pediatr Cardiol.* 2005;26(5):683–685.

45. Reidy JF, Sowton E, Ross DN. Transcatheter occlusion of coronary to bronchial anastomosis by detachable balloon combined with coronary angioplasty at same procedure. *Br Heart J.* 1983; 49(3):284–287.

46. Mavroudis C, et al. Coronary artery fistulas in infants and children: a surgical review and discussion of coil embolization. *Ann Thorac Surg.* 1997;63(5):1235–1242.

47. Okubo M, Nykanen D, Benson LN. Outcomes of transcatheter embolization in the treatment of coronary artery fistulas. *Catheter Cardiovasc Interv.* 2001;52(4):510–517.

48. Kassaian SE, et al. Transcatheter closure of a coronary fistula with an amplatzer vascular plug: should a retrograde approach be standard? *Tex Heart Inst J.* 2008;35(1):58–61.

49. Qureshi SA, Tynan M. Catheter closure of coronary artery fistulas. *J Interv Cardiol.* 2001;14(3): 299–307.

50. Kung GC, et al. Retrograde transcatheter coil embolization of congenital coronary artery fistulas in infants and young children. *Pediatr Cardiol.* 2003;24(5):448–453.

51. Behera SK, et al. Transcatheter closure of coronary artery fistulae using the amplatzer duct occluder. *Catheter Cardiovasc Interv.* 2006;68(2):242–248.

52. Khan MD, et al. Neonatal transcatheter occlusion of a large coronary artery fistula with amplatzer duct occluder. *Catheter Cardiovasc Interv.* 2003;60(2): 282–286.

53. Subramanyan R, Agrawal A, Abhyankar A. Transcatheter closure of a large coronary artery fistula with amplatzer duct occluder: a new approach. *Indian Heart J.* 2001;53(4):493–495.

54. Holzer R, et al. Percutaneous closure of a giant coronary arteriovenous fistula using multiple devices in a 12-day-old neonate. *Catheter Cardiovasc Interv.* 2003;60(2):291–294.

55. Kilic H, et al. Transcatheter closure of congenital coronary arterial fistulas in adults. *Coron Artery Dis.* 2008;19(1):43–45.

56. Armsby LR, et al. Management of coronary artery fistulae: patient selection and results of transcatheter closure. *J Am Coll Cardiol.* 2002;39(6): 1026–1032.

57. Brenot P, et al. Endovascular treatment of coronary arterial fistulae in children and adults. *Arch Mal Coeur Vaiss.* 2007;100(5): 373–379.

58. Kabbani Z, et al. Coil embolization of coronary artery fistulas: a single-centre experience. *Cardiovasc Revasc Med.* 2008;9(1):14–17.

59. Kharouf R, Cao QL, Hijazi ZM. Transcatheter closure of coronary artery fistula complicated by myocardial infarction. *J Invasive Cardiol.* 2007; 19(5):9.

60. Dorros G, et al. Catheter-based techniques for closure of coronary fistulae. *Catheter Cardiovasc Interv.* 1999;46(2):143–150.

61. Perry SB, et al. Transcatheter closure of coronary artery fistulas. *J Am Coll Cardiol.* 1992;20(1):205–209.

62. De Wolf D, et al. Entrapment of a guide wire during percutaneous occlusion of a coronary artery fistula. *Acta Cardiol.* 1998;53(5):287–289.

63. McMahon CJ, et al. Coronary artery fistula: management and intermediate-term outcome after transcatheter coil occlusion. *Tex Heart Inst J.* 2001;28(1):21–25.

64. Chessa M, et al. Transcatheter closure of congenital ventricular septal defects in adult: mid-term results and complications. *Int J Cardiol.* 2009;133(1):70–73.

65. Carminati M, et al. Transcatheter closure of congenital ventricular septal defects: results of the European registry. *Eur Heart J.* 2007;28(19): 2361–2368.

66. Diab KA, et al. Device closure of muscular ventricular septal defects in infants less than one year of age using the Amplatzer devices: feasibility and outcome. *Catheter Cardiovasc Interv.* 2007;70(1): 90–97.

67. Fu Y, et al. Transcatheter closure of perimembranous ventricular septal defects using the new Amplatzer Membranous VSD occluder: results of the U.S. Phase I trial. *J Am Coll Cardiol.* 2006;47(2):319–325.

68. Bass JL, et al. Initial human experience with the Amplatzer perimembranous ventricular septal occluder device. *Catheter Cardiovasc Interv.* 2003; 58(2):238–245.

69. Thanopoulos BD, Rigby ML. Outcome of transcatheter closure of muscular ventricular septal defects with the Amplatzer ventricular septal defect occluder. *Heart* 2005;91(4):513–516.

70. Arora R, et al. Transcatheter closure of congenital muscular ventricular septal defect. *J Interv Cardiol.* 2004;17(2):109–115.

71. Masura J, et al. Percutaneous closure of perimembranous ventricular septal defects with the
eccentric Amplatzer device: multicenter follow-
up study. *Pediatr Cardiol.* 26(3):216–219.

72. Wang J, et al. Transcatheter closure of moderate
to large patent ductus arteriosus with the
Amplatzer Duct Occluder. *Catheter Cardiovasc
Interv.* 2007;69(4):572–578.

73. Ebeid MR, Masura J, Hijazi ZM. Early experience
with the Amplatzer Ductal Occluder for closure
of the persistently patent ductus arteriosus.
J Interv Cardiol. 2001;14(1):33–36.

74. Faella HJ, Hijazi ZM. Closure of the patent ductus
arteriosus with the Amplatzer PDA device: immediate results of the international clinical trial.
Catheter Cardiovasc Interv. 2000;51(1):50–54.

SECTION

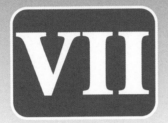

VII

Electrophysiology Procedures

33

Implantable Devices

AVI FISCHER AND ANDRE D'AVILA

C ardiac rhythm device therapy has become more accepted and widespread over the last two decades. It is important to recognize that there are potential complications that may occur both during the implant procedure and follow-up. Experience and technique are important in reducing the risk of complications, but every implanting physician will at some point deal with a complication. There are complications that are not device-specific and may occur with any of the devices implanted and complications unique to specific devices such as implantable cardioverter defibrillators (ICDs) and cardiac resynchronization (CRT) devices. Understanding and appreciating the potential complications is important so that appropriate discussions can take place with the patient and family prior to the implant procedure. While complications are rare and unwanted, the reality is that every implanting physician has complications.

■ VENOUS ACCESS–RELATED COMPLICATIONS

There are various routes of access used for placement of endocardial pacing and defibrillator leads including the subclavian, cephalic, jugular and ileofemoral veins (1–3). Most often, a cephalic vein cutdown, direct axillary vein (extra thoracic subclavian vein) puncture, and direct subclavian vein puncture are utilized. Complications may occur during cannulation, manipulation of the lead within the heart, and placement and fixation of a permanent lead. Inherent in any approach to venous access is the potential for damage to adjacent structures such as neural or arterial structures, excessive bleeding, thrombosis of the vein being manipulated and air embolism. Complications may become evident immediately or in the ensuing hours or even days after implant.

Pneumothorax

Knowledge of venous anatomy is important to reduce the risk of pneumothorax associated with venous access. A direct cephalic vein cutdown has virtually no risk of pneumothorax. When a direct cephalic vein cutdown is not performed and venous puncture is performed via the Seldinger technique, knowledge of the route of the axillary vein and subclavian vein and the relationship of these veins to the clavicle, first rib, and apex of the lung is crucial to minimize the risk of pneumothorax associated with blind puncture. The axillary vein is an extrathoracic structure that terminates at the lateral margin of the first rib; if access is obtained in an extra thoracic location, there is no risk of pneumothorax. Contrast venography may aid in identifying the desired vein and for identifying branches such as the cephalic vein, axillary vein, and subclavian vein (Fig. 33-1). It has been reported that the incidence of pneumothorax associated with subclavian puncture by experienced implanters is approximately 1% (4).

Pneumothorax may manifest during the implant procedure or as late as 48 hours after implantation. It is crucial to be able to identify the occurrence of pneumothorax during the implant. Aspiration of air during the attempted venous puncture may raise the suspicion of pneumothorax, but this is neither sensitive nor specific (1). Signs and symptoms of pneumothorax during the procedure include agitation, chest pain, respiratory distress, hypoxia, hypotension, and tachycardia. Symptoms that arise during the procedure should prompt assessment of blood pressure, pulse, oximetry, and even blood gas analysis. Use of fluoroscopy can quickly identify the presence of pneumothorax during the implant, and chest radiography after the procedure can assist in identifying pneumothorax after completion of the implant (Fig. 33-2).

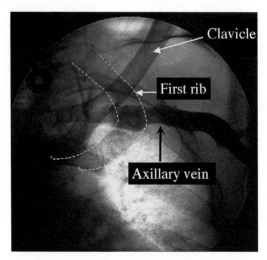

FIGURE 33-1. Contrast venogram performed in the anteroposterior projection demonstrating anatomy of the subclavian system and important landmarks. The axillary vein can be seen crossing the first rib.

Depending on the size of pneumothorax and the amount of lung involved, placement of a chest tube may be required. A chest tube is often considered if more than 10% of the lung volume is involved and if persistent respiratory compromise is present. Use of high-flow 100% oxygen delivered by facemask may help shrink the size of the pneumothorax and facilitate its resolution.

Hemothorax

This complication, although rare, is known to occur if the subclavian vein is lacerated by the access needle or if a larger-bore dilator or sheath is inadvertently introduced into the subclavian

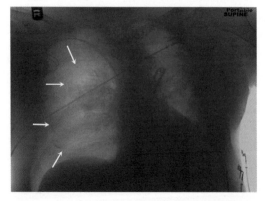

FIGURE 33-2. Anteroposterior chest radiograph in the supine position demonstrating a large right-sided pneumothorax after permanent pacemaker placement. The *arrows* point to the visibly collapsed lung.

artery and then removed. As a result of the laceration or arterial puncture, bleeding occurs into the surrounding tissues and even into the thorax itself. Compression over the site of the laceration to stop the bleeding must be performed; rarely, vascular surgical assistance is required to identify the location of the laceration and repair the damaged vascular structure. If a large sheath is inserted into the artery, strong consideration for surgical repair should be considered and the sheath left in place (1). The possibility of endovascular repair with balloon tamponade or stent graft repair has been reported (5,6). When hemothorax is identified, chest tube placement is often required.

Air Embolism

When introducing leads through a sheath placed in a central vein, air may enter the venous system (7). Air enters the venous system as it is sucked into the sheath during inspiration when intrathoracic pressure is negative. Air embolism may lead to chest pain, hypoxia, hypotension, and even respiratory distress. Often air bubbles can be seen traveling through the right heart ultimately dissipating. The use of sheaths with a one-way hemostatic valve, leg elevation, and having the patient Valsalva when the sheath is open to air minimize this risk. Although the sequelae of air embolism in the venous system are transient, supportive measures such as supplemental oxygen and inotropic support are often utilized.

Miscellaneous Access-Related Complications

As all the veins utilized for access are adjacent to other critical structures, a variety of other potential complications should not be forgotten. Rarely as a result of the proximity of the veins to their corresponding arteries, inadvertent puncture of both the vein and adjacent artery may result in formation of an arteriovenous fistula (8). Other adjacent structures that have the potential for being damaged during venous access include the thoracic duct, regional nerves including the brachial plexus, and even rarely a left internal mammary artery graft (9). All of these complications are quite rare, but the implanter must be aware not only of these structures but also of potential injury to these structures.

■ ARRHYTHMIAS

Tachyarrhythmias

A frequent complication during manipulation of leads and/or guidewires during device implantation is the development of supraventricular or ventricular tachyarrhythmias. These arrhythmias are usually transient and self-limited, terminating either spontaneously or with change in the guidewire or lead position. Occasionally, tachyarrhythmias may sustain and require intervention such as defibrillation. For this reason, it is advocated that all patients be monitored, attached via transcutaneous pads to an external defibrillator, and life-support equipment be present in the room during device implantation.

The most common supraventricular tachyarrhythmias to occur as a result of lead manipulation within the atrium are atrial tachycardia, atrial flutter, and atrial fibrillation. Both atrial flutter and tachycardia can often be pace-terminated by overdrive pacing through the pacing system analyzer (PSA) or with further manipulation of the lead against the wall of the right atrium. Atrial fibrillation when sustained may require cardioversion. The routine use of transcutaneous pacing and defibrillation pads during the implant procedure facilitate cardioversion should it be necessary.

Ventricular tachyarrhythmias are also frequently seen during lead manipulation and premature ventricular contractions (PVCs) during manipulation of the ventricular lead are often used to confirm the lead position as being right ventricular (RV) (rather than in the coronary sinus). Similar to supraventricular tachyarrhythmias, ventricular tachyarrhythmias are often transient and usually do not require treatment. Occasionally manipulation of the guidewire or lead in the ventricle induces sustained ventricular tachycardia. This occurs more frequently during implantation of ICD leads and in patients with significant structural heart disease. As is the case with supraventricular tachyarrhythmias, further lead manipulation in the ventricle, overdrive pacing, and defibrillation may be necessary to terminate a sustained arrhythmia.

Bradyarrhythmias

Bradyarrhythmias that occur during device implantation are frequently transient and self-limited. In particular, patients with intermittent atrio-ventricular (AV) block and those with a left bundle branch block (LBBB) are prone to mechanical trauma to the right bundle, resulting in complete AV block. Care must be exercised when implanting CRT devices, where the presence of a LBBB is almost universal. Having the lead attached to the PSA with backup pacing readily available when crossing the tricuspid valve will aid in preventing asystole should AV block occur with lead manipulation. In addition to AV block, a common mechanism of bradycardia during lead placement is overdrive suppression of a ventricular escape focus during threshold testing. Reducing the pacing rate gradually via the PSA will allow the escape focus to reappear in the event that suppression occurs with threshold testing. In the patient at high risk for development of AV block or asystole during the procedure, a temporary transvenous pacemaker can be placed prior to the procedure. A rare phenomenon has been reported during placement of CRT devices, where profound and irreversible bradycardia and hypotension is seen after coronary sinus cannulation. Speculation as to the precise mechanism exists, and it is believed to be a result of C fiber stimulation in the posterior left atrium, leading to the Bezold–Jarisch reflex (10). Supportive measures with inotropic and vasoactive agents may be required in addition to advanced cardiac life-support.

Arrhythmias in the Postimplantation Period

As a result of irritation at the lead tip–myocardial interface, PVCs may occur in the early period after implantation. These PVCs often have a morphology similar to the paced complexes and are referred to as *tip extrasystoles*. Rarely do these extrasystoles require treatment and they often subside within 24 hours after implantation. Recently, there have been reports of ICD leads being "proarrhythmic," leading to recurrent sustained ventricular tachyarrhythmias days and weeks after implantation. In some instances, ablation and even lead extraction may be necessary to abolish the tachyarrhythmias (11).

■ LEAD PLACEMENT–RELATED COMPLICATIONS

Acute Perforation

Perforations may occur during lead implantation, and the true incidence is probably greater than reported. The incidence varies widely depending on the series and type of leads evaluated. Many perforations go unrecognized as clinical sequelae might not occur when perforations reseal spontaneously. In a review of routine computed tomography scans obtained in patients with implantable cardiac rhythm devices, asymptomatic but radiographically apparent lead perforation was present in 15% of patients (12). Perforation may occur with placement of the RV lead as well as with the right atrial lead; rarely coronary venous perforations occur with left ventricular (LV) lead placement during a CRT device implant. Several findings may suggest the presence of a perforation during implant, and the implanting physician should be aware of these signs and symptoms. Poor sensing and capture thresholds, an extremely distal lead tip location on fluoroscopy, chest pain, a right bundle branch block (RBBB) morphology during RV lead pacing, and contrast outlining the cardiac borders after venography in the case of LV lead placement should raise the suspicion of perforation. Anodal pacing compared with cathodal pacing may help determine whether the lead tip has perforated; cathodal pacing will not capture myocardium, whereas anodal pacing will capture if the lead tip is through the myocardium (13). Progressive hypotension and tachycardia along with changing contours of the cardiac silhouette under fluoroscopy indicate the possibility of cardiac tamponade as a result of perforation. When signs and symptoms of perforation occur, cardiac tamponade should be considered present until ruled out by echocardiography. In addition to tamponade, reports of right-sided pneumothorax have been reported with right atrial lead perforation (14). Older age, female gender, steroid use, recent RV infarction, and the use of stiff stylets increase the risk of perforation. Coronary sinus perforation rarely causes tamponade due to the fact that intravenous pressure (pressure within the coronary veins) is considerably lower than RV pressure. As a result, blood flows into the proximal portion of the vein rather than into the pericardial space.

Management of acute lead perforation depends on the clinical course. If perforation is thought to have occurred, echocardiography should be performed to identify the presence or absence of a pericardial effusion. Acutely, tamponade may occur with accumulation of even small amounts of fluid in the pericardial space.

If signs and symptoms of tamponade are present, pericardiocentesis may be required if echocardiography is not readily available. The use of echocardiography to identify the presence of a pericardial effusion is essential, and in the absence of tamponade, the size of the effusion can be followed. Placement of a pigtail catheter into the pericardial space will prevent recurrent hemodynamic compromise and allow for monitoring of drainage. Timing of removal of the pigtail catheter depends on the presence or absence of reaccumulating fluid. A slow pericardial leak may occur as a result of perforation with symptoms occurring only days after the implant. As a result of the perforation, signs and symptoms of pericarditis may occur within 5 to 7 days and nonsteroidal anti-inflammatory agents may be required for analgesia.

The use of anticoagulants in the postoperative period often becomes an issue and care should be used when initiating or continuing anticoagulation in patients with suspected and especially confirmed perforation. Thrombolytics and IIb/IIIa antagonists should be considered contraindicated in the immediate postoperative period regardless of the presence of perforation.

■ CHRONIC PERFORATION

Occasionally, patients are found during routine follow-up to have lead perforation (Fig. 33-3). The presence of recurrent pericardial effusions, pericarditis, poor sensing, and pacing thresholds as well as lead position on chest radiograph may raise the suspicion of a lead perforation. Pericardial effusions should be drained when present and symptoms of pericarditis treated. Lead repositioning should be performed under hemodynamic monitoring in a facility and location capable of treating tamponade and cardiac surgery backup should be considered. Often a chronic lead can be repositioned, but depending on the age of the lead, the entire lead may need to be removed if manipulation and repositioning is difficult. When this occurs, new venous access should be obtained for placement of a new lead prior to removal of the old lead.

Lead Placement into the Systemic Circulation

There are several ways in which a transvenous pacing lead can enter and be fixed into the left

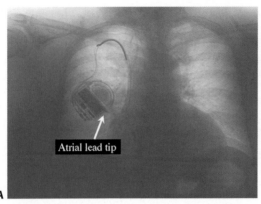
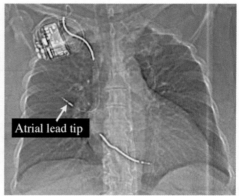

FIGURE 33-3. (**A**) Anterioposterior chest radiograph (taken several years after implant) from a patient referred for a "nonfunctional" atrial lead. The patient has a dual-chamber implantable cardioverter defibrillator implanted on the right. The atrial lead is clearly extracardiac. The patient offered no complaints. (**B**) Scout image from a subsequent computed tomography scan with intravenous contrast performed in the same patient to better define the course of the atrial lead. The course of the atrial lead was through the right atrial wall into the parenchyma of the inferior right upper lobe. No pneumothorax or hemorrhage was present along the tract of the lead. The lead was removed without complication and a new atrial lead placed.

heart (15). Cannulation of an artery rather than a vein, with retrograde passage of a lead across the aortic valve into the left ventricle, is one possibility. The presence of a tortuous and "uncoiled" aorta whose course is more rightward than typical may lead to mistaken placement of the lead into a systemic chamber. Knowledge of the typical course of anatomic structures in the thorax is critical to early identification of such errors. Advancement of the guidewire used for venous access into the IVC confirms the vascular structure as being venous and that the right heart will be used for lead placement. Lead placement into the LV may not be readily apparent on the anteroposterior radiographic image; however, lateral or oblique views will identify the ventricular lead in a posterior location characteristic of the LV. In addition, the morphology of the paced QRS complex will have a characteristic RBBB pattern.

The right atrium is separated from the left ventricle by the membranous septum, and the right and left ventricles are separated by the muscular septum. Inadvertent passage of a lead through these structures is possible with placement of a lead via the venous system into the systemic ventricle. In addition, communications within the cardiac chambers such as an atrial septal defect (ASD) are other potential sources of lead placement into systemic chambers (15,16).

Early recognition of systemically placed leads along with lead repositioning are critical as the thromboembolic risk associated with systemic leads is high even for patients treated with antiplatelet agents (17). Long-term anticoagulation may be necessary in a chronically implanted lead found to be located in the systemic circulation (16,18). Cardiac surgery intervention should be considered for chronic LV leads, as percutaneous lead extraction is more complex and the thromboembolic consequences of removal of leads present in the systemic circulation are more serious (18).

Lead Dislodgement

A common complication of transvenous lead placement is lead dislodgement. The rate of dislodgement of atrial leads tends to be slightly higher than ventricular leads. Dislodgements are thought to correspond to implanter experience, with less experienced operators having higher dislodgement rates (19). With current lead design, the dislodgement rate is less than 2% to 3%; however, some experienced operators believe that the rate should be even lower (19). Generally, dislodgement is the result of poor initial placement with subsequent migration prior to stabilization of the lead via fibrosis and thrombus formation. Dislodgement can be either "macrodislodgement," which is readily visible on

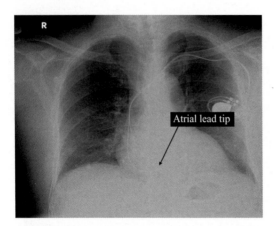

FIGURE 33-4. Anterioposterior chest radiograph taken the day after pacemaker implantation revealing a macrodislodgement of the right atrial lead.

radiographic images (Fig. 33-4), or "microdislodgement" with no clear radiographic evidence of lead migration but pacing and sensing thresholds indicative of lead tip migration (Fig. 33-5). Ensuring that the leads have adequate slack, anchoring the leads with the suture sleeves and limiting elevation and extreme flexion and extension of the ipsilateral upper extremity for several weeks after implant help reduce the inci-

dence of dislodgement. Most important, however, is ensuring that a stable position is obtained at implant.

Recognition of lead dislodgement should result in repositioning of the lead. The presence of ectopy, changing or worsening sensing or pacing thresholds, and even loss of capture or sensing should raise the suspicion that the lead has migrated. Chest radiography should be obtained and compared with previously obtained radiographs. Repositioning of acutely implanted leads is usually not difficult, as the leads have not had sufficient time to fibrose to the endothelium and endocardium. Worsening function of a chronically implanted lead may ultimately require placement of a new lead as mobilizing and repositioning chronic leads can be challenging.

Coronary sinus lead dislodgement is one of the difficulties faced when treating patients with CRT devices (Fig. 33-6). Although rates of dislodgement have been significantly reduced through improved lead technology and design, coronary venous leads continue to have a higher dislodgement rate than RA and RV leads. Loss of LV capture can be readily discerned on the surface electrocardiogram and the morphology of QRS

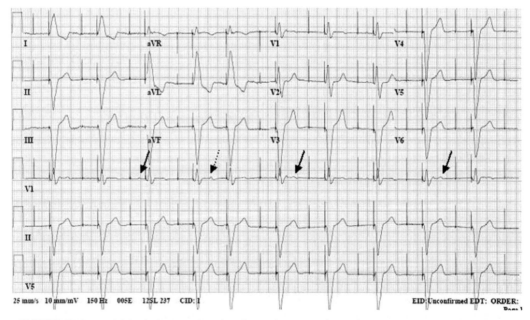

FIGURE 33-5. Twelve-lead electrocardiogram obtained in a patient with a dual chamber pacemaker and microdislodgement of the atrial lead. No P wave is present after delivery of an atrial pace. P waves can be seen (*solid arrows*) and intermittently sensed (*hatched arrow*) with subsequent right ventricular (RV) pacing. (Note the early RV pace after the sensed P wave.)

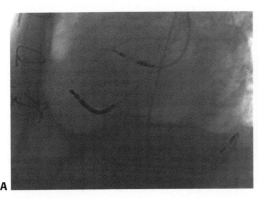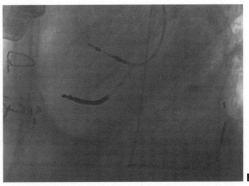

A   B

FIGURE 33-6. Lateral radiographs of a patient with dislodgement of the left ventricular (LV) lead in a cardiac resynchronization defibrillator (CRT-D) system. (**A**) Image taken the day after implant (note suboptimal slack or "J" on the atrial lead). The patient returned for follow-up several months later without improvement in symptoms. (**B**) There was no capture with LV pacing as a result of dislodgement of the LV lead. The patient subsequently underwent replacement of the LV lead.

complex during pacing should be sufficient to diagnose dislodgement of an LV lead. Occasionally, dislodgement manifests as diaphragmatic or extra-cardiac stimulation. Rarely, ventricular ectopy and even ventricular arrhythmias may be the result of coronary venous lead dislodgement. Unfortunately, LV leads are not easily repositioned without support from the sheaths and guides employed during implantation and invariably the dislodged lead must be removed and another LV lead implanted.

Lead Damage

Leads can be damaged by a variety of instruments and tools employed during the implant. Scissors, scalpels and electrocautery can damage the outer insulation present on the leads. Polyurethane leads in particular can be damaged by suture material placed directly on the lead rather than on an anchoring sleeve. On rare occasions, the stylet itself may penetrate the conductor and insulating material in the lead if the angle at which it enters the lead is oblique.

When replacing a generator, pulling and tension placed on the lead close to the terminal pin where the lead enters the header of the device may lead to uncoiling and damage to the conducting elements. Freeing the leads from surrounding capsule rather than "pulling" on the leads prevents unnecessary tension and potential damage. Regardless of the cause, when damage to a lead is recognized, the lead should be discarded or abandoned and a new lead used.

■ THE PULSE GENERATOR POCKET

The importance of creating an appropriately sized pocket in the proper location cannot be overstated as the location and size of the pocket must ensure comfort and mobility of the ipsilateral shoulder and arm. The pulse generator pocket should be made to easily accommodate the pulse generator and leads. Too small a pocket may result in erosion and too large a pocket in device migration. The pocket should be made in the prepectoralis fascia beneath the adipose layer. A pocket made in the wrong plane of tissue (subcuticular) above the adipose layer may lead to chronic pain as the pulse generator presses on the undersurface of the skin. Revision of the pocket and placement in the correct tissue plain will relieve this discomfort. The pulse generator should be placed in a location inferior to the clavicle and medial to keep it from moving into the anterior axillary fold and causing discomfort with arm movements. Late complications such as erosion and migration are often the result of initial suboptimal pocket placement. Potential pulse generator pocket complications include ecchymosis, hematoma, migration, erosion, pain, infection, and rarely dehiscence.

Ecchymosis

Local ecchymosis is common after device implantation even in patients not treated with anticoagulants or antithrombotic agents. Most often observation alone is sufficient even for large ecchymoses as long as the ecchymotic area is not rapidly expanding. Substantial bruising may be seen when devices are implanted in patients treated with agents such as aspirin, warfarin, and clopidogrel, thus care must be taken to achieve adequate hemostasis. Unfractionated and/or low-molecular-weight heparin should be discontinued in all patients prior to device implantation and ideally not administered for at least 24 hours postoperatively. Low-molecular-weight heparin in particular will almost always lead to pocket hematoma formation and thus should not be used at all postoperatively.

When excessive bleeding or oozing is encountered during the implant procedure and electrocautery is ineffective, use of commercially available preparations that aid in local coagulation may be needed. There are a variety of compounds and preparations available, and none appears to be more effective than the other.

Pocket Hematoma Formation

Management of hematoma formation in the pulse generator pocket depends on the sequela associated with bleeding into the pocket. One should remember that with every opening of a pocket, the rate of infection increases. Hematoma evacuation should be considered for continued bleeding (particularly arterial), vascular compromise to the overlying tissue (impaired capillary refill), extreme pain despite analgesics, and threatened dehiscence of the incision. Aspiration is not advised, as sterility will be compromised by introduction of a needle and thus the incidence of infection increased. One of the most effective means of dealing with a pocket hematoma is the use of a pressure dressing applied over the pulse generator pocket.

Pocket Pain

Immediately after device implantation, it is normal for patients to experience local pain and discomfort. This generally subsides in several days and can be treated with mild analgesics. When pain at the implant site is present chronically, there are several possibilities that should not be overlooked. Pocket infection may present with chronic pain even in the absence of other signs of infection and as is the case with pocket

hematomas, needle aspiration is not advised. Antibiotics may be used and if the pocket is opened and explored, cultures should be taken and swabs of the local tissue should be sent for microbiology analysis. In addition to infection, chronic pain may indicate improper positioning of the pulse generator pocket, and rarely allergy to the pulse generator or components exposed in the pocket. There are a number of components present in the pocket (titanium, nickel, cadmium, chromate, polyurethane, and silicone to name a few) to which allergies have been identified. In addition, suture material may cause an allergic reaction (Fig. 33-7). As the diagnosis of "allergy" is difficult to make, it should not be considered until infection is ruled out.

Erosion

Erosion is caused by pressure necrosis or most commonly infection. Generally discomfort, discoloration, and thinning of tissue overlying the device occur prior to overt erosion. Overlying tissue becomes stretched, tense, and thin over the device and ultimately a portion of the generator or leads protrudes through the skin (Fig. 33-8). Identification of impending erosion during the stages before the skin is broken allows for salvage of the pacing system by repositioning of the hardware. Once erosion has occurred, the system is considered contaminated, and the generator and leads must be

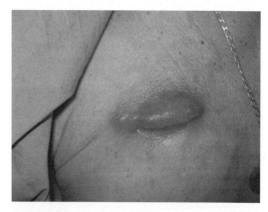

FIGURE 33-7. Photograph taken 5 days after pacemaker implantation. A large blister can be seen over the incision site as a result of "allergy" to the suture material used for closure of the skin. The blister ultimately resolved with no further sequela. (See color insert.)

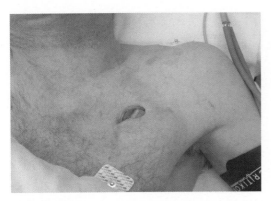

FIGURE 33-8. Erosion of a pacemaker. Note the lack of erythema and the presence of clean margins. The patient offered no complaints. (Photograph courtesy of Joshua M. Cooper, MD.) (See color insert.)

removed. When erosion is present for some time, the skin margins may appear clean and uninfected with little or no erythema or purulence, but this is not the case and the device and pocket should be treated as if it is actively infected. While local debridement, irrigation and/or antibiotics are often attempted this approach is generally not accepted and does not work. Current guidelines recommend removal of both the generator and any existing leads in the event of pocket infection. Features that make erosion more likely to occur include lack of sufficient subcutaneous tissue, improper pocket location (too superficial), extra hardware such as adapters and abandoned leads, irritation by the patient or irritation/rubbing by clothing overlying the device.

Infection

There has been a significant increase in the incidence of cardiac rhythm device infections worldwide (20). The incidence varies widely and depends on the type of device (ICDs have a higher incidence than pacemaker), the experience of the implanting physician, the site of implantation, and the underlying medical conditions of the patient (21,22). One-third to one half of infections affect new implants; the remainder during generator replacement or lead revision (23). Infections are generally classified as localized pocket infections, isolated lead infection, isolated valve infection, or a combination (24). Acute bacterial infection usually presents within weeks of the implant and is usually secondary to

Staphylococcus aureus that adhere to the insulation of pacing hardware. Pus formation in the generator pocket is not uncommon and dehiscence of the incision may occur. Antibiotics are rarely curative and removal of the infected hardware is required. Depending on the indications for the implanted device, reimplantation can be performed immediately if the blood has been "sterilized" with antibiotics or at a later date (with temporary pacing if needed) until a sufficient course of antibiotics has been administered. More slowly, growing bacteria such as *S. epidermidis* often lead to device and/or pocket infection months to years after implantation (Fig. 33-9).

Sepsis and endocarditis may result from pocket or lead infection and generally occur later than isolated pocket infection. The source of infection may be from introduction of organisms during the implant or from metastatic spread. Transesophageal echocardiography is helpful in identifying vegetations present on leads and cardiac valves (Fig. 33-10), and blood cultures can identify the offending organism. The presence of a vegetation mandates removal of all the hardware after initiation of antibiotics. The appropriate antibiotic regimen is determined by the organisms cultured from either the blood or the hardware. Recurrent sepsis in a device patient after completion of an appropriate course of antibiotics without an etiology should prompt consideration of removal of the device and leads.

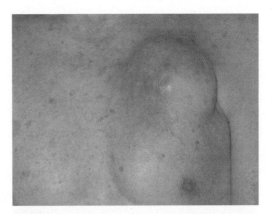

FIGURE 33-9. Photograph of a "pocket infection". Erythema is visible and the pocket is fluctuant. The entire pacing system (generator and leads) required removal. (Photograph courtesy of Joshua M. Cooper, MD.) (See color insert.)

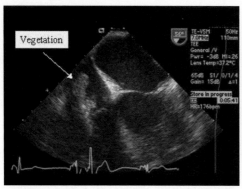
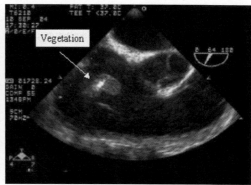

FIGURE 33-10. Transesophageal echocardiographic images of vegetations seen on a defibrillator lead. *Arrows* point to large mobile and pedunculated vegetations.

Dehiscence

Wound dehiscence is rare and occurs within days or weeks after implant usually secondary to stress on the suture line from hematoma or fluid collection within the pocket. When dehiscence occurs in the absence of an underlying cause, surgical technique is responsible. To avoid contamination and infection, immediate intervention needs to occur. Exploration and irrigation followed by closure is usually sufficient to prevent long-term complications. To reduce the risk of dehiscence of the entire incision and suture line, some operators advocate the use of interrupted sutures for the deep layers.

■ VENOUS THROMBOSIS

Acute Thrombosis

As a result of placement of leads through the subclavian vein, thrombus may form on or around the leads and cause venous occlusion (25) (Fig. 33-11). Studies have demonstrated a high rate of asymptomatic thromboses that not surprisingly are related to the number of leads inserted in the vein (26). Symptomatic thrombosis usually presents within days to weeks after implant and is marked by a painful, swollen upper extremity. Extension of the thrombus may occur and include the innominate vein, the superior vena cava (SVC), or even contralateral veins. Clinically significant pulmonary embolism as a result of the thrombus has been reported, but this phenomenon is rare (27). Contrast venography will reveal the location of the thrombus but is rarely performed. More often,

Doppler ultrasosnography is used to identify the presence of thrombus. Rarely, SVC syndrome may manifest if thrombosis extends to the SVC and causes occlusion.

When the thrombus leads to significant symptoms, there are several treatment options. Use of heat and extremity elevation may be used to reduce swelling and allow for collateralization to occur. Other therapies that allow for dissolution of the thrombus or recanalization of the vessel include anticoagulants such as heparin and warfarin as well as thrombolytic agents such as streptokinase or tissue plasminogen activator. Data suggest that rapid improvement in symptoms is seen with the use of thrombolytics without an increased risk of bleeding complications (1). The role of long-term anticoagulation in these patients remains controversial.

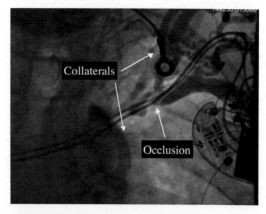

FIGURE 33-11. Contrast venogram performed in a patient with a dual-chamber pacemaker and a venous occlusion. Venous collaterals are present.

Asymptomatic thrombosis is not uncommon and the incidence of venous occlusion seems to be increasing (25,28). It is not necessary to treat an asymptomatic occlusion. The incidence of venous occlusion found at generator change or device replacement is 9% to 12% (29,30). There have been no significant risk factors found, but the rise in venous occlusions seen is in part attributed to more multichamber devices being implanted.

Chronic Venous Occlusion

In most patients, venous occlusion becomes apparent during the process of obtaining venous access for a device upgrade and/or when additional leads are placed as a result of lead failure. When faced with an occlusion, alternative routes of venous access may be required to gain access to central veins. When partial venous occlusion is present, venoplasty has been used, with the lead placed immediately, as thrombosis of the vein often occurs as a result of the endothelial damage associated with the procedure. Obtaining contralateral access with tunneling across the chest has been used, but this method is not advised because of the potential for bilateral upper extremity occlusion. Extraction of functional leads has been employed to gain access to central veins in the presence of venous occlusion (31) to upgrade devices. A variety of techniques and tools exist

to accomplish this (25,31). Rarely, in patients with very limited venous access, implantation via femoral veins with abdominal generator placement may be required (2).

■ LOSS OF CAPTURE

For any pacemaker or ICD system to perform properly, each individual component needs to function, and proper connection of the system (leads to the generator) is an integral element. The most common method for lead connection into a device is via a set screw in the generator header. The terminal pin must be inserted properly into the connector block and the lead tip placed distally before tightening the set screw (Fig. 33-12). In the event that the lead is not seated properly in the connector block, intermittent contact may be present, causing loss of capture and/or inappropriate sensing of electrical signals causing inhibition of pacemaker output or, in the case of an ICD, inappropriate therapies. Equally important is confirming that the terminal pin of each lead is placed into the correct terminal on the device header (Fig. 33-13). A full device interrogation, with evaluation of the lead connections as well as sensing and pacing thresholds after the system is placed into the pocket before closing the incision insures proper connections and function of the system and minimizes inadvertent errors.

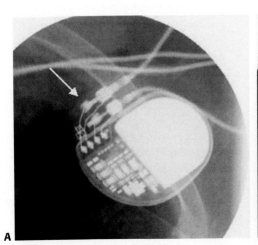
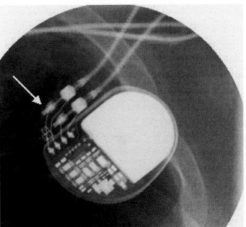

A   B

FIGURE 33-12. Radiographic images of pacemaker generator with the atrial lead not completely inserted in the connector block (**A**, *arrow*) and after advancement of the lead through the connector block (**B**, *arrow*). The ventricular lead is appropriately advanced in both images.

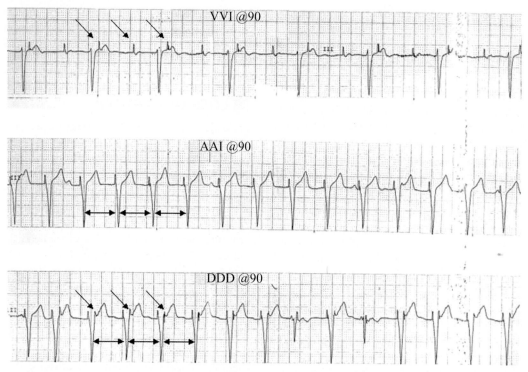

FIGURE 33-13. Telemetry recordings immediately after device implantation in a patient with reversal of atrial and ventricle leads in the device header. The top tracing demonstrates atrial pacing and capture (*arrows*) with VVI pacing. The middle tracing demonstrates ventricular capture (*horizontal arrows*) with AAI pacing. P waves can be seen "marching through" and unaffected by ventricular pacing and capture. The bottom tracing reveals DDD pacing—ventricular pacing and capture (*horizontal arrows*) followed by atrial pacing and capture (*arrows*) at the programmed atrio-ventricular interval. The patient required opening of the pocket to place the lead terminal pins into the correct location in the device.

■ SUMMARY

While the technique of cardiac rhythm device implantation has evolved and become simpler and safer, it is still an invasive procedure fraught with complications even with the most experienced implanter. Knowledge of the patient's cardiovascular history and anatomy as well as awareness of the potential complications possible at every step of the procedure is critical. The potential for problems exists beyond the immediate perioperative period, throughout the longevity of the device.

References

1. Brinker J, Midei M. Techniques of pacemaker implantation and removal. In: Ellenbogen K, Wood M, eds. *Cardiac Pacing and ICDs.* 3rd ed. Malden, MA: Blackwell Science; 2002:216–284.

2. Ching CK, Elayi CS, Di Biase L, et al. Transiliac ICD implantation: defibrillation vector flexibility produces consistent success. *Heart Rhythm.* 2009;6(7):978–983.

3. Ellestad MH, French J. Iliac vein approach to permanent pacemaker implantation. *Pacing Clin Electrophysiol.* 1989;12(7, pt 1):1030–1033.

4. Aggarwal RK, Connelly DT, Ray SG, et al. Early complications of permanent pacemaker implantation: no difference between dual and single chamber systems. *Br Heart J.* 1995;73(6):571–575.

5. Oude Ophuis AJ, van Doorn DJ, van Ommen VA, et al. Internal balloon compression: a method to achieve hemostasis when removing an inadvertently placed pacemaker lead from the subclavian artery. *Pacing Clin Electrophysiol.* 1998;21(12):2673–2676.

6. Hilfiker PR, Razavi MK, Kee ST, et al. Stent-graft therapy for subclavian artery aneurysms and fistulas: single-center mid-term results. *J Vasc Interv Radiol.* 2000;11(5):578–584.

7. Rotem CE, Greig JH, Walters MB. Air embolism to the pulmonary artery during insertion of transvenous endocardial pacemaker. *J Thorac Cardiovasc Surg.* 1967;53(4):562–565.

8. Finlay DJ, Sanchez LA, Sicard GA. Subclavian artery injury, vertebral artery dissection, and arteriovenous fistulae following attempt at central line placement. *Ann Vasc Surg.* 2002;16(6):774–778.

9. Chou TM, Chair KM, Jim MH, et al. Acute occlusion of left internal mammary artery graft during dual-chamber pacemaker implantation. *Catheter Cardiovasc Interv.* 2000;51(1):65–68.

10. Punnam SR, Holiday J, Janes R, et al. Hemodynamic collapse during left ventricular lead implantation. *Pacing Clin Electrophysiol.* 2007;30(9):1112–1115.

11. Lee JC, Epstein LM, Huffer LL, et al. ICD lead proarrhythmia cured by lead extraction. *Heart Rhythm.* 2009;6(5):613–618.

12. Hirschl DA, Jain VR, Spindola-Franco H, et al. Prevalence and characterization of asymptomatic pacemaker and ICD lead perforation on CT. *Pacing Clin Electrophysiol.* 2007;30(1):28–32.

13. Occhetta E, Bortnik M, Marino P. Ventricular capture by anodal pacemaker stimulation. *Europace.* 2006;8(5):385–387.

14. Ho WJ, Kuo CT, Lin KH. Right pneumothorax resulting from an endocardial screw-in atrial lead. *Chest.* 1999;116(4):1133–1134.

15. Van Gelder BM, Bracke FA, Oto A, et al. Diagnosis and management of inadvertently placed pacing and ICD leads in the left ventricle: a multicenter experience and review of the literature. *Pacing Clin Electrophysiol.* 2000;23(5):877–883.

16. Ghani M, Thakur RK, Boughner D, et al. Malposition of transvenous pacing lead in the left ventricle. *Pacing Clin Electrophysiol.* 1993;16(9):1800–1807.

17. Sharifi M, Sorkin R, Lakier JB. Left heart pacing and cardioembolic stroke. *Pacing Clin Electrophysiol.* 1994;17(10):1691–1696.

18. Sharifi M, Sorkin R, Sharifi V, Lakier JB. Inadvertent malposition of a transvenous-inserted pacing lead in the left ventricular chamber. *Am J Cardiol.* 1995;76(1):92–95.

19. Hayes DL, Friedman PA. *Implantation-Related Complications: Cardiac Pacing, Defibrillation and Resynchronization.* 2nd ed. West Sussex, UK: Wiley-Blackwell; 2008:202–233.

20. Cabell CH, Heidenreich PA, Chu VH, et al. Increasing rates of cardiac device infections among Medicare beneficiaries: 1990–1999. *Am Heart J.* 2004;147(4):582–586.

21. Uslan DZ, Sohail MR, St Sauver JL, et al. Permanent pacemaker and implantable cardioverter defibrillator infection: a population-based study. *Arch Intern Med.* 2007;167(7):669–675.

22. Sohail MR, Uslan DZ, Khan AH, et al. Infective endocarditis complicating permanent pacemaker and implantable cardioverter-defibrillator infection. *Mayo Clin Proc.* 2008;83(1):46–53.

23. Choo MH, Holmes DR Jr, Gersh BJ, et al. Permanent pacemaker infections: characterization and management. *Am J Cardiol.* 1981;48(3):559–564.

24. Duval X, Selton-Suty C, Alla F, et al. Endocarditis in patients with a permanent pacemaker: a 1-year epidemiological survey on infective endocarditis due to valvular and/or pacemaker infection. *Clin Infect Dis.* 2004;39(1):68–74.

25. Fischer A, Love B, Hansalia R, Mehta D. Transfemoral snaring and stabilization of pacemaker and defibrillator leads to maintain vascular access during lead extraction. *Pacing Clin Electrophysiol.* 2009;32(3):336–339.

26. Pauletti M, Di Ricco G, Solfanelli S, et al. Venous obstruction in permanent pacemaker patients: an isotopic study. *Pacing Clin Electrophysiol.* 1981;4(1):36–42.

27. Pasquariello JL, Hariman RJ, Yudelman IM, et al. Recurrent pulmonary embolization following implantation of transvenous pacemaker. *Pacing Clin Electrophysiol.* 1984;7(5):790–793.

28. Smith MC, Love CJ. Extraction of transvenous pacing and ICD leads. *Pacing Clin Electrophysiol.* 2008;31(6):736–752.

29. Lickfett L, Bitzen A, Arepally A, et al. Incidence of venous obstruction following insertion of an implantable cardioverter defibrillator: a study of systematic contrast venography on patients presenting for their first elective ICD generator replacement. *Europace.* 2004;6(1):25–31.

30. Bracke FA, Meijer A, Van Gelder LM. Symptomatic occlusion of the access vein after pacemaker or ICD lead extraction. *Heart.* 2003;89(11):1348–1349.

31. Gula LJ, Ames A, Woodburn A, et al. Central venous occlusion is not an obstacle to device upgrade with the assistance of laser extraction. *Pacing Clin Electrophysiol.* 2005;28(7):661–666.

34

Complications of Atrial Fibrillation Ablation

CARLO PAPPONE AND VINCENZO SANTINELLI

urrently, catheter ablation can be considered as an effective treatment among patients with symptomatic atrial fibrillation (AF), but both feasibility and safety of the procedure are strongly required (1–9). Because of its complexity as well as the significant length of time needed to successfully ablate all targeted areas in the left atrium, it is mandatory to define an acceptable risk–benefit ratio and how to avoid many of the serious complications. Although complications rates of catheter ablation of AF are declining (1–3), they may nullify any mid-to-long term benefit of the procedure. There are mechanical complications resulting from catheter manipulation within the cardiac chambers, cardioembolic complications (stroke and transient ischemic attacks), and complications arising from the effects of radio frequency (RF) applications in the left atrium (pericardial effusion/tamponade). The most frequent acute complications arise from vascular access, transseptal puncture, and left atrium navigation and ablation, while incessant new-onset atypical atrial tachycardias are the most frequent late complications. An evolving and better understanding of the procedure-related risks has helped in limiting complication rates by changing ablation approaches to avoid RF applications within the pulmonary veins (PV) or just at the PV ostia, ensuring appropriate anticoagulation during the procedure with accurate monitoring, by using 3D electroanatomic mapping systems for an accurate reconstruction of intracardiac structures, and by recognizing complications promptly both during and after the procedure. Hopefully, improved techniques and operator experience in the future

years will result in further improvement of both the efficacy and safety of catheter ablation of atrial fibrillation and will allow continued growth of this procedure (Fig.s 34-1 and 34-2). At present, CARTO-guided left atrial circumferential ablation (48.2% of patients) and LASSO-guided ostial electric disconnection (27.4%) are the most commonly used techniques (1–3). Death is a very rare complication (0.03%), and in our experience on the basis of more than 15,000 procedures this fatal complication has never occurred. A detailed list of the different complications of circumferential pulmonary vein ablation (CPVA) with their relative incidence is reported in Tables 34-1 to 34-4. Pre-procedural imaging techniques are routinely performed in our department to evaluate the left atrial size, anatomy, and function as well as to exclude the presence of atrial thrombus. During the procedure, while fluoroscopy remains a useful modality for guiding both transseptal catheterization and catheter navigation, several imaging modalities have been developed to improve 3D navigation and ablation within the cardiac chambers (Fig. 34-2). Postoperative imaging is used to monitor the heart function as well as to exclude potential complications like pericardial effusion or pulmonary vein stenosis. Although transthoracic echocardiography and fluoroscopy are mandatory for all patients in the context of AF ablation, the use of other imaging modalities depends on the single-center experience. There must be a balance between irradiation reduction and procedural duration, improvement in catheter manipulation, cost-effectiveness ratio, and potential adverse effects of each imaging procedure.

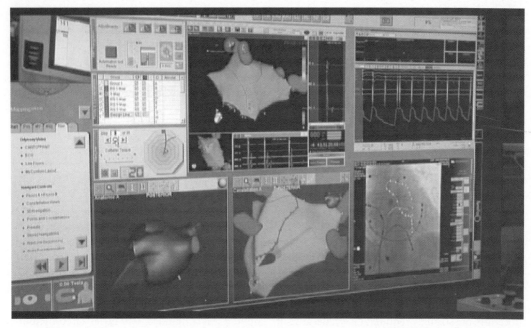

FIGURE 34-1. The past decade has been characterized by a tremendous growth in technology, which has resulted in enhanced success and reduced complications of ablation procedures. The modern electrophysiology laboratory integrates traditional and new technologies, which allow 3D reconstruction of cardiac anatomy and superimposition of anatomical and electrical maps.

VASCULAR COMPLICATIONS

Peripheral vascular complications are usually considered as minor complications and include hematoma, arteriovenous fistula, and femoral pseudoaneurysm. Major vascular complications of the procedure are rare and include retroperitoneal hematoma, hemothorax, subclavian hematoma, and extrapericardial PV perforation. Vascular complications are detected during ablation by invasive blood pressure monitoring, oxygen saturation, and after ablation by pressure monitoring and hemoglobin monitoring. Management of vascular complications consists of an aggressive approach to repair them while limiting anticoagulation (low ACT).

TRANSSEPTAL PUNCTURE

Transseptal puncture is required in patients undergoing AF ablation. Although this approach is safe in the majority of cases (> 99%), potential complications may occur even in experienced hands. In up to 1% of cases transseptal puncture is not feasible, and the main reason for an unsuccessful puncture is related to fossa ovalis/atrial septum anatomy. The majority of the general population does not have a patent

foramen ovale. Therefore, a transseptal puncture for access into the LA is required in most patients undergoing catheter ablation of AF. Techniques, imaging modalities, and complications of

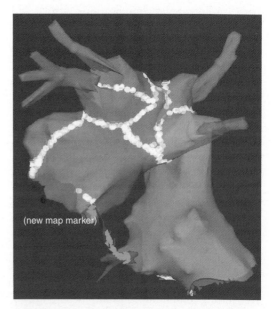

(new map marker)

FIGURE 34-2. 3D navigation and ablation. Overimposition of 3D reconstruction and electrical map allowing "3D navigation and ablation" within the left atrium.

TABLE 34-1 Complications Rates of Catheter Ablation of Atrial Fibrillation

Death	0(0%)	
Pericardial effusion	38(0.23%)	
Stroke	18(0.11%)	Major complication rate 0.38% over 0.38% over 8,682 AFib patients treated with CPVA or CPVA-M*
TIA	25(0.15%)	
Tamponade	31(0.19%)	
Atrial-esophageal fistula	1(0.006%)	
PV stenosis	0(0%)	
Incisional LA tachycardia	1138(6.99%)	
Transient ERAF	2805(17%) ⟶	Minor complication preventable with the CPVA-M*

CPVA, circumferential pulmonary vein ablation; CPVA-M, circumferential pulmonary vein ablation-modified; LA, left atrial; ERAF, early recurrence atrial fibrillation. *Overall complication rate including post CPVA left atrial (LA) tachycardia 7.30%.
Single-center experience including 8,682 patients with atrial fibrillation treated with CPVA or CPVA-M* (San Raffaele Hospital, Milan, Italy.)

TABLE 34-2 Major Complication Rates in the First Worldwide Survey on Catheter Ablation for Atrial Fibrillation

Complication Type	No. of Patients	% of Patients
For all types of procedures		
(*n* = 8745 patients)		
Periprocedural death	4	0.05
Tamponade	107	1.22
Sepsis, abscesses, or endocarditis	1	0.01
Pneumothorax	2	0.02
Hemothorax	14	0.16
Permanent diaphragmatic paralysis	10	0.11
Femoral pseudoaneurysm	47	0.53
Arteriovenous fistulae	37	0.42
Valve damage	1	0.01
Aortic dissection	3	0.03
For procedures involving left atrial ablation		
(*n* = 7154 patients)		
Stroke	20	0.28
Transient ischemic attack	47	0.66
PV stenosis		
No. with > 50% stenosis		
Acute	23	0.32
Chronic	94	1.31
No. with closure		
Acute	2	0.03
Chronic	15	0.21
Patients with symptoms		
Acute	3	0.04
Chronic	41	0.57
Patients undergoing intervention		
Percutaneous	51	0.71
Surgical	2	0.03
Grand total	524	5.9

(From Cappato R, Calkins H, Chen SA, et al. Worldwide survey on the methods, efficacy and safety of catheter ablation for human atrial fibrillation. *Circulation.* 2005;111:1100–1105.)

| TABLE 34-3 | Major Complications in the Overall Population from the Second Worldwide Survey of Catheter Ablation for Atrial Fibrillation |

Type of Complication	No. of Patients	Rate, %
Death	25	0.15
Tamponade	213	1.31
Pneumothorax	15	0.09
Hemothorax	4	0.02
Sepsis, abscesses, or endocarditis	2	0.01
Permanent diaphragmatic paralysis	28	0.17
Total femoral pseudoaneurysm	152	0.93
Total arterio-venous fistulae	88	0.54
Valve damage/requiring surgery	11/7	0.07
Atrium-esophageal fistulae	6	0.04
Stroke	37	0.23
Transient ischemic attack	115	0.71
PV stenoses requiring intervention	48	0.29
Total	741	4.54

(From Cappato R, Calkins H, Chen SA, et al. Updated worldwide survey on the methods, efficacy, and safety of catheter ablation for human atrial fibrillation. *Circ Arrhythm Electrophysiol*. 2010;3:32–38.)

transseptal puncture are described in detail in Chapter 19. In brief, using the standard Brockenbrough approach and fluoroscopy, a "jump" is seen when pulling the transseptal sheath down the septum, indicating the position of the foramen ovale. The needle position in relation to the septum can be further assessed by observing its relationship with catheters marking the His bundle and coronary sinus (CS), using orthogonal planes. Injection of contrast onto the septum may help in evaluating the exact location of the needle before advancing the dilator and the sheath. This method provides useful information to safely perform transseptal puncture in most cases, but variations in the septal anatomy or adjacent structures may increase the risk of complications. Transesophageal echocardiography (TEE) can help to localize the septum, with tenting seen when the needle and sheath are pushed onto the foramen. The problem with using TEE is that it makes airway management difficult, and it usually requires general anaesthesia. To overcome this problem, intra-cardiac echocardiography (ICE) is routinely used in some centres to facilitate an accurate definition of the region. Transseptal puncture may be associated with puncture of adjacent structures such as aortic root, right atrial posterior wall, coronary sinus, and circumflex artery. Perforation of the aortic root and posterior wall by the needle only is usually "benign" while inadvertent advancement of the Mullins introducer into the aortic root is a major and serious complication which requires an aggressive management and usually surgical removal. Cardiac perforation with tamponade is rare occurring in about 0.1% of cases (Fig. 34-3).

■ COMPLICATIONS DURING NAVIGATION AND ABLATION

Embolization

Evaluation for the potential presence of atrial thrombus is required prior to AF ablation for patients at risk since catheter movements may dislodge a thrombus, thus leading to embolic complications. Current guidelines suggest that patients with AF at the time of the procedure should have TEE performed within 48 hours of

TABLE 34-4 **Comparison of Entry Criteria, Outcome, and Complications in the 2 Surveys of Worldwide Experience Reports on Catheter Ablation for Atrial Fibrillation**

	Previous Survey	Current Survey
Period Investigated	1995–2002	2003–2006
No. of centers enrolled	90	85
No. of patients	8745	16, 309
No. of patients per center	97	192
No. procedures	12,830	20, 825
No. procedures per patient	1.5	1.3
Male, %	63.8	60.8
Lower and upper age limit for entry	18–82	15–90
Proportion of centers (%) performing ablation of:		
Paroxysmal AF	100	100
Persistent AF	53.4	85.9
Long-lasting AF	20	47.1
Success rate,%, median		
Free of AADs	52.0	70.0
With AADs	23.5	10.0
Overall	75.5	80.0
Proportion of centers (%) using as exclusion		
Left atrial size upper limit	46.3	31.8
Prior heart surgery	65.1	23.5
Lower cut-off limit of LVEF	64.3	22.4
Overall complication rate, %	4.0	4.5
Iatrogenic flutter	3.9	8.6

(From Cappato R, Calkins H, Chen SA, et al. Updated worldwide survey on the methods, efficacy, and safety of catheter ablation for human atrial fibrillation. *Circ Arrhythm Electrophysiol.* 2010;3:32–38.)

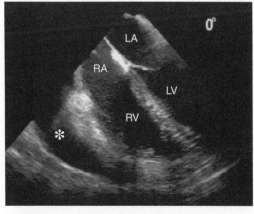

FIGURE 34-3. Left cardiac perforation. *New pericardial effusion.

the procedure regardless of whether they have been anticoagulated with warfarin or not. For low-risk lone paroxysmal AF with prior anticoagulation, there is some uncertainty about the utility of performing routine thrombus detection. In this case, TTE can be used to risk-stratify patients before performing TEE with a very high negative predictive value. Catheter ablation of AF requires multiple RF lesions arranged in an accurate geometrical pattern. Multiple burns and extensive endothelial injury potentially increase the risk of acute and subacute thrombosis. Large surface catheters increase lesion volume mostly by making the lesion longer rather than thicker. Conventional ablation catheters achieve a maximum lesion depth of 5 to 6 mm. RF energy is generally safe and the fibrosis induced by RF energy is completed at 8 weeks after the procedure and is not associated with clinical side effects. The thickness of the atrial wall is usually superior to the maximal thickness generated by RF lesions and limited and short RF applications are at very low risk of thrombosis. The left atrial wall is very thin and is surrounded by critical anatomical structures, which may be damaged by heat. RF applications may be delivered to structures that may react with acute and chronic fibrosis. Navigation and ablation may be associated with potential complications, which include embolization, perforation, PV stenosis, circumflex artery occlusion, and esophageal perforation. Embolization may be caused by preexisting thrombus dislodgment. Multiple successive burns may cause tip carbonization. In addition, extensive endocardial damage is a potential thrombogenic substrate. Finally, multiple transseptal punctures may increase the risk of air embolization. Transesophageal echocardiography before the procedure to rule out even laminar not mobile thrombi is the best way to prevent potential embolization in the majority of cases. Ablation must be performed on anticoagulation, and heparin doses are titrated by ACT with values between 250 and 350. Effective anticoagulation should be maintained in the post-operative period. Tip carbonization is a consequence of excessive heating at the tip-tissue interface and it is commonest with 4-mm tip catheters. Larger 8-mm tip catheters still require anticoagulation. Irrigation technology advancement will further reduce embolic complications. In our experience "dragging while ablating" may reduce the risk of carbonization. Long consecutive RF applications on the same spot should be avoided. Homogeneous irrigation with a specifically designed catheter can reduce complications while enhancing lesion formation. Proximal irrigation protects this part from charring while delivering energy with the lateral side of the ablation tip catheter, and it allows a rapid performance of the lesion. In the near future, heparin-free procedures may be performed with new catheters.

Perforation

Left atrial perforation is usually related to catheter manipulation rather than to RF applications while posterior wall perforation is generally due to RF delivery. Cardiac perforation with tamponade is the most frequent complication, but its rate appears to be comparable to values commonly observed during CA of other arrhythmogenic substrates (9,10). This complication is usually associated with a rapid hemodynamic deterioration. Close availability of surgical facilities for management is mandatory. Cardiac tamponade due to right-sided perforation usually becomes clinically manifest in the first hour after the procedure. Continuous invasive monitoring of blood pressure, ACT, and oxygen saturation is recommended during the procedure. Pericardiocentesis is the treatment of choice and gas analysis of the blood aspirated from the pericardium indicates the site of perforation. "Arterial" blood is diagnostic of left-sided perforation. Management of this complication consists of an aggressive approach to drain blood from the pericardial space, associated with reversal of anticoagulation and drainage for 48 hours. It is not possible to lose a patient for a pericardial tamponade in 2010! The recent introduction of use of "fluid" magnetic catheters has virtually eliminated the risk of cardiac perforation (Fig. 34-4).

Pulmonary Vein Stenosis

One of the most serious complications of catheter ablation of AF is the development of PV stenosis. This complication is due to RF delivery on the PV ostia and was mainly related to the focal or perimetral approach as initially described by Haissaguerre et al. (5) However, at present, its prevalence is declining by at least threefold as RF delivery inside the PVs is avoided in all current approaches and precise 3D reconstruction of atrial geometry and PV ostia is performed (1–3). Since pulmonary vein isolation represents the cornerstone of all ablation strategies for both paroxysmal and persistent AF, to minimize or avoid PVs stenosis, an accurate knowledge of an individual's PV anatomy may be useful particularly when using circular or balloon catheters. Most patients have four PVs, two superior and two inferior with independent ostia. However, there are variations in PV anatomy, such as left common ostium (up to 83% of patients), right common ostium (up to 40%), and a separate origin for the right middle PV (up to 27% of patients). Prior knowledge of the diameter of the

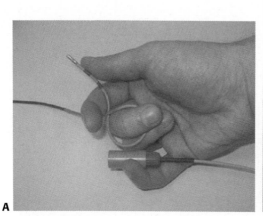
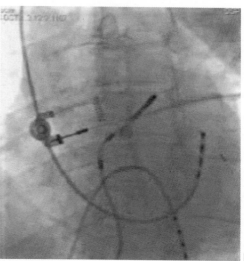

FIGURE 34-4. The development of "fluid" magnetic flexible catheters for ablation (**A**) has reduced substantially the risk of cardiac perforation during ablation procedures, which require the insertion and manipulation of multiple catheter (**B**).

PVs ostia may be useful in the sizing of circular mapping catheters or balloon catheters, since a close approximation of the balloon to the PV ostia is essential for successful PV isolation. Although TEE can evaluate PV diameters, computed tomography (CT) scanning or magnetic resonance imaging (MRI) represent the gold standard. Using these imaging tools the characteristic oval anatomy of the left-sided PVs may be accurately recorded, with a superior–inferior diameter larger than the anterior–posterior one, while the right-sided PVs appear more circular. Additionally, CT or MRI may provide useful information on all anatomical targeted sites. If stenosis occurs in multiple PVs it may be a severe complication causing significant morbidity. PV angioplasty and stenting are associated with very high restenosis rates, while PV dilatation is associated with significant increase in lung flow and improvement of symptoms. The clinical presentation of PVs stenosis varies widely. Most patients are symptomatic and symptoms include dyspnea or hemoptysis or may mimic bronchitis. Because of the variability in symptoms, clinicians must consider this potential complication in all patients after catheter ablation of AF. Diagnostic tests include magnetic resonance angiography and CT while echocardiography does not usually provide adequate assessment. Progression of stenosis is unpredictable and may be rapid. There is discordant data in the literature concerning the incidence of iatrogenic PV stenosis after AF abla-

tion, varying from 0% to 42%. This can be explained by the lack of a standard definition of PV stenosis, the different imaging modalities used to diagnose PV stenosis, and the inhomogeneity in follow-up. Pulmonary vein stenosis tends to occur immediately after the ablation. In most patients, there will be a progressive narrowing of the stenosis, although acute PV stenosis can rarely heal spontaneously. Of note, some patients without acute/peri-procedural narrowing will still have significant PV stenosis revealed by later imaging. If significant restenosis is identified by preablation and postablation angiography or by MRI, a corrective intervention is required promptly because of the potential for progression to total occlusion. Importantly, about half of the PV stenoses require interventional treatment, a strategy that does not necessarily abolish symptoms. This complication can be minimized or avoided by creating circumferential lesions greater than 1.5 cm outside PV ostia as performed by circumferential pulmonary vein ablation (CPVA), which is our approach (4,6–8). In our experience, impedance mapping may be useful to accurately identify the PV/LA junction in order to avoid PV stenosis while assessing lesion formation (11).

Circumflex Artery Occlusion

Ablation of the left inferior PV–mitral valve isthmus may damage the circumflex artery (Fig. 34-5).

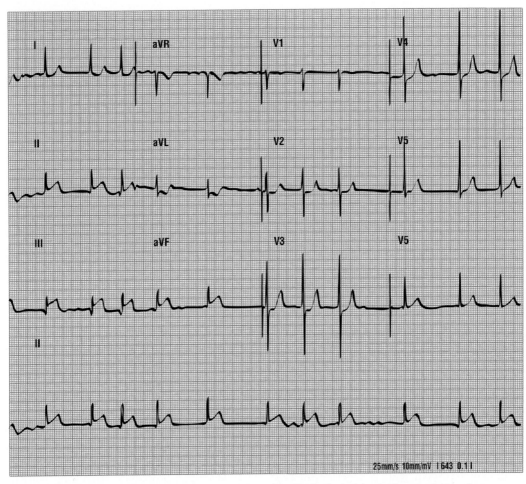

FIGURE 34-5. Electrocardiogram showing ST-segment elevation in the inferior leads, secondary to damage to left circumflex artery.

High blood flow protects the artery wall from heat damage. Acute circumflex artery occlusion has been reported as a complication in surgical series with use of unipolar RF applications but never following RF catheter ablation. However, endothelial heat injury and medial proliferation may result in chronic circumflex artery damage. Catheter manipulation on the endocardial side of the left AV groove or transseptal puncture may cause circumflex spasm.

Esophageal Perforation

Atrioesophageal fistulae were not reported in the first worldwide survey of catheter ablation of AF (1) and presented with a 0.04% rate in the second worldwide survey, with 71% of events leading to death (3). Esophageal fistula as a complication of catheter ablation of AF was first reported by our

group (12) (Figs. 34-6 and 34-7). Previous cases have been reported in patients undergoing surgical ablation of AF by unipolar RF applications on the posterior wall of the left atrium. At present, several cases have been reported after catheter ablation (3). The close proximity of the esophagus to the posterior left atrial wall makes it vulnerable to RF-induced lesions (12,13) (Fig. 34-8). The thickness of the posterior atrial wall is variable, but may be very little. The clinical presentation is late, usually days or even weeks after the procedure (Table 34-5). Symptoms are the consequence of massive air embolism and sepsis. Stroke is usually the first embolic manifestation and may be heralded by fever, chest pain, and other symptoms initially suggestive of pericarditis. In the two cases that we initially reported from a two-center experience, including 4360 patients undergoing CPVA (overall incidence of

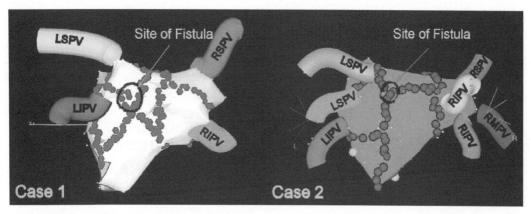

FIGURE 34-6. Three-dimensional anatomic maps of left atrium (LA) and pulmonary veins (PVs) from a posteroanterior view in two patients who developed atrioesophageal fistula. Red tags indicate sites at which radiofrequency energy was applied, generally for a total of 20 to 30 seconds at each site. Approximate location of atrioesophageal fistula that later occurred in cases 1 (**left**) and 2 (**right**) is circled. LIPV, left inferior PV; LSPV, left superior PV; RIPV, right inferior PV; RMPV, right middle PV; and RSPV, right superior PV. (From Pappone C, Oral H, Santinelli V, et al. Atrioesophageal fistula as a complication of percutaneous transcatheter ablation of atrial fibrillation. *Circulation.* 2004;109:2724–2726.) (See color insert.)

esophageal perforation = 0.05%), the initial symptoms were fever and chest pain, both occurring at post procedure day 2 and 3. Importantly, in both patients the TTE was unremarkable. Acute embolization to other targets may follow (heart, kidney) with septic shock. Mortality rates are higher than 50% and survivors experience major consequences. Early diagnosis is mandatory, given that there have been cases of full recovery following emergency surgical intervention. In addition, there has also been a case report of succesful recovery following placement

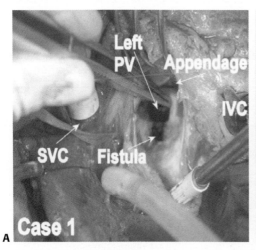
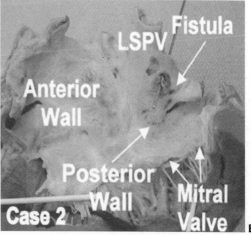

FIGURE 34-7. Anatomic demonstration of atrioesophageal fistulas. (**A**) Case 1: Intraoperative photograph taken from patient's right side with head to left, highlighting atrioesophageal fistula arising medial to left PV ostia. Two distinct ostia cannot be seen because veins are empty and walls have collapsed. (**B**) Case 2: Formalin-fixed LA was incised near left superior PV and opened in book fashion, with anterior wall on left and posterior wall on right. Probe passes through fistula, which was on posterior wall near left superior PV. IVC, inferior vena cava; SVC, superior vena cava; and LSPV, left superior PV. (From Pappone C, Oral H, Santinelli V, et al. Atrioesophageal fistula as a complication of percutaneous transcatheter ablation of atrial fibrillation. *Circulation.* 2004;109:2724–2726.) (See color insert.)

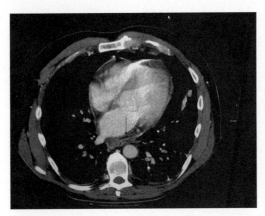

FIGURE 34-8. CT scan of the chest, obtained on presentation of a patient to the emergency department with severe chest pain and fever. There is air and fluid in the pericardium *(arrow)* anterior to the esophagus. (From Vijayaraman, Netrebko P, Geyfman V, et al. Esophageal fistula formation despite esophageal monitoring and low-power radiofrequency catheter ablation for atrial fibrillation. *Circ Arrhythm Electrophysiol.* 2009;2:e31–e33.)

of an esophageal stent (14). The late occurrence (3–10 days postablation) of a febrile state with or without neurological symptoms, chest pain (16), or dysphagia should prompt suspicion of an atri-oesophageal fistula which should be excluded by contrast-enhanced spiral CT. Transesophageal echocardiogram should be avoided because, if a fistula is present, instrumentation of the esopha-

gus may cause rapid deterioration and even death. Careful titration of the combination of output, number, location and duration of pulses is critical. Lines of lesion should not be excessively wide and posterior lines should be placed on the roof of the LA.

■ POSTPROCEDURE ACUTE COMPLICATIONS

The possibility to tailor RF applications, energy settings, irrigation rates in vulnerable areas contributes to minimize post-procedure late complications. Pericardial tamponade must be excluded in patients with postprocedural hypotension, but in our experience this complication is very rare if one uses a careful titration of RF power and duration delivery particularly in challenging areas thus reducing tissue boiling and endocardial rupture. Symptoms of pericardial effusion usually become manifest several hours following the procedure and for this reason, all patients should have a repeat TTE prior to discharge following the procedure, especially if there is hemodynamic compromise. Transthoracic echocardiogram is the study of choice as it is easily and rapidly performed and invaluable in the follow-up of the effusion. Only a few patients have required pericardiocentesis for cardiac tamponade while small, nonhemodynamically significant pericardial

	TABLE 34-5	Time of Initial Symptom Onset, Symptoms Upon Presentation and Result of Diagnostic Tests in 2 Patients Presenting with Esophageal Perforation

Post-procedure Day of Presentation	Symptoms	Diagnostic Test
Case 1		
Day 3	Fever, pleuritic chest pain, elevated white cell count, seizure	Head CT—Patchy bilateral infarcts
Day 12	Chest pain and ST-segment elevation	TTE—Air bubbles in the LA CT—atrioesophageal fistula and pneumomediastinum
Case 2		
Day 2	Fever, chest pain	TTE—Unremarkable
Week 3	Profound weakness, rigors, seizure	Blood cultures positive for - hemolytic streptococci, micrococcus species, and nonhemolytic streptococci. TTE—no evidence of valvular or LA vegetations. TEE—1.2-cm pedunculated mass on the posterior wall of the LA.

effusion may develop in up to 4% of patients. Pericarditic discomfort may occur during the first days and nonsteroidal anti-inflammatory agents are usually an adequate treatment.

■ LATE ARRHYTHMIC COMPLICATIONS

Early recurrences of AF after the index procedure usually occur within the first 2 months, but in half of the cases they are a transient phenomenon not requiring a redo procedure (4,6–8). If recurrence of persistent AF or monthly episodes of symptomatic paroxysmal AF occur beyond the first month after ablation or new-onset incessant highly symptomatic left or right atrial flutter is present, then a second procedure is scheduled at 6 months after the index procedure. A maximum of three ablation procedures per patient are allowed. Atypical atrial flutter of new onset (iatrogenic) is a serious arrhythmic complication after catheter ablation of AF representing a challenge for curative treatment (7,15). With a significantly larger number of patients with persistent or long-standing AF undergoing catheter ablation, iatrogenic left atrial flutter appears to be a more frequent complication regardless of the operator experience. Initially, this iatrogenic arrhythmic complication has been reported in a minority of cases (about 4%), but its prevalence is increasing ($>$ 8%) as catheter ablation is increasingly being offered to sicker AF patients with left ventricular dysfunction and larger atria. More frequently the arrhythmia has been observed in centers using 3D-guided compartmentalization strategies (up to 14%) than in centers exclusively performing ablation of the triggering substrate or PV electrical disconnection alone using the Lasso catheter (3). In our approach (CPVA) if all end points are successfully achieved in the index procedure, postablation atrial tachycardias (ATS) may develop in less than 5% of patients (7), and usually they are macro or microreentrant gap-related rather than focal tachycardias (Figs. 34-9 to 34-14). We have found that a slight modification of the CPVA approach (CPVA-M) with the addition of ablation lines on the posterior wall and the mitral isthmus can reduce the incidence of AT after PV ablation (7) (Fig. 34-15; and Tables 34-6 and 34-7). These ATs should initially be treated conservatively, with medical therapy and cardioversion. Only incessant ATs in symptomatic patients require a repeated procedure to optimize ablation therapy, which will lead to a cure in most cases. Ablation should be tailored to the arrhythmia mechanism rather than performing empiric lesion lines. Close inspection of the 12-lead ECG with P-wave morphology and axis evaluation should be done initially since continuous activation suggests a macroreentrant mechanism, whereas a clear isoelectric baseline between P waves suggests a focal mechanism. We routinely perform both activation and voltage maps combined with entrainment pacing maneuvers to optimize the ablation therapy (7,15). Usually, the activation map reveals earliest and latest activations in different colors relative to the reference site within a time window equal to the tachycardia cycle length. The commonest postablation AT is macroreentrant ($>$ 80% of the cycle length) peri-mitral annular tachycardia (Fig. 34-10), but PV or septum may be involved in the reentry circuit (Figs. 34-11 to 34-14). Entrainment with post-pacing intervals (PPI) $\approx$ tachycardia cycle length (TCL) from three or more than three sites around the superior and inferior mitral annulus, with an activation time around the mitral annulus $\approx$ to the AT cycle length strongly suggests a mitral annular AT. Like the right atrial isthmus-dependent flutter, the narrowest area of the circuit is between the LIPV and the mitral annulus, and the most appropriate approach is to perform reablation of the mitral isthmus looking for residual gaps. For focal microreentrant ATs ($<$80% of the cycle length) originating from reconnected PV ostia, ablation of sites with earliest activation that demonstrate concealed entrainment will usually be successful. Frequently, voltage maps show areas of preserved voltage at the site of earliest activation suggesting areas not previously targeted or incompletely ablated during the index procedure. Reentry around left or right PVs can be demonstrated by proximal and distal coronary sinus, left atrial roof, and septal pacing. Their management requires the use of 3D activation maps for delineating the tachycardia course, and for deploying a lesion line connecting anatomic obstacles to interrupt AT circuits (Figs. 34-9 to 34-14). RF applications are delivered after critical isthmuses have been identified by detailed

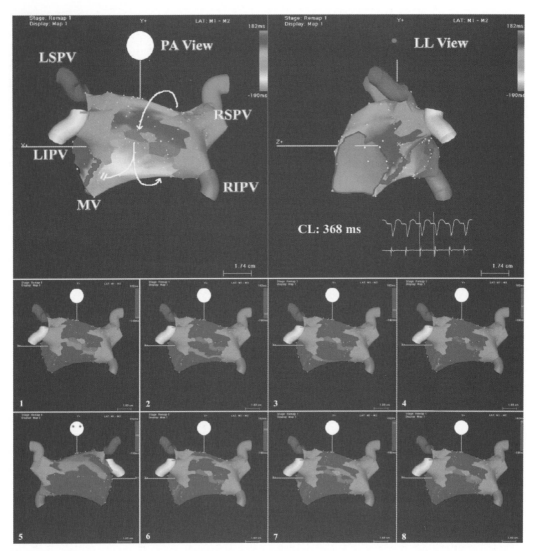

FIGURE 34-9. Single-loop reentry around a previously ablated area. After ablation and block at the mitral isthmus (*dark red line*), a new single-loop tachycardia, now with a cycle length of 368 ms, was induced. The critical isthmus was identified at the posterior wall, between two previously ablated areas. Ablation at this site eliminated the tachycardia. Propagation maps for each of the two tachycardias are shown as an inset in the lower part of each panel. LL, left lateral; LIPV, left inferior pulmonary vein; LSPV, left superior pulmonary vein; MV, mitral valve; PA, postero-anterior; RIPV, right inferior pulmonary vein; RSPV, right superior pulmonary vein. (Reprinted from Mesas CE, Pappone C, Lang CC, et al. Left atrial tachycardia after circumferential pulmonary vein ablation for atrial fibrillation: Electroanatomic characterization and treatment. *J Am Coll Cardiol.* 2004;44:1071–1079, with permission from Elsevier.) (See color insert.)

electroanatomic maps and concealed entrainment. Usually, few RF applications on the critical isthmus are sufficient to eliminate such tachycardias and their inducibility, but in some cases a further ablation line is required. Successful ablation is defined as termination of tachycardia during ablation and noninducibility of the same tachycardia morphology with burst pacing and/or programmed pacing.

■ ATRIAL REMODELING AFTER ABLATION

The assessment of potential consequences of RF ablation on the LA contractility is important for a potential relationship to thromboembolic risk. After ablation, we evaluate carefully the left atrial transport function before and after the procedure and serially during the long-term

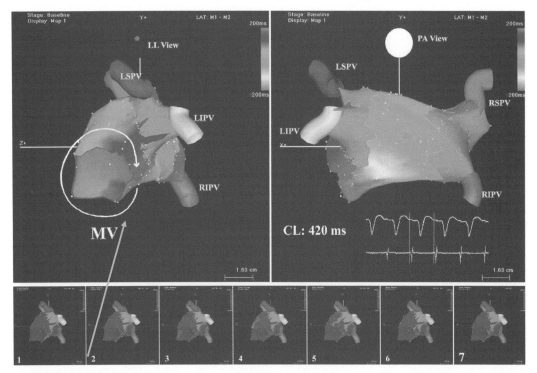

FIGURE 34-10. Activation maps in pulmonary artery (PA) and left anterior oblique (LAO) views of patient #13 showing re-entry using the mitral isthmus. The tachycardia cycle length (CL) was 420 ms. (Reprinted from Mesas CE, Pappone C, Lang CC, et al. Left atrial tachycardia after circumferential pulmonary vein ablation for atrial fibrillation: Electroanatomic characterization and treatment. *J Am Coll Cardiol.* 2004;44:1071–1079, with permission from Elsevier.)

follow-up. In our experience, usually 6 months after ablation LA diameters decrease and LA contractile function may improve but the magnitude of this benefit mainly depends on the atrial dimensions before ablation. In patients without recurrences and with improved atrial transport and function (reverse atrial remodeling) we discontinue chronic anticoagulation therapy.

■ CATHETER ABLATION COMPLICATION RATE: WORLDWIDE EXPERIENCE

Recently, 2 extensive worldwide surveys from early experiences of catheter ablation of AF have offered an unique opportunity to better understand, prevent, and treat AF ablation procedure-related complications (Tables 34-2 to 34-4) (1,3). The published literature has reported a lot of data, many of which are from experienced centers, which necessarily do not reflect the true frequency of potential procedure-related com-

plications. A total of 32 deaths, which corresponds to a prevalence of about one death per 1,000 patients or 0.7 deaths per 1,000 procedures have been reported. Deaths were due to bleeding, thromboembolism, or collateral injury. The first worldwide survey of catheter ablation has found a high number of complications, at 6% (Table 34-2) (1). Since these data were from early catheter ablation strategies, a higher rate of complications should be expected because of "the learning curve." It is conceivable that most complications were due to early catheter ablations than to later ones. In the second worldwide survey of catheter ablation of AF (3), the overall major complication rate was lower at 4.5% than in the first one (Table 34-3) (1). The rate of pulmonary vein stenosis greatly decreased, and in all probability this was due to the move away from ablating within the pulmonary veins toward ablating outside of them at least 1 cm away from PV ostia. Other major complications included cardiac tamponade as well as transient ischemic attacks, stroke, and

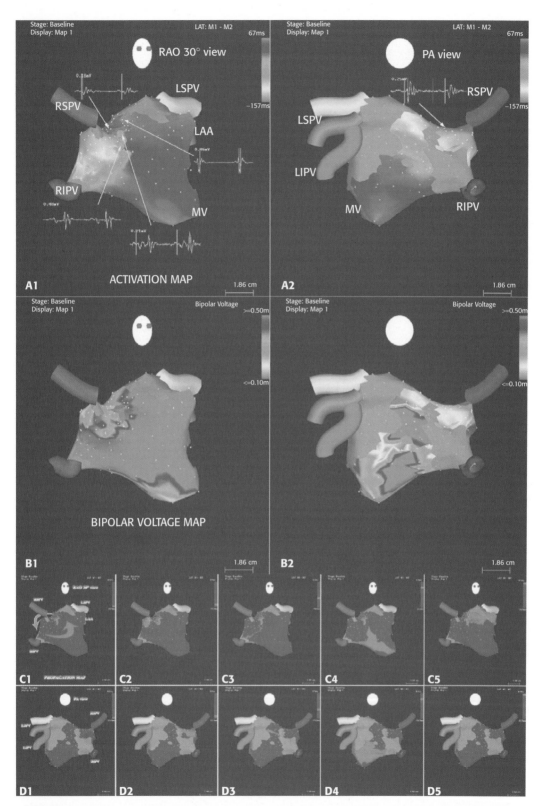

FIGURE 34-11. (**A1 and A2**) Activation maps illustrating a case of single-loop reentry around a previously ablated area at the septal aspect of the right pulmonary veins (Patient #9) in right anterior oblique (RAO) and posteroanterior (PA) views. A line of block with double potentials (**blue tags**) and an electrically silent area (**gray surface**)

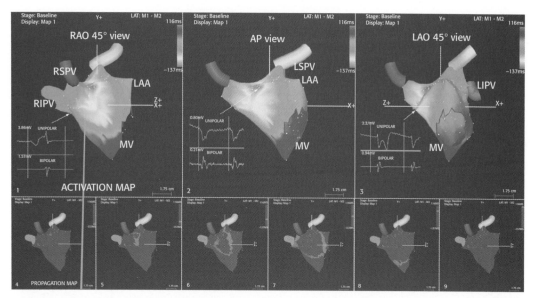

FIGURE 34-12. Three-dimensional reconstruction of the left atrium from a patient with a focal tachycardia originating on the interatrial septum anterior to the ostium of the right superior pulmonary vein (RSPV) (Patient #6). **(Panels 1 to 3)** Activation map during tachycardia, with earliest activation displayed in red and latest in **violet**. Local unipolar electrogram with a QS pattern is shown in **panel 2,** corresponding to the site of successful ablation. **(Panels 4 to 9)** Propagation map in right anterior oblique (RAO) showing centrifugal spread from site of earliest activation. AP, anteroposterior; LAA, left anterior appendage; LAO, left anterior oblique; LIPV, left inferior pulmonary vein; LSPV, left superior pulmonary vein; MV, mitral valve; RIPV, right inferior pulmonary vein. (Reprinted from Mesas CE, Pappone C, Lang CC, et al. Left atrial tachycardia after circumferential pulmonary vein ablation for atrial fibrillation: Electroanatomic characterization and treatment. *J Am Coll Cardiol.* 2004;44: 1071–1079, with permission from Elsevier.)

death. It is possible that many of these centers were still in the learning curve. Currently, there are increasing numbers of patients with comorbid conditions—including structural heart disease and congestive heart failure—who are candidates for catheter ablation. Since procedure-related complications in some cases may be life-threatening, minimizing their occurrence represents an important goal. A careful manipulation of catheters with close monitoring of RF applications and safe energy settings, certainly will minimize potential complications such as cardiac tamponade, which still represents a

major cause of death. Its recognition followed by immediate perdicardiocentesis avoids tamponade-related death. Cardiac surgery "back-up" should be available for patients with persistent bleeding. Subclavian vein access should be avoided since AF ablation procedure needs an aggressive anticoagulation. The risk of cerebrovascular events, including stroke, can be further reduced by appropriate anticoagulation both during and after the procedure. Esophageal injury is an extremely rare but potentially devastating complication of AF ablation, which in many cases ($> 80\%$) results in major morbidity

FIGURE 34-11. (*Continued*) can be seen at the superior segment of the septal line in **A1**. The circuit uses two gaps closely positioned at the superior and middle segments of the line. Single, fragmented bipolar electrograms can be seen at these sites. **(B1 and B2)** Voltage map in the same views showing recovery of the maximum bipolar voltage in the ablated areas. A wide area of high voltage (**violet**) can be seen over the septum in **B1**. **(C1 to C5 and D1 to D5)** Propagation map in RAO and PA showing the spread of activation. LAA, left anterior atrium; LIPV, left inferior pulmonary vein; LSPV, left superior pulmonary vein; MV, mitral valve; PA, posteroanterior; RIPV, right inferior pulmonary vein; RSPV, right superior pulmonary vein. (Reprinted from Mesas CE, Pappone C, Lang CC, et al. Left atrial tachycardia after circumferential pulmonary vein ablation for atrial fibrillation: Electroanatomic characterization and treatment. *J Am Coll Cardiol.* 2004;44:1071–1079, with permission from Elsevier.)

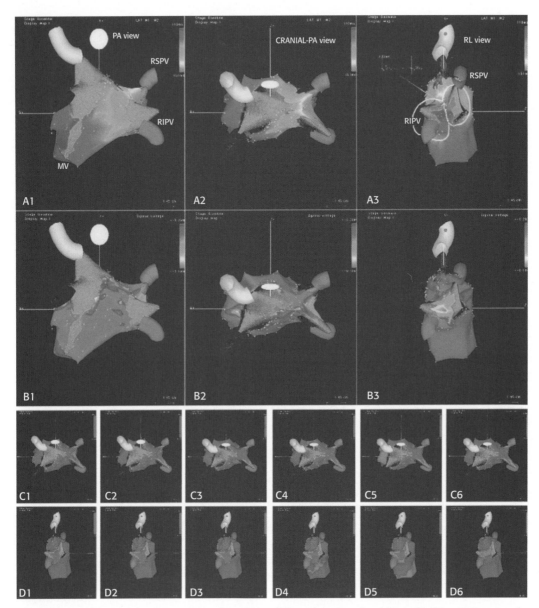

FIGURE 34-13. Activation (**A1 to A3**), voltage (**B1 to B3**), and propagation (**C1 to C6, D1 to D6**) maps of macroreentrant left AT with critical isthmus between right superior and right inferior PVs. (Reprinted from Pappone C, Manguso F, Vicedomini G, et al. Prevention of iatrogenic atrial tachycardia after ablation of atrial fibrillation: A prospective randomized study comparing circumferential pulmonary vein ablation with a modified approach. *Circulation.* 2004;110:3036–3042, with permission from Elsevier.)

or death. Real-time visualization of the esophagus with barium or a radio-opaque marker, and avoidance of RF energy applications over the esophagus, may be useful to minimize esophageal injury. If esophageal injury is suspected, a prompt diagnosis with immediate intervention is required for the patient's survival. Data collection of procedure-related complication rates according to the AF type

(paroxysmal versus persistent/long-standing AF) and the use of the newest ablation tools and technologies or better energy sources are lacking. In addition, consideration should be given to the fact that additional lesions or additional targets within the left or right atrium beyond pulmonary veins isolation are necessary in persistent or long-standing AF. Hopefully, in the future years, with increased experience and

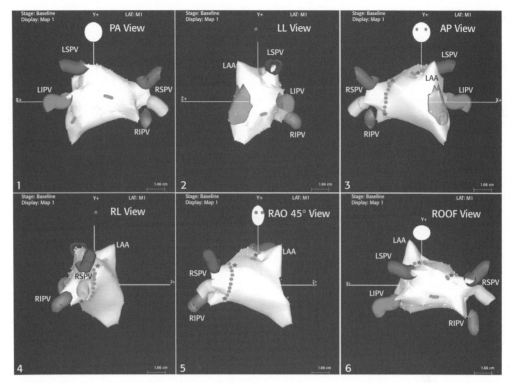

FIGURE 34-14. Three-dimensional solid geometry maps of the left atrium in different views, showing the location of the involved gaps (**red points**) and foci (**blue stars**). Most of the gaps and all three foci are located over the septal aspect of the right veins and the anterior aspect of the left superior pulmonary vein (LSPV) ostium. AP, anteroposterior; LAA, left anterior atrium; LL, left lateral; LIPV, left inferior pulmonary vein; PA, posteroanterior; RAO, right anterior oblique; RIPV, right inferior pulmonary vein; RL, right lateral; ROOF, cranial view; RSPV, right superior pulmonary vein. (Reprinted from Mesas CE, Pappone C, Lang CC, et al. Left atrial tachycardia after circumferential pulmonary vein ablation for atrial fibrillation: Electroanatomic characterization and treatment. *J Am Coll Cardiol.* 2004;44:1071–1079, with permission from Elsevier.) (See color insert.)

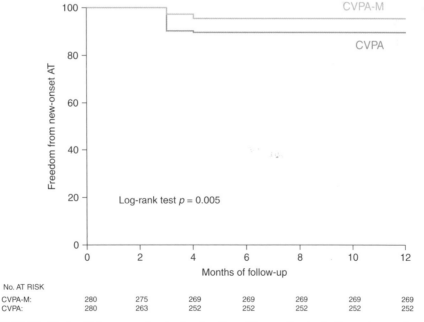

FIGURE 34-15. Kaplan-Meier curves showing freedom from AT according to whether patients underwent CPVA or CPVA-M. (From Pappone C, Manguso F, Vicedomini G, et al. Prevention of iatrogenic atrial tachycardia after ablation of atrial fibrillation: A prospective randomized study comparing circumferential pulmonary vein ablation with a modified approach. *Circulation.* 2004;110:3036–3042.)

TABLE 34-6 **Characteristics of Patients Who Developed New-Onset AT After CPVA or CPVA-M**

Variable	CPVA (n = 28)	CPVA-M (n = 11)	P
Mean age, y	59.6 ± 5.8	59.6 ± 5.2	1.00
Male, n (%)	16 (57)	7 (64)	0.77
Mean duration of AF, y	7.4 ± 1.8	7.1 ± 1.5	0.63
Mean left atrial diameter, mm	42.1 ± 4.4	41.0 ± 5.0	0.51
Mean left atrial ablated area, %	42.3 ± 6.8	37.4 ± 7.6	0.06
Cardiovascular diseases, n (%)			0.16
None	12 (43)	9 (82)	
Coronary artery disease	5 (18)	0 (0)	
Dilated cardiomyopathy	10 (36)	2 (18)	
Hypertrophic cardiomyopathy	1 (4)	0 (0)	
AF, n (%)			1.00
Paroxysmal	2 (7)	1 (9)	
Chronic	29 (93)	10 (91)	
AT mechanism, n (%)			0.66
Macroreentry	23 (82)	8 (73)	
Focal	5 (18)	3 (27)	
Inducibility, n (%)			0.002
Single extrastimulus	16 (57)	0 (0)	
Double extrastimuli	4 (14)	5 (46)	
Burst pacing	8 (29)	6 (54)	
Complete vagal denervation, n (%)	18 (64)	7 (64)	1.00
AF recurrence, n (%)	2 (7)	1 (9)	1.00

Data are mean ± SD when appropriate.
(From Pappone C, Manguso F, Vicedomini G, et al. Prevention of iatrogenic atrial tachycardia after ablation of atrial fibrillation: a prospective randomized study comparing circumferential pulmonary vein ablation with a modified approach. *Circulation.* 2004;110:3036–3042.)

TABLE 34-7 **Cox Regression Model for the Development of AT Post Catheter Ablation for Atrial Fibrillation in 560 Patients Who Underwent CPVA or CPVA-M**

Covariates	Regression Coefficient	P	Adjusted HR	95% CI
Procedure (0/1 = CPVA-M/CPVA)	1.34	<0.001	3.84	1.86–7.89
Gaps in >1 PV (absent/multiple = 0/1)	3.25	<0.001	25.19	11.01–57.30
Gaps in 1 PV (absent/single = 0/1)	2.43	<0.001	11.33	5.02–25.55
AF (paroxysmal/chronic = 0/1)	3.10	<0.001	22.28	6.72–73.87

HR, hazard ratio.
(From Pappone C, Manguso F, Vicedomini G, et al. Prevention of iatrogenic atrial tachycardia after ablation of atrial fibrillation: a prospective randomized study comparing circumferential pulmonary vein ablation with a modified approach. *Circulation.* 2004;110:3036–3042.)

further thechnological advancements, complication rates of catheter ablation of AF will continue to decline, while short term and long success rates will continue to improve.

References

1. Cappato R, Calkins H, Chen SA, et al. Worldwide survey on the methods, efficacy and safety of catheter ablation for human atrial fibrillation. *Circulation.* 2005;111:1100–1105.

2. Cappato R, Calkins H, Chen SA, et al. Prevalence and causes of fatal outcome in catheter ablation of atrial fibrillation. *J Am Coll Cardiol.* 2009;53: 1798–1803.

3. Cappato R, Calkins H, Chen SA, et al. Updated worldwide survey on the methods, efficacy, and safety of catheter ablation for human atrial fibrillation. *Circ Arrhythm Electrophysiol.* 2010;3:32–38.

4. Pappone C, Oreto G, Rosanio S, et al. Atrial electroanatomic remodeling after circumferential radiofrequency pulmonary vein ablation: Efficacy of an anatomic approach in a large cohort of patients with atrial fibrillation. *Circulation.* 2001;104:2539–2544.

5. Haissaguerre M, Jais P, Shah DC, et al. Spontaneous initiation of atrial fibrillation by ectopic beats originating in the pulmonary veins. *N Engl J Med.* 1998;339:659–666.

6. Pappone C, Santinelli V, Manguso F, et al. Pulmonary vein denervation enhances long-term benefit after circumferential ablation for paroxysmal atrial fibrillation. *Circulation.* 2004;109:327–334.

7. Pappone C, Manguso F, Vicedomini G, et al. Prevention of iatrogenic atrial tachycardia after ablation of atrial fibrillation: A prospective randomized study comparing circumferential pulmonary vein ablation with a modified approach. *Circulation.* 2004;110:3036–3042.

8. Oral H, Pappone C, Chugh A, et al. Circumferential pulmonary vein ablation for chronic atrial fibrillation. *N Engl J Med.* 2006;354:934–941.

9. Hindricks G. The Multicentre European Radiofrequency Survey (MERFS): Complications of radiofrequency catheter ablation of arrhythmias. The Multicentre European Radiofrequency Survey (MERFS) Investigators of the working group on arrhythmias of the European society of cardiology. *Eur Heart J.* 1993;14:1644–1653.

10. Calkins H, Yonk P, Miller JM, et al, for the Atakr Multicenter Investigator Group. Catheter ablation of accessory pathways, atrioventricular nodal re-entrant tachycardia, and the atrioventricular junction: Final results of a prospective, multicenter clinical trial. *Circulation.* 1999;99: 262–270.

11. Lang CC, Gugliotta F, Santinelli V, et al. Endocardial impedance mapping during circumferential pulmonary vein ablation of atrial fibrillation differentiates between atrial and venous tissue. *Heart Rhythm.* 2006;3:171–178.

12. Pappone C, Oral H, Santinelli V, et al. Atrioesophageal fistula as a complication of percutaneous transcatheter ablation of atrial fibrillation. *Circulation.* 2004;109:2724–2726.

13. Scanavacca MI, D'Avila A, Parga J, et al. Left atrial-esophageal fistula following radiofrequency catheter ablation of atrial fibrillation. *J Cardiovasc Electrophysiol.* 2004;15:960–962.

14. Bunch TJ, Nelson J, Foley T, et al. Temporary esophageal stenting allows healing of esophageal perforations following atrial fibrillation ablation procedures. *J Cardiovasc Electrophysiol.* 2006;17: 435–439.

15. Mesas CE, Pappone C, Lang CC, et al. Left atrial tachycardia after circumferential pulmonary vein ablation for atrial fibrillation: Electroanatomic characterization and treatment. *J Am Coll Cardiol.* 2004;44:1071–1079.

16. Vijayaraman, Netrebko P, Geyfman V, et al. Esophageal fistula formation despite esophageal monitoring and low-power radiofrequency catheter ablation for atrial fibrillation. *Circ Arrhythm Electrophysiol.* 2009;2:e31–e33.

INDEX

Note: Page numbers followed by f indicate figures; those followed by t indicate tables.